Complications of Head and Neck Surgery

Edited by

Mark C. Weissler, M.D.
Associate Professor
Division of Otolaryngology/
Head and Neck Surgery
University of North Carolina
School of Medicine
Chapel Hill, North Carolina

Harold C. Pillsbury III, M.D.
Chief of Otolaryngology
Division of Otolaryngology/
Head and Neck Surgery
University of North Carolina
School of Medicine
Chapel Hill, North Carolina

1995
Thieme Medical Publishers, New York
Georg Thieme Verlag, Stuttgart • New York

Thieme Medical Publishers, Inc.
381 Park Avenue South
New York, New York 10016

Complications of Head and Neck Surgery
Mark C. Weissler, M.D.
Harold C. Pillsbury III, M.D.

Library of Congress Cataloging-in-Publication Data

Complications of head and neck surgery / [edited by] Mark C. Weissler,
    Harold C. Pillsbury.
        p.   cm.
    Includes bibliographical references and index.
    ISBN 0-86577-529-X.—ISBN 3-13-100621-8
    1. Head—Surgery—Complications.   2. Neck—Surgery—Complications.
    I. Weissler, Mark C.   II. Pillsbury III, Harold C.
    [DNLM: 1. Head—surgery.   2. Neck—surgery.   3. Intraoperative
Complications.   4. Postoperative Complications. WE 705 C7391 1995]
RD521.C66   1995
617.2'101—dc20
DNLM/DLC
for Library of Congress   94-39974
                                                                  CIP

Printed in the United States of America.

5   4   3   2   1

TMP ISBN 0-86577-529-X
GTV ISBN 3-13-100621-8

This text is dedicated to my parents Ann and Joe; to my teachers, particularly Dr. Jack Gluckman, without whose assistance I could never have experienced the wealth of complications which allowed me to adequately edit this text; to my students and residents whose constant attempts to cause complications give me daily food for thought on this subject; and to my wife Ann, my daughter Kate, and my son Sam, who are the only ones who seem able to uncomplicate my life.

Mark C. Weissler, M.D.

This book is dedicated to my wife Sally and my sons, Matthew, Benjamin, and Thomas, who have been wonderful reminders of what is really important in life.

Harold C. Pillsbury III, M.D.

Contents

Contributors vii
Foreword xi
Preface xiii
Acknowledgments xv

1. General Considerations of the Perioperative Period 1
   Mark C. Weissler, M.D.

2. Coagulation and Hemostasis 5
   Wendell G. Yarbrough, M.D., Mark C. Weissler, M.D.

3. Deep Venous Thrombosis and Pulmonary Embolism 31
   Gregory F. Hulka, M.D., Mark C. Weissler, M.D.

4. Postoperative Fever 44
   C. Gaelyn Garrett, M.D., Mark C. Weissler, M.D.

5. Complications of Laryngoscopy, Bronchoscopy, and Esophagoscopy 56
   Kyle L. Bressler, M.D., Michael E. Dunham, M.D., Lauren D. Holinger, M.D.

6. Complications of Laser Surgery 64
   Elie E. Rebeiz, M.D., Stanley M. Shapshay, M.D.

7. Complications of Sinonasal Surgery 74
   William R. Wilson, M.D.

8. Complications of Endoscopic Sinus Surgery 90
   Kim R. Jones, M.D., Ph.D.

9. Complications of Surgery for Neoplasms of the Oral Cavity, Pharynx,
   and Cervical Esophagus 94
   Jack L. Gluckman, M.D., F.A.C.S., Markus Gapany, M.D.

10. Complications of Laryngeal Surgery 107
   Carl E. Silver, M.D., David H. Henick, M.D.

11. Complications of Neck Surgery 122
   William W. Shockley, M.D., Chapman T. McQueen, M.D., Gregory N. Postma, M.D.

12. Use of Prophylactic Antibiotics in Otolaryngology 159
   Anna M. Pou, M.D., Jonas T. Johnson, M.D.

13. Complications of Salivary Gland Surgery 172
   Michael J. Kaplan, M.D.

14. Complications of Thyroid and Parathyroid Surgery 184
   Jesus E. Medina, M.D., F.A.C.S., Edgar M. Boyd, Jr., M.D.

15. Complications of Radiotherapy for Head and Neck Neoplasms 194
   James T. Parsons, M.D., William M. Mendenhall, M.D., Rodney R. Million, M.D.

16. Complications of Chemotherapy in the Treatment of Head and Neck Cancer 230
Stephen A. Bernard, M.D.

17. Complications of Aesthetic Facial Surgery 248
Fred J. Stucker, M.D., F.A.C.S., Robert F. Aarstad, M.D., Denis K. Hoasjoe, M.D., F.R.C.S.(C)

18. Complications of Reconstructive Flaps 279
Richard F. Debo, M.D., Paul A. Levine, M.D.

19. Complications of Surgery for Facial Fractures 290
Robert H. Mathog, M.D.

20. Complications of Middle Ear and Mastoid Surgery 323
Thomas L. Eby, M.D., F.A.C.S.

21. Complications of Cranial Base Surgery 336
Jeffrey L. Wilson, M.D., Dan G. Deschler, M.D., Michael J. Kaplan, M.D., Harold C. Pillsbury III, M.D.

22. Rehabilitation of Facial Nerve Injury 352
Lawrence P.A. Burgess, M.D., F.A.C.S., Richard L. Goode, M.D., F.A.C.S.

23. Complications of Anesthesia for Otolaryngology–Head and Neck Surgery 371
Eileen P. Tyler, M.D.

24. Complications of Head and Neck Imaging 389
Mauricio Castillo, M.D., Patricia A. Hudgins, M.D.

25. Complications in the Critical Care Unit 401
William R. Blythe, M.D., Fuad Ramadan, M.D., David Smith, M.D., Samir M. Fakhry, M.D., F.A.C.S.

Index 422

Contributors

Robert F. Aarstad, M.D.
Assistant Professor
Department of Otolaryngology–Head and Neck Surgery
Louisiana State University
Shreveport, LA

Stephen A. Bernard, M.D.
Associate Professor
Department of Medicine
University of North Carolina
Chapel Hill, NC

William R. Blythe, M.D.
Resident in Otolaryngology–Head and Neck Surgery
Department of Surgery
University of North Carolina School of Medicine
Chapel Hill, NC

Edgar M. Boyd, Jr., M.D.
Head and Neck Oncologic Surgery Fellow
Department of Otorhinolaryngology
University of Oklahoma Health Sciences Center
Oklahoma City, OK

Kyle L. Bressler, M.D.
Children's Memorial Hospital
Chicago, IL

Lawrence P.A. Burgess, M.D., F.A.C.S.
Major, Medical Corps
Assistant Chief, Otolaryngology–Head and Neck Surgery
Associate Professor, USUHS
Department of the Army
Headquarters, Tripler Army Medical Center
Oahu, HI

Mauricio Castillo, M.D.
Clinical Associate Professor
Director of Neuroradiology
Department of Radiology
University of North Carolina School of Medicine
Chapel Hill, NC

Richard F. Debo, M.D.
Fellow, Head and Neck Surgical Oncology
Department of Otolaryngology–Head and Neck Surgery
University of Virginia
Charlottesville, VA

Dan G. Deschler, M.D.
Department of Otolaryngology–Head and Neck Surgery
University of California, San Francisco
San Francisco, CA

Michael E. Dunham, M.D.
Children's Memorial Hospital
Chicago, IL

Thomas L. Eby, M.D., F.A.C.S.
Chief of Otolaryngology
Veterans Administration Medical Center
Birmingham, AL
Associate Professor of Surgery
Division of Otolaryngology–Head and Neck Surgery
Department of Surgery
University of Alabama at Birmingham School of
  Medicine

Samir M. Fakhry, M.D., F.A.C.S.
Assistant Professor
Department of Surgery
University of North Carolina School of Medicine
Chapel Hill, NC

Markus Gapany, M.D.
Department of Otolaryngology–Head and Neck Surgery
University of Cincinnati Medical Center
College of Medicine
Cincinnati, OH

C. Gaelyn Garrett, M.D.
Division of Otolaryngology–Head and Neck Surgery
University of North Carolina School of Medicine
Chapel Hill, NC

Jack L. Gluckman, M.D., F.A.C.S.
Professor and Chairman
Department of Otolaryngology–Head and Neck Surgery
University of Cincinnati Medical Center
College of Medicine
Cincinnati, OH

Richard L. Goode, M.D., F.A.C.S.
Professor of Surgery
Division of Otolaryngology–Head and Neck Surgery
Stanford University Medical Center
Stanford, CA

David H. Henick, M.D.
Fellow in Head and Neck Surgery
Albert Einstein College of Medicine
Montefiore Medical Center
Bronx, NY

Denis K. Hoasjoe, M.D., F.R.C.S.(C)
Assistant Professor
Department of Otolaryngology–Head and Neck Surgery
Louisiana State University
School of Medicine
Shreveport, LA

Lauren D. Holinger, M.D.
Professor and Head
Pediatric Otolaryngology
Head, Section of Bronchoesophagology
Children's Memorial Hospital
Chicago, IL

Patricia A. Hudgins, M.D.
Associate Professor of Radiology
Emory University Hospital
Atlanta, GA

Gregory F. Hulka, M.D.
Department of Otolaryngology–Head and Neck Surgery
University of Cincinnati School of Medicine
College of Medicine
Cincinnati, OH

Jonas T. Johnson, M.D.
Professor
Departments of Otolaryngology and Radiation Oncology
Vice Chairman, Department of Otolaryngology
Director, Division of Head and Neck Oncology and
  Immunology
University of Pittsburgh School of Medicine
Pittsburgh, PA
Department of Otolaryngology
Eye and Ear Institute of Pittsburgh
Pittsburgh, PA

Kim R. Jones, M.D., Ph.D
Division of Otolaryngology–Head and Neck Surgery
University of North Carolina School of Medicine
Chapel Hill, NC

Michael J. Kaplan, M.D.
Department of Otolaryngology–Head and Neck Surgery
University of California, San Francisco
San Francisco, CA

Paul A. Levine, M.D.
Professor and Vice Chairman
Department of Otolaryngology–Head and Neck Surgery
Director, Head and Neck Surgical Oncology
University of Virginia
Charlottesville, VA

Robert H. Mathog, M.D.
Professor and Chair
Department of Otolaryngology–Head and Neck Surgery
Wayne State University
Detroit, MI

Chapman T. McQueen, M.D.
Division of Otolaryngology–Head and Neck Surgery
University of North Carolina School of Medicine
Chapel Hill, NC

Jesus E. Medina, M.D., F.A.C.S.
Professor and Chairman
Department of Otorhinolaryngology
University of Oklahoma Health Sciences Center
Oklahoma City, OK

William M. Mendenhall, M.D.
Department of Radiation Oncology
Shands Cancer Center
University of Florida
Gainesville, FL

Rodney R. Million, M.D.
Department of Radiation Oncology
Shands Cancer Center
University of Florida
Gainesville, FL

James T. Parsons, M.D.
Professor
Department of Radiation Oncology
University of Florida College of Medicine
Gainesville, FL

Harold C. Pillsbury III, M.D.
Thomas J. Dark Distinguished Professor of Surgery
Professor and Chief
Division of Otolaryngology–Head and Neck Surgery
University of North Carolina School of Medicine
Chapel Hill, NC

Gregory N. Postma, M.D.
Division of Otolaryngology–Head and Neck Surgery
University of North Carolina School of Medicine
Chapel Hill, NC

Anna M. Pou, M.D.
Resident, Department of Otolaryngology
Eye and Ear Institute of Pittsburgh
Pittsburgh, PA

Fuad Ramadan, M.D.
Fellow, Critical Care Service for Surgery
Department of Surgery
University of North Carolina School of Medicine
Chapel Hill, NC

Elie E. Rebeiz, M.D.
Assistant Professor
Department of Otolaryngology–Head and Neck Surgery
Tufts University School of Medicine
Boston, MA

Stanley M. Shapshay, M.D.
Professor and Chair
Department of Otolaryngology–Head and Neck Surgery
Tufts University School of Medicine
Boston, MA

William W. Shockley, M.D.
Division of Otolaryngology–Head and Neck Surgery
University of North Carolina School of Medicine
Chapel Hill, NC

Carl E. Silver, M.D.
Chief, Head and Neck Surgery
Montefiore Medical Center
Bronx, NY

David Smith, M.D.
Fellow, Critical Care Service for Surgery
Department of Surgery
University of North Carolina School of Medicine
Chapel Hill, NC

Fred J. Stucker, M.D., F.A.C.S.
Department of Otolaryngology–Head and Neck Surgery
Louisiana State University
Medical Center
Shreveport, LA

Eileen P. Tyler, M.D.
Clinical Assistant Professor
Department of Anesthesiology
University of North Carolina School of Medicine
Chapel Hill, NC

Mark C. Weissler, M.D.
Division of Otolaryngology–Head and Neck Surgery
University of North Carolina School of Medicine
Chapel Hill, NC

Jeffrey L. Wilson, M.D.
Division of Otolaryngology–Head and Neck Surgery
University of North Carolina School of Medicine
Chapel Hill, NC

William R. Wilson, M.D.
Professor and Division Chief
Otolaryngology–Head and Neck Surgery
Department of Surgery
The George Washington University Medical Center
Washington, DC

Wendell G. Yarbrough, M.D.
Division of Otolaryngology–Head and Neck Surgery
University of North Carolina School of Medicine
Chapel Hill, NC

Foreword

This textbook is a much welcomed and indispensable addition to our medical library. It begins in the preoperative period, ends with complications in the critical care unit, and expertly covers complications involving the entire scope of otolaryngology–head and neck surgery.

Any surgeon who undertakes major surgery of the head and neck must, in all conscience, be prepared to cope with potential avoidable and unavoidable complications. This text will greatly assist us with the elimination of avoidable complications and the management of those that are unavoidable.

The quality of teaching set forth in this text is commendable. The contributors to *Complications of Head and Neck Surgery*, all experienced and knowledgeable doctors, are to be praised. The illustrations deserve a special note. Their fine quality supports the entire text, they nicely clarify the details, and in themselves are an artistic pleasure.

This book should appeal to head and neck surgeons, otolaryngologists, plastic surgeons, general surgeons, maxillofacial surgeons, and radiotherapists. It is a teaching text for the inexperienced surgeon as well as a refresher for those more experienced. I welcome it as an addition to my library.

William W. Montgomery, M.D.
Department of Otolaryngology
Harvard Medical School
Massachusetts Eye & Ear Infirmary
Boston, MA

Preface

Even the best technical and most experienced surgeons will encounter complications. Many complications can be avoided, some can be minimized through proper handling, and those that develop full blown must be treated appropriately. Avoiding complications is largely based on a thorough knowledge of the physiology and pathophysiology of health and disease, a sound knowledge of surgical anatomy, a knowledge of the complications most commonly faced in a particular situation, and a humble appraisal of one's own ability to improve the lot of a patient in a particular circumstance. "Do no harm" remains a valid admonition.

In this textbook we begin with several chapters dealing with basic information pertinent to all operations: the perioperative period, hemorrhage and coagulation, deep venous thrombosis and pulmonary embolism, and postoperative fever. We then move on to chapters dealing more specifically with the operative procedures commonly performed by otolaryngologists/head and neck surgeons. We cover those complications most commonly associated with a particular type of operative procedure and explain how those complications can be avoided, recognized, and treated when they arise.

We have included illustrations by an exceptional artist, Mr. Anthony Pazos, tables, and diagrams.

We sincerely hope that this text will benefit otolaryngologists and their patients by assisting them to avoid, recognize, and treat the inevitable complications that will arise.

Mark C. Weissler, M.D.
Harold C. Pillsbury III, M.D.

Acknowledgments

I would like to acknowledge the assistance of Ms. Hope Merritt in the preparation of this manuscript, Mr. Tony Pazos for his great artistic ability, Mr. Jim Costello for his foresight and willingness to participate, and my wife Ann, without whose constant support I could accomplish little.

Mark C. Weissler, M.D.

This text would not have been possible without the dedication and persistence of Ms. Hope Merritt, who brought it to fruition.

Harold C. Pillsbury III, M.D.

1 General Considerations of the Perioperative Period

Mark C. Weissler, M.D.

PREOPERATIVE CONSIDERATIONS

Complications are better avoided than treated. Often the ultimate success or failure of an operative procedure is determined by events that occur preoperatively. The responsible physician must have an overall plan that includes considerations of patient parameters, an understanding of the disease process being treated, and a concept of what long-term goals are realistic and in the patient's best interest. Table 1–1 outlines the important considerations during the preoperative period.

Table 1–1. Preoperative Considerations.

Airway status
  Is the airway tenuous and will it require special considerations at the beginning of the case?
    Awake intubation
    Tracheotomy under local
Nutritional status and hydration
Preoperative studies in order?
  CXR
  Other radiological studies
  Liver function tests
  Arterial blood gases, if appropriate
  Bleeding studies
Appropriate staging and understanding of extent of disease
Overall plan for patient care and contingency plans
Prophylaxis of thromboembolic complications

Airway Status

During any case, whether under local anesthesia with sedation or under general anesthesia, the airway must be secure. Head and neck surgery requires special attention to the airway because all too often the procedures which are performed, whether a tonsillectomy and adenoidectomy or a composite resection, result in temporary airway impairment from bloody secretions, edema, or transferred soft tissue. In addition, the disease processes being treated often impair the airway. Patients with laryngeal or pharyngeal cancers may have direct airway impairment from the bulk of the tumor. Patients with obstructive sleep apnea may have redundant prolapsing soft tissue. A marginal airway which is fine while the patient is awake and alert and sitting up may suddenly become inadequate when the patient is sedated and supine. One should constantly try to anticipate airway difficulties preoperatively so that they do not become airway emergencies during the case. It is crucial that vital equipment to secure the airway be available if problems arise. In cases in which it is anticipated that securing the airway may be difficult, a rigid bronchoscope and equipment to perform a tracheotomy should be immediately available.

Children or adults with an altered mental status, whether from sedation, acute central nervous system (CNS) trauma, or chronic global CNS dysfunction, are a particularly high-risk group of patients for airway compromise. Children with chronic global CNS dysfunction lack an effective reflexive ability to compensate for minimal impairment of the airway. They are particularly prone to suffer airway problems on arousal from general anesthesia after any manipulation of the upper aerodigestive tract, and particularly if there are bloody secretions in the airway.

Nutritional Status and Hydration

Patients with advanced head and neck cancers frequently present with poor nutritional status. Tumor may obstruct the alimentary tract or pain may prevent adequate alimentation. Although it is rarely feasible to delay surgery to replete nutritional deficiencies completely in cancer patients, much can be accomplished to improve hydration and nutritional status by simply passing a small feeding nasogastric tube and beginning enteral feeding for a week or so preoperatively.

Are Preoperative Studies in Order?

It is important to check all preoperative studies, and to do this in time to make important changes in the overall therapeutic plan prior to an extensive operation. Chest x-rays must be checked for evidence of second primary or metastatic disease in cancer patients. The preoperative films of the lesion should be thoroughly reviewed and understood. Liver function tests should be checked for evidence of metastatic disease in oncology patients. Patients with clinical evidence of significant lung disease should have preoperative arterial blood gas analysis performed on room air as a baseline for evaluating postoperative pulmonary function. In some cases, preoperative pulmonary function tests may be in order to assist one in determining whether a patient is likely to tolerate a procedure if that procedure is likely to result in increased postoperative aspiration of secretions. Bleeding studies should be checked and in order.

Appropriate Staging and Understanding of Extent of Disease

In all patients, but especially those undergoing oncologic head and neck surgery, it is imperative that the surgeon have the fullest understanding of the precise extent of local and regional disease prior to planning definitive resection. Only through an understanding of the extent of disease can a surgeon formulate a plan for appropriate surgical removal. Knowledge of the extent of disease is gleaned from the clinical examination, radiological evaluation, and endoscopy. These examinations complement each other. Some aspects of the clinical exam (such as the determination of vocal cord mobility) can only be performed adequately on the awake patient and so are best performed in the clinic.

Overall Plan for Patient Care and Contingency Plans

The surgeon should enter the operating room with a general overall plan of treatment and contingency plans based on intraoperative findings. For instance, when entering the operating room with a patient with a large obstructing pharyngeal cancer with airway compromise and questionable involvement

of the prevertebral fascia on preoperative computed tomography (CT) scan, the plan might be something like that shown in Figure 1-1. One should try to anticipate situations which are likely to arise during the operation and make plans to deal with them before they occur. Otherwise a quagmire of indecision is likely to ensue, from which the patient is likely to suffer. Will a skin graft or other flap be required for closure? Might a tracheotomy be necessary? If so, the patient should be appropriately prepped and draped. It is far easier to prep and drape appropriately at the beginning of a case than to break in the middle of a case to prep and drape other areas.

Prophylaxis of Thromboembolic Complications

In patients deemed at risk of thromboembolic complications, thought should be given to some manner of reducing the risk of developing clots intraoperatively. This might entail subcutaneous heparin, compression hose, or pneumatic compression stockings.

INTRAOPERATIVE CONSIDERATIONS

To Paralyze or Not?

(See Table 1–2 for an overview of intraoperative considerations.) The use of paralyzing agents can be helpful but also can cause problems. During intubation, paralysis will relax the patient and assist with intubation; however, it can also bring the airway situation to a head. Once the patient is paralyzed and spontaneous respiration ceases, the anesthesiologist or surgeon must be able either to mask ventilate or intubate the patient with an endotracheal tube or rigid

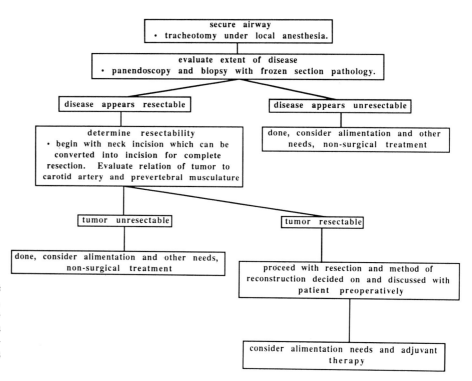

Figure 1–1. Diagram showing the overall plan, with contingencies, which must be formulated preoperatively for a particular patient with a large pharyngeal tumor which is compromising the airway and which is questionably resectable.

Table 1–2. Intraoperative Considerations.

To paralyze or not
Prophylactic antibiotics
Plans for postoperative alimentation
    Nasogastric (NGT)
    Gastrostomy
Plan for skin incisions
    Methylene blue
    Old incisions
    Carotid protection
Monitoring
    Central or swan-ganz line
    Arterial line (a-line)
    Nerve monitoring
    Other monitoring
    Foley catheter

bronchoscope, or be prepared to secure the airway surgically. Rigid esophagoscopy and rigid bronchoscopy require paralysis for their safe performance. Exposure of intraoral neoplasms is often aided by adequate paralysis intraoperatively.

While working around cranial nerves such as the facial nerve, hypoglossal nerve, recurrent laryngeal nerve, and spinal accessory nerve, a nerve stimulator may aid in identification and preservation. This device is only useful in the nonparalyzed patient. What is most important intraoperatively, however (rather than whether the patient is paralyzed or not), is that the anesthesiologist and surgeon communicate on the status of paralysis at a given time. If a previously nonparalyzed patient is given a paralyzing agent intraoperatively and the surgeon is unaware of this, he or she may be lulled into a false assumption when a previously stimulatable structure is no longer stimulatable. Knowledge of the state of paralysis is what is most important.

Prophylactic Antibiotics

Prophylactic antibiotics are of value in resections of head and neck neoplasms in which the mucosa of the upper aerodigestive tract is breached. They are most effective, however, when delivered prior to the beginning of the case, and the surgeon must remember to ask if this has been done.

Plans for Postoperative Alimentation

Patients undergoing extensive head and neck surgery are often blessed by the fact that they continue to have a normal lower gastrointestinal tract which can be used for postoperative nutritional support. It is important to consider this preoperatively, because postoperative placement of a nasogastric tube may be difficult, dangerous, or impossible for fear of disrupting mucosal suture lines. For this same reason, nasogastric tubes should be secured well. We prefer suturing them to the membranous nasal septum in addition to taping them. In patients who will be undergoing surgical

procedures which are likely to delay or preclude postoperative oral alimentation for several months or indefinitely, consideration should be given to a gastrostomy. Gastrostomies can now be placed in a variety of ways by general surgeons, interventional radiologists, and gastroenterologists. The use of an enteral route for nutrition is preferred over parenteral routes whenever possible.

Plan for Skin Incisions

Skin incisions should be planned with a number of factors in mind. Recent biopsy incisions should be excised if they have been potentially contaminated with cancer. One should consider all possible incisions which might be necessary in a given case—for instance, in the opposite neck, or splitting the lower lip—so that all flaps can be made with an adequate base for blood supply. The use of some way to mark the skin preoperatively so that appropriate parts of the flaps can be brought back together at the end of the case can be useful in complex skin incisions. Methylene blue is a temporary dye which works well for this. It can be applied with simple needle punctures.

Monitoring

The need for a variety of monitoring devices should be considered preoperatively. If the patient has significant heart dysfunction, a Swan-Ganz line might be indicated. If dissection around important motor nerves is to be performed, then some form of nerve monitoring—either with a nerve stimulator or electromyographic (EMG) nerve integrity monitor—might be useful. If the procedure might be lengthy or if major blood loss or body fluid shifts are anticipated, then a Foley catheter and possibly a central venous line is necessary.

POSTOPERATIVE CONSIDERATIONS

Monitoring

(See Table 1–3 for an overview of postoperative considerations.) Patients undergoing head and neck surgery often require close monitoring of their airway postoperatively. Often the degree of monitoring necessary falls somewhere between that available in an intensive care unit and that available on a hospital ward. If available, an intermediate care unit is often adequate. Some patients who might not seem appropriate for intensive observation on the surface (such as patients with obstructive sleep apnea, elderly patients with bilateral anterior and posterior nasal packing, and children with global neurological dysfunction undergoing upper airway surgery such as tonsillectomy and adenoidectomy) can benefit most from such monitoring. Caregivers can be lulled into a false sense of security in dealing with these patients postoperatively because of the "minor" nature of the procedures performed. On occasion, the surgeon might meet resistance in admitting

Table 1–3. Postoperative Considerations.

Monitoring
Postoperative CXR or other radiological studies
Labs
    Hematocrit
    Electrolytes
    Arterial blood gas
    Calcium
    Bleeding studies

such patients to intensive observation but should remain firm in his or her conviction. If bed shortages are possible, the availability of such monitored beds should be determined preoperatively.

Postoperative Chest X-rays or Other Radiological Studies

Postoperative chest x-rays (CXR) are indicated on all patients undergoing tracheotomy, low-neck procedures, or difficult endoscopic procedures when the surgeon suspects that the esophagus or tracheobronchial tree might have been breached. Nasogastric tube placement should also be confirmed radiologically before beginning tube feedings, and placement of central venous catheters should be confirmed before interpreting data derived from them.

Labs

BLEEDING STUDIES

Postoperative laboratory data should be individualized. If the operative procedure has been lengthy and the patient has received large amounts of fluid or blood, coagulation studies should be checked as well as the hematocrit and electrolytes. If damage to the parathyroid glands is possible, then postoperative calcium levels should be followed although they will not fall immediately. It is good to check a baseline immediately postoperatively so that trends can be followed. Calcium levels must be interpreted in light of the serum albumin level (subtract 0.8 mg/dL from serum calcium for every 1 g/dL decrease in serum albumin) or, more simply, ionized calcium levels can be followed as a more direct measure of physiologically available calcium.

SUMMARY

The successful practice of surgery is predicated on attention to detail. Careful preoperative planning, meticulous execution of surgical technique, and vigilant postoperative care are all essential to a successful outcome. The surgeon must attempt to foresee potential pitfalls, complications, and contingencies and have plans to deal with them when and if they arise. He or she must be flexible enough to change plans when indicated and resilient enough to respond to adverse outcomes appropriately without being paralyzed by them. Both indecision and blind adherence to a therapeutic plan gone wrong can lead to catastrophe. Throughout, the patient and his or her representatives must be included in the process. It is good to remember that the treatment of the disease and the treatment of the patient, while generally running in parallel, may sometimes diverge. In such instances, the treatment of the patient should take precedence. This may become especially poignant in the face of adverse outcomes, when the physician's ego may be threatened and he or she may become consumed with the battle against the disease while forgetting the patient in whom this battle will occur.

2 Coagulation and Hemostasis

Wendell G. Yarbrough, M.D., Mark C. Weissler, M.D.

COAGULATION

The process of coagulation of blood is vital to maintenance of the circulatory system and to survival. The system is designed with checks and balances to control clot propagation while at the same time allowing for rapid control of bleeding when necessary. The mechanism of coagulation actually begins with platelets and the formation of a cellular plug, as discussed later in this chapter. In this section we will discuss the process of fibrin deposition and the biochemical mechanism that allows for rapid activation of blood clotting, known as the coagulation cascade.

Coagulation Cascade

The process of coagulation, which has as its goal the conversion of soluble fibrinogen to insoluble fibrin, is referred to as a cascade because each enzyme in the system activates another enzyme, which then activates another enzyme until a fibrin clot is formed. The cascade allows a single activated protein at the beginning to cause activation of many enzymes, at the end resulting in amplification of the initiating stimulus and rapid clotting.

The coagulation factors are named in roman numerals for the order of their discovery, not for their position in the coagulation cascade. All proteins except VIII, which is synthesized by endothelial cells, are synthesized in the liver.[1] Table 2–1 lists the roman numeral designation of the coagulation factors and their common nomenclature. All factors except III, V, and VIII are enzymes and all except XIII, a transaminase, are serine proteases.[1] Factors III, V, and VIII are cofactors that accelerate enzymatic reactions and are critical to coagulation. Further classification of coagulation factors groups II, VII, IX, and X because they are all dependent on vitamin K for proper function. All of these factors contain a unique amino acid (gamma carboxyglutamic acid) that allows them to attach to the phospholipid surface of platelets (platelet factor 3, PF3) or the phospholipid component of factor III in the presence of calcium, which dramatically increases their activity.[1] Deficiencies of vitamin K and decreased activity of factors II, VII, IX, and X are frequently

Table 2–1. Nomenclature of Coagulation Factors

Factor I	Fibrinogen
Factor II	Prothrombin
Factor III	Tissue thromboplastin
Factor IV	Calcium
Factor V	Labile factor
Factor VI	Not assigned
Factor VII	Stable factor
Factor VIII	Antihemophilic factor
Factor IX	Christmas factor
Factor X	Stuart-Prower factor
Factor XI	Plasma thromboplastin antecedent
Factor XII	Hageman factor
Factor XIII	Fibrin-stabilizing factor
Fitzgerald factor	High-molecular-weight kininogen
Fletcher factor	Pre-kallikrein

caused by high-dose antibiotics, parenteral feedings, and liver diseases.[1] There are many congenital deficiencies of coagulation factors, which will be discussed later in this chapter.

The classic division of the coagulation cascade into intrinsic and extrinsic pathways is based on the fact that all components of the intrinsic cascade are contained in the blood, whereas the initial step of the extrinsic pathway requires the extrinsic factor III (tissue thromboplastin) not normally found in blood. Both systems require calcium and a phospholipid surface which is supplied by platelets for the intrinsic system and factor III for the extrinsic system.[1] The extrinsic and intrinsic pathways converge into the common pathway with the activation of factor X, which converts prothrombin to thrombin (II to IIa). Thrombin is the focal point of the cascade because it is the factor that converts fibrinogen to fibrin. Additionally, thrombin potentiates coagulation by activating factors V, VIII, and XIII. Thrombin also acts as a downregulator of coagulation by activating protein C, which inactivates coagulation factors and activates the fibrinolytic system.[1]

Figure 2–1 outlines the steps of the coagulation cascade. The extrinsic cascade is activated by release of tissue thromboplastin (III) from the blood vessel wall. The extrinsic

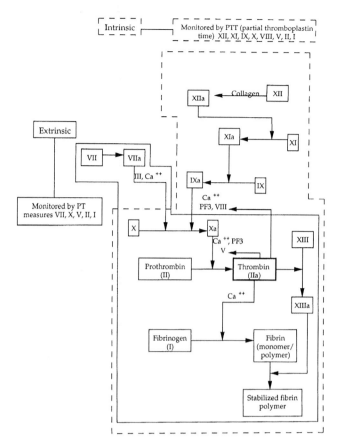

Figure 2–1. Schematic representation of the intrinsic (dashed line) and extrinsic (solid line) and common (both dashed and solid lines) pathways of the coagulation cascade.

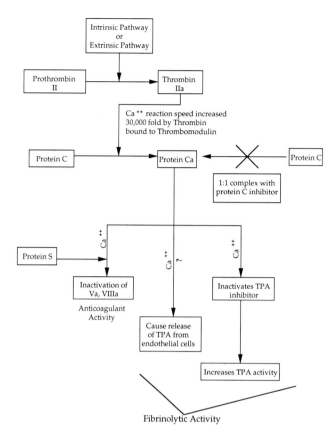

Figure 2–2. Schematic representation of initiation of the anticoagulant system and the fibrinolytic system by thrombin.

pathway quickly provides a small amount of thrombin to initiate coagulation and to accelerate the intrinsic pathway through activation of factors V and VIII.[1] The intrinsic pathway begins when factor XII is partially activated by exposure to collagen. High-molecular-weight kinninogen is required for full activation of XII. The intrinsic system proceeds until the complex of calcium, VIII, and IXa on the cell surface of platelets (PF3) activates factor X.[1]

Figures 2–2 and 2–3 outline the complex relationship between thrombin, coagulation inhibitors, and the fibrinolytic system. Thrombin initiates fibrinolysis by activating protein C, which in turn causes increased activity of tissue plasminogen activator (TPA). TPA activates plasmin, which is the enzyme responsible for degradation of fibrin and fibrinogen. Additionally, both protein C and plasmin inactivate factors V and VIII to inhibit the coagulation cascade.

Testing of coagulation will be discussed fully later in this chapter, but in brief, the intrinsic pathway is monitored by the partial thromboplastin time (PTT). This test measures factors XII, XI, IX, and VIII and the common pathway enzymes X, II, and I (fibrinogen). The prothrombin time (PT) measures the extrinsic system enzyme factor VII in addition to the common pathway enzymes.

CLINICAL EVALUATION OF HEMOSTASIS

The proper preoperative hemostatic evaluation is a topic that is hotly debated. When considering how extensive an evaluation to perform, cost containment as well as time and resource constraints must be weighed against the prevalence of clinically occult hemostatic disorders and the risk of blood loss with the planned procedure. Because a history is widely acknowledged as the single best test for preoperative hemostatic evaluation, its use is a mandatory first step regardless of philosophy regarding laboratory testing.[2]

Several authors state that testing of the coagulation cascade using the activated partial thromboplastin time (aPTT) and prothrombin time should not be obtained preoperatively in patients with a negative history because these tests do not predict surgical bleeding.[3–5] Similarly, some authors state that with a negative history, testing of platelet function via the bleeding time is of no benefit preoperatively.[6–8] On the other hand, authors favoring laboratory testing note that the history can be misleading for several reasons, including (1) poor history taking by the physician, (2) inaccurate history given by the patient, (3) recent development of a bleeding dyscrasia, and (4) patient without previous major hemostatic

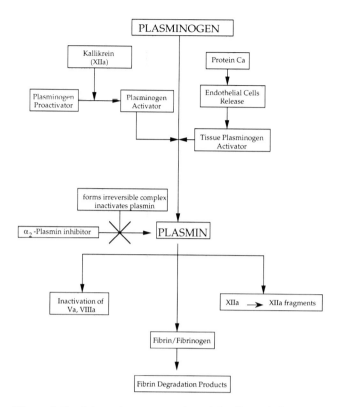

Figure 2–3. Schematic representation of the fibronolytic system with plasmin as its central component.

challenge.[2,9] The fact that history may be unreliable is confirmed by reports that 12% to 50% of potentially serious hemostatic defects are missed by history alone.[10,11] Additionally, it is estimated that 50% of previously undiagnosed bleeding disorders are discovered at the time of a surgical procedure.[12,13] These considerations and the experience of clinicians have led to the endorsement of minimalistic approaches by some and pleuralistic by others. Those who favor the combined use of history and laboratory testing for all but the most trivial procedures do so fully realizing that false positive test results will outnumber discoveries of significant hemostatic defects; however, they also are cognizant of the potentially disastrous operative course of patients with undiagnosed abnormalities of coagulation.

A combined history and laboratory evaluation that attempts to minimalize cost while maximizing the chance of detecting a coagulation defect that would otherwise result in clinically significant blood loss is suggested. The use of a stepped management plan with increasing laboratory use based on the patient's history and likelihood of procedural blood loss is favored.[9] Using the bleeding history discussed next, Rapaport has outlined four groups of patients with increasing risk of surgical bleeding and has suggested increasingly intensive preoperative evaluation.[9]

- *Group 1:* Patients with negative histories, with or without previous surgery, who are to undergo minor procedures such as biopsy. For this group, no laboratory testing is recommended.

- *Group 2:* Patients with negative histories, including prior surgery, and the planned procedure is major. For this group, an aPTT and a platelet count is recommended.

- *Group 3:* All patients with a possible hemostatic defect based on history and all patients who are to undergo procedures that impair hemostasis, such as cardiac surgery with the use of extracorporeal circulation. Patients in this group should have a platelet count and bleeding time to assess platelet function. The coagulation cascade is evaluated by PT and aPPT. If the aforementioned tests are normal, it is also necessary to evaluate fibrinolysis and clot stability (factor XIII deficiency). Screening tests for abnormal fibrinolysis and clot stability are performed by clotting 0.2 mL of plasma with 0.1 mL of $CaCl_2$, and then incubating the clots with saline or 5 M urea, respectively. If all tests are negative, then no further evaluation is required.

- *Group 4:* Patients with a likely or certain hemostatic defect based on history regardless of the planned surgery. The same evaluation as for group 3 is recommended; however, if these tests are negative, additional tests measuring factor VIII and IX coagulant activity and bleeding time after 600 mg of aspirin (to detect von Willebrand's disease or a mild qualitative platelet disorder) are suggested. Also, a thrombin time to test for dysfibrinogenemia and the level of plasma alpha$_2$-antiplasmin is recommended. If surgery cannot be delayed, the bleeding time after aspirin administration can be replaced by a qualitative evaluation of platelet function.

Part of the challenge of implementing this system for preoperative hemostatic evaluation is determining which procedures are major and which are minor. Estimated blood loss and involvement of large vessels obviously contribute to this decision, as does the vascularity of the region or tumor. Other less obvious considerations relate to the hemostatic challenge that the procedure presents. For example, tonsillectomy and adenoidectomy are generally considered minor procedures; however, these procedures represent major hemostatic challenges because they create raw mucosal surfaces that depend solely on intact platelet function and the coagulation cascade for control of hemorrhage. On the other hand, biopsies of skin or superficial subcutaneous tissues are closed and often covered with a pressure dressing. Excessive hemorrhage in these cases will increase the pressure and help control the bleeding. As with any system of preoperative hemostatic evaluation, some cases do not clearly fit into any of these artificially created categories.

We recommend consultation of a hematologist and a full hemostatic evaluation for patients in group 2 with prolonged aPTT or low platelet count and for any patient in groups 3 or 4.

History

An adequate coagulation history will detect roughly 75% of serious hemostatic defects and is the single most important and sensitive part of a preoperative evaluation.[10,14] Having acknowledged the significance of a good history, it is important to realize that up to 25% of heritable factor deficiencies may be missed by history alone due to variable expression or spontaneous mutations.[14] A good bleeding history must include a general medical history, including medications that the patient is currently taking.[2,9] Medications frequently affect platelet function and are often overlooked by both the patient and clinician. The patient must be specifically asked about nonsteroidal anti-inflammatory drugs because many patients do not consider over-the-counter drugs as important. An operative history including minor procedures and dental extractions is also mandatory. The operative history should concentrate on any unexpected or excessive bleeding, including bleeding greater than 24 hours after surgery.[2,9] Mucosal bleeding or spontaneous bleeding are often signs of vascular or platelet abnormalities; however, frequent epistaxis is not worrisome unless there are other complaints.[2] Finally, a family history can often detect heritable bleeding dyscrasias. In cases of positive family histories, the patient's bleeding history following surgical challenges is very important; if the patient has not had significant hemostatic challenges, then laboratory workup is mandatory. A general hemostatic questionnaire is outlined in Table 2-2.

Laboratory Tests of Hemostasis

There are a multitude of laboratory tests of platelet function and of the coagulation cascade. The surgeon must often decide which of these tests to obtain to maximize the probability of detecting an occult hemostatic defect without obtaining useless information. We will discuss the most commonly ordered laboratory tests.

PROTHROMBIN TIME

The PT is the best screening test for abnormalities of the extrinsic and common limbs of the coagulation pathway (Fig. 2-1).[15,16] It is performed by measuring the clotting time of plasma with the ideal concentration of tissue thromboplastin. Decreased levels of factors I (afibrinogenemia), II, V (parahemophilia), VII (hypoproconvertinemia), and X result

Table 2-2. Clinical History of Hemostasis

1. Have you ever bled for an abnormally long time after biting or cutting your tongue, cheek, or gums?
2. Do you spontaneously develop bruises larger than 4 to 5 cm (silver dollar) in diameter without any known cause?
3. Have you had prolonged bleeding after minor procedures such as biopsies or teeth extractions? Has bleeding recurred the day after a minor procedure?
4. Do you take any medications for headaches, arthritis, colds, menstrual cramps, or any medicine to thin your blood, including aspirin?
5. Do you have any relatives with bleeding disorders?
6. Do you have any medical problems that have required a doctor's care within the last 5 years?

in a prolonged PT.[1] Congenitally low levels of these factors are rare conditions, but acquired deficiency of active factors II, VII, and X are common and caused by liver disease, coumadin therapy, or vitamin K deficiency. Disseminated intravascular coagulation, high-titer lupus anticoagulant, and high-dose heparin therapy will also prolong the PT, but low-titer lupus anticoagulant and low-dose heparin will not.[1,15,16]

PARTIAL THROMBOPLASTIN TIME

The PTT is a test that measures abnormalities of the intrinsic pathway of coagulation. The test is performed by adding a platelet substitute (phospholipase A) so that platelet activity is not tested.[15] A modification of the PTT is addition of an activator that maximizes contact activation and increases the sensitivity and reproducibility of the test. The aPTT is used more commonly than the PTT.

Abnormalities of the most common heritable coagulation cascade deficiencies are measured by the aPTT. Decreased levels of factors I (afibrinogenemia), II, V (parahemophilia), VIII:C (hemophilia A), VIII:vWF (von Willebrand's disease), IX (Christmas disease = hemophilia B), X, XI, and XII all result in a prolonged aPTT.[1] The aPTT is more sensitive to deficiencies of factors earlier in the intrinsic cascade (XII, XI, IX, VIII, X) and can be normal with deficiencies of thrombin or fibrinogen.[15] Both blocking inhibitors such as the lupus anticoagulant and specific factor inhibitors will prolong the aPTT.[15] A mix helps to distinguish low factor levels from inhibitors and is discussed later.

Although the aPTT is the single most sensitive laboratory test for coagulation defects, it must be interpreted with knowledge of its limitations. It lacks sensitivity to mild deficiencies of single clotting factors and to hemostatic defects due to coumadin. Slight prolongations of aPTT are of questionable significance because most procedures on patients with mild prolongations have been uneventful.[15] On the other hand, several authors have not correlated increasing hemorrhagic risk with the degree of prolongation of the aPTT, suggesting that any prolongation of the aPTT should be investigated.[10] The most common cause of a prolonged aPTT is coagulation inhibitors; these will be discussed later in this chapter.

THROMBIN TIME

The thrombin time (TT) measures the interaction between exogenously added thrombin and fibrinogen. It is most commonly used as part of a disseminated intravascular coagulation screen or when both PT and aPTT are prolonged, but it is also sensitive for afibrinogenemia and dysfibrinogenemia. It is the most sensitive test for the presence of heparin.[1]

BLEEDING TIME

The bleeding time (BT) is the single best screening test for platelet function, but it has been criticized because in some studies it does not correlate with surgical bleeding.[8] Other authors recommend BT as a routine preoperative test because it screens for von Willebrand's disease and platelet dysfunction, which are two of the most prevalent occult hemostatic defects.[14] In addition to detecting platelet defects, the BT is also prolonged with decreased levels of factor V and vascular disorders (ie, osteogenesis imperfecta, hereditary hemorrhagic telangiectasia). The test is performed by inflating a blood pressure cuff to 40 mm Hg and then making a standardized cut using a template on the inner surface of the forearm. Blood is removed from the edge of the drop using filter paper until bleeding has stopped.

MISCELLANEOUS TESTS

Activated Clotting Time. The activated clotting time (ACT) is a commonly used test for assessing heparinization of patients intraoperatively.[16] Whole blood is mixed with diatomaceous earth, which activates the intrinsic coagulation cascade. Standard practice suggests that the ACT should be prolonged three to four times normal before cardiopulmonary bypass is begun.[16] If accurate levels of heparin are needed, then standardization curves can be calibrated.

Blood Smear. The blood smear is included in this section because it is of importance in assessing platelet function. Platelet morphological abnormalities are seen with some quantitative platelet disorders. Also, examination of the smear may reveal schistocytes and thrombocytopenia, which may suggest disseminated intravascular coagulation or thrombotic thrombocytopenia.[17]

Mixes. Mixing of patients' plasma with an equal volume of normal plasma is a standard test for the identification of coagulation inhibitors, such as the lupus anticoagulant, and for confirming the presence of specific factor deficiencies. The aPTT is the test most frequently prolonged in these situations, but mixes with the PT may be performed as well. If the prolongation of the aPTT or PT is due to decreased levels of a specific factor, then the mix should correct to normal.[15] On the other hand, if an inhibitor of coagulation is responsible for the prolonged aPTT or PT, the mix will not correct or only partially correct.[15] When the mix corrects, factor levels should be obtained to identify which factor is deficient. If the mix does not correct in patients without bleeding symptoms, then waiting 1 to 2 months and repeating the test will often allow for a transient inhibitor to clear.[18,19] If surgery cannot be delayed, then further workup for identification of the inhibitor should be undertaken. Inhibitors of coagulation will be discussed later in this chapter.

PLATELET DISORDERS AND THEIR TREATMENT

Platelets are an essential component, arguably the most important, of the coagulation system. Every aspect of coagulation, from the initial cellular plug to the coagulation cascade

as well as the eventual endothelial repair, depends on adequate platelet numbers and function. Metabolic and congenital disorders affect platelet function and numbers, but drug or alcoholic perturbation is far more commonly seen in surgical practice. Eventually, most surgeons will treat patients with platelet disorders; therefore, a rudimentary knowledge of platelet function and treatment of platelet defects is required.

Function

Platelets are anuclear cellular fragments that bud from the cytoplasm of megakaryocytes in the bone marrow. Seventy percent of platelets circulate whereas 30% are reserved in the microcirculation or spleen. The average life span of platelets is 9 to 12 days, at which time they (along with deformed platelets) are removed from the circulation by macrophages in the spleen and liver.[1,21] Defects in platelet life span or abnormal sequestration in the spleen or liver can lead to thrombocytopenia, with resultant hemorrhagic complications.

Even when there is no trauma to the endothelia, platelets are necessary to maintain vascular integrity and prevent hemorrhage into the soft tissues in the form of purpura and petechiae. Platelets maintain the endothelia by incorporating themselves into the endothelial wall in a manner that can be equated to "feeding" the endothelial cells.[1,21] When the endothelia is disrupted as with surgery or trauma, platelets perform two vital functions at the center of the effort to control hemorrhage. First, exposure of subendothelial tissue, such as connective tissue, causes platelets to adhere to the site of the injury and to each other. The plug formed depends on a protein expressed on the cell surface of platelets known as von Willebrand's factor, abbreviated VIII:vWF, which denotes that it is a component of the factor VIII complex. VIII:vWF is bound to the platelet cell surface by both protein Ib and the IIb/IIIa protein complex.[1,21] Bound VIII:vWF mediates platelet adherence to connective tissue through an unknown mechanism. Quantitative and/or qualitative decrease of VIII:vWF is seen in von Willebrand's disease, discussed later in this chapter. Once exposed to subendothelial tissues, platelets release the stored contents of granules from their cytoplasm into the surrounding tissues. There are several platelet disorders caused by failure to synthesize, release, or respond to granule contents, but these are relatively rare and will not be discussed.[20] Granules in functioning platelets contain many chemotactic factors, as well as adenosine diphosphate (ADP), calcium, fibrinogen, and epinephrine, all of which speed platelet aggregation.[1,21] Calcium stimulates a phospholipase to cleave phospholipids from the platelet membrane providing the building blocks for prostaglandins. The primary prostaglandin synthesized by platelets is thromboxane A2 (TXA_2), which causes vasoconstriction and further increases platelet aggregation.[1,21] Therefore, the platelet rapidly provides vasoconstriction and a cellular plug at the site of endothelial injury in a process known as primary hemostasis.

The second function of platelets is to stabilize the initial plug by contributing to the coagulation cascade. Glycoproteins IIb and IIIa on the cell surface of platelets bind fibrinogen, which serves to increase platelet aggregation and provide a high concentration of the final substrate of the coagulation cascade.[21] Platelets also provide a catalytic surface for the coagulation reactions to occur by exposing cell surface phospholipids (platelet factor 3 = PF3) that allow coagulation factors to form complexes on the platelet membrane. The platelet surface provides high concentrations of coagulation substrates and enzymes and a protective surface that shields the factors from plasma inhibitors. The importance of the platelet in the coagulation cascade is attested to by the fact that the complex of Va, Xa, and calcium on the platelet membrane generates thrombin 278,000 times faster than factor Xa alone.[21] The result of the coagulation cascade catalyzed by platelets is the rapid deposition of fibrin strands, which then entrap platelets forming a meshwork that is able to stop hemorrhage.[1]

Figure 2–4 shows the complex interactions of platelets with the vessel wall and with the factors of the coagulation cascade. Ultimately these interactions result in formation of a cellular plug and a fibrin clot.

Idiopathic Thrombocytopenic Purpura/Autoimmune Thrombocytopenia

Although this group of diseases is commonly referred to as idiopathic thrombocytopenic purpura (ITP), this term is somewhat outdated, less encompassing, and less descriptive than the terminology we will use; namely, autoimmune thrombocytopenia (AITP). Three categories of AITP based on duration of thrombocytopenia and associated autoimmune diseases are (1) idiopathic thrombocytopenic purpura (ITP),

a chronic disease of unknown cause with an insidious onset affecting predominantly young adults with a 3 to 1 female predominance; (2) secondary autoimmune thrombocytopenia, whose disease course resembles ITP but is associated with an autoimmune disease, malignancy, or other immunomodulatory disease or treatment; and (3) acute postviral autoimmune thrombocytopenia, a disorder usually seen in children following a viral infection, with thrombocytopenia lasting less than 6 months (Table 2–3). A chronic form of acute postviral autoimmune thrombocytopenia lasting more than 6 months rarely occurs and cannot be distinguished from ITP.[22]

Although the causes of AITP are unknown, it is known that all three of the aforementioned syndromes are associated with autoantibodies to platelets.[23,24] The mechanism for formation of the antibodies is unknown, although hypotheses include molecular mimicry (with viral markers resembling platelet cell surface markers), anti-idiotype antibodies (where secondary antibodies are made to antibodies formed against viral markers), and exposure of previously hidden markers on the platelet surface.[23]

CLINICAL COURSE AND TREATMENT

Patients with AITP typically present with petechiae, cutaneous purpura, and/or mucosal bleeding such as epistaxis, bleeding gums, hematuria, melena, or menorrhagia, all of which are due to thrombocytopenia. Mucosal bleeding is associated with lower platelet counts, and these patients are at increased risk for severe hemorrhage, including cerebral hemorrhage, leading some experts to treat all patients with mucosal bleeding.

Diagnosis is primarily clinically based with supporting laboratory findings of an isolated thrombocytopenia without other abnormalities in the complete blood count or coagulation tests. Splenomegaly is not a characteristic of AITP, and its presence suggests another diagnosis. The presence of platelet autoantibodies further support the diagnosis of AITP but is not necessary in all cases. Drug-induced thrombocytopenia, posttransfusion purpura, and clumping of

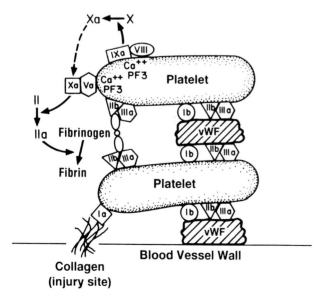

Figure 2–4. Schematic representation of complex interaction of platelet cell surface with von Willebrand's factor, coagulation factors, blood vessel wall, and collagen. Ia, Ib, IIb, and IIIa represent proteins on the platelet cell surface.

Table 2–3. General Clinical Features of AITP

GENERAL CLINICAL FEATURES OF AITP		
	Acute	*Chronic*
Peak age indidence	2–8 years	20–40 years
Sex incidence	F = M	3F:1 M
Onset	Sudden	Insidious
Duration	<6 months (usually weeks)	>6 months (often years)
Associated disorders	Preceding viral infection	(i) Idiopathic (ii) Secondary; multiple, including autoimmune, cancer, HIV, chemotherapy, radiation therapy

From Waters.[13]

platelets due to ethylenediaminetetraacetic acid (EDTA; an anticoagulant in blood collection tubes) should be distinguished from AITP. A history of a recent viral infection or of a concomitant autoimmune disease helps distinguish ITP from secondary AITP or acute postviral AITP.

The treatment of AITP varies depending on the extent and chronicity of the thrombocytopenia, the severity of the bleeding, and the lifestyle of the patient. Patients with chronic AITP (ITP, secondary AITP) have traditionally been treated with steroids followed by splenectomy, if necessary. Removal of the spleen abolishes a major source of autoantibody production as well as abolishing the primary site of platelet destruction.[23] Following this treatment course, 80% of patients will obtain a permanent remission. Ten percent of patients will relapse after an initial response, and 10% will not respond.[23] Intravenous IgG treatment has recently been shown to increase the response rate to steroids as well as the likelihood of remission after splenectomy. Some patients who do not respond to splenectomy will respond to intravenous IgG therapy. IgG is thought to block the reticuloendothelial system by competing for binding sites on macrophages that would normally bind to and destroy platelets covered in antibodies.[25]

If a patient with chronic AITP requires surgery, preoperative intravenous IgG is recommended and has been shown to increase the safety of surgery by increasing platelet counts.[23] If platelet counts cannot be increased with IgG therapy, platelet transfusion may be necessary.[23]

Acute postviral thrombocytopenia is managed differently because of the excellent prognosis and extremely rare incidence of severe hemorrhage.[22] The disease is one of childhood in greater than 90% of cases and usually follows a viral infection.[25] The autoantibody responsible for the acute form is IgM, which explains the short duration of illness of 3½ weeks on average.[23,25] Because of the benign nature of acute postviral thrombocytopenia, a noninterventionist strategy with limitation of activity, avoidance of nonsteroidal anti-inflammatory drugs, and weekly platelet counts is effective and avoids expensive hospitalization and intravenous therapy. Only if the child is over 10 years of age or has severe hemorrhage is a treatment protocol similar to that described for chronic AITP suggested.[23] If surgery is required in a patient with postviral thrombocytopenia, intravenous IgG should be given and offers the same therapeutic benefits described for chronic AITP.[23,25]

To summarize, chronic AITP usually responds well to intravenous steroid and/or IgG therapy often followed by splenectomy. Acute postviral thrombocytopenia usually is self-limited, requiring only behavior modification and weekly platelet counts. If any patient with AITP is to undergo surgery, intravenous IgG is recommended to increase platelet counts with a concomitant decrease in the risk of bleeding.

Thrombotic Thrombocytopenic Purpura

Thrombotic thrombocytopenic purpura (TTP) is a rare (1/10^6 population), life-threatening disorder characterized by the pentad of change in neurological status, microangiopathic hemolytic anemia, thrombocytopenia, fever, and renal dysfunction.[22] The fever is usually low grade and the renal disorder is usually mild. Cerebral involvement is rarely catastrophic and usually fluctuates.[22,26-29] The presence of schistocytes, spherocytes, anisocytosis, and pleocytosis in the face of thrombocytopenia (usually <40,000) should suggest a diagnosis of TTP if disseminated intravascular coagulation (DIC) has been excluded. Definitive diagnosis is made only with pathologic evaluation of tissue. Gingival biopsies and bone marrow biopsies are diagnostic in 15% and 30% of cases, respectively, but because no other easily obtainable tissue makes the diagnosis more frequently, both biopsies are usually done.[30]

The pathogenesis of TTP is not completely understood, but recent advances are unraveling the mechanisms involved. Pathologic examination of involved tissues reveals small arterial and arteriolar thromboses composed mainly of platelets.[30] Fibrin and coagulation factor levels are not abnormal, distinguishing TTP from DIC. Studies have shown that plasma from patients with TTP causes platelet aggregation, which is enhanced by the presence of von Willebrand's factor (VIII:vWF). Abnormalities in VIII:vWF multimers associated with active disease further suggest a role for this molecule in the pathogenesis of TTP.[26-28] Other investigators have found a decreased level of prostacyclin stimulatory factor in the plasma of patients with TTP. Absence of adequate levels of this factor leads to decreased endothelial production of prostacyclin (PGI$_2$), which is the most potent natural inhibitor of platelet aggregation.[27]

CLINICAL COURSE AND TREATMENT

Untreated, the mortality from TTP may reach 90%, and even with maximal treatment death rates into the 1970s were reported as high as 70%.[26,30] Findings of platelet aggregation factors in the plasma of patients with TTP have led to changes in treatment protocols to include plasma infusions, plasmapharesis, and antiplatelet agents. These strategies have improved survival to between 70% and 90%.[22,27] Standard protocol is to begin plasma transfusions immediately at a rate of 6 to 8 units daily in adults.[27] An improvement in neurological status occurs in 60% to 70% of patients within 48 to 72 hours. If no response to plasma is seen in 48 hours, then plasmapharesis should be initiated.[27] Due to slightly improved response rates of 60% to 80%, some authors favor institution of plasmapharesis upon diagnosis of TTP.[27] After return of platelet counts to normal and remission of neurological symptoms, plasma infusions or plasmapharesis may be stopped with the understanding that relapses occur in a small percentage (<10%) of patients who may require long-term therapy.[22,27,29] Antiplatelet medications do not affect survival when administered alone, but there is a suggestion of increased survival when administered concommitantly with plasma infusions or plasmapharesis.[22,27] Control of chronic or relapsing TTP may be improved with long-term use of antiplatelet agents.[22,27]

Despite the often severe thrombocytopenia seen in patients with TTP, platelet transfusions should be avoided. Platelet transfusions have been associated with progression of the disease, consistent with the pathogenesis of platelet thrombosis.[27] Also, heparin should not be administered because it has never been shown to improve survival and in some reports is associated with decreased survival.[22]

Platelet Dysfunction in Renal Disease

Uremic patients have varying degrees of platelet dysfunction that is reversible with hemodialysis, peritoneal dialysis, or renal transplant.[31] Serum levels of guanidinosuccinic and hydroxyphenolic acids are elevated in patients with renal insufficiency, and they have been implicated as etiologic agents of platelet dysfunction in these patients. These acids have been shown to decrease the availability of phospholipids (PF3) on the surface of platelets that are important as a catalyst to the coagulation cascade.[31] A functional defect in the interaction between proteins (IIb, IIIa) on the platelet membrane and von Willebrand's factor (VIII:vWF) has also been observed in uremic patients.

The standard therapy of bleeding disorders in patients with renal failure continues to be dialysis. Increased levels of high-molecular-weight multimers of VIII:vWF in the plasma after dialysis correlate with correction of bleeding times.[31] Twenty-five percent of patients' bleeding times corrected within 24 hours of dialysis. Six days of dialysis corrected 70% of patients' bleeding times.[31] When quicker correction of bleeding abnormalities is required, cryoprecipitate and DDAVP (1-deamino-8-D-arginine vasopressin) have been effective.[32-34] Infusion of cryoprecipitate causes maximal shortening of the bleeding time between 1 and 12 hours after infusion, with significant improvement within 4 hours.[32] The effect of cryoprecipitate vanishes 24 to 36 hours after infusion, with return of bleeding times to pretransfusion baseline.[32]

Administration of 10 bags of cryoprecipitate carries the risk of transfusion-mediated infections equal to that of transfusion with 10 units of packed red blood cells. Due primarily to the infectious risks of administering cryoprecipitate, correction of bleeding time in uremic patients with DDAVP has gained widespread use.[31-34] The effect of DDAVP with intravenous infusion is almost immediate, and the therapeutic effect lasts on average 4 hours. The standard dose of DDAVP is 0.3 μg/kg administered intravenously. Side-effects are ususaly mild, with facial flushing, transient headaches, and mild decreases in systolic or diastolic blood pressure being most common. These side-effects can usually be controlled by decreasing the rate of infusion.[34] Mechanically, DDAVP is thought to cause its therapeutic effect by stimulating platelets to release stores of VIII:vWF.[33] Blood concentrations of the large-molecular-weight multimers of VIII:vWF correlate with the shortening of bleeding time, and it is thought that these large forms of VIII:vWF promote platelet adhesion and aggregation better than the smaller multimers.[33] Because storage pools of VIII:vWF are decreased after administra-

tion of DDAVP, additional doses generally do not have as good a clinical response as the first dose.[34] When patients become less responsive to DDAVP and control of bleeding is still required, cryoprecipitate is a therapeutic alternative.

Miscellaneous and Drug-Induced Thrombocytopenia

The etiology of an isolated thrombocytopenia must be explored before an elective surgical procedure can be performed. A careful history frequently reveals the etiology of the thrombocytopenia to be related to drugs or alcohol. Both clinically insignificant and significant thrombocytopenia is associated with pregnancy.[35,36] Differentiating these causes of thrombocytopenia from AITP allows proper preoperative management of patients.

DRUG-INDUCED THROMBOCYTOPENIA

Over 100 drugs have been shown to cause immune-mediated destruction of blood cells, including platelets.[37] Many mechanisms have been expounded to explain how certain drugs lead to specific destruction of platelets. The most popular theory proposes that antibodies are made in response to a new antigen formed by the interaction of a drug or its metabolites with the cell membrane of platelets. The antibody formed may act independently or require that the drug be present to bind and destroy platelets. Heparin is the most studied drug that causes immune thrombocytopenia; however, quinine, quinidine, and gold are also frequently associated with drug-induced platelet destruction.[37,38] The dose or route of administration is not related to the onset or severity of the thrombocytopenia. Without previous exposure to the drug, at least a 6-day lag period between onset of thrombocytopenia and administration of the drug is expected.

Patients with immune-mediated thrombocytopenia frequently present with fever, chills, arthralgias, the abrupt onset of moderate to massive petechiae, hematomas, or mucosal bleeding not related to trauma.[37] The bleeding, especially if mucosal, may be severe or life threatening. The best treatment is immediate cessation of the causative agent. Because antibodies responsible for the thrombocytopenia have been shown to persist for years, the patient should never receive the drug again.[37] For patients with more severe or life-threatening bleeds, therapy parallels that of AITP. As with the treatment of AITP, steroids and high-dose IgG are the cornerstones of treatment. A favorable response to a single course of therapy is consistent with drug-induced thrombocytopenia rather than AITP.[34]

ETHANOL-RELATED THROMBOCYTOPENIA

Over 80% of chronic alcoholics admitted for detoxification have a mild to moderate thrombocytopenia that will begin to resolve within days of abstention.[39] Ethanol is directly toxic to platelets and megakaryocytes, causing a 50% reduction in platelet survival as well as decreased platelet production.[37]

Even before the onset of thrombocytopenia, ethanol causes a qualitative decrease in platelet function mainly due to decreased stores of ADP and decreased production of thromboxane A_2 (TXA_2) resulting in prolongation of bleeding times. The relationship of hemorrhage in alcoholics to the adverse effects of ethanol on platelets is unknown.

Withdrawal from alcohol has been associated with deep venous thrombosis and pulmonary embolism. The increased risk in chronic alcoholics is not understood but may relate to a rebound thrombocytosis seen in almost all heavy drinkers, which lasts up to 3 weeks after cessation of alcohol consumption.[39]

THROMBOCYTOPENIA IN PREGNANCY

Autoimmune thrombocytopenia, disseminated intravascular coagulation, thrombotic thrombocytopenic purpura, and drugs can all lead to thrombocytopenia in pregnant patients. Discussion will be limited to thrombocytopenic conditions unique to pregnancy because the other disease processes have been discussed previously.

Pregnancy is associated with increased platelet activation and consumption, accounting for thrombocytopenia in about 8% of normal pregnant patients.[35,36] Pregnancy-associated thrombocytopenia (PAT) is by definition mild (100 to 150 $\times 10^9$ platelets per liter) and is not associated with fetal thrombocytopenia or any increased risk to the mother or fetus.[35,36] No treatment is necessary for PAT if the mother has no history of bleeding disorders.[36]

In contrast, thrombocytopenia associated with pre-eclampsia, which occurs in 16% to 50% of pre-ecclamptic women, may be severe (below 50×10^9 per liter) and has been associated with neonatal mortality as high as 60%.[20,25,35,40] Recently, early diagnosis and delivery (the only effective treatment) has dramatically decreased neonatal and maternal mortality.[40] Within 4 days of delivery, maternal platelet counts rise and are greater than 100×10^9 per liter in 98% of patients.[25] The pathogenesis of pre-eclampsia is unknown, but platelet production of increased amounts of thromboxane A_2 (TXA_2) has been implicated. Low-dose aspirin inhibits cyclo-oxygenase, the enzyme responsible for TXA_2 production, and has been shown to prevent pre-eclampsia in high-risk patients.[41]

COAGULATION DISORDERS AND TREATMENT

Hemophilia A

Hemophilia A is an X-linked inherited disorder of coagulation that affects roughly 1/10,000 of the male population.[1,15] Factor VIII coagulation activity is decreased in these patients, and the clinical manifestations of the disease relate directly to the level of factor VIII activity.[1,42] Severe hemophilia is described as factor VIII coagulation activity of less than 1%, moderate 3% to 5%, and mild 5% to 12%.[1] Severely affected patients will present with hemarthroses, hematomas,

hematuria, and bleeding from the mucosal surfaces of the nose and mouth.[15] Patients with mild disease will not have spontaneous bleeding but will have severe hemorrhage with surgery or trauma.[15] With the advent of factor concentrates that patients are able to self-administer, even severe hemophiliacs can attain fairly normal daily activities.

To understand the hemostatic defect in hemophilia A, a basic understanding of factor VIII is needed. Factor VIII is a glycoprotein that normally circulates as a complex of two proteins encoded on separate genes.[1] The nomenclature applied to the complex is outlined in Table 2–4. The smaller portion of the complex is responsible for the clotting activity and is referred to as VIII:C. The larger subunit varies in size due to the formation of multimers and is responsible for the von Willebrand activity (VIII:vWF), which is measured by aggregation of platelets from test plasma. The activity of the VIII complex that results in aggregation of platelets in the presence of the antibiotic ristocetin, is referred to as VIIIR:RCo.[1] Antibodies have been developed that recognize and differentiate antigens of the VIII complex usually responsible for coagulant activity and for von Willebrand activity. The antigenic presence of the two portions of the VIII complex as identified by antibodies is referred to as VIII:Ag (coagulant antigen) and vWF:Ag (von Willebrand antigen). The antigenic presence does not imply function because the antigens can be present but the activity absent. Low levels of VIII:C result in hemophilia A, and low levels of VIII:vWF result in von Willebrand's disease.

TESTING FOR HEMOPHILIA A

The activity of VIII:C can be measured in plasma and has a wide normal range varying from 50% to 200%. One hundred percent is designated as normal and is 1 unit of activity per milliliter of plasma. The classic laboratory evaluation of patients with hemophilia A reveals a prolonged activated partial thromboplastin time with normal prothrombin time and bleeding time. VIII:vWF and VIIIR:RCo are normal whereas VIII:C is usually 1% to 15%.[1] Levels of VIII:Ag normally parallel levels of VIII:C.

Table 2–4. Nomenclature for the Factor VIII Complex

VIII:C	Procoagulant activity of the factor VIII complex that is deficient in hemophilia A.
VIII:vWF	von Willebrand activity of the factor VIII complex that is deficient in von Willebrand's disease.
VIII:Ag	Antigenic property of the portion of the factor VIII complex normally responsible for the coagulant activity of factor VIII.
vWF:Ag	Antigenic property of the factor VIII complex normally associated with the von Willebrand activity of factor VIII.
VIIIR:RCo	Activity of the factor VIII complex that supports aggregation of platelets by the antibiotic ristocetin, referred to as ristocetin cofactor activity.

TREATMENT OF HEMOPHILIA A

Patients with hemophilia A are usually treated with VIII:C concentrates. Before concentrates were available, cryoprecipitate was used but dosing was difficult due to the high volumes often required and the inability to calculate the exact dose due to variations in VIII:C concentration from sample to sample. Since the mid-1980s, increased awareness of infectious risks has dictated that factor concentrates be free of hepatitis B virus and human immunodeficiency virus (HIV) contamination. Screening of donors and blood products, as well as monoclonal antibody purification and treatment of factor VIII with solvents and detergents, has yielded safe products for treatment of hemophilia. Dosage can be calculated by the knowledge that in patients without inhibitors, administration of 1 unit of VIII:C per kilogram of body weight reslts in an increase of 0.02 units per milliliter.[13] For major surgery, the VIII:C level should be corrected to 0.8 to 1.0 units per milliliter (80% to 100%) during surgery and then maintained at 0.3 to 0.5 units per milliliter (30% to 50%) for 10 to 14 days.[13] The half-life of VIII:C in patients with hemophilia is 6 to 10 hours, so replacement of factor is usually performed at 8 to 12 hours; however, factor VIII assays should be used to guide replacement.[1,13,42]

Alternate therapy for mild or moderate hemophiliacs includes the use of desmopressin (DDAVP). DDAVP has been successful in raising the VIII:C level two- to threefold.[43] The mechanism is thought to be stimulation of endothelial cells to release von Willebrand factor, which serves as a carrier for the coagulant portion of VIII in the blood.[43] The dose and administration are 0.3 µg/kg subcutaneously or intravenously. The effect is usually seen within 30 to 60 minutes and lasts 4 hours. Three to four repeat doses can be given but may be less effective than the original.

Mild to moderate hemophiliacs undergoing minor procedures such as dental extractions may also be treated with epsilon-aminocaproic acid (EACA, Amicar) or tranexamic acid.[42] Both of these agents decrease fibrinolysis by inhibition of plasminogen activation. The standard dose is 4 g Amicar by mouth (PO) every 4 to 6 hours for 7 to 10 days or 0.25 mg/kg tranexamic acid PO 3 to 4 times a day. These agents should not be used if the patient has hematuria due to an association with upper urinary tract obstruction.

INHIBITORS OF FACTOR VIII IN HEMOPHILIA

Inhibitors of factor VIII occur in roughly 10% of all hemophiliacs but affect severe hemophiliacs more commonly than patients with mild or moderate disease.[1,42,44] In general, increased exposure to infused factor VIII increases the risk of developing an inhibitor; however, after 50 to 100 exposure days the risk begins to diminish.[44] Inhibitors are quantitated by adding a known quantity of VIII:C to sample serum and then analyzing for VIII:C activity after 1 hour.[1] For every 1/2-unit decrease in VIII:C activity, one Bethesda unit of inhibitor is present.[1] Treatment of hemophiliacs with inhibitors depends on the titre and the amnestic response of

the patient. Roughly 25% of hemophiliacs will be low responders, and 75% will be high responders. The amnestic response of a high responder will occur in 2 to 4 days and render standard therapy with factor VIII concentrates ineffective in all patients except those with low titres.[1] For patients with high titre inhibitors, prothrombin complex (factor IX concentrates), which contains factors II, VII, IX, and X, is clinically effective about 50% of the time. The usual dose is 75 to 100 U/kg every 8 to 12 hours. Activated prothrombin complex concentrates (Autoplex, FEIBA) that contain activated factors II, VII, IX, and X are effective about 65% to 75% of the time. Both of these treatments for hemophiliacs with inhibitors have complications of thromboembolic disease and disseminated intravascular coagulation.[42] Recombinant activated factor VII may be beneficial to patients unresponsive to other therapies and is currently under investigation.

HEMOPHILIA B (CHRISTMAS DISEASE)

Hemophilia B is discussed here because it is clinically indistinguishable from hemophilia A. It has an X-linked recessive inheritance profile like hemophilia A, but its incidence is roughly one tenth that of hemophilia A (1 per 100,000 male population).[15] Only testing for specific factor activity distinguishes hemophilia B from hemophilia A. As with factor VIII, 30% of IX activity is required for normal hemostasis following surgery or trauma.[15] Appropriate treatment with factor IX concentrates (prothrombin complex concentrates) is calculated by assuming that infusion of 1 U/kg raises the factor IX level by 1%. The goal is usually less than 50% correction because of the increased risk of thromboembolic disease and disseminated intravascular coagulation. Because of the risk of thromboses, simultaneous low-dose heparin is sometimes given.

von Willebrand's Disease

Decreased levels or an abnormal multimer pattern of von Willebrand factor (vWF) are present in patients with von Willebrand's disease (vWD). Classically, patients with vWD present with a congenital (autosomal recessive) bleeding disorder, with increased activated partial thromboplastin time, increased bleeding time, and decreased plasma concentrations of VIII:C and VIII:vWF.[45-47] The preceding discussion of the factor VIII complex indicates that the larger portion of the complex is the vWF (Table 2-4). vWF is important for aggregation of platelets to one another and for adhesion of platelets to the endothelial surface (Fig. 2-2).[1]

CLINICAL MANIFESTATIONS AND LABORATORY TESTS

vWD is one of the most common hemostatic disorders, and its severity varies from patient to patient even within the same family.[45,47] To a lesser extent, the severity of the disease can also vary within the same patient from time to time.[47] Administration of nonsteroidal anti-inflammatory drugs will sometimes cause the first clinical symptoms in patients with mild disease and should be avoided due to increased hemorrhagic risk.[46] Severe recessive (type III) vWD is rare and is clinically hard to distinguish from hemophilia. More commonly vWD presents with mucosal bleeding or bleeding following trauma or surgery.[46] If vWD is suspected, laboratory evaluation of the patient should be undertaken prior to any surgical procedure. Table 2–5 lists the typical laboratory results of patients with hemophilia and vWD.

As with the clinical manifestations of vWD, the laboratory evaluation of any patient can vary from time to time, making the diagnosis difficult.[47] Because of the variability of clinical symptoms and laboratory results, negative laboratory tests must be repeated if clinical suspicion is high. The aPTT is variably prolonged depending on the VIII:C concentration. If VIII:C is less than 30%, then prolongation of the aPTT will result. All patients will have a prolonged BT at some time; however, a normal BT does not rule out the diagnosis.[14] In most patients, VIIIR:RCo is reduced as measured by the aggregation of platelets in the presence of ristocetin. However, some subtypes (IIb and platelet) have increased aggregation of platelets with low concentrations of ristocetin. VIII:C and VIII:vWF are decreased even though vWF:Ag may be normal. Like many factor disorders, the antigenic expression can be normal due to production of a nonfunctioning protein. In the case of vWD, multimeric examination of vWF is important to distinguish the different subtypes of the disease. Also important for differentiation of vWD subtypes is the measurement of ristocetin-induced platelet aggregation. Differentiation of subtypes is important in treatment and will be discussed later. Table 2–6 lists the subtypes of von Willebrand's disease.

Type I vWD accounts for 70% to 80% of patients with this disorder. In this subtype, all multimers of vWF are present but at decreased levels.[43] Type II accounts for roughly 10% to 15% of patients, with type IIa being the most common within this category.[43] In type II disease, vWF:Ag may be normal but there is an absence of the high-molecular-weight multimers.[42,43] Type III vWD is distinguished by almost complete absence of vWF of any form with very low vWF:Ag. Platelet type vWF is also known as pseudo-vWD because it is due to a defect of protein Ib on the surface of platelets, causing abnormally high affinity binding of vWF. Platelet type vWD is a primary platelet disorder but is mentioned because of its clinical similarity to true vWD.

Table 2–5. Laboratory Evaluation of Patients with von Willebrand's Disease and Hemophilia

	VON WILLEBRAND'S DISEASE	HEMOPHILIA
VIII:C	Decreased or normal	Decreased
VIII:vWF	Decreased	Increased or normal
vWF:Ag	Decreased or normal	Increased or normal
Bleeding time	Increased	Normal

Table 2–6. Classification of von Willebrand's Disease

TYPE	VIII:vWF	VIII:C	MULTIMER PATTERN
Ia	Decreased	Decreased	All multimers decreased
Ib	Decreased	Decreased	All multimers decreased, large multimers relatively decreased
Ic	Decreased	Decreased	All multimers decreased, abnormal triplet pattern
IIa	Decreased	Decreased	Large and midsized multimers decreased
IIb	Decreased	Decreased	Large multimers decreased, greater than normal aggregation of platelets with low concentration of ristocetin
IIc	Decreased	Decreased	Large multimers decreased, abnormal triplet pattern
IId	Decreased	Decreased	Large multimers decreased, abnormal triplet pattern
III	Decreased	Decreased	All multimers absent
Platelet	Decreased	Decreased	Large multimers decreased, greater than normal aggregation of platelets with low concentration of ristocetin

TREATMENT OF vWD

The goal of therapy in vWD is to correct VIII:C, VIIIR:RCo, and the BT. Cryoprecipitate and plasma have been used to correct clinical bleeding as well as normalize laboratory tests because they contain adequate amounts of VIII:C and VIII:vWF.[46] These blood products carry the risk of infectious transmission, and recently the use of desmopressin (DDAVP) has shown efficacy for most patients with vWD.[42,43] (For a more in-depth discussion of DDAVP, see the preceding section "Platelet Disorders and Their Treatment.") DDAVP is the treatment of choice for type I vWD and acts by causing a two- to threefold increase in VIII:vWF and VIII:C.[43,46] Type II and III vWD do not respond to DDAVP because in type II the vWF released by platelets and endothelial cells is abnormal and in type III there is little or no vWF to be released.[42,47] In types IIb and platelet vWD, not only does DDAVP fail to shorten BT, it also causes severe but transient thrombocytopenia.[43] The mechanism of thrombocytopenia in type IIb vWD is by binding of the abnormal vWF to platelets, which causes their agglutination.[34] Because multimeric workup of vWD is often laborious, most authors have suggested a preoperative test dose of DDAVP with mesurement of BT to distinguish responders from nonresponders.[34,43]

The treatment of choice for types II and III vWD is the intermediate purity factor VIII concentrate (Humate-P), which contains adequate amounts of VIII:vWF. This product contains a vWF profile similar to normal plasma, whereas the other intermediate purity products are relatively deficient in the high-molecular-weight multimers.[46] Humate-P has been shown to correct the bleeding time to the normal range, with results lasting from 2 to 78 hours after infusion.[46] In some patients, the BT remains prolonged despite normal levels of VIII:C and VIII:vWF after infusion.[46] Studies have shown that patients with normal VIII:C and VIII:vWF tolerate surgical procedures without excessive bleeding despite the prolonged BT; therefore, it may not be necessary to correct the bleeding time if VIII:C and VIII:vWF are normalized.

Inhibitors to vWF can develop in patients with vWD or myeloproliferative disorders. The inhibitor is an antibody that can result in severe and even life-threatening hemorrhage. Treatment parallels that of hemophilia with inhibitors. Infusion of activated prothrombin complex concentrates has been effective, as have protein-A columns and plasmapharesis, both of which remove gamma globulin from the plasma.[46]

Liver Disease

The defects of coagulation associated with liver failure (LF) are basically the same whether the cause is cirrhosis, acute hepatitis, chronic hepatitis, or toxicity. Because the liver produces all coagulation factors (excluding von Willebrand's factor) and it also is responsible for manufacturing the important anticoagulants protein C, protein S, and antithrombin III, it is not surprising that patients with LF have abnormal coagulation. The liver also produces the important fibrinolytic enzyme, plasminogen, as well as the inhibitors of fibrinolysis, alpha$_2$-antiplasmin, and plasminogen activator inhibitor. The changes in the aforementioned and fibrinolytic enzymes are confounded by the fact that patients with LF also have thrombocytopenia and decreased platelet function as well as vitamin K deficiency. With so many facets of the coagulation and fibrinolytic systems affected, it is surprising that LF patients do not have hemorrhagic episodes more frequently than they do. Bleeding in patients with LF is usually due to an anatomic defect (varices, peptic ulcer disease, gastritis, etc.), which is then exacerbated by the coagulation defect.[48]

PLATELET ABNORMALITIES IN LIVER FAILURE

Thrombocytopenia with platelet counts of less than 100,000 per milliliter is common in LF. Reduced platelet survival with increased splenic sequestration appears to be the primary mechanism of thrombocytopenia.[49] If low-grade disseminated intravascular coagulation (DIC) is present, further reduction of platelet count and funtion is expected due to increased consumption and the coating of the platelet with fibrin degradation products, which alters metabolism of membrane fatty acids and platelet function. If the patient with LF consumes ethanol, further deterioration of platelet function, as discussed earlier in this chapter, will occur.

In addition to thrombocytopenia, patients with LF also have a qualitative platelet defect, as evidenced by decreased platelet aggregation and reduced ATP and serotonin release.[49] The size (volume) of platelets in LF is decreased, which could explain the diminished aggregation because smaller platelets do not function as well as larger platelets. Abnormal arachidonic acid metabolism with low production of thromboxane

A$_2$ (TXA$_2$) may further explain the functional platelet abnormalities.[49]

The defects of primary hemostasis in LF due to thrombocytopenia and qualitative platelet defects have been correlated with clinical bleeding and must be addressed in LF patients who are bleeding or require surgery.[49]

COAGULATION CASCADE DEFECTS IN LIVER FAILURE

Patients with LF do not absorb vitamin K well due to cholestasis and are unable to store vitamin K in the liver. As a result, LF patients have vitamin K deficiency.[48] Additionally, decreased production of all coagulation factors, except von Willebrand's factor, is seen in LF. The severity of the LF correlates with decreasing levels of these proteins. As mentioned before, all coagulation factors will be decreased; however, decreased levels of the vitamin-K-dependent factors seem to occur first.[49]

LABORATORY EVALUATION

The minimal laboratory studies that should be obtained for patients with LF include PT, aPTT, platelet count, and fibrinogen level.[48] The PT will almost always be elevated due to low levels of factors II, IX, X, and VII which are compounded by vitamin K deficiency.[42,49] Factor VII levels are especially sensitive to LF due to its extremely short half-life.[42,49] Most patients will also have a prolonged aPTT and mild thrombocytopenia with normal fibrinogen. Prolongation of the aPTT is not as sensitive to LF as prolongation of the PT; therefore, it may be normal with mild disease. A low fibrinogen level suggests that intravascular coagulation may be occurring and a workup for DIC, as discussed later, is needed.

The severity of LF and the amount of functioning liver mass have been correlated with abnormal coagulation tests.[49] Survival of patients with LF has been correlated with decreased prothrombin activity and factor VII levels.[49] Factor VII levels of 38% or less can identify patients who will die of LF within 2 months.

TREATMENT

Due to the high incidence of vitamin K deficiency in LF, administration of a single parenteral dose of vitamin K is recommended as an initial step in LF patients with acute hrmorrhage. Replacement of coagulation factors is accomplished most safely by using fresh frozen plasma (FFP), which contains all coagulation factors.[48] Despite its relative safety, administration of FFP may precipitate hepatic encephalopathy and/or cause fluid overload in patients with severe LF. Prothrombin complex concentrates should be avoided because they contain only the vitamin-K-dependent factors and may contain some activated factors. The platelet defect must also be addressed in bleeding LF patients, even if platelet counts are normal. Platelet aggregation tests can confirm qualitative platelet defects in LF. If platelet function is abnormal, treatment with desmopressin (DDAVP), as described earlier in this chapter, or platelet concentrates is necessary.

The use of heparin in LF with intravascular coagulation is controversial. Some authors have reported improvement of coagulation abnormalities and decreased risk of hemorrhage with low-dose heparin therapy.[49] Others have noted that heparin therapy is hazardous in patients with LF due to erratic metabolism of heparin, with possible hemorrhagic episodes related to overdosage.

Disseminated Intravascular Coagulation

DIC is by far the most frequent and serious acquired defect of coagulation.[42] Excessive surgical bleeding in patients without hereditary coagulation defects is most likely due to DIC.[47] In DIC, the usual balance between coagulation and fibrinolysis is lost. In the normal state, damage to vascular endothelia is followed by an orderly and localized progression from platelet adhesion and coagulation to resolution of clot and vascular repair.[42,48] In certain pathologic situations, the balance between coagulation and fibrinolysis as well as the ability to keep the coagulation cascade localized is lost. Coagulation under these circumstances results in consumption of coagulation factors and platelets due to widespread formation of fibrin thromboses throughout the microcirculation, with simultaneous activation of the fibrinolytic system. The clinical symptoms in DIC depend on the balance between thrombosis and fibrinolysis. Symptoms range from diffuse hemorrhage to diffuse thrombosis with tissue ischemia. In many patients, both thromboses and hemorrhage occur simultaneously at different body sites.[1,42]

PATHOGENESIS AND CLINICAL MANIFESTATIONS

Many disease processes are associated with DIC, and a partial list is given in Table 2-7 according to the proposed mechanism of action.[1,42] Associated factors such as slowed microvascular blood flow and vasoconstriction contribute to the pathogenesis of DIC; however, these factors alone will not produce DIC.[42] An inciting event is necessary to initiate DIC through one or several different mechanisms. Sepsis is a common cause of DIC and is thought to initiate coagulation primarily by causing platelet release of thromboplastin, although some bacterial endotoxins also damage endothelia and others act as pseudo-thrombin and directly convert fibrinogen to fibrin.[42] Malignancies are thought to initiate DIC via thromboplastin release, as are fat emboli and hemolysis.[42] It is important to note that once DIC has been initiated, it is self-perpetuating because the microthrombi further slow blood flow and increase acidosis.[1,42]

Clinical manifestations of DIC can be divided into immediate and late. Immediate signs include hypotension due to obstruction of the microcirculation as well as vasoconstriction and fever. Simultaneously, an occult or clinically obvious coagulation defect develops.[42] Bleeding symptoms,

Table 2-7. Primary Mechanism of Disease States Causing DIC

Thromboplastin release
  Sepsis
  Malignancies (especially mucin secreting adenocarcinomas)
  Hemolysis
  Fat emboli
  Placental abruption
  Amniotic fluid bolus
Endothelia damage (intrinsic pathway activation)
  Sepsis
  Acidosis
  Vasculitis
  Burns
  Anaphylaxis
  Crush injuries
  Rickettsial diseases (Rocky Mountain spotted fever)
Directly convert fibrinogen to fibrin
  Snake venom
  Bacterial toxins
Contact of blood with foreign material
  Extracorporeal circulation

when present, are from three unrelated sites, which may include petechiae, purpura, and venipuncture bleeding.[1] The initial symptoms may lead to death even with adequate management of the patient. If the patient survives these initial symptoms, late manifestations of DIC will appear. The late complications of DIC range in severity depending on the extent of the episode of DIC and the nature of the underlying cause. Late manifestations may result in death and are due to tissue and organ failure secondary to ischemic damage from microvascular obstruction.[42] Commonly affected organ systems include lungs, liver, kidneys, heart, pancreas, and the gastrointestinal tract.[42] Care of the patient with these complications is supportive.

LABORATORY DIAGNOSIS

All measurable coagulation factors—including I, II, V, VII, XI, XII, and the antithrombotic enzyme antithrombin III—are usually depleted in patients with DIC.[42,47] However, fibrinogen may be normal or increased due to its rapid synthesis by the liver.[1,42] Examination of the peripheral blood smear is an easy and inexpensive first step in diagnosis. The smear will reveal schistocytes and thrombocytopenia, suggesting the diagnoses of thrombotic thrombocytopenic purpura or DIC.[17] Diagnosis is further assisted by the use of a DIC battery, which includes PT, aPTT, fibrinogen level, and platelet count.[47] If all four tests are abnormal, DIC has been confirmed (assuming that the patient does not have chronic liver failure).[47] Addition of the test to detect fibrin degradation products (FDPs) will confirm the diagnosis if only three of the four tests are abnormal. In patients with chronic liver disease, diagnostic criteria for DIC include PT > 25 seconds; platelet count < 50,000 per milliliter; decreased fibrinogen; and FDPs > 40 micrograms per milliliter.[47]

TREATMENT

Treatment of DIC is aimed at increasing sluggish blood flow, correcting hemostatic defects, and (most importantly) correcting the underlying cause. Maintenance of adequate arterial systemic blood pressure through the use of crystalloid or blood products is essential. Correction of hemostatic defects through the use of platelet and FFP infusions is often necessary. Platelet counts should be kept at 100,000 per milliliter.[47] Cryoprecipitate is often helpful in replenishing factors I (fibrinogen) and VIII, whereas prothrombin complex (factor IX concentrates) is helpful in replenishing vitamin-K-dependent factors.[1] Drug therapy with phenoxybenzamine hydrochloride 1 mg/kg body weight can reduce arteriolar spasm, particularly in the lungs, and has been effective in preventing DIC.[42] The most effective therapy for DIC is removal of the underlying cause, and the most dramatic recoveries occur when the inciting event (such as sepsis or retained dead fetus) can be corrected.

Controversy still exists concerning the use of anticoagulants or fibrinolytic agents in DIC. Heparin is useful in patients with hypercoagulable state, but indications for its use in acute DIC are not clearly established.[50] Theoretically, heparin should decrease coagulation through its action on antithrombin III. However, in patients with DIC, antithrombin III levels are usually decreased and the patients are often acidotic, which decreases the efficacy of heparin. Also, heparin has no effect on thrombi that have already formed and has not been found to change clinical outcome.[1,42] The use of fibrinolytic therapy is helpful if major vessels are occluded; however, bleeding tendencies, especially in patients who have recently had surgery, will worsen.[1] Fibrinolytic therapy has also been useful in preventing adult respiratory distress syndrome associated with DIC. If fibrinolytic therapy results in serious bleeding, it should be stopped. Initiation of fibrinolytic therapy requires frequent monitoring of coagulation parameters, including PT, aPTT, fibrinogen levels, platelet count, and FDPs.[42]

In conclusion, DIC is best managed with supportive care, replacement of coagulation factors and platelets, and (most important) correction of the underlying condition. Fibrinolytic therapy may be useful in preventing the late complications of DIC but must be used with caution to prevent excessive hemorrhage. All contraindications to fibrinolytic therapy, such as central nervous system hemorrhage or internal hemorrhage, should preclude this therapy. Recent surgery may delay initiation of fibrinolytic therapy.

Inhibitors of Coagulation

In general, there are two types of inhibitors that result in prolongation of the commonly used coagulation tests: blocking inhibitors such as the lupus anticoagulant (LA), and specific factor depressants. Blocking inhibitors interfere with an entire coagulation reaction but are usually not associated with clinical or excessive surgical bleeding.[13,18,51] Specific factor inhibitors are rare except when associated with congenital factor deficiencies that have required replacement. The specific factor inhibitors are associated with clinically significant bleeding and require perioperative therapy to control hemorrhage.[18]

LUPUS ANTICOAGULANTS

The term *lupus anticoagulant* is somewhat of a misnomer for the antiphospholipid antibodies that cause prolongation of all phospholipid-dependent coagulation tests.[51] It is a misnomer because the antibodies which are IgG subclass occur with many disease states other than lupus—including viral illnesses, vascular diseases, and malignancies—and have been associated with use of many medications, including penicillin and its derivatives, chlorpromazine, quinidine, and hydralazine.[18,52,53] More importantly, designation of these antibodies as anticoagulants is misleading because they are not associated with bleeding in patients.[13,51,54] In fact, they are associated with venous and arterial thrombosis and strokes in up to 42% of patients with systemic lupus erythematosus (SLE), leading some authors to recommend the use of anticoagulants perioperatively in these patients.[13,53-55] The cause of the hypercoagulable state associated with LA is unknown but may be related to inhibition of prostacyclin synthesis.[51]

The prevalence of LA in the general population is estimated to be between 0.6% and 2% but may be higher in children with viral illnesses or who are taking penicillin or one of its derivatives.[51,52,55] As stated previously, patients with LA are not at risk of bleeding unless other coagulation defects exist simultaneously. Both thrombocytopenia and hypoprothrombinemia have been associated with LA; therefore, a platelet count and PT to rule out these disorders is mandatory in the preoperative evaluation of these patients.[55]

The laboratory hallmark of LA is a prolonged aPTT that does not correct when the affected plasma is mixed with normal plasma.[54] To rule out specific factor inhibitors, tests for anti-VIII and anti-XI must be performed because these are the most common specific factor inhibitors.[53] Inhibitors of factors V, VII, IX, X, and XII can also result in a prolonged aPTT, but these inhibitors are extremely rare and testing for them is not always necessary.[53] Additionally, an enzyme-linked immunosorbent assay (ELISA) is available that will detect roughly 70% of LA.[54] A platelet neutralization procedure that uses a platelet suspension to absorb the antiphospholipid antibodies before measuring the aPTT will result is shortening of the aPTT in plasma with LA, but not in plasma with specific factor inhibitors.[53]

No treatment is necessary for LA preoperatively, with the possible exception of anticoagulants in patients with SLE. If surgery can be delayed, a 2-month waiting period will allow for correction of transient LA that is common in children and in patients without concurrent autoimmune diseases. If the aPTT remains prolonged despite the waiting period or the surgery is imminent, then identification of the inhibitor as an LA assures that surgery can be performed without risk once the platelet count and prothrombin activity (PT) have been checked.[53]

SPECIFIC FACTOR INHIBITORS

Specific factor inhibitors frequently cause severe bleeding and are associated with autoimmune disorders, ulcerative colitis, hypersensitivity reactions to penicillin, and the postpartum state.[1,52] The most common subset of patients with specific factor inhibitors are hemophiliacs, with a 10% incidence of factor VIII inhibitors.[42,44,52] Regardless of the cause of anti-VIII antibodies, treatment for correction of bleeding tendencies preoperatively requires the administration of increased doses of factor VIII, factor IX, or activated prothrombin complex.[1,42] All of these treatment modalities are expensive and were discussed in more detail earlier in this chapter in relation to hemophilia A. Acquired inhibitors of VIII not associated with hemophilia are not usually responsive to factor VIII concentrate infusions but may respond to DDAVP.[15,43] Prednisone, cytoxan, plasmapharesis, and gamma globulin are effective in some of these patients.[15,42]

Five percent of patients with hemophilia B (factor IX) deficiency will develop inhibitors to factor IX. Similar to factor VIII inhibitors in hemophilia A, the factor IX inhibitor in hemophilia B arises after exposure to factor IX (blood, plasma, factor IX concentrates); however, unlike inhibitors of factor VIII, factor IX inhibitors tend to decrease after 4 to 6 months if there is no further exposure.[44] Patients with low titre inhibitors may be treated with high-dose factor IX, but high titre inhibitors often require activated prothrombin complex therapy.[15,44]

Acquired inhibitors of factors V, VII, IX, X, and XI have been described but are extremely rare.[15,44,53]

SICKLE HEMOGLOBINOPATHIES

Sickle cell hemoglobinopathies include all diseases that have the common pathology of intracellular polymerization of hemoglobin beta chains. Sickle cell anemia is the most common of these disorders, but similar clinical courses are seen with sickle-C disease and sickle-beta thalassemia.[56] All of these disorders have at least one B hemoglobin allele mutation, resulting in an amino acid change from glutamate to valine at position 6 of the protein. Sickle cell trait with one hemoglobin S (Hb S) and one hemoglobin A (Hb A) does not result in physiologic sickling or in clinical disease. Sickle hemoglobin (Hb S) under conditions of low oxygen tension polymerizes, resulting in change of the red blood cell (RBC) shape to sickle and target forms. The abnormally shaped blood cells are rapidly cleared from the circulation, resulting in a decreased RBC lifespan and a chronic hemolytic anemia.[56]

Clinical manifestations of sickle cell anemia are multiple and vary from patient to patient. Repeated vaso-occlusive injuries to organs result in morbidity and mortality. Active intervention has increased survival from 85% to 99% in the first decade of life.[57] Approximately 60% of sickle cell anemia patients survive to age 40, whereas 80% of sickle-C patients survive to age 50.[56,58] Sickle-C disease is the mildest of the sickle hemoglobinopathies, but even these patients can suffer significant morbidity.[59] With increased survival, morbidity

from long-term organ damage is manifesting itself in all forms of the disease.[56] The causes of morbidity and mortality and the surgical management of these patients will be discussed.

Central Nervous System

Six percent to twenty-five percent of sickle cell patients will experience neurological sequellae due to their disease, with the mean age of first stroke being 8 years of age.[57] No effective therapy has been established except for long-term transfusion therapy. Even with transfusions, 10% of patients will have more strokes. If transfusions are halted, 50% of patients will have additional cerebral vascular accidents.[57]

Reticuloendothelial

Sickle cell anemia results in functional asplenia very early in life due to chronic vaso-occlusion. Because of the lack of splenic function, infections with polysaccharide encapsulated organisms (S. pneumoniae, H. influenza) occur at an incidence of 400× that in the normal population. Prophylactic antibiotic therapy and immunizations have decreased the incidence of and mortality from these infections.[56-58] In some patients, before the spleen has involuted, a rapid enlargement of the organ with a sudden drop in hematocrit and thrombocytopenia occurs. This life-threatening complication requires immediate volume support/transfusion and often splenectomy.[56]

Renal

Renal disease is common in patients with sickle cell anemia, who usually present with vaso-occlusive damage primarily in the hyperosmotic regions. The vascular insult results in papillary necrosis with hematuria and damage to the counter-current multiplier system with resultant hyposthenuria. Because of the hyposthenuria, urine osmolarity in sickle cell patients is not a good indication of hydration status. Despite the frequency of renal pathology, only 4% of adult patients develop renal failure.[56,57]

Hepatobiliary

Painful enlargement of the liver due to intrahepatic sickling is a rare event, but due to chronic hemolytic anemia pigmented gallstones frequently lead to cholecystitis.[56,57]

Musculoskeletal

Sickle cell crises are painful events related to vaso-occlusion of the bone marrow. These events are not life threatening; however, they require hospitalization for analgesia and hydration and are a major source of morbidity in some patients. Repeated episodes may led to avascular necrosis, primarily of the femoral head.[56]

Pulmonary

The acute chest syndrome is a life-threatening complication often seen after a febrile illness consisting of hypoxia, fever, leukocytosis, and an abnormal chest x-ray.[56] Pulmonary infections are particulary dangerous because of the associated hypoventilation and hypoxia that can lead to massive sickling and vaso-occlusion.

Cardiovascular

Due to chronic anemia, patients with sickle cell anemia have a high output state that is usually well tolerated. By adult life, most patients will have left ventricular hypertrophy and often right ventricular hypertrophy from increased pulmonary vascular resistance related to ventilation perfusion mismatches.[56]

Preoperative Management

For children with sickle cell disease, a pediatric anesthesiologist and a hematologist knowledgable of sickle cell disease and its complications should be consulted prior to surgery. Although intraoperative management is clear with avoidance of hypoxia, acidosis, hypothermia, and hypovolemia being standard, preoperative management is still a topic of debate.[56,60] Most authors agree that some minor procedures in which minimal blood loss is expected can be performed without preoperative transfusion. Due to reports of severe complications even with minor procedures, some authors suggest simple transfusion to attain a hemoglobin concentration of 10 g/dL to provide a safety net.[56,60] Lowering the percentage of cells with Hb SS lowers the risk of intravascular occlusion, but increasing the hematocrit past 45% increases viscosity and the possibility of vaso-occlusion.[60]

In procedures for which expected blood loss is high or compromise of ventilation secondary to postoperative neurological status, aspiration, pain, or immobility is likely, preoperative transfusion is suggested.[60] If possible, transfusion of 15 mL/kg packed red blood cells beginning 1 month prior to the procedure boosts the hemoglobin to 10 g/dL while decreasing the Hb SS from 100% to 65%. Two weeks after the initial transfusion, a repeat transfusion is given to maintan the total hemoglobin. Because endogenous erythropoiesis was suppressed by the initial transfusion, the percentage of Hb SS cells usually drops to below 40% after the second transfusion. A third transfusion immediately preoperatively is optional.[56]

Regardless of transfusion status, all patients should be admitted to the hospital the night prior to surgery for hydration at one and one half times maintenance requirements.[56] Patients should not have an acute illness prior to surgery, especially one involving the respiratory system.

Postoperative Management

Prior to extubation, the patient should be awake, ventilating, and oxygenating without assistance. A postoperative chest x-ray assessing atelectasis, collapse, and edema is suggested.[56] Any desaturation or increased oxygen need mandates transfer to an intensive care unit for vigorous pulmonary toilette and reintubation if necessary.[56] Analgesia is important to allow adequate pulmonary clearing. Drugs such as parenteral nonsteroidal anti-inflammatory drugs offer good analgesia without the risk of sedation and hypoventilation.

Postoperatively the patient should be well hydrated; however, overhydration can lead to pulmonary edema with desaturation and intravascular sickling. Careful monitoring of urine output usually is sufficient to follow volume status, but central venous or pulmonary capillary wedge pressure monitoring should be implemented if necessary.

Future Directions

The lifespan of patients with sickle cell hemoglobinopathies has been extended due to aggressive early diagnosis and therapy. However, the morbidity, expense, and long-term sequellae of the disorder and its treatment are still major problems. New treatment approaches designed to decrease morbidity include chemotherapy to increase the fetal hemoglobin (Hb F) content (with a decrease in sickling tendency) and bone marrow transplantation or genetic engineering to cure the disease. The last option is not yet feasible, but the first two options are readily available.

Increasing expression of the Hb F gene decreases the concentration of Hb S and therefore sickling tendency. Some patients naturally express Hg F levels of 20%, which are associated with benign disease. Preliminary data show that chemotherapy can attain levels of Hg F of 20% and decrease vaso-occlusive creses by 50%.

Bone marrow transplantation carries a significant risk of graft versus host disease, neoplasms from chronic immunosuppression, and mortality.[58,61] These risks must be weighed carefully against the morbidity and mortality associated with sickle cell anemia. Part of the dilemma surrounding transplantation is the fact that some Hb SS patients do very well whereas others suffer early strokes and death. At present, these groups cannot be separated. If it were possible to determine which patients would do poorly, the decision of whether or not to transplant would be much easier.

ACUTE AND CHRONIC ANTICOAGULATION

Anticoagulant therapy is used for various medical conditions, including rheumatic heart disease, deep venous thrombosis, chronic atrial fibrillation, and recurrent pulmonary embolism. Patients with prosthetic heart valves and arrhythmias are at risk for arterial embolization and require lifelong anticoagulation. Likewise, some form of anticoagulation is mandated for circulatory assistance with an intra-aortic balloon pump as well as when extracorporeal circulation, such as cardiac bypass and hemodialysis, is required.[62]

Due to the relatively high incidence of postoperative hemorrhagic complications in anticoagulated patients and the high likelihood of treating such patients, surgeons must have a working knowledge of anticoagulant therapy. Additionally, surgeons should feel comfortable with the option of pre- and postoperative anticoagulant prophylaxis for patients at increased risk of thrombotic complications. Heparinlike compounds and coumarin derivatives are the drugs used most frequently for anticoagulation in the United States and will be the primary drugs discussed here. Heparin is used for acute anticoagulation, whereas Coumadin is used for chronic anticoagulation.

Heparin

Heparin is a negatively charged molecule (mol wt < 3000 to 30,000 d) that has many pharmacological actions, including anticoagulation, adherence to endothelia, decrease of vascular permeability as induced by vasoactive agents, and decreased platelet adherence and aggregation.[63-65] Heparin, for medical use, is derived from bovine lung or porcine intestinal mucosa.[64] The two preparations have never proven to differ in efficacy, but their side-effect profiles reveal increased immune-mediated thrombocytopenia with the bovine preparation.[66]

ACTION

The anticoagulation effect of heparin is due primarily to its interaction with the hepatic anticoagulant protein, antithrombin III, which naturally but slowly binds and inactivates several clotting factors. A pentasaccharide sequence of heparin has been identified as the antithrombin III binding site, and when this pentasaccharide is present, the heparin molecule will reversibly bind antithrombin III with high affinity.[63] When heparin complexes with antithrombin III, the antithrombin III molecule changes conformation, allowing for much faster inactivation of several serine proteases in the coagulation cascade (factors XIIIa, XIa, Xa, IXa, and IIa).[63,64] The overall result of inhibiting these serine proteases is to slow the clotting reaction and decrease the amount of IIa (thrombin) available to split fibrinogen to fibrin. Xa and IIa (thrombin) are the most clinically important coagulation factors inhibited by the heparin-antithrombin III complex. Inhibition of factor Xa is necessary but not sufficient for heparin's antithrombotic activity.[63] The anti-IIa and anti-Xa functions can be separated partially by fractionating the heparin molecules by size.

The separation of the anti-Xa and anti-IIa effects of heparin has raised the possibility of separating the therapeutic effects of heparin from the hemorrhagic side-effects. When discussing the properties of heparin, it is useful to understand the meaning of the terms *anticoagulation, antithrombosis,* and *antihemostasis.* Anticoagulation is the ability of heparin to alter the coagulation tests performed in a laboratory (primarily aPTT). Antithrombosis is the desired effect of heparin to prevent intravascular thrombosis, whereas antihemostasis is an undesired effect of heparin to cause hemorrhage.

Animal studies and in vitro testing have suggested that the antihemostatic and anticoagulant effects of heparin can be separated from the antithrombotic effects.[67,68] For instance,

low-molecular-weight (LMW) heparin does not prolong the aPTT (has no effect on thrombin = IIa) but is a potent inhibitor of factor Xa. This same low-molecular-weight fraction of heparin (mol wt = 4000 to 6000 d) when administered to rabbits in comparable doses to unfractionated heparin did not adversely affect hemostasis but decreased thrombosis to a greater extent than unfractionated heparin.[68] The reason low-molecular-weight heparin can inhibit thrombosis without affecting hemostasis in animals is not fully understood; however, proposed mechanisms expound the facts that LMW heparin does not have anti-IIa properties or adversely affect platelet function.[67,68]

Naturally, the idea of separating heparin's antithrombotic function from its undesired antihemostatic action was received with great excitement in the surgical community, where the risk of deep venous thrombosis and pulmonary embolism must be weighed against the increased risk of hemorrhagic side-effects. Human studies on patients with deep venous thromboses have proven that the efficacy of LMW heparin is equal to unfractionated heparin in resolving thromboses.[69] Results of initial studies examining the use of LMW heparin for surgical prophylaxis have been mixed, showing efficacy at least comparable to unfractionated heparin but with a dose-dependent increase in hemorrhagic complications with no clear advantage over conventional heparin.[70-72] The goal of antithrombosis without increased hemorrhage is still being investigated and deserves further attention.

PHARMACOKINETICS DOSE AND CINICAL USE

Heparin is the therapeutic agent used most commonly for acute anticoagulation. It is the drug of choice for extracorporeal circulation (hemodialysis, cardiopulmonary bypass), intra-aortic balloon pump, deep venous thrombosis, postoperative prophylaxis for deep venous thrombosis, pulmonary embolism, postprocedure coronary artery balloon recanalization, and DIC.[50,64] Despite its widespread applications, there are many contraindications to the use of heparin, including coagulation defects (either platelet or factor defects), clinical bleeding (gastric ulcer, postsurgical), hypertension, thrombocytopenia secondary to heparin administration, and allergy secondary to heparin.

Appropriate dosage of heparin is related to its half-life and the desired effect. The dose for any patient is either set empirically, in the case of prophylaxis, or changed based on the results of laboratory tests evaluating anticoagulation. The half-life of heparin is roughly 90 minutes but increases with increasing doses. After being cleared from plasma by either binding endothelial cells or being taken up by the reticuloendothelial system, heparin is eliminated by both renal and hepatic pathways. One third of a standard dose of heparin is cleared by the body in a single pass.[64]

Standard therapy for pulmonary embolism or deep venous thrombosis is to load the patient with 5000 to 10,000 units of heparin intravenously (IV) and begin a constant infusion of 10 to 15 U/kg/h. In patients with extensive thrombosis, higher doses are often necessary due to the rapid clearance of heparin in these patients.[64] Six to eight hours after the continuous infusion has begun, the aPTT should be checked and the dosage of heparin changed to achieve a 1.5-fold increase in the aPTT. After each change in dosage, a similar protocol should be followed until the dose has stabilized. Once the heparin dose is constant, daily aPTT and every second or third day platelet and hematocrit should be checked.[64] A decrease in the hematocrit may require discontinuation of heparin or a dosage reduction. Thrombocytopenia or a large drop in the platelet count is an indication for cessation of heparin therapy.

Perioperative DVT occurs in 25% to 50% of patients over 40 undergoing general surgical procedures.[72–74] The risk of DVT increases with age, length of procedure, and obesity and in patients with a malignancy, chronic obstructive pulmonary disease, or diabetes mellitus.[72] The risk of fatal pulmonary embolism related to DVT following general surgical procedures has been found to be roughly 1% in patients over 40 years of age. Low-dose heparin (5000 units subcutaneously every 12 hours) therapy in a large prospective randomized trial decreased the incidence of fatal pulmonary embolism 10-fold.[64]

Standard heparin protocols to reduce the risk of perioperative deep venous thrombosis and pulmonary embolism call for 5000 U of heparin 2 hours preoperatively and then every 12 hours for 1 week or until the patient is fully ambulatory, whichever comes last.[73,74] This dosage is given subcutaneously and has proven efficacious for prevention of deep venous thrombosis without increasing the risk of major hemorrhagic complications peri- or postoperatively.[73,74] The incidence of wound hematoma is increased with low-dose heparin therapy.[73,74]

COMPLICATIONS OF HEPARIN

As a drug, heparin has a low therapeutic ratio primarily because the derangement in clotting time is logarithmically related to the heparin dose. This relationship ensures that small doses of heparin have a small effect on clotting time whereas large doses prolong the clotting time indefinitely.[64] The primary complications of heparin therapy are hemorrhagic.

Bleeding due to heparin can have varied etiologies related to both the multiple actions of heparin, overdosage, and patient considerations such as gastrointestinal ulceration or trauma. As stated previously, patients with mucosal ulcerations (gastric or duodenal ulcers) should not be treated with heparin due to the possibility of catastrophic bleeding that is difficult to control. Overdosages of heparin with extreme prolongation of aPTT are associated with increased risk of hemorrhage. Close monitoring of coagulation tests is necessary even with established doses of heparin because of the often unexpected and unexplained change in a patient's requirement for heparin.

Moderate hemorrhage associated with trauma, mucosal ulcerations, or heparin overdosage can often be managed by temporary cessation of heparin therapy. Due to the short half-life of heparin, normal coagulation is usually restored in 4

to 6 hours. In patients with life-threatening or uncontrollable hemorrhage, protamine sulfate, a highly basic material that binds and inactivates heparin, can be administered. The dosage of protamine sulfate is calculated based on the fact that 1 mg of protamine sulfate neutralizes approximately 100 U of heparin.[64] The plasma concentration of heparin can be extrapolated based on the activated clotting time or estimated, assuming a half-life of 90 minutes for intravenous heparin.[16,64] Due to the inaccuracies of determining plasma heparin concentration and the short half-life of heparin, it is recommended that only one half the calculated dose be given initially and further dosages be determined based on the initial response. Protamine has several serious side-effects, including hypotension and paradoxical bleeding, and should not be used for reversal of heparin's effects unless bleeding cannot be controlled by other methods.

Bleeding in patients receiving heparin therpay can also be related to an immune-mediated thrombocytopenia. Heparin-induced thrombocytopenia is relatively common, occurring in 5% of patients receiving heparin.[66] The platelet count can decrease at any point during treatment; however, approximately 90% of patients will not experience thrombocytopenia until 6 days after the initiation of therapy.[66] This type of bleeding cannot be treated with protamine sulfate. The only treatment is immediate cessation of heparin and supportive care if necessary. Withdrawal of heparin is curative, but platelet counts may not respond for several days. Immune-mediated thrombocytopenia can be prevented by checking platelet counts at least every 3 days and discontinuing heparin therapy if a consistent drop is noted.[64] Thrombocytopenia can be induced or perpetuated by very small doses of heparin, including standard flushes of intravenous lines. If heparin-induced thrombocytopenia is suspected, intravenous lines should be flushed with citrate or saline instead of heparin.

Coumadin

Coumadin and its derivatives are the only available oral anticoagulants. Warfarin or Coumadin is the most commonly prescribed drug of this class in the United States. Due to ease of administration, oral anticoagulants are typically preferred when long-term treatment is required as with prosthetic heart valves, chronic atrial fibrillation, and rheumatic heart valvular disease.

ACTION

All coumadinlike drugs act through interfering with synthesis of the vitamin-K-dependent coagulation factors (II = prothrombin, VII, IX, and X) in the liver. Vitamin K is a required cofactor for carboxylation of the glutamic acid residues of factors II, VII, IX, and X. Carboxylation allows these factors to bind calcium, which is necessary for activity. Coumadin blocks carboxylation by preventing reduction of the epoxide form of vitamin K, thereby locking vitamin K in the oxidized form and functionally stopping the production of active coagulation factors.[64]

PHARMACOKINETICS DOSE AND CLINICAL USE

Coumadin is rapidly but variably absorbed from the gastrointestinal tract. Once in the plasma, Coumadin is highly protein bound; however, the amount of free and bound drug varies greatly from patient to patient. Only the free form of Coumadin is active.[64] Any drug that competes with Coumadin for protein binding can significantly increase the free fraction and the risk of hemorrhagic complications. Several drugs are known to displace Coumadin from its protein binding site, and when administered simultaneously dosage adjustment of Coumadin is necessary. Drugs that increase or decrease coumadin concentration are given in Table 2–8.

The standard regimen for beginning Coumadin therapy is to administer 5 mg daily and adjust the dose until full anticoagulation, as measured by a 1.5- to 2.0-fold increase in the prothrombin time, is attained.[75] Recent data have shown decreased hemorrhagic complications with adequate anticoagulation when a 1.5-fold increase in the PT is used as the goal rather than the more prolonged PT recommended in the past.[64]

Upon initiation of Coumadin therapy, PT increases due to depletion of factor VII, which has the shortest half-life of the vitamin-K-dependent factors. Initially, the prolongation of PT does not imply that the patient is functionally anticoagulated. In fact, during the initial administration of Coumadin, the patient may be hypercoagulable. Protein C, also vitamin K dependent, has a half-life comparable with factor VII and its depletion before depletion of factors IX and X can cause increased thrombus formation. During this window of protein C inactivation with functioning factors IX and X, which lasts 4 to 5 days, it is important to protect against hypercoagulability. The most common method to protect the patient against thromboembolism is to anticoagulate the patient with heparin for 4 to 5 days until active factors IX and X have been replaced with inactive analogs.[64]

Table 2–8. Drugs that Interfere with Coumadin Action.

INCREASE EFFECTIVENESS OF COUMADIN	DECREASE EFFECTIVENESS OF COUMADIN
Allopurinol	Barbiturates
Amiodarone	Carbamazepine
Aspirin	Ethanol (chronic abuse)
Allochloral hydrate	Griseofulvin
Athacrynic acid	Rifampin
Cimetidine	
Disulfiram	
Ethanol (acute intoxication)	
Metronidazole	
Phenylbutazone	
Phenytoin	
Sulfonamides	

From Platt and Nightingale.[109]

Of great concern to surgeons is how to manage a patient on Coumadin who requires a surgical procedure. Some minor procedures can be performed without taking the patient off Coumadin, but for the majority of procedures reversal of anticoagulation is necessary. In a series of patients on Coumadin who underwent surgical procedures, no increase in thrombotic complications was noted when anticoagulation was stopped for an average of 6.6 days.[76] Cessation of Coumadin 3 days before the date of surgery usually resulted in return of the PT to normal or within 20% of normal and was only rarely associated with bleeding complications or wound hematomas. When surgery was performed with the PT prolonged more than 20% greater than normal, a 10% incidence of bleeding complications was seen.[76] If the clinical situation demands anticoagulation closer to the time of surgery, then anticoagulation therapy can be switched to heparin 3 to 5 days preoperatively. As discussed earlier in this chapter, anticoagulation with heparin can be reversed more easily due to its short half-life.

COMPLICATIONS OF COUMADIN

The most frequent complications associated with anticoagulation with Coumadin are bleeding and persistent or recurrent thromboembolism.[64,76] Thromboembolism is associated with inadequate anticoagulation in high-risk patients; however, 10% to 15% of high-risk patients taking adequate doses of Coumadin will experience thromboembolism usually within 3 years of initiating treatment.[76]

As might be expected, hemorrhagic complications are associated with an increase in the free fraction of Coumadin with concurrent increase in the PT and are usually related to inappropriate dosage or drug-drug interactions (Table 2–8).[77,78] The bleeding rates for patients receiving Coumadin have been as high as 28.7% with major bleeding episodes as high as 8.1%, but these data reflect higher doses than currently recommended.[77] Bleeding is typically from the gastrointestinal tract, skin, or urinary tract and is often associated with underlying risk factors such as cancer, surgery, or mucosal ulcerations.[77] Minor bleeding can be controlled with change in coumadin dosage or oral vitamin K administration. More significant bleeding or unavoidable emergency surgery requires more rapid reversal of Coumadin's effects by using parenteral vitamin K. Coagulation defects begin to correct within 3 to 4 hours after high-dose vitamin K administration, but maximal effects of vitamin K administration take up to 8 hours. Once anticoagulation has been reversed with vitamin K, it may take a long time to anticoagulate the patient with Coumadin again. For patients who require anticoagulation but are having bleeding complications, vitamin K in small doses (1 to 2 mg) administered intravenously usually corrects PT to therapeutic ranges within 8 to 21 hours with control of hemorrhage while allowing continued anticoagulation.[78]

A rare but occasionally fatal side-effect of Coumadin administration is skin necrosis. Typically, this adverse effect is localized to the breasts, flanks, and other fatty areas of women and is not life threatening. Areas of blackened thrombosed skin appear 3 to 5 days after the initiation of therapy.[64] Partial deficiency of protein C is associated with this complication and has led to the hypothesis that skin thrombosis is secondary to a rapid depletion of functional protein C. Life-threatening skin necrosis is more likely to occur in patients with protein C deficiency and deep venous thrombosis. Therapy for this rare complication is immediate cessation of anticoagulant therapy.

Other Agents
DEFIBROTIDE

Defibrotide is a relatively new drug with antithrombotic and fibrinolytic action but without any measurable anticoagulant effect. It is a polydesoxyribonucleotide of mammalian origin that is thought to work by increasing the synthesis and release of tissue plasminogen activator (tPA) and prostaglandins from endothelial cells. Double-blind, placebo-controlled trials have proven defibrotide's efficacy in resolution of thrombophlebitis.[80] Even more important to surgeons, the drug has shown efficacy similar to heparin for perioperative prophylaxis against deep venous thrombosis in patients undergoing gynecological or general surgical procedures. Furthermore, there have been no detectable side-effects and no increase in hemorrhage by any measure. [81,82]

DIHYDROERGOTAMINE

The ergotamines are a class of drugs that exert vasoconstrictive effects primarily on veins and venules while exerting minimal effects on arteries and arterioles. The combination of dihydroergotamine with heparin administered subcutaneously has been shown to decrease significantly the formation of DVT compared to heparin alone. A possibly serious complication of ergotamines is arterial vasoconstriction in the face of sepsis. Investigators have suggested discontinuation of dihydroergotamine in the presence of hypotension, sepsis, or infection. A positive effect of dihydroergotamine was a decrease in postoperative blood loss supposedly due to its vasoconstrictive effects.[72] Due to the positive effects of dihydroergotamine in combination with heparin to decrease DVT formation and decrease blood loss, further investigation of this and other drug combinations is warranted.

SYNTHETIC PENTASACCHARIDE, DERMATAN SULFATE, AND OTHER HEPARINOIDS

These agents have proven useful in separating the anti-IIa and anti-Xa functions of heparin. The synthetic pentasaccharide has potent anti-Xa but no anti-IIa activity. Conversely, dermatan sulfate acts through heparin cofactor II to inhibit IIa while not affecting Xa. Likewise, in initial studies other heparinoids have shown good antithrombotic properties without antihemostatic effects.[62] Heparinoids, alone or in combination, may prove useful in prevention of DVT without increasing hemorrhage. Furthermore, some of these agents could be used in patients with allergies to heparin or heparin-induced thrombocytopenia.[62]

ASPIRIN AND NONSTEROIDAL ANTI-INFLAMMATORY DRUGS

The role of platelets in hemostasis and coagulation is vital. As discussed in some detail earlier in this chapter, platelets interact directly with the vascular endothelia to control hemorrhage. Further, normal platelets are essential for proper function of the coagulation cascade. On the other hand, platelets are also implicated in disease processes and are critical in promoting thrombosis, which leads to myocardial infarction and cerebrovascular accidents. Because of the relatively high incidence of vaso-occlusive disease in the U.S. population, several therapeutic options that modulate platelet activity have been developed. Unfortunately, these treatments frequently put patients at higher risk of hemorrhagic complications during and around the time of surgery. Compounding the problem is the fact that many patients routinely take antiplatelet medications such as aspirin (ASA) and other nonsteroidal anti-inflammatory drugs (NSAIDs) for treatment of disorders ranging from headaches to arthritis. Because of the widespread use of these compounds and the increased operative and perioperative risk to patients taking them, a working knowledge of these drugs is necessary.

Nonsteroidal anti-inflammatory medications, including ASA, are used by many patients for a wide variety of medical problems. Recent studies proving benefit of daily ASA in preventing secondary myocardial infarction and strokes in patients with transient ischemic attacks, and the suggestion that low daily dosage of ASA may prevent primary myocardial infarction, have increased the use of these drugs.[83,84]

Inhibition of platelet function by NSAIDs is due to inactivation of the enzyme cyclo-oxygenase, which is responsible for prostaglandin I_2 (PGI_2) and thromboxane A_2 (TXA_2) synthesis. In the platelet, inhibition of TXA_2 synthesis is the primary effect of NSAIDs with concomitant inhibition of platelet aggregation and vasoconstriction. In the vascular endothelium, NSAIDs' effect is due primarily to inhibition of PGI_2 synthesis, which results in increased platelet aggregation and vasoconstriction.[84] The net effect of NSAIDs is to alter the balance between the thrombogenic effect of inhibition of PGI_2 synthesis and the antithrombotic effect of inhibition of TXA_2. The balance favors the antithrombotic effect for reasons that are not fully understood but may include the ability of endothelia but not platelets to synthesize new cyclo-oxygenase after inhibition by ASA.[84] Some studies have proven that preoperative use of ASA increases the risk of perioperative bleeding, resulting in increased transfusion requirements and reoperation for bleeding.[85,86] Even "minor" procedures such as electrocoagulating biopsy of colonic polyps have resulted in massive bleeding in patients on low-dose ASA.[87] On the other hand, other investigators have not been able to correlate increased perioperative bleeding to ingestion of ASA.[88]

When determining the safety of NSAIDs for perioperative use, it is important to realize that ASA irreversibly inactivates cyclo-oxygenase while all other NSAIDs are reversible inhibitors. In general, ASA results in longer inhibition of platelet function because a single dose of ASA inactivates the platelet cyclo-oxygenase for the lifetime of the platelet.[21] In general, 20% of platelets are needed for normal hemostasis and 10% of platelets are replaced with new platelets daily.[21] Using these guidelines, stopping ASA 2 days before surgery theoretically should allow adequate recovery of platelet function.[89] In practice, 4 or 5 days off of ASA preoperatively is required for normal hemostasis because ASA inactivates the cyclo-oxygenase in megakaryocytes in addition to that in platelets.[21,84,90] The proper timing of preoperative discontinuation of NSAIDs other than ASA depends on the half-life of each drug. Sulindac and nonacetylated salicylates do not appreciably affect platelet function and are preferred in patients who cannot discontinue therapy.[89] Ibuprofen does prolong bleeding time at 2 hours after ingestion; however, at 24 hours it no longer affects bleeding time, platelet adhesiveness, or platelet aggregation.[91]

In conclusion, ASA should be discontinued 4 to 5 days preoperatively to avoid hemorrhagic complications from surgery. Other NSAIDs generally do not inhibit platelet function for as long as ASA and should be stopped 5 to 6 half-lives before surgery. For example, discontinuation of ibuprofen (half-life = 2.5 hours) 24 hours preoperatively allows for normalization of platelet function. Drugs that inhibit platelet function, including NSAIDs, should be avoided in patients with other hemostatic disorders.

COMPLICATIONS OF TRANSFUSION

The use of blood components and derivatives is unavoidable and indeed is often lifesaving. A study by McCulloch et al examining the use of blood during head and neck surgery revealed that maxillectomies followed by composite resections and laryngectomies were associated with the highest blood loss.[92] This study demonstrated that roughly 65% of these patients were eligible for, and would have had their blood needs met by, autologous blood donations.[92] The avoidance of transfusions except when medically necessary and the use of autologous blood are recommended and will further decrease the risk of transfusion complications.

Transfusion-related complications are typically categorized as early and late complications. This division is somewhat artificial in that the time period dividing early from late is unclear. Complications of transfusion will be discussed as immediate (hemolytic transfusion reaction) and late (all others). Also, immunomodulation secondary to transfusion, a topic that has been ignored by otolaryngologists until recently, will be discussed.

Immediate Complications of Transfusion

Hemolytic reactions can be either immediate or late with varying degrees of clinical severity. Immediate hemolytic transfusion reactions are usually due to A, B, O-incompatible blood transfusions. These reactions are particularly severe because the anti-A or anti-B IgM antibodies responsible for the reaction are preformed and already circulating in the patient's blood. Additionally, the IgM antibody is capable of fixing complement, which results in intravascular lysis of the foreign red blood cells.

The intravascular lysis of cells and massive activation of complement results in the clinical symptoms of fever, chills, dyspnea, nausea, vomiting, chest pain, hypotension, and pain at the infusion site.[1] Laboratory features include the presence of free hemoglobin in the plasma which is filtered by the kidneys, resulting in hemoglobinuria. Catabolism of the plasma hemoglobin by the liver results in an elevated bilirubin, which is usually unconjugated. Lysis of the red cells results in an elevated lactate dehydrogenase (LDH), which is a useful marker (although nonspecific) of intravascular hemolysis. In the anesthetized patient having an immediate hemolytic transfusion reaction, the initial symptoms may be related to DIC with hypotension, shock, and generalized oozing.[1]

Treatment of hemolytic transfusion reactions is immediate cessation of transfusion followed by supportive care. Diuresis is of utmost importance to allow for clearance of hemoglobin without damage to the kidneys. Management of DIC is the same as discussed earlier in this chapter.

Delayed hemolytic transfusion reactions are clinically mild compared to immediate reactions. The primary symptom is a decrease in hematocrit with or without a fever that occurs 2 to 21 days after transfusion.[93] As opposed to acute hemolytic transfusion reactions, delayed reactions are associated with extravascular destruction of red blood cells; therefore, renal failure is uncommon and usually reversible.[1,93] After a delayed hemolytic transfusion reaction has occurred, the patient must be observed closely for an acute hemolytic transfusion reaction if retransfusion is necessary.[93] Severe acute reactions can follow clinically mild late reactions with further transfusions even if the blood is compatible in vitro.[93]

Late Complications of Transfusion

Recently, the infectious complications of transfusion—namely, hepatitis, human immunodeficiency virus (HIV), and the human T-cell lymphotropic viruses (HTLV-I, HTLV-II)—have captured the attention of patients, the public, and the press. The infectious risks of transfusion relate directly to the number of units transfused (or the equivalent for blood derivatives) and to the contamination of the blood supply. Blood products are usually divided into blood components and blood derivatives. Blood components are whole blood, packed red blood cells (pRBC), cryoprecipitate, platelets, and fresh frozen plasma (FFP). Blood derivatives (albumin, gamma globulin, and coagulation factors) have undergone more extensive processing and are usually derived from multiple units of blood. These blood products account for the vast majority of transfusions in the United States. A list of available blood components, their primary use, and the infectious risk associated with each is presented in Table 2–9.

To assure as safe a supply of blood products in the United States as possible, there is a four-tiered system to decrease the risk of infectious disease transmission via blood products. First, blood transfusions are limited to patients who absolutely require transfusion, with the use of autologous blood when possible. Second, selection of safe donors via an all-volunteer donor pool with the addition of confidential self-exclusion limits has yielded HIV infection among blood donors to 1/40 to 1/80 the rate in the general population.[94,95] Third, laboratory testing detects the vast majority of infected blood units. Presently blood is screened for syphilis, hepatitis B and C viruses, HIV types 1 and 2, HTLV-I, and HTLV-II. Finally, pooled blood products routinely undergo processing to inactivate viruses.[94] We will discuss hepatitis B virus (HBV) and hepatitis C virus (HCV) separately. Human immunodeficiency virus, HTLV-I, and HTLV-II will also be discussed.

HEPATITIS B

Hepatitis B infection is a well-known risk to the surgeon from either needle sticks or exposure to blood or body fluids during surgery. Patients who require transfusion are also at risk for contracting hepatitis B, but efforts to decrease the risk of transfusion-related hepatitis B have been successful. In fact, the incidence of clinical hepatitis B among recipients of blood products is now equal to the incidence of hepatitis B in the general population.[94] Roughly 1% of blood donors are positive for markers of hepatitis B, which is roughly 100 times greater than the incidence of positive testing for HIV among blood donors.[96] Despite the relatively high incidence of markers for the disease in blood donors, the risk of contracting hepatitis B from a transfusion is small and is predicted to be about 1 in 200,000 per unit.[94]

Unlike HIV infection, which is expected in every case to lead to disease and death, infection with HBV leads to clinical disease in only 50% of infected persons, and only 3% to 4% will require hospitalization.[94] Nevertheless, the disease when contracted is serious and can be life threatening. Surgeons and other health care workers at risk of infection should be vaccinated against HBV. Despite widespread calls for vaccination among at-risk populations, only 10% have been vaccinated.[97] Two options are currently available—a recombinant-yeast and plasma-derived vaccine—both of which are safe and effective in preventing hepatitis B.[97] The American Academy of Pediatrics has recommended vaccination of all children against hepatitis B, but data are incomplete at this time to determine if the vaccine given early in life will provide lifelong protection. Roughly 2% to 5% of normal individuals will not mount an adequate response to the hepatitis B vaccine after a single course.[97] Forty percent of nonresponders will mount an adequate response with a second course, but 60% will never respond adequately. Presently, there is no alternative vaccine for nonresponders.

HEPATITIS C

Hepatitis C accounted for the vast majority (>90%) of what had been referred to as non-A, non-B hepatitis (NANBH) prior to the discovery of the HCV in 1989.[98–101] Roughly 90% of all cases of transfusion-related hepatitis are attributable to this virus.[98,100] Recently developed screening tests have dramatically decreased the risk of contracting hepatitis C from a transfusion. In 1986, the risk of contracting hepatitis C was 1 in 500 per unit; now the risk is 1 in 6000 per unit.[102]

Hepatitis C as a disease has been described as indolent by some, but others have suggested that longer observation is

Table 2–9. Human Blood Products

PRODUCT	PRECAUTIONS/CONTENTS	INFECTIOUS RISK
Whole blood	A,B,O identical + compatibility testing/contains all coag factors but labile factors (V, VII) deteriorate within 24 hours	Risk of 1 donor/unit
Packed red blood cells	A,B,O compatible + compatibility testing/contains negligible platelets and coagulation factors	Risk of 1 donor/unit
Platelet concentrates	A,B,O compatible/contains 5×10^{10} platelets, 6–8 units increases platelet count by >30,000–40,000/μL	Risk of 1 donor/unit
Platelet, hemapharesis	A,B,O compatible/contains 3×10^{11} platelets, 1 unit increases platelet count by >30,000–40,000/μL	Risk of 1 donor/unit (1 unit equal to 6 units platelet concentrate)
Fresh frozen plasma	A,B,O compatible/contains all coagulation factors including 200 units VIII and factor V	Risk of 1 donor/unit
Cryoprecipitate	A,B,O compatible/contains factors VIII, XIII, 1 (fibrinogen), and von Willebrand factor	Risk of 1 donor/unit
Factor VIII concentrates	Type of viral inactivation/contains high levels of factor VIII	Safe if monoclonal antibody purified or solvent/detergent inactivated
Recombinant factor VIII	None/contains high levels of factor VIII	Safe

needed to assess the true nature of the disease. After infection, an incubation period of 2 to 26 weeks is followed by a clinically mild disease with lower peaks of liver function tests than with hepatitis B.[101,102] The liver function tests then fluctuate with periods of normal laboratory evaluation followed by mild elevations of liver function tests.[101] This pattern of varying liver function tests, which may last months to years, makes the diagnosis of complete recovery difficult.[101] Likewise, disappearance of antibodies to HCV does not absolutely imply complete recovery, further complicating the diagnosis of cure.[101]

Regardless of the means of infection, roughly 50% of individuals infected will develop chronic active hepatitis (CAH).[100,101] Of patients with CAH, 50% will have progressive disease and 50% will have stable disease.[101] Data have shown that regardless of mode of transmission, 25% of patients infected with HCV will develop cirrhosis.[101] Age is a prognosticator in that patients younger than 50 years develop cirrhosis at a rate of 19%, whereas patients older than 50 years have a 40% chance of developing cirrhosis.[101] The clinical course of cirrhosis due to HCV is mild compared to alcohol-related cirrhosis, with the majority of patients being asymptomatic or only mildly symptomatic for years.[101] Despite the relatively mild course of HCV-associated cirrhosis, 10% of patients will develop decompensated cirrhosis or portal hypertension over an 8-year period.[101] Even though death related to liver disease is increased, absolute mortality from all causes is not increased in patients with transfusion-related hepatitis C followed for an average of 18 years.[103] This could imply that patients who require transfusion have shortened life expectancies, which will mask the relatively late negative effect of hepatitis C on mortality, or that hepatitis C is a relatively mild disease that has little effect on long-term survival. Even longer follow-up is necessary to discover which of these implications is correct.

HIV, HTLV-I, AND HTLV-II

These three viruses are grouped together because of their rarity, because they are all retroviruses, and because the results of infection with each can be disastrous. HIV is the infectious agent responsible for the acquired immunodeficiency syndrome (AIDS). HTLV-I and HTLV-II are associated with leukemia and, in the case of HTLV-I, a myelopathy (tropical spastic paraparesis).[94,104] Public concern over transfusion has justifiably centered on the risk of contracting HIV. Although the risk of HIV is at least 10 times less than the risk of getting hepatitis C, the difference is that all cases of HIV infection are now thought to lead eventually to AIDS and death.

The prevalence of HIV-positive blood donors is much less than the prevalence of HIV in the general population. The relatively low incidence of 1 in 10,000 donors positive for HIV has been attributed to the voluntary donor system with confidential self-exclusion.[96] Serological screening of blood products reduces the risk of contracting AIDS from a trans-

fusion to between 1 in 60,000 per unit and 1 in 225,000 per unit.[94,104] Using tests presently available, the blood supply cannot be totally free of HIV contamination because of the window period in which donors are infectious but have not yet developed antibodies.[104] Ninety-five percent of patients infected with HIV will develop antibodies within 5 months; however, the window period is shorter than this period and is estimated to last a median of 2.1 months.[104] During these 2 months, blood collected from a person infected with HIV is contagious but testing of the blood will not indicate that the blood should be discarded.

HTLV-I and HTLV-II infections do not always lead to disease. In fact, only 4% of patients infected with HTLV-I will develop T-cell leukemia or tropical spastic paraparesis.[94] The disease spectrum associated with HTLV-II infection has not been defined fully, but it appears to be associated with a low risk of T-cell hairy-cell leukemia and a neurodegenerative syndrome.[104] Prior to the institution of serological screening of donated blood in 1988, the risk of contracting these viruses was 1 in 8500 per unit.[104] After routine screening of blood for these viruses was begun, the rate declined to 1 in 69,000 per unit.[94,104]

Immunomodulation Secondary to Blood Transfusions

For years, the positive effect of blood transfusions on solid tissue transplant survival has been known.[105] Survival of allografts improve with transfusion of donor-specific or random blood, implying that the immune system is somehow altered by transfusion.[105] The mechanism of immunomodulation is not completely understood; however, experimental evidence has suggested that T lymphocytes, natural killer cells, and macrophages are all affected by a single transfusion of blood.[105,106]

Recent studies have shown that the immunosuppression caused by blood transfusion can be deleterious to the survival of cancer patients. Patients with lung, colon, breast, and other tumors have decreased survival if they have been transfused.[105] Likewise, blood transfusions in patients with head and neck squamous cell carcinoma are significantly related to recurrence of disease and decreased survival.[106,107] Multivariate analysis has shown that transfusion and margin status are the only independent predictors of recurrence, suggesting that transfusion status is more important than primary size or nodal status as a predictor of recurrence.[106] Of the two studies performed on head and neck squamous cell carcinoma, one shows no effect of multiple transfusions whereas the other shows a dose-related effect, with patients who received more blood having poorer results.[106,107]

Prevention of transfusion-related immunosuppression is best achieved by avoiding transfusions except when absolutely necessary. The second option is to transfuse autologous blood because the autologous blood does not have the immunosuppressive effects of random homologous blood. Finally, because the immunosuppressive component of blood is thought to be related to leukocyte contamination, washed blood that has had the contaminant white cells removed may allow transfusion without increased risk of recurrence or decreased survival.[105,106] The risk of washed blood in head and neck surgery has not been defined clearly at this time. Other experimental therapies to block the immunosuppressive effect of transfusion are the use of prostaglandin synthetase inhibitors and immunomodulatory drugs such as cyclophosphamide.[105]

Massive Transfusion

Massive transfusions occur for multiple reasons, including trauma, pelvic fractures, surgical procedures, and bleeding due to DIC. The massively transfused patient is defined as a patient who has received 10 units of blood in 24 hours or more than 1 blood volume in 24 hours.[108] Complications due to massive transfusion include metabolic disorders relating to the citrate load and hypothermia, as well as acute respiratory distress syndrome and disorders of coagulation.

Continued bleeding after control of the inciting event in patients requiring massive transfusions may be due to underlying causes or due to coagulation defects secondary to the transfusions. Massive transfusion is associated with thrombocytopenia in 89% of patients.[108] Additionally, platelet aggregation has been shown to be decreased in animal models of massive transfusion. Despite the high incidence of thrombocytopenia and the possible association of qualitative platelet defects, routine platelet transfusions have not been shown to decrease blood loss.[108] Massive transfusions are also associated with factor deficiencies due to a dilutional decrease followed by a coagulopathy that is directly related to the length of hypotension.[108] Studies have indicated that routine administration of FFP in massively transfused patients is not indicated and that efforts to limit the time of shock are more important for adequate hemostasis.[108]

Pulmonary dysfunction in massively transfused patients who have withstood shock is an unavoidable complication. The acute respiratory distress syndrome is thought to be due to activated neutrophils and/or prostaglandins formed as a reaction to the disease process.[108] Studies invoking the use of drugs that decrease prostaglandin synthesis or affect neutrophil function may clarify whether these agents help prevent pulmonary dysfunction.

Many physicians are concerned that hypocalcemia following transfusion of large quantities of citrated blood will affect hemostasis. In fact, cardiac function will be adversely affected due to hypocalcemia long before the coagulation system.[108] However, if the patient is hypothermic, hepatic function (which normally can metablize the amount of citrate in 20 U of whole blood every hour) is diminished. Hypocalcemia in hypothermic patients is seen most often in association with hypothermic cardiac surgical procedures, but can occur in any hypothermic patient. Treatment with calcium chloride effectively increases cardiac output and blood pressure in patients with citrate toxicity, which is necessary until the liver metabolizes the excess citrate.[108]

REFERENCES

1. PiHiglio DH, Sacher RA, eds. *Clinical Hematology and Fundamentals of Hemostasis.* Philadelphia: FA Davis Co.; 1987.
2. Borzotta AP, Keeling MM. Value of the preoperative history as an indicator of hemostatic disorders. *Ann Surg.* 1984;200(5):648–652.
3. Eisenberg JM, Clarke JR, Sussman SA. Prothrombin and partial thromboplastin times as preoperative screening tests. *Arch Surg.* 1982;117:48–51.
4. Suchman AL, Mushlin AI. How well does the activated partial thromboplastin time predict postoperative hemorrhage? *JAMA.* 1986;256(6):750–753.
5. Kaplan EB, Sheiner LB, Boeckmann AJ, et al. The usefulness of preoperative laboratory screening. *JAMA.* 1985;253(24):3576–3581.
6. Barber A, Green D, Galluzzo T, et al. The bleeding time as a preoperative screening test. *Am J Med.* 1985;78:761–764.
7. Lind S. Prolonged bleeding time. *Am J Med.* 1984;77:305–312.
8. Lind S. The bleeding time does not predict surgical bleeding. *Blood.* 1991;77(12):2547–2552.
9. Rapaport SI. Preoperative hemostatic evaluation: Which tests, if any? *Blood.* 1983;61(2):229–231.
10. Kitchens CS. Prolonged activated partial thromboplastin time of unknown etiology: A prospective study of 100 consecutive cases referred for consultation. *Am J Hematol.* 1988;27:38–45.
11. Janvier G, Winnock S, Freyburger G. Value of the activated partial thromboplastin time for preoperative detection of coagulation disorders not revealed by a specific questionnaire. *Anesthesiology.* 1991;75(5):920–921.
12. Rareshide EH, Amedee RG. Hemostasis in the surgical patient. *Louisiana State Med J.* 1991;143:7–10.
13. Waters AH. Autoimmune thrombocytopenia: Clinical aspects. *Semin Hematol.* 1992;29(1):18–25.
14. Bolger WE, Parsons DS, Potempa L. Preoperative hemostatic assessment of the adenotonsillectomy patient. *Otolaryngology-Head and Neck Surg.* 1990;103(3):396–405.
15. Sirridge MS, Shannon R, eds. *Laboratory Evaluation of Hemostasis and Thrombosis.* 3rd ed. Philadelphia: Lea & Febiger; 1983.
16. Reich DL. Monitoring hemostasis in the perioperative period: Anticoagulation control. *J Cardiothoracic Vasc Anesth.* 1991;5(6):4–7.
17. Clodfelter RL. The peripheral smear. *Emerg Med Clin North Am.* 1986;4(1):59–74.
18. Schmidt JL, Yaremchuk KL, Mickelson SA. Abnormal coagulation profiles in tonsillectomy and adenoidectomy patients. *Henry Ford Hosp Med J.* 1990;38(1):33–35.
19. Burk CD, Miller L, Handler SD, et al. Preoperative history and coagulation screening in children undergoing tonsillectomy. *Pediatrics.* 1992;89(4):691–695.
20. Weiss HJ, Rogers J. Thrombocytopathia due to abnormalities in platelet release reaction: Studies on six unrelated patients. *Blood.* 1972;39(2):187–196.
21. Webster MWI, Chesebro JH, Fuster V. Platelet inhibitor therapy: Agents and clinical implications. *Hematol/Oncol Clin North Am.* 1990;4(1):265–289.
22. Petitt RM. Thrombotic thrombocytopenic purpura: A thirty year review. *Semin Thromb Hemost.* 1980;6(4):350–355.
23. Buchanan GR. Overview of ITP treatment modalities in children. *Blut.* 1989;59:96–104.
24. Kaplan C, Morinet F, Cartron J. Virus-induced autoimmune thrombocytopenia and neutropenia. *Semin Hematol.* 1992;29(1):34–44.

25. Lusher JM, Warrier I. Use of intravenous gamma globulin in children and adolescents with idiopathic thrombocytopenic purpura and other immune thrombocytopenias. *Am J Med.* 1987;83(suppl 4A):10–16.

26. Kelton JG, Moore JC, Murphy WG. Studies investigating platelet aggregation and release initiated by sera from patients with thrombotic thrombocytopenic pupura. *Blood.* 1987;69(3):924–928.

27. Machin SJ. Clinical annotation: Thrombotic thrombocytopenic purpura. *Br J Haematol.* 1984;56:191–197.

28. Chediak J, Eldridge J, Bergmann F, et al. Further evidence of von Willebrand factor involvement in thrombotic thrombocytopenia purpura. *Thrombosis and Haemostasis.* 1988;60(1):13–17.

29. Rarick MU, Espina B, Mocharnuk R, et al. Thrombotic thrombocytopenic purpura in patients with immunodeficiency virus infection: A report of three cases and review of the literature. *Am J Hematol.* 1992;40:103–109.

30. Berkowitz LR, Dalldorf FG, Blatt PM. Thrombotic thrombocytopenic purpura: A pathology review. *JAMA.* 1979;241(16):1709–1710.

31. Jubelirer SJ. Hemostatic abnormalities in renal disease. *Am J Kidney Dis.* 1985;5(5):219–225.

32. Janson PA, Jubelirer SJ, Weinstein MJ, et al. Treatment of the bleeding tendency in uremia with cryoprecipitate. *N Engl J Med.* 1980;303(23):1318–1322.

33. Mannucci PM, Remuzzi G, Pusineri F, et al. Deamino-8-D-Arginine vasopressin shortens the bleeding time in uremia. *N Engl J Med.* 1983;308(1):8–12.

34. Mannucci PM. Desmopressin: A nontransfusional form of treatment for congenital and acquired bleeding disorders. *J Am Soc Hematol.* 1988;72(5):1449–1455.

35. Janes SL. Thrombocytopenia in pregnancy. *Postgrad Med J.* 1992;68:321–326.

36. Burrows RF, Kelton JG. Incidentally detected thrombocytopenia in healthy mothers and their infants. *N Engl J Med.* 1988;319(3):142–145.

37. Salama A, Mueller-Eckhardt C. Immune-mediated blood cell dyscrasias related to drugs. *Semin Hematol.* 1992;29(1):54–63.

38. Walls JT, Curtis JJ, Silver D, et al. Heparin-induced thrombocytopenia in open heart surgical patients: Sequelae of late recognition. *Ann Thorac Surg.* 1992;53:787–791.

39. Girard DE, Kumar KL, McAfee JH. Hematologic effects of acute and chronic alcohol abuse. *Hematol/Oncol Clin North Am.* 1987;1:321–333.

40. Horowitz HI, Cohen BD, Martinez P, et al. Defective ADP-induced platelet factor 3 activation in uremia. *Blood.* 1967;30(3):331–340.

41. Wallenburg HCS, Makovitz JW, Dekker GA, et al. Low-dose aspirin prevents pregnancy-induced hypertension and pre-eclampsia in angiotensin-sensitive primigravidae. *Lancet.* 1986;i:1–3.

42. Hardaway RM, Adams WH. Blood clotting problems in acute care. *Acute Care.* 1988–1989;14–15:138–207.

43. Mannucci PM. Desmopressin (DDAVP) for treatment of disorders of hemostasis. *Prog Hemostasis Thrombosis.* 1986;8:19–45.

44. Shapiro SS, Hultin M. Acquired inhibitors to the blood coagulation factors. *Semin Thromb Hemost.* 1975;1:336–385.

45. Barbui T, Baudo F, Ciavarella N, et al. Spectrum of von Willebrand's disease: A study of 100 cases. *Br J Haematol.* 1977;35:101–112.

46. Aledort LM. Treatment of von Willebrand's disease. *Mayo Clin Proc.* 1991;66:841–846.

47. Bloom AL. The von Willebrand syndrome. *Semin Hematol.* 1980;17(4):215–227.

48. Handin RI. Coagulation disorders. In: Braunwald E, Isselbacher KJ, Petersdorf RG, Wilson JD, Martin JB, Fauci AS, eds. *Harrison's Principles of Internal Medicine.* 11th ed. New York: McGraw-Hill; 1987:1475–1480.

49. Violi F, Ferro D, Quintarelli C, et al. Clotting abnormalities in chronic liver disease. *Dig Dis.* 1992;10:162–172.

50. Sack GH, Levin J, Bell WR. Trousseau's syndrome and other manifestations of chronic disseminated coagulopathy in patients with neoplasms: Clinical, pathophysiologic, and therapeutic features. *Medicine.* 1977;56(1):1–37.

51. Shapiro SS, Thiagarajan P. Lupus anticoagulants. *Prog Henost. Thromb.* 1982;6:263–285.

52. Orris DJ, Lewis JH, Spero JA, et al. Blocking coagulation inhibitors in children taking penicillin. *J Ped.* 1980;97(3):426–429.

53. Kornberg A, Silber L, Yona R, et al. Clinical manifestations and laboratory findings in patients with lupus anticoagulants. *Eur J Haematol.* 1989;42:90–95.

54. Hart RG, Kanter MC. Hematologic disorders and ischemic stroke. *Stroke.* 1990;21(8):1111–1121.

55. Love PE, Santoro SA. Antiphospholipid antibodies: Anticardiolipin and the lupus anticoagulant in Systemic Lupus Erythematosus (SLE) and in non-SLE disorders. *Ann Int Med.* 1990;112:682–698.

56. Ware RE, Filston HC. Surgical management of children with hemoglobinopathies. *Ped Surg.* 1992;72(6):1223–1236.

57. Vichinsky EP. Comprehensive care in sickle cell disease: Its impact on morbidity and mortality. *Semin Hematol.* 1991;28(3):220–226.

58. Smith JA. What do we know about the clinical course of sickle cell disease? *Semin Hematol.* 1991;28(3):209–212.

59. Piomelli S. Sickle cell diseases in the 1990s: The need for active and preventive intervention. *Semin Hematol.* 1991;28(3):227–232.

60. Banerjee AK, Layton DM, Rennie JA, et al. Safe surgery in sickle cell disease. *Br J Surg.* 1991;78:516–517.

61. Beutler E. Bone marrow transplantation for sickle cell anemia: Summarizing comments. *Semin Hematol.* 1991;28(3):263–267.

62. Messmore HL. Clinical efficacy of heparin fractions: Issues and answers. *CRC Critical Rev Clin Lab Sci.* 23(2):77–94.

63. Holmer E, Söderberg K, Bergqvist D, et al. Heparin and its low molecular weight derivatives: Anticoagulant and antithrombotic properties. *Haemostasis.* 1986;16(suppl 2):1–7.

64. Perry MO. Anticoagulation: A surgical perspective. *Am J Surg.* 1988;155:268–276.

65. Hirsh J. Heparin induced bleeding. *Nouv Rev Fr Hematol.* 1984;26:261–266.

66. King DJ, Kelton JG. Heparin-associated thrombocytopenia. *Ann Int Med.* 1984;100:535–540.

67. Holmer E, Mattsson C, Nilsson S. Anticoagulant and antithrombotic effects of heparin and low molecular weight heparin fragments in rabbits. *Thromb Res.* 1982;25:475–485.

68. Carter CJ, Kelton JG, Hirsh J, et al. The relationship between the hemorrhagic and antithrombotic properties of low molecular weight heparin in rabbits. *Blood.* 1982;59(6):1239–1245.

69. Holm HA, Ly B, Handeland GF, et al. Subcutaneous heparin treatment of deep venous thrombosis: A comparison of unfractionated and low molecular weight heparin. *Haemostasis.* 16(suppl 2):30–37.

70. Bergqvist D, Burmark US, Frisell J, et al. Prospective double-blind comparison between Fragmin and conventional low-dose heparin: Thromboprophylactic effect and bleeding complications. *Haemostasis.* 1986;16(suppl 2):11–18.

71. Kakkar VV, Kakkar S, Sanderson RM, et al. Efficacy and safety of two regimens of low molecular weight heparin fragment (Fragmin) in preventing postoperative venous thrombolism. *Haemostasis.* 1986;16(suppl 2):19–24.

72. Sasahara AA, DiSerio FJ, Singer JM, et al. Dihydroergotamine-heparin prophylaxis of postoperative deep vein thrombosis: A multicenter trial. *JAMA.* 1984;251:2960–2966.

73. Kiil J, Kiil J, Axelsen F, et al. Prophylaxis against postoperative pulmonary emblism and deep-vein thrombosis by low-dose heparin. *Lancet.* 1978;1:1115–1116.

74. Kakkar VV, Corrigan TP, Fossard DP. Prevention of fatal postoperative pulmonary embolism by low doses of heparin: An international multicentre trial. *Lancet.* 1975;2:45–51.

75. Hirsh J, Poller L, Deykin D, et al. Optimal therapeutic range for oral anticoagulants. *Chest* 1989;95(2):5S–11S.

76. Tinker JH, Tarhan S. Discontinuing anticoagulant therapy in surgical patients with cardiac valve prostheses. *JAMA.* 1978;239(8):738–739.

77. Levine MN, Raskob G, Hirsh J. Hemorrhagic complications of long-term anticoagulant therapy. *Chest.* 1989;95(2): 26S–36S.

78. Perry DJ, Kimball DB. Low dose vitamin K for excessively anticoagulated prosthetic valve patients. *Military Med.* 1982;147:836–837.

79. Alving BM, Comp PC. Recent advances in understanding clotting and evaluating patients with recurrent thrombosis. *Am J Obstet Gynecol.* 1992;167(4):1184–1191.

80. DiPerri T, Vittoria A, Messa GL, et al. Defibrotide therapy for thrombophlebitis-controlled clinical trial. *Haemostasis.* 1986;16(suppl 1):42–47.

81. Ciavarella N, Ettorre C, Schiavoni M, et al. Effectiveness of defibrotide for prophylaxis of deep venous thrombosis in gynecological surgery: A double-blind, placebo-controlled clinical trial. *Haemostasis.* 1986;16(suppl 1):39–41.

82. Mozzi E, Chiurazzi D, Germiniani R, et al. Effectiveness of defibrotide for prophylaxis of deep venous thrombosis after general surgery: A double-blind, placebo-controlled clinical trial. *Haemostasis.* 1986;16(suppl 1):36–38.

83. Hirsh J. The clinical role of antiplatelet agents. *Drug Therapy.* 1981;49–60.

84. Hirsh J, Salzman EW, Harker L, et al. Aspirin and other platelet active drugs: Relationship among dose, effectiveness, and side effects. *Chest.* 1989;95(suppl 2):12S–18S.

85. Goldman S, Copeland J, Moritz T, et al. Starting aspirin therapy after operation: Effects on early graft patency. *Circulation.* 1991;84(2):520–526.

86. Kitchen L, Erichson RB, Sideropoulos H. Effect of drug-induced platelet dysfunction on surgical bleeding. *Am J Surg.* 1982;143:215–217.

87. Dyer WS, Quigley EMM, Noel SM, et al. Major colonic hemorrhage following electrocoagulating (hot) biopsy of diminutive colonic polyps: Relationship to colonic location and low-dose aspirin therapy. *Gastrointest Endoscopy.* 1991; 37(3):361–364.

88. Ferraris VA, Swanson E. Aspirin usage and perioperative blood loss in patients undergoing unexpected operations. *Surg Gyn Ob.* 1983;156:439–442.

89. Miller LG, Prichard JG. Current issues in NSAID therapy. *Primary Care.* 1990;17(3):589–601.

90. Reymond MA, Marbet G, Radü EW, et al. Aspirin as a risk factor for hemorrhage in patients with head injuries. *Neurosurg Rev.* 1992;15:21–25.

91. McIntyre BA, Philip RB, Inwood MJ. Effect of ibuprofen on platelet function in normal subjects and hemophiliac patients. *Clin Pharmacol Ther.* 1978;24(5):616–621.

92. McCulloch TM, Glenn MG, Riley D, et al. Blood use in head and neck tumor surgery: Potential for autologous blood. *Arch Otolaryngol Head Neck Surg.* 1989;115:1314–1317.

93. Solanki D, McCurdy PR. Delayed hemolytic transfusion reactions: An often-missed entity. *JAMA.* 1978;239(8):729–731.

94. Dodd RY. The risk of transfusion-transmitted infection. *N Engl J Med.* 1992;327(6):419–420.

95. Alter HJ, Epstein JS, Swenson SG, et al. Prevalence of human immunodeficiency virus type 1 p 24 antigen in US blood donors—an assessment of the efficacy of testing in donor screening. *N Engl J Med.* 1990;323:1312–1317.

96. Starkey JM, MacPherson ML, Bolgiano DC, et al. Markers for transfusion-transmitted disease in different groups of blood donors. *JAMA.* 1989;262(24):3452–3454.

97. Katkov WN, Dienstag JL. Prevention and therapy of viral hepatitis. *Semin Liver Dis.* 1991;11(2):165–174.

98. Dodd RY, Popovsky MA, et al. Antibodies to hepatitis B core antigen and the infectivity of the blood supply. *Transfusion.* 1991;31(5):443–449.

99. Czaja AJ. Chronic hepatitis C virus infection—a disease in waiting? *N Engl J Med.* 1992;327(27):1949–1950.

100. Tremolada F, Casarin C, Tagger A, et al. Antibody to hepatitic C virus in post-transfusion hepatitis. *Ann Int Med.* 1991;114:277–281.

101. Genesca J, Esteban JI, Alter JH. Blood-borne non-A, non-B hepatitis: Hepatitis C. *Semin Liver Dis.* 1991;11(2):147–164.

102. Donahue JG, Muñoz A, Ness PM, et al. The declining risk of post-transfusion hepatitis C virus infection. *N Engl J Med.* 1992;327(6):369–373.

103. Seeff LB, Buskell-Bales Z, Wright EC, et al. Long-term mortality after transfusion-associated non-A non-B hepatitis. *N Engl J Med.* 1992;327(27):1906–1911.

104. Nelson KE, Donahue JG, Muñoz A, et al. Transmission of retroviruses from seronegative donors by transfusion during cardiac surgery: A multicenter study of HIV-1 and HTLV-I/II infections. *Ann Int Med.* 1992;117(7):554–559.

105. Waymack JP, Alexander JW. Blood transfusions as an immunomodulator—a review. *Comp Immum Microbiol. Infect Dis.* 1986;9(2/3):177–183.

106. Jones KR, Weissler MC. Blood transfusion and other risk factors for recurrence of cancer of the head and neck. *Arch Otolaryngol Head Neck Surg.* 1990;116:304–309.

107. Johnson JT, Taylor FH, Thearle P. Blood transfusion and outcome in stage III head and neck carcinoma. *Arch Otolaryngol Head Neck Surg.* 1987;113:307–310.

108. Rutledge R, Sheldon GF, Collins ML. Massive transfusion. *Crit Care Clin.* 1986;2(4):791–805.

109. Platt DR, Nightingale CH. Warfarin drug interactions. *Infect Surg.* 1986;91–98.

3 Deep Venous Thrombosis and Pulmonary Embolism

Gregory F. Hulka, M.D., Mark C. Weissler, M.D.

Each year practically every medical journal features articles concerning the thromboembolic diseases of venous thromboses and pulmonary emboli. Generally, the articles review the numerous advances in diagnosis, management, and prevention of these disorders. Some treatment methods are based on standard regimens and are relatively easy to perform, whereas others are complicated and difficult to perform and presently have little clinical application. In this chapter, new methods as well as standard treatment protocols will be covered, and rational approaches toward diagnosis and treatment will be described.

Although the clinical entities of deep venous thromboses and pulmonary emboli are approached much differently from a diagnostic standpoint, their treatment plans are similar in many aspects.

DEEP VENOUS THROMBOSIS

Presentation

A high index of suspicion is essential for the appropriate diagnosis of deep venous thrombosis. Certainly, patients on orthopedic services should frequently be checked for deep venous thromboses because the incidence in this group of patients is high. However, deep venous thromboses can and do occur in other patient populations. As otolaryngologists, we are fortunate in that our paitents are usually ambulatory within 24 to 48 hours postoperatively, thus reducing the incidence of deep vein thrombosis. Smaller vessel thromboses are still common in all surgical patients, but fortunately they are much less significant clinically. The most common clinical manifestations of deep venous thrombosis include localized tenderness, pain, and swelling over the lower extremities. Physical exam, although helpful, is not always a reliable means of diagnosis. Frequently patients that are lying in bed for long periods of time will not demonstrate a significant amount of swelling in the affected extremity despite extensive thrombotic disease, and a positive Homan's sign (slight pain at the back of the knee or calf when the ankle is slowly and gently dorsiflexed with the knee bent) is not necessarily found in all patients with deep venous thrombosis.

Several risk factors have been identified as predisposing patients to deep venous thromboses: age greater than 40, surgery lasting longer than 30 minutes, a previous history of deep venous thrombosis or pulmonary emboli, prolonged immobilization, paralysis, malignancy, obesity, varicose veins, and estrogen use. The type of surgical procedure is also important because patients with manipulation of venous structures or the lower extremity have a much higher incidence of deep venous thrombosis. Some authors prefer to divide patients into low-, medium-, and high-risk categories based on how many of these risk factors are present in a given patient; however, the most important point is to keep a high clinical suspicion in patients with any of these factors (Table 3-1).

Table 3-1. Risk Factors for the Development of Deep Venous Thrombosis

Age > 40
Surgery lasting longer than 30 minutes
Previous history of deep venous thrombosis or pulmonary embolism
Prolonged immobilization
Paralysis
Malignancy
Obesity
Varicose veins
Estrogen use
Surgical procedures involving manipulation of venous structures or the lower extremity

From Raskob and Hull.[22]

Etiology

The etiology of deep venous thrombosis is not fully understood; however, the risk factors mentioned previously do seem to increase the likelihood significantly. Internal vascular injury, stasis, and hypercoagulability are the chief factors contributing to deep venous thrombosis in surgical patients, but other surgical factors also seem to be important. Stasis of the circulating blood during surgery in the supine position as well as the vasodilatory effects of anesthetic agents seem to increase the venous capacitance, thus decreasing the blood flow such that the likelihood of coagulation is increased. Trauma to the vessels of the lower extremity, although rare in otolaryngology patients, can occur, particularly when obtaining fibular grafts. Although this procedure does not directly manipulate the deep veins, it does allow for the

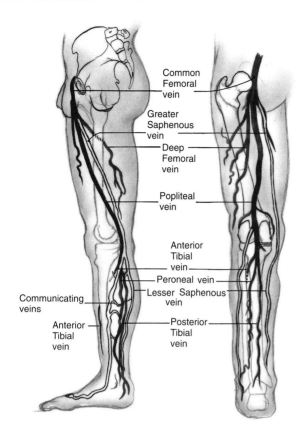

Figure 3–1. The deep veins of the lower extremity.

propagation of clots within the veins of the distal lower extremity, particularly the lateral saphenous, posterior tibial, and communicating veins (Fig. 3–1).

Diagnosis

As previously mentioned, physical exam is often unrewarding and is not accurate in the diagnosis of deep venous thrombosis. In fact, in approximately 50% of patients undergoing an evaluation for suspected thrombosis, clinical diagnosis will be incorrect. Included in the differential for deep venous thrombosis are ruptured synovial cysts, ruptured calf muscles, arthritis, and cellulitis. Preferably, any tests for evaluation of deep venous thrombosis would be noninvasive. Certainly any test involving disruption or irritation of the venous system should be avoided because it could lead to the development of thrombosis itself.

Impedance Plethysmography

Impedance plethysmography is performed with the patient in a supine position with the legs elevated at an angle of approximately 15 degrees. The knees are bent at 30 degrees and the hip is rotated externally. The basic concept of this test is that following the release of venous congestion, venous emptying of a lower extremity is usually rapid; however, if the veins are obstructed, they empty more slowly. With the patient's legs elevated in the manner described earlier, the venous volume within the legs should be minimal. Electrodes

are then placed around the calf of the leg, and these are used for measuring the volume of the lower extremity. A thigh cuff is then inflated to 45 cm water pressure for 45 seconds and is then deflated. In a normal leg, there will be rapid decrease in the venous volume upon deflation of the thigh cuff. However, a falsely positive test can result from inappropriate leg position, thigh compression by the uninflated cuff, the patient's clothing, circumferential dressings or bandages on the extremity, and electrode misplacement. A single negative finding after multiple repositionings and multiple tests is considered a negative result for the entire test. If used routinely by well-trained individuals, this test can have a sensitivity and specificity of up to 95% for proximal deep venous thrombosis. However, in considering more distant thrombi, this test leaves much to be desired because of collateral vasculature allowing for better venous run off. Impedance plethysmography is often used in combination with other tests, specifically portable Doppler.

Portable Continuous Wave Doppler

For this test, patients are placed in a reverse Trendelenburg position. Using a 5-MHz Doppler instrument, deep veins to be investigated are identified by their location in reference to an accompanying artery. The leg distal to the point of auscultation is then compressed, and the effect on the vein being examined is assessed. Deep venous thrombosis is suspected if there is altered venous hemodynamics as a result of partial or total venous occlusion, or if there is absence of flow in the vein being examined. It is important during this portion of the exam to be aware of the normal phasic changes in venous flow based on respiration. At peak inspiration, there is increased abdominal pressure and subsequently venous flow may cease, only to resume again with expiration. This can lead to misdiagnosis of deep venous thrombosis during the inspiratory cycle. False negatives also exist, particularly when there are nonobstructing thromboses or if there are deep veins that are thrombosed that are simply not running in acompaniment with an artery. Continuous wave Doppler testing is often combined with other tests, particularly impedance plethysmography.

Duplex Imaging

Duplex imaging has become the standard method of evaluation for deep venous thrombosis at most institutions. It is a relatively easy study to perform and has a sensitivity and specificity that in well-trained hands is above 95% for proximal disease. It also has the potential to be a portable examination, allowing for much more convenient testing of the patients. The term *duplex* comes from combining high-resolution, real-time, b-mode ultrasonography (for imaging of the actual vein) with pulse Doppler sampling, which helps determine flow. This combination can provide a gray-scale imaging of vasculature in its relation to the surrounding tissues as well as demonstrate flow patterns. This method of testing also allows for more direct visualization than previously mentioned tests, which are based on physiological changes in venous hemodynamics under variances of pressure and position. Because the Doppler allows for examination of vessels at given locations, it allows for a more extensive determination of the extent and anatomic level of any obstruction. It can also help identify thrombus that is nonobstructing and would otherwise be missed by noninvasive tests. These tests are performed with the patient in the reverse Trendelenberg position, and all the veins are examined from the groin to the proximal tibial vessels. Visualization of the thrombus, low compressibility of the venous lumen by the probe, and either no signal or the presence of abnormal Doppler signal are all considered positive test results. A high degree of correlation has been found to exist between Duplex scans and venography.[1,2]

Triplex Scanning

In addition to the examination performed by duplex imaging, triplex imaging allows for measuring the flow through the vessel. Usually, the flow is indicated by various colors on a monitor, which are proportionate to the direction and velocity of the flow. By adding color flow examination, it is possible to understand better the hemodynamic changes that occur in the venous system, both acutely (at the time of venous thrombosis) and over time as flow patterns change and venous outflow patterns evolve.

Phleborheography

Phleborheography is an indirect measurement made to evaluate deep venous thrombosis. It measures respiratory venous waves and the free movement of venous blood at different levels in the lower extremities. When the deep veins are obstructed, the waves are absent, and compression of the foot or distal leg results in the backup of venous blood. The test is performed by placing four cuffs, one each at the foot, lower calf, upper calf, and thigh. The function of the lower cuffs is to measure changes in respiratory waves and blood volume. They also provide the venous compression distally. This test has limited usefulness because it cannot detect calf disease or nonocclusive thrombosis. Placement of the cuff should be in many positions to be sure that the appropriate venous obstruction is obtained.

Venography

Ascending contrast venography is only briefly mentioned here. For a long time it was the standard test for detection of deep venous thrombosis, but since the advent of the newer noninvasive methods it is rarely performed. In this study, contrast agents are placed into the veins of the lower extremities and the images are then obtained of the entire leg's venous system. Although this method of evaluation is excellent for detecting calf thrombosis and deep venous thrombosis, it presents many problems. The dye load used in venography can lead to deterioration of renal function and, perhaps most significantly, the dye itself can lead to thrombophlebitis and

subsequent clot formation. This test is also extremely difficult to perform in terms of the variability in technique and amount of dye used, pain caused to the patient, and amount of time it takes to perform the examination.

TREATMENT OF DEEP VENOUS THROMBOSIS

Once the diagnosis of deep venous thrombosis has been established, anticoagulation remains the standard treatment. Most commonly, the initial treatment consists of the immediate use of heparin followed by the addition of warfarin.

Heparin Therapy

Unless there are specific contraindications, continuous administration of intravenous heparin should be initiated as soon as the diagnosis of deep venous thrombosis has been established. Treatment regimens are targeted to achieve a partial thromboplastin time (PTT) of approximately 1.5 to 2 times the control value.[3] Immediate intravenous boluses of 5000 to 15,000 units are given initially, followed by a constant infusion rate of approximately 500 to 1500 units per hour thereafter. It is important to achieve a PTT value of 1.5 times or greater the control value within the first 24 hours because the risk or recurrence of thromboembolic phenomena is much greater if this is not achieved.[4] Because one of the major complications of heparin therapy is progressive thrombocytopenia, the platelet count should be checked daily during the first 4 to 5 days of therapy. Any downward trend should alert the physician to the possibility of thrombocytopenia. Similarly, patients who have recently undergone surgery are also at risk for episodes of bleeding. Because of this, all wounds should be carefully observed for the development of hematoma or oozing from the edges. Other sources of bleeding, such as gastrointestinal (GI) ulcers or colonic polyps, should also be watched for. The incidence of heparin-induced thrombocytopenia was about 10% in one study.[5] Therefore, platelet counts were recommended every day or every other day as long as heparin therapy continued. In the situation of spontaneous bleeding that presents a great risk to the patient, such as intracranial bleeding or intestinal bleeding that is not controllable, the effect of heparin should be neutralized with the use of protamine sulfate (recommended doses include initial intravenous [IV] boluses of 5000 units, followed by an IV drip of 800 units per hour).

It is generally recommended that warfarin be started concomitantly with the heparin. During the time that heparin therapy is started, the patient should be kept at strict bed rest with leg elevation and application of heat to the leg until symptoms such as pain and swelling of the leg resolve.

Warfarin Sodium (Coumadin)

Warfarin sodium therapy is usually initiated within 24 hours of heparin therapy initiation. Although maintenance doses of warfarin are usually 2.5 to 7.5 mg per day, initial doses consist of 5 to 10 mg per day for approximately 3 days. Prothrombin time (PT) is followed until it increases to 1.5 times, but not greater than two times, the normal value. Once the appropriate prothrombin time has been achieved for 24 hours, which is usually at least 4 days after the initiation of Coumadin therapy, heparin may be discontinued. There are two important points to consider when using both heparin and warfarin. First heparin can slightly lengthen the prothrombin time and subsequently give a false increase in the prothrombin time when warfarin is initiated. This must be considered prior to the discontinuance of heparin therapy. Second, Coumadin can cause a transient hypercoagulable state, and therefore it is important that heparin therapy be continued for at least 5 days after initiation of Coumadin therapy. During this time, heparin is overlapped to prevent the further propagation of deep venous thrombosis during this hypercoagulable state, which normally occurs within the first 24 to 72 hours after initiation of warfarin therapy.

Usually, warfarin sodium is prescribed for a 3- to 6-month period following the initial diagnosis of deep venous thrombosis. This time period is extended in the situation in which the patient has risk factors, such as a malignant process which is still present in the patient or is expected to continue and subsequently increase the chance of recurrence.

Warfarin therapy is not without its complications. As with heparin therapy, hemorrhage is again the most common and potentially disastrous complication of therapy. In patients who are on continuous warfarin therapy, clinic visits should include questions about subtle signs of bleeding, such as blood in the stool or urine, dark stools, and arthralgias, which may indicate bleeding within joint spaces. In the case of severe bleeding following treatment with warfarin sodium, fresh frozen plasma is used to neutralize the effect of warfarin. Vitamin K1 can block the effect of warfarin, but it does not act as quickly as fresh frozen plasma.

Warfarin acts by altering the synthesis of factors 2, 7, 9, and 10 in the liver. This is achieved by warfarin competing with vitamin K, which is essential in the final step of production of these coagulation factors in the process of adding the gamma carboxyglutamic acid chain to their corresponding precursors. Once warfarin has been taken, it is completely absorbed by the gastrointestinal tract with a half-life of approximately 42 hours. Its inactive metabolites are excreted in both the urine and stool. There can be some resistance to warfarin therapy in patients who have impaired gastrointestinal absorption. These include patients using cholestyramine resins, excessive amounts of certain antacids, or liquid paraffin laxatives. On the other hand, because warfarin is 97% protein bound, drugs that displace albumin-bound compounds increase the bioavailability and therefore the action of warfarin.

Relative excesses or deficiencies in vitamin K will also change the effectiveness of warfarin therapy. Massive amounts of vitamin K compete with warfarin and subsequently decrease its effectiveness. Conversely, patients with a deficiency in vitamin K will show a relative sensitivity to warfarin therapy.

Another frequently unrecognized complication of warfarin therapy is warfarin necrosis, which presents as an erythematous patch on the skin which can progress to a dark hemorrhagic area followed by infection and occasionally gangrene. More than 90% of affected patients are female. Usually beginning 2 to 5 days after starting warfarin therapy, this complication is typically found in the lower half of the body and the adipose tissues of the breasts and legs. This is thought to result from a relatively rapid fall in protein C levels at the initiation of warfarin therapy and results in a hypercoagulable state. If this clinical picture is seen, prompt heparinization is necessary. This is another justification for overlapping the warfarin and heparin therapy because continuing the heparin for 5 to 7 days prevents this complication.

An absolute contraindication to warfarin therapy is pregnancy because fetal abnormalities are common when this drug is used. Infants may exhibit stippled epiphyses, subtle nose deformities, and punctate calcifications as well as other bony abnormalities. Central nervous system and ocular abnormalities, and even death resulting from fetal hemorrhage, may occur. Contraindications to anticoagulant therapy are listed in Table 3–2.

Table 3–2. Contraindications to Anticoagulation

ABSOLUTE CONTRAINDICATIONS	RELATIVE CONTRAINDICATIONS
Cerebral or subarachnoid hemorrhage	Gastrointestinal hemorrhage
Malignant hypertension	Recent stroke
Serious active bleeding	Recent surgery
Recent spinal cord, brain, or eye surgery	Hepatic failure
	Renal failure
	Bacterial endocarditis
	A bleeding tendency
	Active gastrointestinal bleeding

Fibrinolytic Agents

Fibrinolytic agents are usually reserved for patients whose clot extends proximally above the origin of the deep femoral vein. Agents used for thrombolytic therapy include streptokinase, urokinase, and tissue plasminogen activator. With the use of these agents, the incidence of pulmonary embolism can be kept down to a level of approximately 5%.

As with most medical therapies, several different dosage strategies for streptokinase have undergone trials. Streptokinase is usually given as a single large dose (around 250,000 units) administered over less than 1 hour, followed by a maintenance dose of 100,000 units per hour intravenously. This can be continued for various lengths of time but is usually given for about 5 hours. Other protocols include much larger doses (up to 500,000 units) given as the initial dose, followed by even larger numbers of units per hour given over 5 or more hours. Usually, the regimen is repeated every day for 3 to 5 days. Some individuals prefer to pretreat patients with hydrocortisone to minimize systemic side-effects of streptokinase. Laboratory testing of these patients by examination of partial thromboplastin times and levels of fibrinogen is performed to confirm that a fibrinolytic state has been achieved.

Urokinase is also used for treatment of deep thrombosis. Treatment regimens again are variable but are typically around 4000 units of urokinase given per kilogram over the first 10 to 20 minutes followed by the constant infusion of approximately 4000 units per kilogram per hour. This is continued for approximately 2 hours. Again, the patients are redosed for up to 5 days; but compared to streptokinase therapy, the dosages on the ensuing days are usually less than on the initial day of treatment, with approximately 4000 units per kilogram per hour given over 1 hour twice a day.

Tissue plasminogen activator is currently undergoing trials at many institutions and will probably replace streptokinase and urokinase in the future.

There are many absolute contraindications to thrombolytic therapy, including the presence of active internal bleeding, evidence of intracranial pathology, or a stroke within the last 2 months. Other contraindications include recent surgery, a history of gastrointestinal bleeding, peptic ulcer disease, visceral malignancy, recent obstetrical delivery, and uncontrolled hypertension. In patients with evidence of a cardiac mural thrombus, the possibility of clot lysis and subsequent embolization must be considered when weighing the benefits of thrombolytic therapy.

In terms of complications, some authors have found that the hemorrhagic complication rate in systemic lytic therapy is approximately three times greater than that with heparin, ranging between 10% and 15%. On the other hand, a higher percentage of patients undergoing systemic lytic therapy have more complete recanalization of the deep venous system when compared to those undergoing anticoagulation alone (50% vs 10% to 25%, respectively). One area where thrombolytic therapy may have a definite advantage over anticoagulant therapy is in the treatment of phlegmasia cerulia dolens and in patients with impending venous gangrene.

Surgical Thrombectomy

A small subsection of the population would benefit from surgical thrombectomy. Generally, these are patients with extremely advanced disease, including the ileofemoral veins as well as the axillary or subclavian vein. Part of the limitation of surgical thrombectomy includes the high incidence of rethrombosis and residual problems with alveolar dysfunction. Postoperatively, these patients are commonly placed on anticoagulants, which also increases their chances of postoperative complications.

Transvenous Vena Caval Filtration

Vena caval filtration in patients with deep venous thrombosis is typically performed on patients who have a history of recurrent deep venous thrombosis with pulmonary emboli, or in patients who pose an unacceptable risk of bleeding complications. It may also be considered in patients that fail standard regimens of anticoagulation therapy. Since 1968, multiple

devices have been developed, all working by the same underlying principle: a filter in the vena cava which allows blood to flow by but causes clots to be trapped within the device. Almost all such devices are placed under local anesthesia and involve catheterization. The characteristics of a good vena caval filter include easy insertion, effectiveness against further emboli, stability in position over time, minimal reactivity with the vessel wall, and absence of total vena caval occlusion.

Of all the filters used, perhaps the most common is the Greenfield filter. It is a cone-shaped filter devised of stainless steel consisting of six legs with small recurved hooks at their distal ends for anchoring within the vessel wall. Approximately 4.5 cm in length, its cone shape tapers toward the proximal end. In reviews performed by the original designer, long-term patency rates are up to 98%, and recurrent embolism rates with its use are approximately 4%. The usual indications for filter placement are (1) documented deep venous thrombosis or pulmonary embolus with contraindication to anticoagulation therapy; (2) recurrent pulmonary embolism despite anticoagulation; (3) deep venous thrombosis without any evidence of acute pulmonary embolism in patients at unusually high risk of embolism or of severe morbidity should embolism occur, such as those with free-floating or poorly adherent thromboses, chronic pulmonary hypertension, or poor respiratory reserve; and (4) a complication of anticoagulation. The preferred approach for insertion of the vena caval filters is the internal jugular vein; and, of the two, the right is used in the majority of patients. In general, the femoral veins are avoided unless absolutely necessary because the potential for dislodging thrombus is much higher by using this site. The filters are usually placed under fluoroscopic guidance and are situated below the level of the renal veins. Indications for placing them above this level include patients who have had renal transplants, renal cell carcinoma with renal vein tumor extension, or infrarenal vena caval thrombosis.

The morbidity associated with the placement of most vena caval filters is minimal. Misplacement of the filters is one of the more common complications and is usually associated with attempted placement superiorly to the renal veins. In one of the larger studies of vena caval filters, one filter accidentally lodged in the right atrium but was removed and replaced in the suprarenal veins.[6] Some patients do experience lower-extremity edema; this is most likely associated with occlusion at the filter resulting in venous stasis. Up to 25% of patients receiving filters who are also treated with anticoagulants can have complications associated with bleeding. However, in one of the larger series reported,[5] no long-term wound complications were noted. In those 469 patients who were followed long term in this study, the incidence of death related to pulmonary embolism was only 3.6%. Almost one third of these deaths were within the first 24 hours after filter insertion and represented underlying preoperative medical problems rather than placement of the filter itself. Notably, however, the overall mortality in long-term follow-up of these patients was 133 out of 469 patients (28%). Of these deaths, 79% took place during the first year after filter insertion, and 27% occurred within the first 2 weeks after filter placement.

Overall, this reflects the effectiveness of the placement of these filters, particularly considering that the group of patients who receive them are at extremely high risk for recurrent embolic phenomena.

Prophylaxis of Venous Thrombosis

One of the most important factors in establishing treatment plans for patients with deep venous thrombosis is identifying those that are at high risk for this disease. Patients in whom venous stasis and subsequent thrombosis are likely include those undergoing surgery of duration greater than 30 minutes, prolonged immobility, pelvic or lower extremity trauma, right ventricular failure, and obesity.[7] Patients with a history of vascular injury or altered coagulability are also at high risk for deep venous thrombosis. Certainly, early ambulation in the postoperative period is a simple and extremely effective method of minimizing stasis, and in general otolaryngology patients have this luxury. However, some patients will require prophylaxis, and measures should be directed toward minimizing stasis and/or reducing the coagulability of blood. There are many methods available for addressing either of these treatment plans, and they are often used in various combinations to increase the effectiveness of prevention of deep venous thrombosis without increasing potential complications.

Mechanical Prophylaxis

Mechanical prophylaxis of deep venous thrombosis is usually directed at reducing venous stasis. The easiest and least cumbersome method in use is early postoperative ambulation, which also benefits wound healing as well as preventing pulmonary complications. However, there is some question as to whether or not this truly reduces the incidence of deep venous thrombosis.[8] Leg elevation is also recommended by some as a simple method of decreasing venous stasis.

Elastic Stockings

Elastic stockings placed on the lower extremity bilaterally function to decrease the volume in the venous system, therefore increasing the relative velocity for the venous blood. Stockings should be worn bilaterally before the operation and for at least 3 days postoperatively. These stockings are designed such that a graduated compressive force is placed on the lower extremity, with the greatest constriction at the foot and with decreased pressure exerted toward the trunk. Up to 60% reduction in deep venous thrombosis can be expected using compression stockings alone.[9] One advantage of the stockings is that they can be worn easily by patients who are not totally ambulatory but are able to move from bed to chair or bathroom.

Pneumatic Compression Hose

The next step in efforts to improve venous drainage is the use of intermittent pneumatic compression devices on the lower extremities. As with elastic stockings and other mechanical devices, these are used effectively in patients who have contraindications to the use of heparin or other anticoagulants, such as neurosurgical patients.

Evidence shows that pneumatic compression induces a local and systemic fibrinolysis in addition to increased venous drainage, both of which act to decrease the incidence of venous thrombosis. At least one study has demonstrated that clot lysis time decreases at a rate that is proportional to the volume of tissue that is compressed by the hose.[10] This has also been well demonstrated by the placement of compression devices on the upper extremities, where a beneficial effect on deep venous thrombosis was also noted.[11] Overall, the use of pneumatic compression devices decreases the rate of deep venous thrombosis by about 50%.[8]

It is not clear exactly when pneumatic compression devices should be applied or how long they need to be left on the patient to maximize effectiveness. Although there is some evidence to suggest that the use of pneumatic compression devices in the operating room and recovery room alone is effective, other evidence suggests that removing the pneumatic compression devices soon thereafter is associated with an increased incidence of late deep venous thrombosis.[12] Therefore, it seems at least 5 days' use of the pneumatic compression hose postoperatively is necessary in patients who are expected to be immobilized for long periods of time.[13]

The pneumatic compression hose can also be used in addition to compression stockings. The addition of compression stockings to patients who are using pneumatic devices adds little inconvenience, and it can further reduce the rate of deep venous thrombosis by up to 5%.[8]

Pharmacologic Prophylaxis

Many different agents have been tried for reducing the incidence of deep venous thrombosis. These include subcutaneous heparin, Dextran 70, aspirin, and dihydroergotamine. Antiplatelet drugs (in particular aspirin) were originally thought to be excellent pharmacological agents for the prevention of deep venous thrombosis. Because of its low cost, low incidence of side-effects, and easy administration, aspirin once appeared to be an excellent choice for prophylaxis. Unfortunately, in rigorous trials it did not appear to prevent deep venous thrombosis. Most of the early studies were discussed in the orthopedic literature, and although there was some decrease in the incidence of pulmonary embolism, there was no decrease in the incidence of deep venous thrombosis.[14]

Low-molecular-weight Dextran has also been used for prophylactic treatment of deep venous thrombosis. It is thought to have two methods of action: (1) decreasing stasis by functioning as a volume expander, and (2) acting as an antiplatelet substance. Because of this second effect, Dextran can be overdosed, resulting in increased bleeding times and subsequent postoperative complications. Because of its high cost, difficulty with administration, significant side-effect of bleeding, and difficulty in monitoring its effectiveness (PT or PTT times do not accurately indicate the relative effectiveness of its action), it is infrequently used for prophylaxis. Recently the National Institutes of Health made a list of recommended prophylaxis for deep venous thrombosis for various surgical patients. Of all categories of patients, the only one for which Dextran was recommended was orthopedic patients.[15]

Another interesting finding in orthopedic patients was that the use of epidural anesthesia prevented deep venous thrombosis when compared to general anesthesia used during surgery for total hip replacements.[16] In those patients receiving epidural anesthesia, the incidence of deep venous thrombosis was only 20% compared to 73% in patients receiving general anesthesia. Additionally, the incidence of pulmonary embolism was reduced from 47% to 13% in the same two groups of patients. Although this finding likely represents the cardiovascular effects of the various anesthetic agents, it speaks against the use of general anesthesia in patients at high risk for deep venous thrombosis who are to undergo procedures for which local anesthesia could be considered.

Heparin Therapy

For some time, low-dose heparin has functioned as the gold standard for prevention of deep venous thrombosis. Heparin acts by complexing with antithrombin III and then potentiates its inhibitory effect on the coagulation cascade. Its use has been subjected to several randomized trials in most surgical fields, and it has been scrutinized by many boards of health. Testing regimens (including various strengths and routes of administration of heparin) have been tried, and use of low-molecular-weight heparin versus standard heparin has been tested. In a recent review of the effects of subcutaneous heparin on pulmonary embolism and deep venous thrombosis, some orthopedic surgery trials were noted not to indicate a reduction in the incidence of deep venous thrombosis with the use of subcutaneous heparin. These studies were criticized for not being large enough to establish a true effect on the rate of deep venous thrombosis.[17] In those orthopedic studies that included radio-labeled fibrinogen for evaluation of pulmonary embolism and proximal thromboses, heparin was found to have a significant effect. There seems to be little difference in the effectiveness of subcutaneous heparin given every 8 hours versus every 12 hours, with reduction in odds of 42% and 49%, respectively. Similarly, little difference was found in incidences of bleeding. Heparin has been recommended by the National Institutes of Health for use as a prophylactic treatment of deep venous thrombosis in all surgical patients except neurosurgical, gynecologic, and obstetric patients. It is a safe, inexpensive, and easily administered form of prophylaxis.

Warfarin Therapy

Warfarin therapy has also been used as prophylaxis of deep venous thrombosis. Two regimens are generally used. The first involves giving 10 mg of warfarin sodium the night before the operation.[18] This is then followed by giving 5 mg the evening following surgery and thereafter 5 mg as a daily dose while checking the prothrombin time. The daily dose is then adjusted until the PT is elevated 1.12 to 1.2 times normal. If the warfarin cannot be given by mouth, it can be administered intramuscularly. The second method of warfarin treatment involves beginning warfarin therapy 10 to 14 days prior to surgery.[19] The warfarin is adjusted such that the PT ratio is in the 1.12 to 1.2 range at the time of surgery. Therapy is then continued until the patient is discharged home. Although these regimens have been shown to be effective in reducing the incidence of deep venous thromboses, they have significant disadvantages. Major postoperative bleeding has been reported in 5% to 10% of these patients.[19,20] Additionally, it is often difficult to achieve the target ratio range and maintain this level. Other complications associated with warfarin therapy include transient hypercoagulability and, although extremely rare, warfarin skin necrosis.

Combination Therapy

Although most of the mechanical and pharmacological methods of combating deep venous thrombosis are successful alone, they are not mutually exclusive. Combinations of treatment methods such as heparin plus stockings, stockings plus compression hose, and other combinations of pharmacological and mechanical treatments have been utilized and studied extensively in various surgical subspecialities. No specific recommendations have been made for otolaryngology patients because these patients are generally at low risk due to their early ambulation and lack of surgical manipulation to the lower extremities. The one exception to this is patients who are undergoing free fibular grafts, who are not allowed early ambulation, and who have had surgical manipulation of the veins of the lower extremity. Although there is no clear-cut answer to the best method of prophylaxis, these patients should probably be treated as high-risk orthopedic patients and receive the combination of Dextran and external compression devices which has shown to be better than Dextran alone.[21] Clearly it would be best not to put the external compression device over the fresh surgical wound.

Other otolaryngology patients still may warrant some method of prophylaxis. Based on a National Institutes of Health recommendation for low-risk general surgical patients, low-dose heparin (5000 units twice a day) should be given subcutaneously as a method of prophylaxis.[15]

PULMONARY EMBOLISM

Pulmonary embolism should not be considered a separate disease from deep venous thrombosis, but rather a resulting complication of it. Unfortunately, there is no typical physical or routine laboratory finding that can cinch the diagnosis of pulmonary embolism. Because of this, it is often difficult to decide which patients are experiencing pulmonary embolic phenomena. This is unfortunate because it is considered the most common preventable cause of death within the hospital and is responsible for at least 100,000 deaths every year in the United States alone.[22] As small deposits of platelets, red cells, and fibrin accumulate in the valve cusp pockets or some of the intramuscular sinuses of the leg veins, the precursors to deep venous thrombosis develop. Left untreated, approximately 20% of the distal venous thrombi will extend into the proximal venous system.[23] As these continue to propagate, they can reach the deep veins of the thigh and extend into the pelvis, where over 95% of pulmonary emboli will originate. Technically, other materials can be considered as sources for emboli, including air, fat, and tumor; however, only under unusual circumstances do these other embolic materials cause pulmonary emboli.

Clinical Features of Pulmonary Embolism

The initial presentation of patients with pulmonary emboli is extremely varied and is associated with an extensive differential diagnosis. In general, the onset of symptoms is acute, and perhaps the best documentation of symptoms was obtained during the urokinase and streptokinase pulmonary embolism trials. The most common symptoms upon presentation included dyspnea (84%), pleuritic chest pain (74%), cough (53%), hemoptysis (30%), and syncope (13%)[24] (Table 3–3). Patients with massive pulmonary emboli were more likely to exhibit these symptoms than patients with submassive pulmonary emboli. Certainly, pulmonary embolism can occur with none of these symptoms, which makes the diagnosis difficult. In massive pulmonary embolus, presentation may be that of cardiovascular collapse and hypotension, whereas small emboli may be associated with confusion, wheezing, and even unexplained arrythmias. Because such an obscure picture is presented, the diagnosis is often one that is considered with the understanding that over half of the patients initially suspected of having pulmonary embolism will eventually be cleared by testing.[25] The diagnosis is also difficult in that sometimes symptoms present over several hours, whereas other patients may exhibit no symptoms at all.[26]

Because of this rather nebulous presentation, attempts at diagnosis are often made using ancillary tests. Serum evaluation including bilirubin, lactic dehydrogenase (LDH), and serum glutamic oxaloacetic transaminase (SGOT) are evaluated by some, but these tests are insensitive and nonspecific. Similarly, blood gases are often obtained, but having a normal PO_2 does not necessarily exclude the diagnosis of pulmonary embolism. An electrocardiogram is often obtained in patients

Table 3–3. Incidence of Presenting Symptoms in 327 Patients with Massive or Submassive Pulmonary Embolism

SYMPTOM	% WITH SYMPTOM
Dyspnea	84%
Pleuritic chest pain	72%
Cough	53%
Hemoptysis	30%
Syncope	14%

Data from the streptokinase and urokinase pulmonary embolism trials.

and can be abnormal in up to 85% of patients with acute pulmonary embolism.[24] The classic S1, Q3, T3 pattern and right-axis shift is observed in only 10% of the patients, and QRS changes and ST segment changes are seen in roughly 50%. Prospectively, chest radiographs are nonspecific and are read as normal in 20% to 30% of patients presenting with pulmonary embolism, although on retrospective review many initially normal chest x-rays are seen to show subtle changes,[27,28] Perhaps the best use of the chest x-ray is for ruling out other causes of symptoms, such as pneumothorax or pneumonia. Up to 50% of patients that do have findings on a chest x-ray will demonstrate elevation of the hemidiaphragm. A parenchymal infiltrate is also seen in another half of these patients. Pleural effusions are seen in about a third of the patients with pulmonary embolism but may be seen more often if decubitous views are also obtained. Less than 1 in 20 patients will demonstrate the classic Hampton's hump—an infarction that takes the form of a pyramidal-shaped infiltrate with a peak toward the hilum. Westermark's sign, an increased radiolucency secondary to decreased vascular filling, is more often diagnosed retrospectively than at the time of the initial reading of the film.

With all this in mind, the diagnosis of pulmonary embolism often cannot be established definitively based on information received from patient history, physical exam, or routine laboratory investigation alone. It is because of this that the lung scan and angiography have become such important tools for the evaluation of pulmonary embolism.

Lung Scanning

VENTILATION SCANS

Perhaps the best prospective evaluation of ventilation-perfusion scans that has been performed is the Prospective Investigation of Pulmonary Embolism Diagnosis (PIOPED) study. As a result of this study, several conclusions can be drawn. A normal or near-normal ventilation-perfusion scan makes a pulmonary embolism highly unlikely. Similarly, a low probability shown by a ventilation-perfusion scan along with a low clinical suspicion for the disease makes pulmonary embolism highly unlikely. When a patient exhibits a high probability from ventilation-perfusion scan and clinical suspicion is extremely high, pulmonary embolism is probable. In all other cases, such as with indeterminate or intermediate lung scans, a ventilation-perfusion scan is of no diagnostic value. It is still recommended as an initial step in the evaluation of patients because it is noninvasive and has minimal complications. For those patients in whom the diagnosis has been neither strongly confirmed nor rejected, pulmonary angiography is the next step.

PERFUSION SCANS

Perfusion scanning was introduced in the early 1960s.[29] The basic principle of perfusion scanning is that microaggregates of albumin or albumin microspheres labeled with technetium-99m (99mtc) which have been injected into the patient traverse the vascular system and are trapped as microemboli in the pulmonary capillary bed. The distribution, based on the presence or absence of blood flow in an area of the lung, will demonstrate areas of perfusion defects upon scanning. It is important to realize, however, that an area of decreased vascularity does not necessarily represent an area of pulmonary embolism. Conditions such as obstructive airway disease, pneumonia, and pleural effusions will result in perfusion defects due to shunting phenomena. The original scans involved anterior-posterior projections only and therefore were highly nonspecific. In the 1970s, multiple images were obtained using a gamma camera. The resulting six- or eight-view lung scans significantly increased specificity and have subsequently become the standard study. The use of single-photon emission computed tomography (SPECT) has introduced the technology of computer tomography with the use of a rotating gamma camera.[30,31] With this, three-dimensional views can be obtained of perfusion defects, and it is thought that this may help decrease the incidence of indeterminate lung scans. Although not in common clinical use today, they may eventually become the standard of care.

To improve further the specificity of perfusion scans, they are done in concert with ventilation scans. Areas of hypoventilation could then be seen and compared to areas of decreased perfusion. The most common technique involves the use of xenon 133 (133 Xe). Initial images are obtained as the patient begins inhaling 133 Xe and every 30 seconds for several minutes as the patient breathes the xenon, allowing for alveolar equilibration. Areas of hypoventilation secondary to obstructive lung disease are decreased in this manner. Once this has been done, results of the ventilation scan are compared to those of the perfusion scan. The most common cause of an abnormal ventilation scan is chronic obstructive pulmonary disease.

Many different approaches to performing ventilation-perfusion scans are taken. Some institutions prefer doing the perfusion scan first, and if it is normal, no further evaluations are performed. When it is abnormal, a ventilation scan is then performed. Other institutions prefer starting with the ventilation scan as the radio-labeled albumin used in a perfusion scan remains in the patient for a relatively long period of time and blurs the picture in the ventilation scan.

The main problem with the ventilation-perfusion scan is the number of indeterminate tests obtained as well as difficulty in actually interpreting the test. Radiologists are becoming more accustomed to reading these scans, and it seems that agreement on interpretation is becoming more frequent, as the recent PIOPED study has shown.[32] A high-probability scan is based on findings of one or more segmental perfusion defects with no corresponding ventilation or chest radiographic abnormalities (the so-called V/Q mismatch). When clinical suspicion is high, no further evaluation may be necessary. Angiography will confirm pulmonary emboli in approximately 95% of these patients.

One of the main limitations of the use of xenon 133 in ventilation scans is that images are only obtained in one projection. This can make comparison difficult, particularly to the

multiple images obtained in perfusion scans. When the perfusion scans are done first, background shadowing from the radio-labeled aggregates within the pulmonary vasculature presents problems. Other agents have been used to try to overcome these limitations. Some have recommended xenon 127 because of its higher photon energies. Unfortunately, xenon 127 is much more expensive than xenon 133, is harder to shield, and is not as easily available. To overcome the limitations of a single view, a radio-labeled aerosol of diethylamine trianamine pentaacetic acid (99mTc-DTPA) has been used. This rapidly deposits uniformly in the lung periphery, and multiple images can then be obtained to compare to the same projections of perfusion scans. Although not widely used at present, it may become more common in the future because of these benefits.

Ventilation-perfusion scans have become one of the key diagnostic tests in evaluation of patients with suspected pulmonary embolism. They must always be interpreted in the light of the overall clinical situation. Highly suspicious scans may be all the diagnostic workup that is necessary in the proper clinical situation. Indeterminate scans are of little value, and further diagnostic testing may be indicated.

Pulmonary Angiography

Pulmonary angiography has long been recognized as the gold standard for the diagnosis of pulmonary embolism. As with any angiography, patients who have an allergy to contrast material should proceed with caution but can usually be evaluated safely with some of the newer contrast agents. Other relative contraindications include right ventricular end diastolic pressure greater than 20 mm of mercury and amiodarone-induced pulmonary toxicity.[33,34] The use of some of the newer contrast agents with low osmolarity has greatly increased the safety of pulmonary angiography. It also appears that some of these low-osmolarity contrast agents increase the comfort of the patient by decreasing some of the burning and heat sensation patients experience, as well as the urge to cough. These advantages have also helped the quality of studies because use of these agents has led to less patient movement and therefore fewer blurred images.[35,36] The quoted morbidity and mortality rate using these newer agents is less than 1%. In the PIOPED study, angiography was felt to contribute to the cause of death in two patients (0.3%), both of whom had multiple underlying, serious medical problems. The procedure itself involves percutaneous cannulation of the right femoral vein and the placement of a sheath through which catheters can be inserted. In general, right atrial, right ventricular, and pulmonary artery pressures are recorded prior to the arteriography. This is done as the catheter is advanced through the right atrium, into the right ventricle, and then out through the pulmonary artery. Usually the right side is evaluated first because this is the direction the catheter normally progresses on its own. Contrast agents are then injected into the main pulmonary arteries (left or right) to obtain the initial views. Following this initial view, if any area is particularly suspicious, more selective angiography can be performed to evaluate subsections of the pulmonary vasculature.

Because many patients undergoing pulmonary angiography are also strongly suspected of having deep venous thrombosis, it may be helpful to choose a vessel other than the femoral veins for placement of the catheter because these may be involved with clot, and introduction of the catheter could cause displacement of the clot and subsequent pulmonary emboli. Many use a brachial vein instead of a femoral vein, but this technique is much more difficult because of the smaller size of the vessel and the difficulty of threading the catheter through more difficult angles. Another complication that has fortunately become much less frequent is accidental perforation of the right heart and pulmonary arteries, previously due to the use of stiff catheters. Most catheters used today are much more pliable, and the risk of this complication has decreased dramatically. Cardiac tamponade is now rarely seen.[37]

The goals of angiography are to identify either the presence of a filling defect, which may represent a clot in situ, or the presence of vascular cutoff, indicating the abrupt cutoff of blood flow by clot to a portion of the lungs. Any of these situations found during angiography is considered positive for pulmonary embolism, and treatment is therefore initiated.

Other Imaging Techniques

An ideal diagnostic test for demonstrating pulmonary embolism would be minimally invasive, thrombus specific, and cause minimal discomfort to the patient. There are two such methods presently under investigation. One involves using antiplatelet antibodies radio labeled with technetium-99, and the other involves antifibrin antibodies. Both have been used for the detection of deep venous thrombosis, but their use has not yet been particularly convincing. They may eventually provide a much more accurate and less invasive test for evaluation of pulmonary embolism.[38]

TREATMENT OF ACUTE PULMONARY EMBOLISM

Anticoagulation

In general, treatment regimens for anticoagulation in patients with pulmonary emboli are the same as for deep venous thrombosis in the legs. This seems to be a rational approach because the vast majority of pulmonary emboli originate from deep venous thrombosis within the leg veins, and the use of anticoagulation will prevent the propagation of the clot within the pulmonary vascular system as well as further propagation of the clots within the veins of the legs or upper extremities. The American College of Chest Physicians and the National Heart, Lung, and Blood Institute (NHLBI) posted a consensus report on treatment of thromboembolism with antithrombotic therapy.[39] The recommendations included a bolus of 5000 to 10,000 units of heparin followed by an infusion rate of 1000 units per hour. The activated partial thromboplastin time is then monitored every 4 to 6 hours and the heparin infusion rate is adjusted to obtain an activated partial thromboplastin time of 1.5 to 2 times the control value. Coumadin therapy is recommended to be started on day 2 or 3 of heparin therapy. Part of the goal is to overlap the heparin therapy and the Coumadin therapy when Coumadin can cause a transient hypercoagulable state. For this reason the heparin is usually continued for approximately 7 to 10 days with an overlap of about 1 week. Coumadin doses begin at 10 mg, and daily maintenance doses are normally between 5 and 10 mg with a goal prothrombin time of 1.2 to 1.5 times the control value. Assuming there are no continuing risk factors for recurrence of thromboembolic phenomena, Coumadin is recommended for at least 3 months of therapy and perhaps indefinitely in patients that are high risk for deep venous thrombosis and subsequent pulmonary embolism.

Some controversy exists as to what are appropriate loading doses and modes of heparin and warfarin administration. Some believe initial intravenous boluses of heparin should be as high as 20,000 units.[40] In the past, warfarin dosages were recommended to be adjusted to 2 to 2.5 times control values for the prothrombin time. In the early 1980s, studies demonstrated convincingly that low doses of Coumadin could prevent venous thromboembolism at an equivalent rate while giving a much lower rate of bleeding complications.[41] Based on this decreased incidence of complications, the figure of 1.2 to 1.5 times the control value is recommended. Another confusing bit of terminology is the INR, or international normalized ratio, used at some institutions for following prothrombin times. A goal in this system is a ratio of 2.0 to 3.0. This number is often confused with the standard PT ratio of 1.2 to 1.5 times hospital laboratory control values.

Unfortunately, with treatment using pharmacological anticoagulation alone, recurrence rates are high. In the early phases of the urokinase pulmonary embolism trial (UPET), 23% of patients treated with heparin developed recurrent pulmonary emboli.[42] Other studies have shown the somewhat lower yet still significant recurrence rates of 17% and 18%.[43,44] Although the high rate of recurrence is not fully understood, it is believed to be secondary to the failure of lysis of the thrombus within the deep veins and subsequent recurrent embolic phenomena originating from the untreated deep venous thrombosis. Additionally, the pulmonary embolus itself may not completely resolve, with some studies showing incomplete resolution in as many as 50% of patients after 4 months of follow-up.[45] Because of this relatively high rate of failure with anticoagulant treatment, other methods of treatment have been sought. Most recently, thrombolytic therapy has become a highly investigated and successful method of managing thromboembolic phenomena.

Thrombolysis

Many patients in the hospital probably undergo small subclinical thromboembolic processes that are never detected by the physician and do not lead to any notable complications. However, in patients with previous histories of cardiopulmonary disease or in cases where the embolus is large enough to be symptomatic, urgent treatment is essential. Pulmonary artery obstruction leads to increased right ventricular afterload when the pulmonary vascular bed is obstructed by 25% or more. There is a compensatory increase in right ventricular and pulmonary artery pressures. As this right ventricular afterload continues to increase, the ventricular chamber becomes dilated and contracts much less efficiently, leading to right ventricular failure and eventually cardiovascular collapse. If the patient already has underlying pulmonary disease, much smaller pulmonary emboli can lead to significant hemodynamic effects. In addition to the direct cardiac effects, emboli cause release of certain humoral factors that can lead to both vasoconstriction and bronchospasm. Serotonin, a potent neural and smooth muscle agonist, is released. This is stored in platelets and can function to mediate bronchospasm in small airways. Thromboxane A_2 is also released and functions as a potent vasoconstrictor and bronchoconstrictor. Because of these reactions, an increased amount of dead space may form within the lung, further decreasing the efficiency of ventilation.

As opposed to anticoagulant therapy, thrombolytics function to dissolve the emboli quickly and therefore return the pulmonary vasculature to normal physiological parameters more quickly. This allows for the return of normal right ventricular function and subsequently helps eliminate any potential for right ventricular failure. Additionally, by lysing the thrombus the vasoactive and bronchoactive substances have less of a chance to function due to their decreased presence. At this time, at least three thrombolytic agents have been used to treat pulmonary emboli: streptokinase, urokinase, and recombinant human tissue-type plasminogen activator (rt-PA). Urokinase has been used the longest and has become the standard agent against which newer clot-dissolving agents are compared. Urokinase converts plasminogen directly to plasmin by cleaving the former. Streptokinase is a protein derived from streptococcus haemolyticus and functions by combining with plasminogen to form a streptokinase-plasminogen activator complex; this complex then converts other plasminogen molecules to plasmin. Streptokinase's main advantage over other treatment methods is that it is much less expensive. However, it often causes more significant side-effects, including nausea, fever, chills, and general malaise. Recombinant human tissue-type plasminogen activator is a product of recombinant technology that functions to activate plasminogen directly to form plasmin. All have been tried in multiple trials and have their own advantages and disadvantages. In general, the primary advantages of any type of thrombolytic therapy include (1) accelerated clot lysis, (2) accelerated pulmonary tissue reperfusion, and (3) improved pulmonary capillary blood volume. The initial reports by the UPET study showed that when urokinase was used and followed by anticoagulation, the percentage of patients who died of disease or had recurrent disease was much less. It should be cautioned that these differences were not statistically significant, but this was thought to be due to the size of the study group. Some of the patients were followed for as long as 7 years after their initial pulmonary embolism. Those patients who received combined therapy with both thrombolytic and anticoagulant agents demonstrated a higher pulmonary capillary blood volume and preservation of the normal pulmonary vascular responses to exercise.[46] Some also feel that patients who have massive pulmonary emboli and continue to have a large clot burden can develop chronic pulmonary hypertension, and by treatment with thrombolytic agents, this devastating complication can be prevented.

Contraindications to the use of thrombolytic agents are similar to those for the use of anticoagulants. These include intracranial and intraspinal disease, recent cranial surgery or head trauma, history of hemorrhage or stroke, and active or recent internal bleeding. Relative contraindications include a history of major surgery or trauma, nonhemorrhagic stroke, uncontrolled severe hypertension, a recent biopsy or invasive procedure in an area inaccessible to external compression, and severe coagulation defects.

Treatment regimens vary from institution to institution. FDA-approved regimens for pulmonary embolism include initial loading doses followed by continuous infusions. For streptokinase, 250,000 international units are given as a loading dose over 30 minutes followed by 100,000 units per hour for the next 24 hours. Urokinase is dosed as 2000 international units per pound as a loading dose given over 10 minutes followed by an infusion of 2000 international units per pound per hour for 12 to 24 hours. Rt-PA is given as a 100-mg continuous peripheral intravenous infusion over 2 hours. Out of these three regimens, the rt-PA regimen appears to have the most rapid onset of action and the best safety profile, probably due to its short period of treatment. It also presents fewer side-effects (fever, chills, and flushing that are so typical of streptokinase). One of the key differences between these regimens and those for myocardial infarction is that heparin therapy is not given concomitantly with the thrombolytic agent. Because all three regimens involve fixed dosages, there is no need to perform laboratory tests during the infusions; nor are dose adjustments necessary. At the conclusion of infusion, a PTT should be obtained, and as long as the value is not more than twice the upper limit of normal, heparin therapy can be restarted and continued without necessitating a loading dose. If it is greater than two times the normal value, it should be rechecked in approximately 4 hours and repeated every 4 hours until the level declines into the acceptable range.

Endovascular Treatment for Pulmonary Embolism

In cases of massive pulmonary embolism, up to 50% of patients will die within 30 minutes and 85% will die within 6 hours.[47] In such urgent situations, patients may not survive long enough to benefit from thrombolytic therapy. In such cases, open embolectomy on cardiopulmonary bypass has been considered traditionally as one of the only chances for survival. Overall survival rates are about 58% and seem to be better when cardiopulmonary bypass is utilized. Notably, the logistics for treatment of patients via open embolectomy are formidable. Such treatment involves the ability to access open-heart facilities quickly, a swift transfer of patients from an angiography suite to the operating room, and rapid diagnosis of the problem. Patients at small hospitals have little chance of survival due to the time required for transfer.

Because of these difficulties, attempts were made to devise a method for transvenous embolectomy. In the late 1960s, a technique was described using a steerable catheter with a radio-opaque suction cup at its tip. Using either the internal jugular vein or the femoral vein, the device is inserted into the vena cava, through the right heart, and into the pulmonary vasculature. Under fluoroscopic viewing, the catheter is advanced. Pulmonary artery pressures are measured prior to the removal of any clot and are used as a basis for comparison after extraction of any emboli. With the catheter in place, small amounts of contrast agents can be injected to delineate the location of the embolus. The small suction cup at the end of the device is placed up against the clot, and at a distal port a syringe is aspirated to apply a vacuum against the clot. Quick return of blood implies that the cup has not been seated adequately against the clot, and it is replaced until suction is obtained. The embolus is then removed through the vein while continuous negative pressure is placed on the syringe.

One of the interesting aspects of this method of treatment is that success is not necessarily measured by the amount of clot removed or by the absolute clearing of the clot from within the vasculature but is determined by the return toward normal physiological parameters, such as pulmonary artery pressure and cardiac output as measured through the catheter itself. As soon as the patient is adequately volume resuscitated, a mean pulmonary artery pressure of 20 mm mercury or less is often used as an endpoint. Another advantage of this technique is that at the endpoint of this procedure, a Greenfield filter or other filter device can easily be placed below the renal veins in the inferior vena cava if so desired.

Initial results of this procedure have been promising. In an original series of 32 patients treated by this method, 78% survived. Seven deaths were attributed to cardiopulmonary arrest related to the contrast injection, four to myocardial infarction thought secondary to the hypotension experienced prior to catheterization, and one to rupture of a vessel by a Swan-Ganz catheter. These results compare favorably to those of open embolectomy. Additionally, this technique is easily set up and does not require moving the patient from the radiological suite to the operating room, as does open embolectomy.

Vena Caval Filter

Vena caval filters are not actually used for the acute treatment of pulmonary embolism but are used in prophylactic treatment for recurrent pulmonary embolism. (See the preceding discussions of prophylaxis and treatment of deep venous thrombosis for information about these filters.)

CONCLUSION

Deep venous thrombosis and pulmonary embolism are among the most common significant postoperative complications with which the surgeon is likely to deal. A thorough knowledge of the pathophysiology, diagnosis, and treatment of these disorders can go a long way toward alleviating unecessary morbidity and mortality.

REFERENCES

1. Dosick SM, Blakemore WS. The role of Doppler ultrasound in acute deep vein thrombosis. *Am J Surg.* 1978;136f:265–268.
2. Langsfeld M, Hershey FB, Thorpe L, et al. Duplex B-mode imaging for the diagnosis of deep venous thrombosis. *Arch Surg.* 1987;122:587–591.
3. Hyers, TM, Hull RD, Weg JG. Antithrombotic therapy for venous thromboembolic disease. *Chest.* 1989;95(suppl 2): 37s–51s.
4. Hull RD, Raskob GE, Hirsh J, et al. Continuous intravenous heparin compared with intermittent subcutaneous heparin in the initial treatment of proximal-vein thrombosis. *N Engl J Med.* 1986;315:1109–1114.
5. Ansell JE, Price JM, Shah S, et al. Heparin-induced thrombocytopenia: What is its real frequency? *Chest.* 1985;88:878–882.
6. Greenfield LJ, Wakefield TW. Prevention of venous thrombosis and pulmonary embolism. *Adv Surg.* 1989;22:301–324.
7. Marshall JC. Prophylaxis of deep venous thrombosis and pulmonary embolism. *Can J Surg.* 1991;34:551–554.
8. Flanc C, Kakkar VV, Clarke MB. Postoperative deep vein thrombosis: Effect of intensive prophylaxis. *Lancet.* 1969; 1:477–478.
9. Colditz GA, Tuden RL, Oster G. Rates of venous thrombosis after general surgery: Combined results of randomized clinical trials. *Lancet.* 1986;2:143–146.
10. Tarnay TJ, Rohr PR, Davidson AG, et al. Pneumatic calf compression, fibrinolysis and the prevention of deep venous thrombosis. *Surgery.* 1980;88:489–496.
11. Knight MTN, Dawson R. Effect of intermittent compression of the arms on deep venous thrombosis in the legs. *Lancet.* 1976; 2:1265–1268.
12. Salzman EW, Ploetz J, Bettmann M, et al. Intraoperative external pneumatic calf compression to afford long-term prophylaxis against deep vein thrombosis in urological patients. *Surgery.* 1980;87:239–242.
13. Butson ARC. Intermittent pneumatic calf compression for prevention of deep venous thrombosis in general abdominal surgery. *Am J Surg.* 1981;142:525–527.
14. Guyer RD, Broth RR, Rothman RH. The detection and prevention of pulmonary embolism in total hip replacement. *J Bone Joint Surg.* 1982;64A:1040–1044.
15. Prevention of venous thrombosis and pulmonary embolism. Consensus Conference NIH. *JAMA.* 1986;256:744–749.
16. Modig J. Thromboembolism and blood loss: Continuous epidural block versus general anaesthesia and controlled ventilation. *Reg Anaesth.* 1982;7:584–588.
17. Collins R, Scrimgeour A, Yusuf S, et al. Reduction in fatal pulmonary embolism and venous thrombosis by perioperative administration of subcutaneous heparin. *NEJM.* 1988;1162–1173.
18. Harris WH, Salzman EW, Athanasoulis C. Comparison of warfarin, low molecular weight dextran, aspirin, and subcutaneous heparin in prevention of venous thromboembolism following total hip replacement. *J Bone Joint Surg.* 1974;56:1552–1562.
19. Francis C, Marder V, Evart C, et al. Two-step warfarin therapy: Prevention of postoperative venous thrombosis without excessive bleeding. *JAMA.* 1983;249:374–378.
20. Kelton JG, Hirsh J. Bleeding associated with antithrombotic therapy. *Semin Hematol.* 1980;17:259–291.

21. Reilly DT. Prophylactic methods against thromboembolism. *Acta Chir Scand Suppl.* 1988;550:115–118.

22. Raskob GE, Hull RD. Diagnosis and management of pulmonary thromboembolism. *Q J Med.* 1990;76:787–797.

23. Kakkar VV, Flanc C, Howe CT, et al. Natural history of post-operative deep-vein thrombosis. *Lancet.* 1969;2:230 233.

24. Bell WR, Simon TL, DeMets DL. The clinical features of sub-massive and massive pulmonary emboli. Am J Med. 1977; 62:355–360.

25. Hull RD, Hirsh J, Carter CJ, et al. Diagnostic value of ventilation-perfusion lung scanning in patients with suspected pulmonary embolism. *Chest.* 1985;88:819–828.

26. Palevsky HI. The problems of the clinical and laboratory diagnosis of pulmonary embolism. *Seminars Nucl Med.* 1991;21: 276–280.

27. Simon M. Plain film and angiographic aspects of pulmonary embolism. In: Moser KM, Stein M, eds. *Pulmonary Embolism.* Chicago: Year Book Medical Publishers; 1973.

28. Talbot S, Worthington BS, Roebuck EJ. Radiographic signs of pulmonary embolism and pulmonary infarction. *Thorax.* 1973; 28:198.

29. Alderson PO, Martin EC. Pulmonary embolism: Diagnosis with multiple imaging modalities. *Radiology.* 1987;164:297–312.

30. Osborne DR, Jaszczak RJ, Greer K, et al. Detection of pulmonary emboli in dogs: Comparison of single photon emission computed tomography, gamma camera imaging and angiography. *Radiology.* 1983;146:493–497.

31. Donaldson RM, Kahn O, Raphael MJ, et al. Emission tomography in embolic lung disease: Angiographic correlations. *Clin Radiol.* 1982;33:389–393.

32. The PIOPED investigators: Value of the ventilation/perfusion scan in acute pulmonary embolism: Results of the prospective investigation of pulmonary embolism diagnosis (PIOPED). *JAMA.* 1990;263:2753–2759.

33. Perlmutt LM, Braun SD, Newman GE, et al. Pulmonary arteriography in the high-risk patient. *Radiology.* 1987;162:187–189.

34. Wood DL, Osborn MJ, Rooke J, et al. Amiodarone pulmonary toxicity: Report of two cases associated with rapidly progressive fatal adult respiratory distress syndrome after pulmonary angiography. *Mayo Clin Proc.* 1985;60:601–603.

35. Fischer HW, Spataro RF, Rosenberg PM. Medical and economic considerations in using a new contrast medium. *Arch Intern Med* 1986;146:1717–1721.

36. Grainger RG. The clinical and financial implications of low-osmolar radiological contrast media [letter]. *Clin Radiol.* 1984; 35:251–252.

37. Goldhaber SZ. Recent advances in the diagnosis and lytic therapy of pulmonary embolism. *Chest.* 1991;99 (suppl 4): 173s–179s.

38. Oster ZH, Som P. Of monoclonal antibodies and thrombus-specific imaging. *J Nucl Med.* 1990;31:1055–1058.

39. Hyers TM, Hull RD, Weg JG. Consensus conference: Anti-thrombotic therapy for venous thromboembolic disease. *Chest.* 1986;89 (suppl 2):26s–35s.

40. Moser K. Venous thromboembolism. *Am Rev Respir Dis.* 1990; 141:235–249.

41. Hull R, Hirsh J, Jay R, et al. Different intensities of anticoagulation in the long term treatment of proximal venous thrombosis. *NEJM.* 1982;307:1676–1681.

42. The Urokinase Pulmonary Embolism Trial: A national cooperative study. *Circulation.* 1973;47(suppl 2):1–108.

43. Wheeler AP, Jaquiss RDB, Newman JH. Physician practices in the treatment of pulmonary embolism and deep venous thrombosis. *Arch Intern Med.* 1988;148:1321–1325.

44. Monreal M, Ruiz J, Salvador R, et al. Recurrent pulmonary embolism. A Prospective study. *Chest.* 1989;95:976–979.

45. Tow DE, Wagner HN. Recovery of pulmonary arterial blood flow in patients with pulmonary embolism. *NEJM.* 1967;276: 1053–1059.

46. Sharma GVRK, Folland ED, McIntyre KM, et al. Long term hemodynamic benefit of thrombolytic therapy in pulmonary embolic disease. *J Am Coll Cardiol.* 1990;15:65A.

47. Greenfield LJ, DeLucia A. Endovascular therapy of venous thromboembolic disease. *Surg Clin N Am.* 1992;72:969–989.

4 Postoperative Fever

C. Gaelyn Garrett, M.D., Mark C. Weissler, M.D.

PATHOPHYSIOLOGY OF FEVER

Regulation of Body Temperature

Body temperature is regulated by the thermoregulatory control center in the preoptic nucleus of the anterior hypothalamus, which maintains the thermal setpoint. This setpoint allows for circadian rhythmicity, with temperatures rising from average predawn values of 97.0°F (36.1°C) or lower to 99.5°F (37.5°C) or higher in the afternoon. This diurnal variation, relatively constant in timing and magnitude for each person, must be taken into consideration when evaluating temperature elevations in patients. Fever will be superimposed on the diurnal flux and, therefore, will be highest in the afternoon or early evening. For this reason, a patient cannot be considered afebrile until he or she has been monitored for 24 hours. Within the range of the circadian rhythm, core body temperature (temperature of blood perfusing the internal organs) is determined by the difference between heat production and heat loss. Approximately 2400 kcal of heat is produced per day, with the metabolic activity of the heart and liver accounting for much of it. Skeletal muscle metabolic activity also contributes during periods of exercise and shivering. Heat is dissipated mainly at the body's surfaces. Loss from the skin via radiation and evaporation accounts for the most, followed by loss from the lungs. Convection and conduction are less important mechanisms of heat loss in the normal state.[1]

Abnormal temperature elevations may occur via two mechanisms: (1) disruption of hypothalamic function, and (2) resetting of the hypothalamic setpoint. The first mechanism results in hyperthermia and the second, fever. The differentiation is important clinically because the treatment approach is different. Hyperthermia is best managed by physical cooling mechanisms such as cooling blankets, whereas fever is best managed by antipyretics such as aspirin and acetaminophen, which lower the thermal setpoint.

Temperature elevation in a surgical patient usually results from a resetting of the thermal setpoint, commonly by release of endogenous pyrogen. Prior to the late 1940s, fever was thought to be a result of exogenous pyrogens released by bacteria. With the work of Dr Paul Beeson in 1948 came the discovery that fever is caused by a product of host inflammatory cells.[2,3] This endogenous pyrogen is released by mononuclear phagocytes and is identical to two other previously identified immunologic mediators. These three substances—lymphocyte-activating factor, leukocyte endogenous mediator, and endogenous pyrogen—are now known commonly as interleukin-1, which is the central mediator of both fever and of the acute-phase host response to infection and inflammation.[4,5]

Release of interleukin-1 (IL-1) by mononuclear phagocytes can be stimulated by a variety of mechanisms, including bacterial endotoxin, exposure to microorganisms, phagocytosis, immune complex formation, and tissue injury. Once released, IL-1 acts directly on the central nervous system and hypothalamus via induction of phospholipases and the release of arachidonic acids from membrane phospholipids. This, in turn, results in increased levels of prostaglandins, especially prostaglandin E. These products of arachidonic acid synthesis most likely modulate the hypothalamic thermoregulatory mechanism, resulting in an increase in the setpoint to fever levels.[1,4] The newly adjusted setpoint results in signals being sent to the posterior hypothalamus to increase heat production and decrease heat loss. Clinically, this is evidenced by cutaneous vasoconstriction and cessation of sweating to decrease heat dissipation. Heat production is increased by muscle contractions, resulting in shivering (Fig. 4–1). Antipyretics such as aspirin reduce fever by inhibiting the synthesis of prostaglandin from achidonic acid.

Consequences of Fever

Fever is a common response to infection in a variety of species. There has been speculation that fever has beneficial effects on the host immune system and indeed, in certain species, this has been shown to be the case. In humans, however, no direct evidence exists to confirm this. Fever itself can have deleterious effects, mostly in the very young and the very old. Febrile seizures can occur in children usually under the age of 6 years. In the elderly with preexisting cardiac or pulmonary disease, fever may cause serious cardiovascular sequelae such as arrhythmias, hypotension, congestive heart failure, or myocardial ischemia. The increased

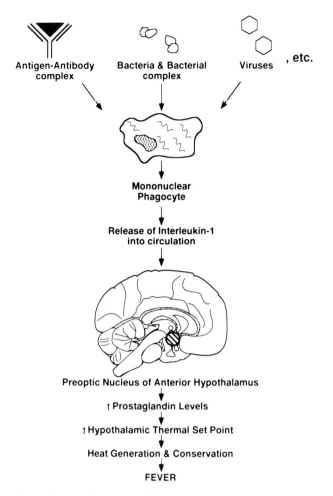

Figure 4–1. Pathogenesis of fever.

demand on the heart is a result of the increased tissue demand for oxygen. Oxygen consumption will increase 7% for each 1°F rise in body temperature. Despite these effects, fever is usually well tolerated in most otherwise healthy patients.

EVALUATION OF POSTOPERATIVE FEVER

The initial question that must be addressed is what constitutes a fever. The most frequently quoted normal human body temperature is 98.6°F (37.0°C). However, temperatures measured above this value do not always signify the presence of fever. As stated previously, there is a diurnal variation of temperature with normal peak values of 99.5°F (37.5°C) and higher in the late afternoon or early evening. The other factor to be considered is how the temperature was taken. Rectal temperatures are about 1 degree higher and axillary temperatures are about 1 degree lower than oral temperatures. Has the patient recently drunk any hot or cold liquids that may affect oral temperatures? On most surgical wards, an oral temperature ≥ 101.3°F (38.5°C) constitutes a fever and deserves a fever evaluation.

Most medical students and surgical interns are taught the most common causes of postoperative fever by thinking of the "six W's" wind, water, wound, walking, wonder drugs,

and woman. *Wind* refers to atelectasis. *Water* refers to urinary tract infection. *Wound* refers to wound infection. *Walking* refers to phlebitis or deep venous thrombosis. *Wonder drugs* refers to febrile reactions to medications. *Woman* refers to endometritis or mastitis. Obviously, this latter cause is common only in postpartum patients and therefore not applicable in head and neck surgery patients. These, of course, are not the only causes of postoperative fever, but they do serve to direct the evaluation.

It is a common practice to evaluate the febrile patient by ordering a battery of tests following the history and physical examination. Usual tests include a complete blood count with differential (CBC), chest radiograph, urinalysis, and pancultures of the urine, sputum, blood, and drainage fluid. One 1983 study examined the cost effectiveness and clinical usefulness of the fever workup in 71 patients who developed a fever following abdominal surgery. Of these 71 patients, 27% had culture-proven infections of some type. For 74% of the patients with infection, the correct diagnosis was made based on the clinical findings and a single confirmatory test. This study concluded that a shotgun approach to determine the source of fever was unnecessary and resulted in excess hospital costs.[6] Appropriate fever evaluation should be aimed at those causes related to the specific procedure and at the most common causes occurring at that specific time in the postoperative period. Any evaluation should begin with a careful history and physical examination, with special attention to specific areas as dictated by the individual circumstance. For example, a patient with a Foley bladder catheter who develops a fever should have a workup to rule out urinary tract infection as a cause. Laboratory tests are used to confirm or deny the most likely causes as determined by the history and physical examination.

This chapter outlines the most common causes of postoperative fever. Also included are some causes related specifically to otolaryngologic/head and neck surgery. It has been subdivided into four time periods relating to the surgery: (1) intraoperative and immediately postoperative, (2) postoperative days 0 to 2, (3) postoperative days 2 to 4, and (4) postoperative days 5 to 10. A fever developing during these periods can be more efficiently evaluated by knowing the most common etiologies of each period. It is hoped that this approach will avoid the expensive shotgun evaluation seen too commonly.

FEVER DURING SURGERY OR IMMEDIATELY POSTOPERATIVE

Malignant Hyperthermia

Malignant hyperthermia (MH) is a potentially fatal syndrome characterized by a generalized hypermetabolic state that occurs in susceptible patients when given a potent inhalational anesthetic drug in combination with a depolarizing muscle relaxant. The physiological defect involves intracellular modulation of calcium in the sarcoplasmic reticulum of skeletal muscle. Symptoms are variable, but any increase in body temperature while in the operating room should alert the anesthesiologist to the possibility of an MH crisis because anesthetics and surgical exposure generally produce hypothermia. It should be cautioned that hyperthermia is not always the presenting symptom and may occur late in the crisis. Therefore, temperatures should be monitored closely during the ensuing hours in an intensive care setting.

Prompt recognition of the syndrome with early intervention is essential to prevent serious morbidity. The diagnosis of MH is usually first suspected in the operating room, with hypercarbia occurring early in the course. The anesthesiologist should aggressively evaluate for the cause of any elevation in end-tidal CO_2. Arterial blood gas samples may also reveal significant hypoxia and acidosis. Serum samples should be sent for electrolytes to identify possible hyperkalemia and hypermagnesemia, myoglobin, lactates, creatinine phosphokinase (CPK), and aldolase. Urine should be checked for myoglobin as well. This syndrome, including appropriate treatment and preventative measures, is discussed in greater detail in Chapter 23 ("Complications of Anesthesia).

Blood Transfusion

Blood tranfusions are relatively rare during most general otolaryngology procedures. Patients undergoing major head and neck operations, however, are at greater risk for needing an intraoperative blood transfusion. Febrile reactions to blood tranfusions usually occur within 4 hours after the transfusion is started and may last up to 36 hours. These reactions are not due to red cell incompatibility but are a result of immune reactions between recipient antibodies and donor leukocytes and platelets. The human lymphocyte antigen (HLA) may be involved. These reactions may be avoided by using leukocyte-poor packed red cells and HLA-compatible platelets if available. Treatment of the febrile reaction is to stop the transfusion and administer an antipyrogen as needed. Even though transfusions are more common intraoperatively or immediately postoperatively, a febrile reaction may occur during other periods after a transfusion is given.

FEVER 0 TO 2 DAYS POSTOPERATIVE

Atelectasis

Atelectasis is the most common cause of early postoperative fever.[7] Most studies have examined the incidence of atelectasis after intrabdominal or cardiothoracic surgery with reported incidences between 2.5% and 70% depending on the clinical diligence and diagnostic criteria used. In a series of patients undergoing major head and neck oncologic resections, the incidence of atelectasis was 65% to 70%.[8] Clinically significant atelectasis commonly occurs on the first to third postoperative day and has been characterized by fever, mild to moderate tachypnea, and tachycardia. Fever, however, is usually the first sign to initiate evaluation. Physical examination reveals decreased breath sounds in the affected

lobes, tubular breathing, and rales. Blood gas analysis is usually not indicated, but when performed it may reveal arterial hypoxemia and pulmonary shunting. Often a chest radiograph is obtained during a fever workup to rule out pneumonia. The appearance of atelectasis radiographically depends on the extent of anatomic involvement. Minimal involvement of the basilar lung segments will appear as linear horizontal densities near the diaphragm. Segmental atelectasis involving sublobar areas of lung most often occurs in the basilar segments as well. Lobar atelectasis involves collapse of complete lobes. Absence of fever does not necessarily exclude the presence of atelectasis postoperatively. One prospective study found that fever was an accurate indicator of radiographic evidence of atelectasis in only 56% of subjects. It concluded that neither the presence nor absence of fever can rule in or out postoperative atelectasis.[9]

An extensive study in 1963 using an animal model attempted to elucidate the cause of atelectasis induced fever. The authors concluded that bacteria in the distal bronchial tree resulted in the production of endogenous pyrogen, which, in turn, resulted in peripherally mediated vasoconstriction and decreased heat loss.[10] A recent theory has speculated that alveolar macrophages may be induced by atelectasis alone to produce interleukin-1, a known endogenous pyrogen.[11] The definite cause, however, remains uncertain.

ETIOLOGY

Intraoperative and postoperative alterations in respiratory function may result in significant pulmonary sequelae manifested in part by elevated body temperature postoperatively. Regardless of the type of surgery, several changes in pulmonary mechanics occur during surgery directly related to general anesthesia and mechanical ventilation. These changes predispose the susceptible patient to postoperative pulmonary complications, the most common of which is atelectasis.[7,12]

A generalized impairment in lung volumes is consistently seen with general anesthesia. Changes include decreased functional residual capacity (FRC), vital capacity (VC), tidal volume, and development of a rapid and shallow breathing pattern. An increase in physiological deadspace and minute ventilation is seen to maintain adequate alveolar ventilation (V_A) and $PaCO_2$. Factors that can decrease V_A include volatile anesthetics, respiratory depressant intravenous drugs, and muscle relaxants. Atelectasis intraoperatively is caused mainly by the shallow breathing associated with decreased lung volumes. As lung volumes decrease toward residual volume, the small distal airways (>0.1 mm diameter) in dependent regions have a tendency to close, resulting in air/gas trapping in the alveoli. As the trapped air/gas is resorbed, atelectasis occurs. Higher concentrations of oxygen in the alveoli will lead to more rapid resorption and increased atelectasis. For this reason, some advocate decreasing the concentration of inspired oxygen as the patient awakens from general anesthesia. Another factor affected by anesthesia or surgical trauma is a decrease in pulmonary surfactant. Once atelectasis develops, this loss makes reexpansion of the involved segment more difficult.

In the early postoperative period, atelectasis develops or persists mainly due to hypoventilation without the normal spontaneous deep breaths that occur approximately every 5 to 10 minutes in normal, healthy individuals. These maximal inhalations to total lung capacity help maintain adequate FRC and RV and prevent air trapping, as described earlier. This hypoventilation postoperatively is secondary to splinting from pain or the use of narcotic analgesics. Obviously, splinting as a cause is seen more commonly in thoracic or upper abdominal surgery.

Several factors have been shown to increase the risk of developing atelectasis after surgery.[13,14] These include smoking, obesity, obstructive lung disease, duration of anesthesia, and the presence of upper respiratory tract infection. Underlying pulmonary disease marked by forced expiratory volume in 1 second (FEV_1) < 1 L, pO_2 < 55 mm Hg, and pCO_2 > 44 mm Hg has been shown to be the principal predictor of pulmonary complications. Other factors affecting closing volume should also be considered. As long as closing volume is less than FRC, air trapping will not occur. Increasing age is marked by decreasing lung elasticity, resulting in closing volumes approaching or exceeding FRC. Positioning of the patient is also important. The supine position reduces FRC and may cause dependent portions of the lung to function below closing volume, thereby increasing the risk of atelectasis.

COMPLICATIONS

In a majority of cases, postoperative atelectasis is transient and clinically insignificant. However, lung segments that are atelectatic are at increased risk for developing consolidation and resulting pneumonia.

MANAGEMENT AND PREVENTION

The prevention and treatment of atelectasis are basically the same, with the goal being maintenance or restoration of FRC. Awareness of associated risk factors may lead to prevention or earlier intervention to minimize morbidity. Appropriate patient positioning is a simple and effective means of improving pulmonary function. The sitting position results in increased FRC as compared to the supine position and promotes lung expansion. Early ambulation is even more effective because the patient will take deeper breaths with the added exertion. Patients who are bedridden should be managed with frequent position changes to alter the portion of the lung that is dependent.

Active encouragement of the patient to breathe deeply during the early postoperative period is the next approach in the prevention or treatment of atelectasis. Incentive spirometry remains the most commonly employed modality. First introduced by Bartlett in 1973, this device requires the patient to inspire forcefully against preset resistances with visual cues when the goal is reached.[12] Optimal results are achieved when the patient has been instructed in its use preoperatively and active bedside encouragement occurs postoperatively.

Proper management of postoperative pain will also decrease the persistence or development of atelectasis. In abdominal or thoracic surgery, intraspinal or epidural narcotics result in significantly increased postoperative FVC and FEV_1 when compared to intravenous or intramuscular narcotics. Unfortunately, these alternate routes of narcotic administration are not appropriate in head and neck surgery. Therefore, judicious use of both intravenous and oral narcotics is indicated to alleviate surgical pain. The goal is to make the patient as comfortable as possible without oversedation. The fear of respiratory depression and hypoventilation following narcotic administration is generally exaggerated.

Necrotizing Wound Infection

Although rare, necrotizing infections of the soft tissues of the head and neck can be devastating. They generally occur in relation to a preexisting infection such as tonsillitis, peritonsillar abscess, or odontogenic processes. Postoperatively, these necrotizing infections occur more frequently after clean-contaminated abdominal surgery; however, contamination with the most commonly implicated pathogens has been noted in the oropharynx as well. Clinically, a fever occurring within the first 48 hours after surgery associated with marked clinical toxicity, as partially evidenced by tachycardia and respiratory distress, should alert the clinician to examine the wound closely. Classic signs include wound edema with gray or purple discoloration. Drainage of a brown or watery fluid may be seen as well as wound crepitus. Infections may be monomicrobial or polymicrobial. Commonly encountered pathogens include *Clostridial* species, aerobic and anaerobic streptococci, and *S. aureus*.

Aggressive wound debridement is essential to ensure patient survival. Removal of all necrotic tissue should be done surgically. Antimicrobial therapy is directed against organisms seen on gram stain of the wound drainage fluid. The presence of gram-positive rods is consistent with a clostridial infection.

Other Causes

Any surgery performed in an infected bed, such as drainage of a neck abscess, may result in fever both during the procedure and shortly after by release of remaining pyrogens. These temperature elevations should resolve quickly unless there is ongoing infection.

Fever can occur transiently after relatively minor procedures such as tonsillectomy and adenoidectomy. In a series of several thousand patients undergoing this operation, 2.6% developed postoperative temperature elevations higher than 101.3 °F (38.5 °C) early after the operation.[15] The majority of these resolved within 24 hours, and less than 0.2% had their discharge delayed as a result of persistent fever. The fever after these clean-contaminated cases is probably a result of surgical stress, the effects of anesthesia, and transient bacteremias. Many surgeons will give prophylactic antibiotics beginning at the time of surgery and continuing for several days after surgery. This is felt to reduce both the incidence of fever and postoperative discomfort. Any fever that persists after 24 hours should be evaluated for other sources of possible infection.

Any fever developing after esophageal endoscopy should alert the clinician to the possibility of an esophageal perforation. One study of 52 patients with esophageal perforations from all causes reported fever > 103.1 °F (39.5 °C) in 83% of patients.[16] Chest or neck pain is also a frequent complaint. Associated signs include tachycardia and subcutaneous crepitance. Prompt diagnosis is essential to prevent serious morbidity or mortality. This topic is covered in greater detail in Chapter 5 ("Complications of Laryngoscopy, Bronchoscopy, and Esophagoscopy").

Toxic Shock Syndrome

Toxic shock syndrome (TSS) is a multisystem disorder that was initially brought to medical attention in 1980, with its occurrence noted in a series of menstruating women using superabsorbent tampons. Since then, this disease has been reported as a complication in a wide variety of surgical procedures, including those in the head and neck. By 1984 more than 25% of cases were not associated with menstruation.[17] Of interest is the comparison made between tampon use and the use of nasal packing following nasal surgery. Indeed, the syndrome was first reported in a patient with nasal packing following a septorhinoplasty in 1982.[18] Since then, further cases of TSS have been reported following nasal cases both with and without nasal packing. It should be recognized, therefore, that TSS can occur after any operation in which *S. aureus* can be a contaminant regardless of the use of absorbent material. An example is a case of TSS reported after an uncomplicated submandibular gland excision.[19]

Several initial published series of TSS noted an association with a specific *Staphylococcus aureus* exotoxin. This toxin has been specified toxic shock syndrome toxin 1 (TSST-1) and has been found in the majority of patients with the syndrome, although less commonly in patients with nonmenstrual TSS. TSST-1 is a known inducer of interleukin-1 synthesis, which is an endogenous human pyrogen. How the TSST-1 exotoxin interacts with the host immune system to produce the syndrome remains unclear.

CLINICAL PRESENTATION

TSS is a rapidly developing, serious multisystem disease that can be fatal if not treated aggressively. Fortunately, the initial reported fatality rate of 13% in 1980 fell to 2.7% by 1984.[17] A high index of suspicion is needed in all postoperative patients who present with fever, hypotension, and erythroderma within the first 48 to 72 hours. The median time for onset of symptoms is 2 days after surgery. The

Centers for Disease Control (CDC) has established guidelines for the diagnosis of TSS (Table 4–1).[20] Initial symptoms commonly include fever > 102.1 °F (38.9 °C), abdominal pain, vomiting, diarrhea, and proximal limb and abdominal myalgia. By definition, hypotension will develop within 72 hours along with a characteristic diffuse, nonpruritic, blanching, macular erythroderma. Other signs include hyperemia of the mucous membranes and mental status changes. Laboratory alterations may indicate renal and liver dysfunction with elevations of serum creatinine, blood urea nitrogen (BUN), total bilirubin, aspartate transaminase (AST), and alanine transaminase (ALT). Thrombocytopenia and leukocytosis with a marked left shift are common. Blood cultures are usually negative. The surgical wound commonly appears unremarkable but upon probing may reveal thin discharge and positive cultures for *S. aureus*. Desquamation of the palms and soles develops late in the clinical course (1 to 2 weeks after onset).

Currently there is no definitive diagnostic test for TSS. Consequently, the diagnosis is based entirely on clinical presentation using the criteria established by the CDC. Other diseases to be considered in the differential diagnosis include Kawasaki disease, staphylococcal scalded skin syndrome, scarlet fever, Rocky Mountain spotted fever, leptospirosis, and Stevens-Johnson syndrome. Of these, Stevens-Johnson syndrome most closely resembles TSS and, therefore, must be considered carefully during the evaluation.

MANAGEMENT

The primary treatment of TSS is supportive care. Initial intervention should be directed at fluid resuscitation and support of blood pressure and intravascular volume. This may be done with either crystalloid or colloid. Persistent hypotension may require treatment with vasopressors and invasive monitoring with arterial lines and central venous pressure catheters. Ventilatory support is indicated in those patients who develop significant pulmonary dysfunction as a result of adult respiratory distress syndrome (ARDS). Dialysis may be needed in patients with acute tubular necrosis.

Patients with nasal packing or splints in place should have them removed immediately after the diagnosis of TSS is suspected. Appropriate wound care includes gentle debridement as needed as well as the application of Betadine-soaked gauze dressing in the opened wound. Surgical drains should also be removed.

With prompt treatment, most patients survive without permanent sequelae. A myriad of conditions have been described as late effects, but these are uncommon. All patients with TSS are at increased risk of developing a recurrence, although it is more common in menstrual TSS. The recurrent episodes are usually not as severe, and they generally occur within several months of the initial episode.

Systemic antistaphylococcal antibiotics have not been shown to alter the course of disease but do reduce the rate of recurrence. Appropriate antimicrobial therapy includes beta-lactamase-resistant penicillins, first-generation cephalosporins, vancomycin, and clindamycin.

Table 4–1. Toxic Shock Syndrome Case Definition

Criteria A

Fever—temperature ≥ 38.9 °C (102 °F)

Rash—diffuse or palmar erythroderma progressing to subsequent peripheral desquamation (hands and feet)

Mucous membrane—nonpurulent conjunctival hyperemia, or oropharyngeal hyperemia, or vaginal hyperemia, or discharge

Hypotension—systolic blood pressure (BP) <90 mm Hg for an adult (<16 yr) or <5th percentile for age for a child; or orthostatic hypotension as shown by a drop in diastolic BP ≥15 mm Hg from recumbent to sitting; or history of orthostatic dizziness

Multisystem involvement
    (≥4 of the following)
    Gastrointestinal—history of vomiting or diarrhea at onset of illness
    Muscular—CPK,* ≥2× ULN† 4–20 days after onset
    CNS—disorientation or alteration in consciousness without focal signs at a time when patient is not in shock or hyperpyrexic
    Renal—BUN or serum creatinine clearance, ≥2× ULN†; and abnormal findings on urinalysis (≥5 WBCs per high-power field [HPF]; ≥1 RBC per HPF; protein, ≥1+); or oliguria defined as urine output <1 mL/kg/h for 24 h
    Hepatic—total serum bilirubin level ≥1.5× ULN†; or SGPT‡ ≥2× ULN†
    Hematologic—thrombocytopenia (platelets <100,000/mm³)
    Cardiopulmonary—adult respiratory distress syndrome; or pulmonary edema; or new onset 2° or 3° heart block; or ECG criteria for myocarditis decreased voltage and ST-T wave chains; or heart failure shown by new onset of gallop rhythm or by increase in size of cardiac silhouette from one chest roentgenogram to another during the course of the illness, or diagnosed by cardiologist
    Metabolic—serum calcium level, ≤7.0 mg/dL with serum phosphate level, ≤2.5 mg/dL and total serum protein level, ≤5.9 mg/dL

Evidence for absence of other causes
    When obtained; negative blood, throat, urine, or CSF cultures
    When obtained; absence of serological evidence of leptospirosis, rickettsial disease, or rubeola
    Evidence for absence of Kawasaki syndrome; no unilateral lymphadenopathy or fever lasting >10 days

Criteria B

At least 2 episodes meeting criteria for fever, rash, mucous membrane, hypotension, and one of the situations under multisystem involvement

From Chesney et al.[20]

*Creatinine phosphokinase.

†Upper limits of normal for laboratory.

‡Serum glutamic pyruvic transaminase level.

FEVER 2 TO 4 DAYS POSTOPERATIVE

Urinary Tract Infection

Urinary tract infection (UTI) associated with urinary bladder catheterization is the most common nosocomial infection, accounting for approximately 40% of all hospital-acquired infections.[21–23] In surgery patients, UTI is the second most common nosocomial infection (27% of all infections) following surgical site infection (37% of all infections), as reported by a large surveillance study by the National Infections Surveillance System between 1986 and 1992.[24] It is a common practice among anesthesiologists and surgeons to have a Foley bladder catheter inserted at the time of surgery. Bladder catheterization allows for precise urine output measurement, providing vital data concerning fluid balance both during an operative procedure and postoperatively. Catheters are also placed in preparation for lengthy operations in which bladder distension might be a problem. Postoperatively, urinary catheters may be placed for patients who have urinary retention or bladder stretch injuries. Most of these situations usually result in catheterization of less than 5 days. Nevertheless, postoperative UTI is still a recognized complication following short-term catheterization.

The reported risk of developing a UTI is 5% to 10% for each day a bladder catheter is in place.[22,23] Therefore, most patients with a catheter in place for 30 days will have bacteriuria. The majority of these infections will be monomicrobial, with polymicrobial infections predominating in long-term (>30 days) catheterization and in those patients more severely debilitated. The most common isolates on urine culture are *E. coli*, *Klebsiella* sp., *Pseudomonas aeruginosa*, and *Proteus* sp.[21,23]

RISK FACTORS

Several risk factors associated with the development of catheter-associated UTI have been identified. One prospective study using multivariate analysis identified increased duration of catheterization, absence of urinemeter drainage, microbial colonization of the drainage bag, diabetes mellitus, absence of systemic antibiotic administration during the period of catheterization, female sex, and elevated serum creatinine.[25] Other studies have included periurethral colonization as an additional predisposing factor to bladder bacteriuria.[23] This is important because migration of bacteria along the catheter is the most likely mechanism of developing a UTI. The reservoir of the offending bacteria appears to include perineal colonization by the patient's own colonic microflora or contamination from the hospital environment.

COMPLICATIONS

Complications of untreated short-term, catheter-associated bacteriuria range from simple fever to, on rare occasions, death. Acute pyelonephritis and bacteremia are intermediate complications. There are currently no data recording the incidence of acute pyelonephritis; however, bacteremia has been reported to occur after catheter insertion in approximately 8% of patients. These usually transient bacteremias are clinically asymptomatic in a majority of patients. The presence of bacteriuria in a catheterized patient is associated with clinical bacteremia (usually gram-negative rod) in 2% to 4% of patients. Some patient deaths have been associated with the presence of catheter-associated bacteriuria. One prospective study using multivariate analysis reported a threefold increase in mortality in catheterized patients who developed bacteriuria when compared to catheterized patients who did not develop bacteriuria.[23]

PREVENTION

Prevention of short-term, catheter-associated bacteriuria is aimed at (1) prevention of urethral catheterization, and (2) prevention of bacteriuria once a patient is catheterized.

Alternatives to urethral catheterization should be considered and implemented when possible. For male patients with either temporary or prolonged urinary incontinence, a condom catheter may be used instead of a Foley catheter. Patients with postoperative urinary retention or delayed ability to void may be managed with intermittent catheterization. Often, only one to two "in-and-out" catheterizations are required before normal bladder function returns. Suprapubic catheterization is another alternative when bladder catheterization is indicated. This minor procedure involves percutaneous introduction of a small catheter through the abdominal wall into the bladder. Most studies comparing the infection rate between suprapubic and transurethral catheterization have found a lower rate of bacteriuria with suprapubic catheters. Complications associated with placement of suprapubic catheters include cellulitis, leakage, and hematoma around the insertion site. These, however, are relatively uncommon.

Once the decision has been made to place a transurethral catheter, the goal is to prevent bacteriuria and subsequent symptomatic UTI. The single best method of accomplishing this is to remove the catheter as soon as possible before bacteriuria develops. Factors that are known to be protective of or at least reduce the risk of infection during the period of catheterization include the use of a closed collecting system in which the tube empties directly into an attached drainage bag. This method was first shown to reduce the incidence of bacteriuria in a landmark study by Kunin and McCormack in 1966.[26] It is important to maintain the integrity of the catheter-collecting tube junction to lessen the risk. The junction between the collecting tube and the drainage bag is another point of possible bacterial contamination. The attachment of a urinemeter has been shown to lower the incidence of bacteriuria, presumably by breaking the urine column between the bag and catheter[23] (Fig. 4–2).

The use of prophylactic antibiotics has been a controversial issue. It is generally accepted that prophylactic antibiotics are of little benefit in preventing UTI when the catheter is in place less than 3 days or longer than 14 days. One study examined the incidence of catheter-associated UTI in patients who received concurrent antimicrobial therapy for unrelated reasons. The results indicated that the use of antibiotics within 48 hours prior to catheter removal increased the likelihood of a negative final urine culture by fivefold.[27] Others are hesitant to use prophylactic antibiotics for fear of inducing resistant strains; however, no studies to date have substantiated this argument. For us, as head and neck surgeons, many of our patients who might require bladder catheterization are on postoperative antibiotics prophylactically to prevent wound infection. This period of antimicrobial coverage frequently occurs concurrently during the usually short period of bladder catheterization.

DIAGNOSIS AND TREATMENT

The diagnosis of a UTI is made on the basis of urinalysis with urine cultures to identify and quantify the bacteria. In general, cultures are considered positive when quantitative growth is greater than 100,000 organisms per milliliter of urine. However, studies have shown that bacteria initially present in urine specimens at concentrations less than 100 organisms per milliliter will, over subsequent days, reach concentrations of at least 100,000 organisms per milliliter.[23]

Pneumonia

Hospital-acquired pneumonia continues to be a serious cause of postoperative morbidity. It is the third leading cause of nosocomial infection in surgical patients after wound and urinary tract infections, but it accounts for more fatalities. In a large (95-hospital) comprehensive 6-year surveillance study by the National Center for Infectious Disease (1993), pneumonia was the second most common nosocomial infection after head and neck surgery.[24] Reviewing all surgical sites (n = 20), pneumonia occurred more frequently in head and neck patients compared to all other sites except thoracic and intracranial. Two studies specifically addressing complications of head and neck surgery reported an incidence of postoperative pneumonia in 10% to 11% of patients.[28,29] From an economic standpoint, development of postoperative pneumonia prolongs hospitalization an average 8 to 9 days.

The diagnosis of pneumonia is usually based on the presence of fever [usually > 101.3 °F (38.5 °C)], a new infiltrate on chest roentgenogram, and increased production of purulent sputum, which on gram stain contains white cells and a specific organism. Cultures are useful mainly to establish antibiotic sensitivities. The pathogen(s) responsible for nosocomial pneumonia vary from hospital to hospital. In tertiary referral centers, gram-negative bacilli and *Staphylococcus aureus* are seen more commonly. Community-based hospitals have fewer gram-negative bacilli and more pathogens typical of community-acquired pneumonias such

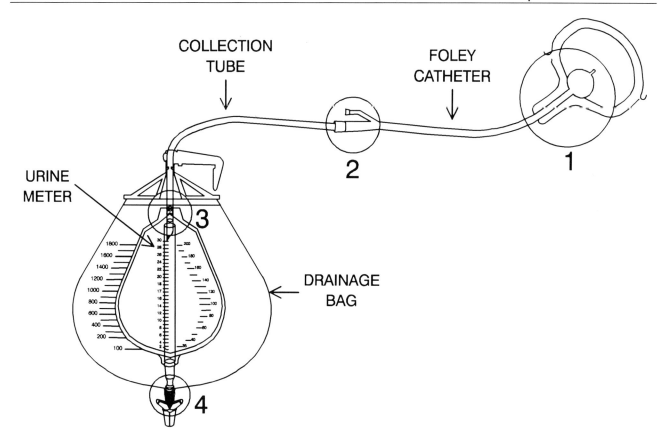

COLLECTION TUBE

FOLEY CATHETER

URINE METER

DRAINAGE BAG

Figure 4-2.   Sites of possible bacterial entry into the urinary tract with the use of an indwelling bladder catheter: (1) Foley catheter/urethral junction; (2) catheter/collecting tube junction; (3) collecting tube/drainage bag junction; (4) drainage bag emptying port.

as *Streptococcus pneumoniae*. Physicians should be aware of the pathogens seen most commonly in their hospitals to guide antimicrobial therapy appropriately.

ETIOLOGY

Colonization of the nasopharynx or tracheobronchial tree with hospital organisms occurs during the first few days after surgery. Colonization with gram-negative bacilli occurs more frequently in hospitalized patients, especially those who are critically ill. A factor that has gained increasing interest is gastric colonization and its subsequent influence on the development of pneumonia. Gastric contents are normally sterile in healthy people due to the presence of hydrochloric acid. This protective state may be altered by advancing age, various gastrointestinal disorders, malnutrition, or medications that alter gastric pH. The oropharynx may then become colonized via retrograde migration. A review of several studies revealed that patients receiving H_2 blockers and/or antacids have a higher incidence of postoperative pneumonia. Patients receiving sucralfate, which acts independently of pH, have lower rates of infection. The presence of nasogastric (NG) tubes has also been implicated in the development of pulmonary infection by increasing reflux and by providing a direct conduit for bacteria to the oropharynx.[30]

Cross colonization via contact with hospital personnel and contaminated hospital equipment is another important source of nosocomial pathogens in patients. Gram-negative bacilli

and *S. aureus* commonly colonize the hands of health care providers. For this reason, among others, it is important to observe infection control guidelines, such as handwashing before and after patient contact and the frequent use of gown and gloves. Hospitals that follow these preventive measures have been shown to have lower rates of pneumonia.[31]

The changes in pulmonary mechanics occurring intraoperatively and postoperatively that contribute to the development of atelectasis also play a role in the development of pneumonia. The incidence of postoperative pneumonia is, however, much less than the incidence of atelectasis. The presence of atelectasis predisposes to the occurrence of pneumonia due to impaired clearance mechanisms and pooled secretions acting as culture media. This usually occurs between postoperative days 4 and 10. However, not all patients who develop atelectasis will develop a pneumonia. The highest incidences of pneumonia are seen following major trauma or extensive surgery. Other associated risk factors include pulmonary edema, smoking, lengthy operations, and a long preoperative hospitalization. Malnutrition was identified as a risk factor for postoperative pneumonia but not for atelectasis in a study by Windsor and Hill (1988). They found that protein depletion was associated with an impairment of respiratory function marked by reduced diaphragmatic muscle mass, generalized respiratory muscle weakness, and reduced maximum voluntary ventilations.[32] Malnourished patients are known to have impaired granulocyte function, increasing their susceptibility to postoperative infection.

A prospective study by Weber et al (1993) identified risk factors specific to patients undergoing head and neck oncologic surgery. These included increasing length of surgery, malnutrition (albumin $<$ 3.5 g/100 cc), greater than 70 packs per year smoking history, and the need for blood transfusion.[29] The increased risk associated with receiving blood transfusions is most likely multifactorial; however, some studies have shown impaired immunity with decreased phagocytic cell function in both humans and animals.

MANAGEMENT

As with most postoperative complications, the most effective means of treating nosocomial pneumonias is to prevent them from developing. Knowing the factors associated with their development guides preventive measures, such as handwashing, mentioned previously. The preventative measures outlined in the section on atelectasis are also applicable for preventing postoperative pneumonia.

Once a pulmonary infection has been diagnosed, treatment should be directed toward organism specific antimicrobial therapy along with measures to maximize pulmonary function. Antibiotic selection is initially aimed at those organisms most likely to be implicated in that specific hospital setting. Because gram-negative bacilli, specifically *Pseudomonas aeruginosa* and *Klebsiella pneumoniae*, and *S. aureus* are most common in tertiary referral centers, broad-spectrum antibiotics covering these organisms are begun until culture results are available. Common practice is to begin double-coverage therapy with a β-lactam and an aminoglycoside to prevent the serious morbidity and mortality associated with these infections. Because of the potential toxic effects of aminoglycosides, some physicians are changing to monotherapy with a broad spectrum, third-generation cephalosporin or extended-spectrum penicillin. Adjustments are then made based on sensitivity data. Nosocomial pneumonia in community hospitals is more frequently due to pathogens associated with community-acquired pneumonia. Accordingly, monotherapy may be sufficient coverage initially.[33]

Maximizing pulmonary function using the same measures outlined for atelectasis is aimed at shortening the course of the illness. Improving pulmonary clearance mechanisms and restoring normal lung volumes are vital to recovery.

Phlebitis

CATHETER RELATED

Most hospitalized patients have some type of intravenous catheter in place. Many surgical patients have central venous catheters inserted intraoperatively that remain in place postoperatively for cardiovascular and fluid monitoring. A review of several studies reported an incidence of catheter colonization in as many as 34% of patients overall, rising to $>$50% of patients with either peripheral or central venous catheters in place more than 4 days.[11] Superficial catheter-induced phlebitis is usually recognized clinically by fever,

tenderness, and clot in the vein proximal to the insertion site. Pain and erythema may also be seen. Bacterial (septic) phlebitis is confirmed by gram stain or culture of the clot. Both septic and nonseptic phlebitis associated with central venous catheters may present with fever and edema of the upper extremity followed by pain and erythema.

The management of both peripheral and central phlebitis is initiated with removal of the affected catheter. When suspected as a source of infection, the catheter tip should be sent for culture. Elevation and heat to the involved site are common modalities to treat both types of peripheral phlebitis. Antibiotic therapy is then begun if septic phlebitis is suspected. Complete resolution of the infection may require excision of the clotted vein segment. Central venous catheter phlebitis may require systemic heparinization after catheter removal. Septic central venous phlebitis is confirmed with blood cultures positive for the same organism grown from the catheter tip. Appropriate antibiotic therapy is then initiated, with adjustments made with sensitivity data.

DEEP VENOUS THROMBOSIS

Phlebitis may develop in the deep veins of the lower extremities unrelated to intravenous catheters. Common signs and symptoms include fever, edema of the extremity, distended veins, localized areas of cutaneous discoloration, and increased heat and tenderness over the involved vein. It is important to note, however, that deep venous thrombosis (DVT) may be present in the absence of symptoms. The occurrence of pulmonary embolism may be the first evidence of a DVT. General risk factors for DVT include stasis, endothelial damage, and hypercoagulability. Inactivity in the postoperative period is the greatest risk to the surgical patient. In addition to preventing atelectasis, early mobility decreases the risk of developing DVT. Once the diagnosis of DVT has been confirmed by appropriate imaging studies, initial therapy consists of systemic heparinization.

Pulmonary Embolism

Fever is usually not the first clinical sign to initiate evaluation for possible pulmonary embolism. Temperature elevations are often seen after significant parenchymal injury has occurred. Presentation of pulmonary embolism may vary from nonspecific complaints such as anxiety and weakness to dyspnea, syncope, and severe substernal chest pain. Initially, physicians may suspect myocardial infarction. Other associated signs and symptoms include hyperventilation, persistent hypoxia despite supplemental oxygen, cough, and tachycardia. Pulmonary embolism may lead to pulmonary artery hypertension with signs and symptoms of acute cor pulmonale. With massive embolism, sustained hypotension, and other signs of shock may occur. Continuous electrocardiogram (ECG) monitoring is indicated.

Diagnosis of pulmonary embolism can only be made with certainty by pulmonary angiography; however, ventilation-perfusion lung scans may suffice because these have lower associated morbidity. Perfusion scanning is highly sensitive, so a negative scan essentially rules out the diagnosis but it also has low specificity. Therefore, guidelines have been developed to aid the clinician. Concomitant ventilatory scans can identify areas of perfusion-ventilation mismatch. Interpretation of ventilation-perfusion scanning is based on certain patterns that are defined as normal, low probability (10%), intermediate probability (30%), and high probability (90%). Equivocal scans may be indications to obtain pulmonary angiography to provide a definitive diagnosis.

Once a diagnosis of pulmonary embolism has been made, a thorough examination of the lower extremities should be performed to identify the source of the embolus. Risk factors for developing postoperative pulmonary embolism are the same as outlined for deep vein thrombosis. The subjects of deep vein thrombosis and pulmonary embolism, including specific management, are discussed in greater detail in Chapter 3 ("Deep Venous Thrombosis and Pulmonary Embolism").

FEVER 5 TO 10 DAYS POSTOPERATIVELY

Wound Infection

Wound infection is the most common nosocomial infection for all surgical sites based on a 6-year review of 42,509 patients developing postoperative infections in the National Nosocomial Infection Surveillance System.[24] Wound infection also accounted for the most postoperative infections after head and neck surgery (37% of 789 infections). Several factors must be considered when interpreting this data, however. The surgery encompassed by the specialty of otolaryngology/head and neck surgery is considerably varied. Many of the procedures are classified as clean contaminated when the aerodigestive tract is entered, such as during a laryngectomy. These operations have a higher incidence of postoperative wound infection when compared to clean procedures such as parotidectomy. This increased incidence, however, has been diminished by the now accepted practice of administering perioperative prophylactic antibiotics.

A fever occurring between 5 and 10 days postoperatively should alert the surgeon to examine the operative site closely to rule out wound infection. Although bacteria most likely contaminate the wound at the time of the initial procedure, it takes several days before bacterial growth is sufficient to produce a clinically evident infection. Examination may reveal erythema, induration, tenderness, edema, and warmth. However, these signs are not always indicative of an infection. Mild erythema and induration are seen with normal wound healing. Progressive erythema and edema of neck flaps may herald the occurrence of infection. Infection may also be indicated by a subcutaneous collection of fluid. Gentle and conservative probing of the wound edge may be diagnostic by revealing the presence of purulent fluid. In wounds where suction drainage is used, the character of the drainage fluid may change. Normally, the drainage will progress from fresh blood just after surgery to serosanguinous or serous fluid.

The quantity should also decrease over 3 to 4 days postoperatively, at which time the drains can usually be removed. With infection, the fluid may appear cloudy or frankly purulent and may increase in output. Cultures should be obtained of the fluid to guide antimicrobial therapy, if indicated. Laboratory data may reveal leukocytosis. The mild leukocytosis commonly noted shortly after an operative procedure should have resolved by this time, and any elevation this late is suspicious for infection. The fever associated with a wound infection is usually less than 102.2°F (39°C) unless an abscess has developed.

RISK FACTORS

The development of a wound infection is the result of several predisposing factors. Many of these relate to the patient's preoperative condition, including nutritional status, overall general health, and whether or not the patient smokes or drinks significant amounts of alcohol. Patients with head and neck cancer frequently suffer from other medical problems associated with heavy tobacco and alcohol use, including cardiac, pulmonary, and liver dysfunction. The effect of prior radiotherapy on the incidence of wound infection in head and neck patients has not been delineated clearly. Several studies have reported higher rates of wound dehiscence, hematoma, and fistula formation in addition to wound infection in patients who have had prior radiotherapy. One study that showed no increased risk in the occurrence of postoperative wound infection did report significantly higher morbidity when it did occur, including longer hospitalization, increased rate of fistulization, and increased need for secondary surgical repair.[34] Intraoperative factors increasing the risk for wound infection include flap reconstruction, advanced disease, prolonged operative time, failure of an air-tight closure, and failure of prophylactic antibiotic administration.

COMPLICATIONS

Most postoperative wound infections can be managed adequately without serious sequelae with local wound care and appropriate antibiotic therapy. Wound infections occurring in the head and neck, however, can add significant morbidity. Procedures with mucosal closures in the neck are at increased risk for fistula formation as a result of postoperative infection. Infection-associated wound breakdown in the neck places the patient at risk for carotid artery rupture.

PREVENTION

Wound infections add significant morbidity to the surgical patient. A 1985 study of patients undergoing major head and neck surgery estimated that hospitalization increased by 2 weeks and that hospital charges increased more than $10,000 in patients who developed a postoperative wound infection.[35] Therefore, the major emphasis should be on preventing wound infections.

The primary factor causing infection in any wound is the presence of a sufficient bacterial innoculum. The accepted concentration of bacteria required to produce a clinical infection is 10^5 organisms/mL.[36] This is important, specifically in head and neck procedures when the oral cavity or pharynx is entered. Saliva, which contains 10^7 aerobic bacteria/mL and 10^8 anaerobic bacteria/mL, will inevitably contaminate the wound bed. In addition, the presence of a preexisting tracheostomy almost ensures that the neck wound will be contaminated with respiratory secretions. It is now an accepted practice to administer prophylactic antibiotics whenever the oral cavity or pharynx is entered (see Chapter 12, "Use of Prophylactic Antibiotics in Otolaryngology").

Appropriate surgical techniques are extremely important in the prevention of postoperative wound infections. This begins with the initial skin preparation with an antibacterial agent such as betadine scrub and solution. Prior to wound closure, irrigation with warm saline is performed to remove clot and debris and to dilute the bacterial concentration. Careful attention to air-tight skin closure and water-tight mucosal closure is essential for the proper function of suction drains and to prevent leakage of oropharyngeal secretions into the wound bed. The use of suction drains is a common practice in surgery of the head and neck to prevent fluid collections (hematoma/seroma) that can become growth media for bacteria and to eliminate dead space and encourage flap healing. Improper drain management can actually increase the risk of wound infection. Drains should be examined often for proper functioning, and they should be removed as soon as previously determined criteria are met.

Drug Fevers

Fever associated with drug therapy usually occurs 7 to 10 days following initial administration and persists for the duration of drug use. Temperature usually returns to normal soon after discontinuing the drug; however, the fever will return if the drug is restarted. Initially, the fever may be low grade. In a series of patients felt to have drug-induced temperature elevation, the fever was spiking in nature and exhibited a normal diurnal rhythm.[37]

Drug-induced fevers may result from several mechanisms, although most are thought to be due to a hypersensitivity reaction. In these instances, the fever cannot be explained by a known pharmacological effect of the drug and is unrelated to dose, and associated signs and symptoms suggest an immunologic etiology. Therefore, it is unusual for fever to be the sole indicator of an allergic drug reaction because patients may experience arthralgias, urticaria, myalgias, gastrointestinal (GI) discomfort, and rashes. Fever may be the first sign of impending severe drug reaction. Certain patients with autoimmune disorder, such as systemic lupus erythematosus (SLE), appear to have a predisposition to developing allergic drug reactions. Other factors thought to increase the risk of developing a drug-induced fever include genetic factors, increased age of the patient, duration of therapy, and route and dose of drug administration.

In addition to hypersensitivity reactions, other possible causes of drug-induced fever include the following mechanisms: (1) administration of drugs contaminated with pyrogens in the intravenous solutions (eg, amphotericin B); (2) infusion-related phlebitis (eg, cephalosporins and vancomycin); (3) direct pharmacological action of drug (eg, release of endogenous pyrogen from injured malignant cells as a result of chemotherapy; (4) interference with normal thermoregulatory mechanisms (eg, synthroid and antihistamines in large doses); and (5) idiosyncratic drug reactions (eg, oxidizing agents in patients with G6PD deficiency).

Diagnosis of drug-induced fever is often a diagnosis of exclusion; however, a high clinical index of suspicion may lead to the appropriate diagnosis prior to obtaining an expensive evaluation for a fever of otherwise unknown origin. A knowledge of the most common drugs associated with fever is helpful. In addition, the presence of associated allergic symptoms would be further evidence of a drug reaction. The definitive diagnosis is made with complete defervescence on discontinuation of the suspected drug and reappearance of fever with reinstitution of therapy. Rechallenge with the suspected agent should be carefully considered, however, because a severe allergic reaction may occur, resulting in serious morbidity.

The list of drugs associated with fever is long and varied, although certain ones are more commonly implicated. Of the drugs cited most frequently, antibiotics that have been administered perioperatively are most suspect for a postoperative fever, although the incidence of true antibiotic-induced fever is low according to two large series.[38,39] Penicillins and cephalosporins had incidences of drug fever in <1% of patients, and these were the most commonly reported. Allergic reactions with associated fever are not as common today, presumably due to the increased purity of the antibiotic preparations. Other drugs commonly associated with drug fever include quinidine, procainamide, antituberculars, methyldopa, and phenytoin. Unless first instituted perioperatively, these drugs would be rare causes of a postoperative fever.

SUMMARY

Fever occurring in the postoperative period is common and, in many cases, inconsequential. A careful history and physical examination often leads to the most likely cause. Knowledge of the more common causes of fever occurring at specific intervals in the postoperative period should lead to a more cost-effective evaluation. The majority of these causes relate to common practices in all surgical fields. However, the incidences of various postoperative infections vary according to the type of surgery. The aim of this chapter is to guide the otolaryngologist/head and neck surgeon in the evaluation of a fever occurring in the postoperative period. It is hoped that the commonly practiced and cost-ineffective shotgun approach can be abandoned in favor of more directed clinical evaluations.

REFERENCES

1. Simon HB. Pathophysiology of fever and fever of undetermined origin. *Medicine.* 1987;7:XXIV.
2. Atkins E, Bodel P. Clinical fever: Its history, manifestations, and pathogenesis. *Fed Proc.* 1979;38(1):57.
3. Bernheim HA, Block LH, Atkins E. Fever: Pathogenesis, Pathophysiology, and Purpose. *Ann Intern Med.* 1979;91:261.
4. Dinarello CA, Wolff SM. Molecular basis of fever in humans. *Am J Med.* 1982;72:799.
5. Dinarello CA. Interleukin-1. *Rev Infec Dis.* 1984;6:51.
6. Freischlag J, Busuttil RW. The value of postoperative fever evaluation. *Surgery.* 1983;94(2):358.
7. Schwieger I, Gamulin Z, Suter PM. Lung function during anesthesia and respiratory insufficiency in the postoperative period: Physiological and clinical implications, *Acta Anaesthesiol Scand.* 1989;33:527.
8. Seikaly H, Kuzon WM, Gullane PJ, et al. Pulmonary atelectasis after reconstruction with pectoralis major flaps. *Arch Otolaryngol Head Neck Surg.* 1990;116:571.
9. Roberts J, Barnes W, Pennock M, et al. Diagnostic accuracy of fever as a measure of postoperative complications. *Heart Lung.* 1988;17:166.
10. Lansing AM, Jamieson WG. Mechanisms of fever in pulmonary atelectasis. *Arch Surg.* 1963;87:184.
11. Burchard KW. Temperature alteration. In: Davis JH, ed. *Clinical Surgery.* St Louis: CV Mosby; 1987.
12. Bartlett RH, Brennan ML, Gazzaniga AB, et al. Studies on the pathogenesis and prevention of postoperative pulmonary complications. *Surg Gynecol Obstet.* 1973;137:925.
13. Williams-Russo P, Charlson ME, MacKenzie CR, et al. Predicting postoperative pulmonary complications. *Arch Intern Med.* 1992;152:1209.
14. Lewis FR. Management of atelectasis and pneumonia. *Surg Clin North Am.* 1980;60(6):1391.
15. Crysdale WS, Russel D. Complications of tonsillectomy and adenoidectomy in 9,409 patients observed overnight. *Can Med Assoc J.* 1986;135:1139.
16. White RK, Morris DM. Diagnosis and management of esophageal perforations. *Am Surg.* 1992;58:112.
17. Wright SW, Trott AT. Toxic shock syndrome: A review. *Ann Emerg Med.* 1988;17:268.
18. Thomas SW, Baird IM, Frazier RD. Toxic shock syndrome following submucous resection and rhinoplasty. *JAMA.* 1982;247:2402.
19. Fornadley JA, Gomez PJ, Crane RT, et al. Toxic shock syndrome following submandibular gland excision. *Head Neck.* 1990;12:66.
20. Chesney PJ, David JP, Purdy WK, et al. Clinical manifestations of toxic shock syndrome. *JAMA.* 1981;246(7):741.
21. Asher EF, Oliver BG, Fry DE. Urinary tract infections in the surgical patient. *Am Surg.* 1988;54:466.
22. Nickel JC. Catheter-associated urinary tract infection: New perspectives on old problems. *Can J Infect Control.* 1991;6(2):38.
23. Warren JW. Catheter-associated urinary tract infections. *Infect Dis Clin North Am.* 1987;1(4):823.
24. Horan TC, Culver DH, Gaynes RP, et al. Nosocomial infections in surgical patients in the United States, January 1986–June 1992. *Infect Control Hosp Epidemiol.* 1993;14:73.
25. Platt R, Polk BF, Murdock B, et al. Risk factors for nosocomial urinary tract infection. *Am J Epidemiol.* 1986;124(6):977.
26. Kunin CM, McCormack RC. Prevention of catherter-induced urinary tract infections by closed sterile drainage. *N Engl J Med.* 1966;307:637.
27. Hustinx WNM, Mintjes-de Groot AJ, Verkooyen RP, et al. Impact on concurrent antimicrobial therapy on catheter-associated urinary tract infection. *J Hosp Infect.* 1991;18:45.
28. McGuirt WF, McCabe BF, Krause CJ. Complications of radical neck dissection: A survey of 788 patients. *Head Neck Surg.* 1979;1:481.
29. Weber RS, Hankins, P, Rosenbaum B, et al. Nonwound infections following head and neck oncologic surgery. *Laryngoscope.* 1993;103:22.
30. Craven DE, Steger K, Barber TW. Preventing nosocomial pneumonia: State of the art and perspectives for the 1990s. *Am J Med.* 1991;91(suppl 3B):44s.
31. Haley RW, Culver DH, White JW, et al. The nationwide nosocomial infection rate: A new need for vital statistics. *Am J Epidemiol.* 1985;121:1258.
32. Windsor JA, Hill GL. Risk factors for postoperative pneumonia—the importance of protein depletion. *Ann Surg.* 1988;208(2):209.
33. Schleupner CJ, Cobb DK. A study of the etiologies and treatment of nosocomial pneumonia in a community-based teaching hospital. *Infect Control Hosp Epidemiol.* 1992;13:515.
34. Johnson JT, Bloomer WD. Effect of prior radiotherapy on postsurgical wound infection. *Head Neck.* 1989;11:132.
35. Mandell-Brown M, Johnson JT, Wagner RL. Cost effectiveness of prophylactic antibiotics in head and neck surgery. *Otolaryngol Head Neck Surg.* 1984;92:520.
36. Davidson AG, Clark C, Smith G. Postoperative wound infection: A computer analysis. *Br J Surg.* 1971;58:333.
37. Tabor PA. Drug-induced fever. *Drug Intell Clin Pharm.* 1986;20:413.
38. Miller RR, Greenblatt DJ, eds. Drug effects in hospitalized patients. *Experiences of the Boston Collaborative Drug Surveillance Program 1966–1975.* New York: John Wiley & Sons, 1976:227–264.
39. Caldwell JR, Cluff LE. Adverse reactions to antimicrobial agents. *JAMA.* 1974;230:77.

5 Complications of Laryngoscopy, Bronchoscopy, and Esophagoscopy

Kyle L. Bressler, M.D., Michael E. Dunham, M.D., Lauren D. Holinger, M.D.

The complications that may result from endoscopic examination in the upper aerodigestive tract are remarkable, considering the usual short duration of these procedures. New technology has brought advanced applications and, with them, the potential for increased complications. Optimal patient care demands that the endoscopist prepare for and avoid these potential pitfalls.

THE ENDOSCOPY SUITE

Ideally, the procedure should be performed in an operating suite or a designated area with full resuscitative capabilities. Occasionally, examinations may need to be performed in the intensive care unit. With the increasing use of fiberoptic endoscopy, more elective procedures are performed outside of the endoscopy suite. Caution must be used in these circumstances, especially in any procedure in which laryngospasm is a possibility.

Proper organization of equipment and personnel is important to avoid complications. Preferably, instruments should be kept surgically clean and stored in glass-enclosed cabinets where they are in clear view of the endoscopist (Fig. 5-1). Wrapping in plastic pouches may cause unnecessary delay in an emergency situation. The wrapping process may also damage the delicate forceps used for biopsies and foreign-body extractions.

A large variety of forceps, bronchoscopes, laryngoscopes, and esophagoscopes are essential, particularly for foreign-body extraction. If a surgeon does not feel comfortable with the variety of instruments available, consideration should be given to transferring the patient to another facility.

EQUIPMENT

Even with proper maintenance, surgical equipment will occasionally fail. For the removal of bronchial foreign bodies, the surgeon should have two sets of instruments in the endoscopy suite. The surgeon should check all equipment immediately prior to use. One should never be caught at a critical point during a procedure without functioning instruments.

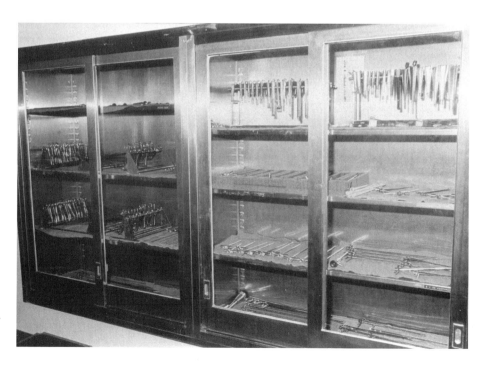

Figure 5-1. Glass-enclosed endoscopy cabinet where instruments are kept surgically clean.

56

Proper lubrication of rigid endoscopes prior to insertion reduces mucosal trauma. Mishandling of equipment can also lead to serious consequences. A good example of this is misplacement of the distal loose end of a plugged-in fiberoptic light cord. If left on a drape, towel, or skin, the heat displaced may result in burns or a fire. With four to five light cords necessary for some procedures, it is easy to overlook the misplacement of one of these cords. Care should be taken to turn all light sources off when not in use.

One of the most important aspects of equipment care is the proper sterilization of instruments. Transmission of infection by means of endoscopes has been well documented.[1-3] The 1980s saw the resurgence of mycobacterial infection, as well as the emergence of the HIV virus, intensifying the need for meticulous instrument cleaning.

Special concern should be given to the flexible endoscopes with suction irrigation capabilities. Recently, it has been shown that even after monitoring for proper care, a significant portion of these scopes will harbor pathogenic organisms.[4] This is the result of the miniaturization of the instruments with resultant narrowing of the individual channels, making them extremely difficult to clean. Without removal of all gross tissue, disinfection or sterilization is impossible. New products with completely disposable patient contact parts are currently undergoing clinical trials. Successful sterilization requires close monitoring of infection control guidelines. Recent actions by the Food and Drug Administration have cast doubt over the effectiveness of commonly used disinfectants.[5]

ANESTHESIA

Communication between the endoscopist and anesthesiologist is a critical factor in avoiding operative complications. Failure to relay information at the beginning of a case may end in an untoward result, especially in those cases involving the airway. An open line of communication will also decrease anesthetic time. One must remember that no particular specialty owns the airway and that complementary skills are often needed to maintain the airway.

Monitoring performed during these procedures has become more extensive in recent years. In addition to the electrocardiogram (EKG), blood pressure cuff, and stethoscope, pulse oximetry and end-tidal CO_2 monitoring have become routine. Although it is tremendously helpful, this information must be correlated with the clinical findings of the patient. A cyanotic patient with a 100% oxygen saturation reading on the pulse oximeter should be considered oxygen deprived until proven otherwise. Hypoxia is a constant concern during examination of the aerodigestive tract, and especially in the pediatric population.[6]

Changing pulse rate or decreasing oxygen saturation can easily be missed in the modern operating room, with its multitude of warning bells and tones. The presence of loud conversation or music in the operating room during airway procedures should be limited. Extra caution should be taken during local cases because the patient may become fearful by comments overheard.

Many endoscopic procedures are performed under local anesthesia. Lidocaine is the preferred anesthetic agent in most cases because of its effectiveness and wide margin of safety. Rarely, however, topical application may result in systemic toxicity with confusion, disorientation, and apprehension. These initial signs may lead to seizures and cardiopulmonary collapse. An important determination to make during a procedure in which a patient becomes more active is whether this is a result of under- or overdosage of anesthesia. A dosage of less than 250 mg in adults is considered safe.[7] The most dangerous area for rapid absorption is the tracheobronchial tree, in which peak concentrations can mimic that of intravenous administration.

TECHNIQUE

Meticulous, gentle technique is the key to avoiding complications during endoscopy. Gentleness begins with proper patient preparation. Because most of the instruments used are rigid metallic objects, pressure trauma is a significant potential problem. Eyelids must be taped close, with proper lubrication applied to prevent corneal abrasions. A surgical towel is used for a head drape.

Dental injury is a common complication. All patients should have their dentition examined carefully prior to endoscopy, with appropriate corrections made. A tooth guard must be used if dentition is present. In small children or edentulous adults, a gauze sponge can be substituted. The teeth should never be used as a fulcrum. This is most commonly a problem with the central maxillary dentition. If a tooth is found to be missing at the end of a procedure, an extensive search should be made to find it, including a chest x-ray and neck films. It should never be assumed that the tooth has been swallowed.

The endoscopist needs to exercise gentle care during patient positioning. Rapid, forceful extension of the cervical spine in elderly patients or those with degenerative disease can result in atlantoaxial instability; neurological impairment may be a secondary complication.[8] If a patient presents with neurological or cervical complaints prior to endoscopy, appropriate consultation should be obtained. Children with Down's syndrome risk atlantoaxial subluxation. Flexion and extension films of the C spine should be obtained prior to the procedure in susceptible individuals.

DIRECT LARYNGOSCOPY

Direct laryngoscopy may serve as both a diagnostic and therapeutic procedure. There are many different types of laryngoscopes suited for different diagnostic and therapeutic purposes. In general, the endoscopist should use a laryngoscope that gives the largest field of vision but that is not too large for the oral cavity. An inappropriate scope can cause

Table 5–1. Laryngoscopy

Complications
  Dental trauma
  Cervical spine injury
  Oral cavity edema
  Cardiac arrhythmias
  Laryngeal disruption
    Vocal cord injury
    Anterior commissure web
    Posterior glottic stenosis laryngospasm
    Laryngeal edema
  Epiglottis injury

oral or pharyngeal edema and dental trauma. If a difficult laryngoscopy is expected, intravenous steroids should be given prior to the start of the procedure.

The larynx is extremely sensitive to stimulation. Cardiac arrhythmias are a well-known risk, especially in hypoxic patients. Two techniques can help decrease the chance of complications. The first is the routine spraying of the larynx with lidocaine prior to any instrumentation. The other is avoidance of hypoxia during the procedure. Efficient use of time can help facilitate the latter, but in the pediatric population and in those with poor pulmonary function, this may not be enough. New laryngoscopes are available through which oxygen can be insufflated, thus decreasing the chance of hypoxia.[9,10]

When possible, operative laryngoscopy should be performed with the aid of a microscope. (Fig. 5–2). Unless involved by the lesion, the underlying muscles should not be violated. Magnification decreases the chance of injury to normal tissue. Special microlaryngeal instruments are available. Various suspension devices are available to fixate the scope during microlaryngoscopy. An instrument stand that attaches to the operating table can support the suspension device and does not require adjustment when changing the table height.

Certain anatomic areas should not be violated during biopsy. Most prominent are the anterior commissure and the posterior glottis. Disrupting the anterior larynx bilaterally can cause web formation. Scarring in the interarytenoid area may cause tethering of the arytenoids (Fig. 5–3), leading to a pseudoparalysis.

Voice change should not be considered a routine finding after laryngeal biopsy for benign lesions. With the field of voice therapy expanding rapidly, many patients are undergoing extensive speech analysis, including stroboscopy, prior to laryngeal procedures.

During or after any laryngoscopy, the physician must always be prepared for the possibility of laryngospasm. Positive pressure is the initial treatment. Paralysis and intubation may be required. Succinylcholine and intravenous access should be available. To reduce the risk of laryngospasm, it is helpful to spray the vocal cords with lidocaine at the beginning and end of the procedure.

Other complications of laryngoscopy include laryngeal edema and severe odynophagia. Odynophagia is usually the result of the tip of the laryngoscope bending the epiglottis and compressing it against itself. Usually, this can be avoided by smooth placement of the laryngoscope blade. Some endoscopes are meant to be placed under the epiglottis, such as the anterior commissure models. Careful technique must be used with these instruments. Often patients with epiglottic trauma must be admitted to the hospital postoperatively for pain control and intravenous fluid administration. Edema is also usually technique related, caused by excessive manipulation. Close airway observation is critical in these patients.

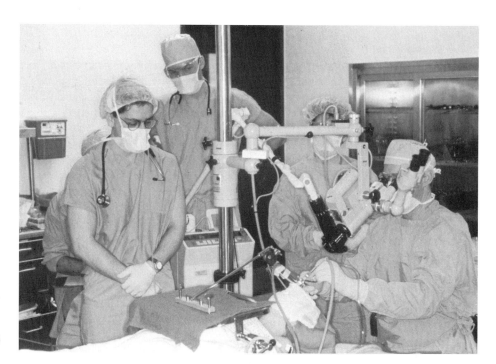

Figure 5–2. Proper laryngoscopy technique. Illustrated is a suspension laryngoscopy with the patient's face draped for a possible laser procedure.

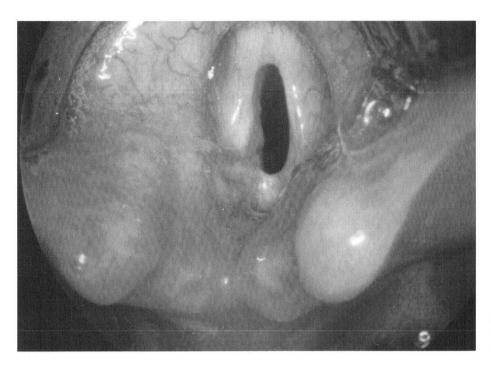

Figure 5–3. Posterior glottic stenosis secondary to disruption of mucosa in the interarytenoid area.

ESOPHAGOSCOPY

Flexible Esophagoscopy

In recent years, the flexible esophagoscope has become increasingly popular, with rigid endoscopy used mainly for foreign-body removal and some biopsies. The use of the flexible esophagoscope has allowed many procedures to be performed under local anesthesia with sedation.

Table 5–2. Esophagoscopy

Complications
   Dental trauma
   Cervical spine injury
   Bleeding
   Pharyngeal/esophageal perforation
   Pneumomediastinum
   Mediastinitis

A perceived advantage of flexible instruments is their safety, when compared with the rigid metal scopes. Although this may be true to a certain extent, flexible esophagoscopy remains a potentially dangerous procedure.[11] Studies have shown perforation rates below 1% for both flexible and rigid esophagoscopy.[12,13] With the lack of tactile feedback, perforation may occur with poor technique. The lack of tactile feedback also becomes a problem when using instruments through the side channel for the flexible endoscopes. Brushes and biopsy forceps may perforate the esophageal wall if not used properly. The instruments must be in direct view at all times.

Rigid Esophagoscopy

Proper technique for rigid esophagoscopy begins with positioning the patient. Most commonly, a shoulder roll is used to extend the neck. This should not be excessively large. Another method used to extend the neck is shown in Figure 5–4. With this head extension technique, the esophagus is in more of a direct line, and thus there is less chance of the instrument perforating the esophageal wall. This technique is riskiest in those patients with degenerative cervical spine disease, and it should be used cautiously in elderly patients.

Two procedures that deserve special attention are esophageal dilation and foreign-body removal. A variety of methods have been used to dilate the esophagus, including hydrostatic, pneumatic, and retrograde techniques. All run a higher risk of perforation than routine esophagoscopy. Dilation should not be performed without first viewing the strictured area endoscopically. Radiographs alone are insufficient. A useful rule of thumb for passing the mercury-filled bougies is to end the dilation after three consecutive sizes have been passed or when blood is first seen on the bougies, whichever occurs first. Dilation should never be attempted in patients taking high doses steroids because of the risk of perforation.[14]

Endoscopic removal of pointed esophageal foreign bodies is especially treacherous. Removal with the rigid esophagoscope is the treatment of choice, with the point-sheath technique the most efficacious.[15] If one is unable to remove the foreign body without sheathing the pointed edge, passage into the stomach is preferred. After removal of esophageal foreign bodies, especially those that have been present for extended periods, a second look to evaluate the area immediately after extraction is not recommended. Granulation tissue may be hiding a severely damaged portion of the wall, and there is a higher risk of perforation.

The risk of esophageal perforation is primarily related to the extent of the lesion for which esophagoscopy is indicated. This is especially true for sharp foreign bodies, esophageal malignancy, and severe caustic ingestions. Other predisposing

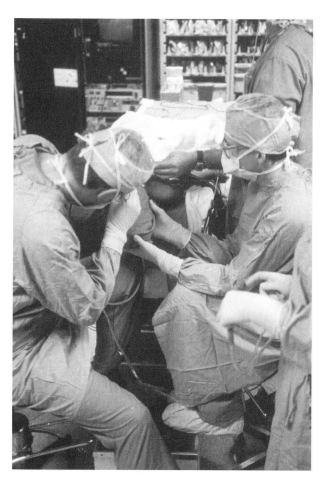

Figure 5–4. Proper esophagoscope technique. An assistant supports the head in an extended position. This gives the endoscopist a direct route into the esophagus.

factors include cervical spine disease and craniofacial anomalies that affect the mandible. Perforations due directly to instrumentation can usually be traced to poor technique.

Cervical esophageal ruptures usually occur in the posterior wall or through the pyriform sinus. Contamination starts in the retropharyngeal space or pretracheal space and can spread into the mediastinum. Thoracic perforations spread directly into the pleural space and/or mediastinum (Fig. 5–5).

The clinical manifestations of esophageal perforation vary with the site and size of the tear. Patients with cervical perforation experience neck pain and swelling, usually associated with neck crepitance. Fever and an elevated white blood count follow within several hours. Thoracic perforation causes immediate severe chest pain, dysphagia, and dyspnea. Fever and sepsis with shock follows rapidly in untreated cases. Physical and radiographic signs of pneumothorax may be present.

Morbidity and mortality due to mediastinitis remains high despite aggressive medical and surgical therapy. Physical signs of mediastinal involvement include asymmetrical chest movement during respiration and an audible rub due to pericardial effusion. Hypotension develops early and is poorly responsive to intravenous fluid hydration.

Plain radiographs of the chest hand neck show free air in the periesophageal soft tissues. The site and extent of the per-

foration can be demonstrated with a contrast esophagram using a water-soluble dye such as Gastographin or dilute barium.

With the possible exception of small cervical perforations, all patients should undergo surgical exploration with repair and drainage of the injury. Cervical injuries are approached through a lateral cervical approach to the retropharyngeal space. The tear should be repaired in two layers and the site should be drained. Thoracic perforations are usually approached through a left thoracotomy. Tube thoracostomy and mediastinal drainage are required. Severe thoracic lesions require a diverting pharyngostomy and a feeding gastrostomy.

Postoperatively, all patients receive intravenous fluids and antibiotics. Oral feedings can be reinstated after a contrast esophagram has documented closure of the perforation without leakage.

BRONCHOSCOPY

Manipulation of the tracheobronchial passages always carries the risk of airway obstruction (Table 5–3). To minimize the chance of complications, a thorough preoperative evaluation is necessary. This must include a history, physical examination, and a chest x-ray. Occasionally, bronchoscopy will be performed as an urgent life-saving technique. The patient may require airway stabilization with intubation.

Flexible bronchoscopy is most commonly performed in adults, with a major complication rate of 0.08%.[16] Rigid bronchoscopy under general anesthesia is now mostly used for foreign-body removal, pediatric endoscopy, and intraoperative evaluations. Although flexible endoscopes are considered safer and cause less trauma to the airway, the same potential dangers exist as with rigid endoscopes.

Before passing a bronchoscope, the larynx should be sprayed with lidocaine to minimize the chance of laryngospasm. Succinylcholine and recusitation equipment should be available. If used to pass the rigid bronchoscope, the laryngoscope should be removed when the bronchoscope has passed into the proximal trachea so that two hands can be used to stabilize the bronchoscope. Gentle manipulation is important because this is both the anatomic and temporal point in rigid bronchoscopy where most of the tissue edema is created (Fig. 5–6).

Biopsies are frequently performed during bronchoscopy. Bleeding usually ceases in a matter of minutes, although occasionally tamponade may be necessary. This is relatively easy with a rigid bronchoscope but is not possible with a flexible instrument. The suction channels on the fiberoptic scopes can be blocked easily, and clouding of the distal lens with blood is a constant problem. Special precautions should be taken during transbronchial lung biopsies and tumor biopsies, especially of bronchial adenomas. A solution of 1/30,000 epinephrine should be available to spray down the bronchoscope to the bleeding site. Pneumothorax is also a risk after transbronchial lung biopsy, and a post biopsy chest x-ray is recommended.[17]

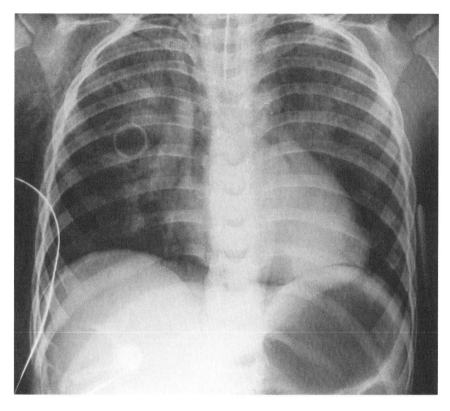

Figure 5–5. Pneumomediastinum following esophagoscopy.

Table 5–3. Bronchoscopy

Complications
  Dental trauma
  Cervical spine injury
  Laryngospasm
  Laryngeal edema
  Airway obstruction
  Bleeding
  Infection
  Pneumomediastinum
  Pneumothorax
  Bacteremia
  Fever
  Bronchospasm
  Cardiac arrhythmias

Fever following fiberoptic bronchoscopy occurs in 10% to 25% of patients.[18] Some of this can be attributed to bacteremia, whereas in other cases, fever may involve the transfer of toxins to the intravascular space. Bacteremia seems to be more common after bronchoalveolar lavage. Unfortunately, this procedure is often performed in immunocompromised patients who are most susceptible to systemic infection. Bacteremia has been linked to meningitis and pneumonia in postbronchoscopy patients.[19,20]

Bronchospasm can be a serious intraoperative and postoperative complication. Fortunately, it is an unusual occurrence in nonasthmatic patients. Believed to be at least partly mediated by efferent vagal pathways, death secondary to bronchospasm after fiberoptic bronchoscopy has been well docu-

mented. Aminophylline, steroids, and/or nebulizer treatments may be required. Tetracaine anesthesia is contraindicated in asthmatics.[21]

Cardiac arrhythmias are most likely to occur during hypoxia and have been reported in 40% of a prospectively studied flexible bronchoscopy group.[22] Topical lidocaine anesthesia during flexible bronchoscopy seems to have a protective effect. Additional precautions include avoiding elective bronchoscopy in patients with recent cardiac events or significant cardiac compromise.

Pediatric bronchoscopy has undergone major advances in recent years as optical systems and anesthetic techniques have improved. Significant challenges remain, however, and the occasional pediatric endoscopist should be extremely cautious.

One of the most significant sequelae after endoscopy in the pediatric age group is subglottic and glottic edema. This is usually the result of the use of instruments that are too large for the airway. In addition, some of the specifications listed on the endoscopes are erroneous and can be misleading.[23]

Poor technique can also contribute to postoperative edema. A bronchoscope should never be passed forcefully through a narrow subglottis. In this situation, a rigid telescope by itself and anesthesia via insufflation should be able to provide an adequate view.

Foreign-body removal during bronchoscopy presents the greatest risk of any airway procedure. Although the removal of these objects is being performed with better lighting and improved equipment, there is still a risk of creating an uncontrolled airway. Backup light cords, light source, suction, and a spare bronchoscope should be present. An extra broncho-

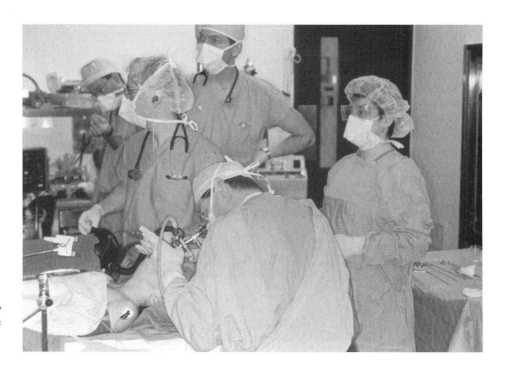

Figure 5-6. Proper bronchoscopy technique. Note the position of the endoscopist and other operating room personnel.

scope is useful for situations in which the foreign body occludes the primary endoscope during removal. A long alligator forceps should be present to grab objects that may lodge in the larynx after being stripped at the vocal cords.

General anesthesia during spontaneous ventilation is the preferred anesthetic technique for foreign-body removal. Supplemental topical anesthesia should also be used. Systemic paralysis and positive-pressure ventilation can cause distal displacement of the foreign body and can lead to complete loss of a marginal airway.

When passing the endoscope for a bronchial foreign body, the suspected normal bronchus should be inspected first. If clear, the involved bronchus should then be entered. Care must be taken not to impact the object further. Once the object is grasped, the bronchoscope should be advanced over the grasping instrument rather than pulling back the forceps into the bronchoscope. If the foreign body becomes dislodged in the trachea, it should be pushed back with a suction tip or other instrument into the bronchus, where it was originally located. This is much safer than attempting to remove an object in the trachea, where it may break into several pieces and potentially lodge in both bronchi. Finally, a finite amount of time should be allotted to remove a foreign body. Considerable edema can result from extensive instrumentation, and it is often wise to return to the endoscopy suite after a course of steroids and antibiotics.

The foregoing information pertains mostly to foreign-body removal with rigid bronchoscopes. Although flexible bronchoscopy has a role in diagnosing pediatric airway abnormalities, it is clearly an inferior method in dealing with foreign bodies.[24] Limiting its use are inadequate suction capability, lack of ventilation, limited forceps selection, and inability to remove impacted foreign bodies.

REFERENCES

1. Webb SF, Vall-Spinosa A. Outbreaks of serratia marcescens associated with the flexible fiberbronchoscope. *Chest*. 1975; 68:703–708.
2. Leers WD. Disinfecting endoscopes: How not to transmit mycobacterium tuberculosis by bronchoscopy. *Can Med Assoc J*. 1980;123:275–280.
3. Birnie GG, Quigley EM, Clements GB, et al. Endoscopic transmission of hepatitis B virus. *Gut*. 1983;24:171–174.
4. Kacmarke RG, Moore RM, McCrohan J, et al. Multi-state investigation of the actual disinfection/sterilization of endoscopes in health care facilities. *Am J Med*. 1992;92:257–261.
5. Sparicidin recall. Food and Drug Administration; 1991.
6. Ledbettr JL, Rasch DK, Pollard TG, et al. Reducing the risks of largnygoscopy in anesthetized infants. *Anesthesia*. 1988; 43(2):151–153.
7. Marsh BR, Ravich WJ. Laryngoscopy, bronchoscopy, and esophagoscopy. In: Johns ME, ed. *Complications of Otolaryngology— Head and Neck Surgery*. Vol 2. Toronto: BD Decker; 1986.
8. Norton JD, Manhala G. Atlanto-axial instability revisited: An alert for endoscopists. *Ann Otol Rhinol Laryngol*. 1982;91: 567–570.
9. Ledbettr JL, Rasch DK, Pollard TG, et al. Reducing the risks of laryngoscopy in anesthetized infants. *Anesthesia*. 1988; 43(2):151–153.
10. Parsons DS. New set of pediatric laryngoscopes. *Ann Otol Rhinol Laryngol*. 1990;99(11):892–895.
11. Shahmir M, Schuman BM. Complications of fiberoptic endoscopy. *Gastrointest Endosc*. 1980;26:86–91.
12. Palmer ED, Witts CW. Survey of gastroscopic and esophagoscopic accidents: Report of Committee of Accidents of the American Gastroscopic Society. *JAMA*. 1957;164:2012–2015.
13. Patterson DJ, Graham DY, Smith JL, et al. Natural history of benign esophageal stricture treated by dilatation. *Gastroenterology*. 1983;85:346–360.
14. Tucker GF Jr, Tucker JA. Complications in endoscopic procedures. In: Conley JJ, ed. *Complications in Head and Neck Surgery*. Philadelphia: WB Saunders; 1979:304.

15. Jackson D. *Bronchoscopy and Esophagoscopy*. Philadelphia: WB Saunders; 1927.

16. Credle WF Jr, Smiddy JF, Elliott RC. Complications of fiberoptic bronchoscopy. *Am Rev Respir Dis*. 1974;109:67–72.

17. Muntz HR, Wallace M, Lusk RP. Pediatric transbronchial lung biopsy. *Ann Otol Rhinol Laryngol*. 1992;101:135–136.

18. Pubin J, Suter PM. Diagnostic bronchoalveolar lavage in patients with pneumonia produces sepsis-like systemic effects. *Intensive Care Med*. 1992;18(1):6–10.

19. Beyt BE, King DK, Glew RH. Fatal pneumonitis and septicemia after fiberoptic bronchoscopy. *Chest*. 1977;72:105–107.

20. Peteira, W, Kovnat DM, Khan MA, et al. Fever and pneumonia after flexible fiberoptic bronchoscopy. *Am Rev Respir Dis*. 1975;112:59–64.

21. Tucker GF Jr, Tucker JA. Complications in endoscopic procedures. In: Conley JJ, ed. *Complications in Head and Neck Surgery*. Philadelphia: WB Saunders; 1979:294.

22. Katz AS, Michelson EL, Stawicki J, et al. Cardiac arrhythmias. *Arch Intern Med*. 1981;141:603–606.

23. Stankiewicz JA, Holinger LD. Endoscopic sizing: An attempt at uniformity. *Laryngoscope*. 1986;96(9):997–1001.

24. Sackner MA. State of the art bronchofibroscopy. *Am Rev Respir Dis*. 1973;111:65–88.

6 Complications of Laser Surgery

Elie E. Rebeiz, M.D., Stanley M. Shapshay, M.D.

Prevention of complications dictates a thorough understanding of the interaction of laser energy with living tissue. With this information, the surgeon understands the therapeutic effects of the laser and is able to predict the potential risks and avoid complications when using lasers in surgery. The surgeon must be well acquainted with the laser being used and its unique soft-tissue effects, which are wavelength specific. Important variables must be considered, such as the energy used (wattage and time of exposure), the different delivery modes available (micromanipulator, fiber, or handpiece), and the diameter of the emanating laser beam (commonly referred to as spot size). Use of medical lasers does not require an in-depth knowledge of the physics and engineering of the laser device. A basic technical background is necessary, however, and a set of operating room laser safety protocols should apply. The surgeon should be familiar with such technical terms as wavelength, power, energy, pulsed and continuous beam, power density, spot size, repetition rate, pulse duration, and focal length for proper communication with technician or nurse. It is also important to document the laser parameters used in each situation and, if possible, photodocument the pathologic process because it is not possible to obtain a pathologic specimen in some procedures, such as photocoagulation of a vascular malformation. Although surgeons tend to be independent by nature, an experienced nurse or an assistant trained in the use of the particular laser and its wavelength should always be present in the operating room to assist the surgeon.

Hazards from laser surgery to the patient, surgeon, and operating room personnel (Table 6–1) can be minimized by following simple safety guidelines, usually taught in laser training courses. A study by Ossoff[1] demonstrated that attendance at a hands-on laser surgery course that stressed safety precautions was associated with a reduced rate of laser-related complications. This was true when a selected group of otolaryngologists who participated in the course was compared with another group of otolaryngologists who were members of a senior otolaryngology society and were surveyed solely on the basis of their society membership.

Many of the lasers used in clinical practice are nonvisible, which increases the risk of injury, especially to the retina.

Table 6–1. Complications of Laser Surgery

Patient
    Burn to skin/mucosa
    Endotracheal tube fire
    Tissue edema
    Pneumothorax
    Delayed healing
    Bleeding
    Scarring
    Ignition of drapes
Operating room personnel
    Burns to skin
    Eye injury
    Contamination from laser plume
    Electric shock

The patient's eyes should always be covered with wet gauze and aluminum foil, and the face is covered with a wet towel. These towels become dry during a lengthy procedure and must be kept moist at all times. Appropriate glasses, specific for each laser wavelength, should be worn by all personnel present in the operating room, and visible signs should always be put on the doors warning incoming personnel about laser use in that room.

The assistants should be trained to put the laser in the standby mode routinely when it is not being used. This will prevent an accident if the operator depresses the foot switch. In this regard, it is important to separate the foot pedal for the electrocautery from the foot pedal for the laser because the surgeon can easily depress the wrong pedal. This creates a fire hazard to surgical drapes and danger for operating room personnel and the patient. Once again, if the laser is put in the standby mode every time it is not in use, it will not be activated by accident. As the surgeon becomes more experienced with laser surgery, however, he or she tends to become more complacent about safety principles.

The rate of complications of laser surgery in the tracheobronchial airway was reviewed in 1984 in a large, multi-institutional study[2] combining centers from the United States and Europe. This report included 1503 procedures

64

using the neodymium:yttrium aluminum garnet (Nd:YAG) laser for bronchoscopy performed in 1156 patients (Table 6–2). More than two thirds of the procedures were performed under general anesthesia with a rigid bronchoscope. Six deaths occurred in this large series, all of which were attributed to hypoxemia resulting from excessive anesthesia, bleeding, or retained secretions (Table 6–2). No instances of fire, tracheal perforations, or massive arterial hemorrhage occurred.

In a survey[3] of laser complications from 229 otolaryngologists, 81 complications were reported by 208 responders. The most common complications were endotracheal explosion (28), laryngeal web (15), and facial burn (9). Prevention of complications was stressed (Table 6–3).

We have used lasers in surgery of the nasal and oral cavities, oropharynx and hypopharynx, larynx, tracheobronchial tree, and facial skin in more than 5000 patients since 1982 without any airway fires, burns, or eye injuries. This is a testimonial to strict adherence to safety protocols and to laser safety training by all personnel.

This chapter focuses on complications of laser surgery in surgery of the head and neck and airway. A brief discussion of complications in otology will be included only for completeness.

OPERATIVE COMPLICATIONS

In otolaryngology, complications are particularly possible in the airway, and firing of the laser beam often occurs in a field filled with anesthetic gases and oxygen. Patients with airway obstruction present a challenge to the anesthesiologist and to the otolaryngologist. The laser is often used to debulk, in an almost bloodless procedure, a large obstructive lesion in the larynx and trachea that would otherwise be unresectable.

Table 6–2. Immediate and Delayed Complications of Laser Bronchoscopy in a Multi-institutional Study of 1503 Cases

COMPLICATION	NUMBER OF PATIENTS
Immediate	
Cardiovascular	7
Bradycardia	3
Cardiac arrest	2
Circulatory collapse	2
Hemorrhage	14
Pneumothorax	3
Delayed	
Cardiovascular	8
Anoxia	3 (2 deaths)
Cardiac arrest	2
Circulatory collapse	1 (1 death)
Myocardial infarction	2 (2 deaths)
Hemorrhage	2 (1 death)

From Dumon et al.[2]

Table 6–3. Complications of CO_2 Laser Surgery

COMPLICATION	NUMBER
Endotracheal explosion	28
Laryngeal web	15
Facial burn	9
Pneumothorax	5
Laryngeal stenosis 4	
Endotracheal cuff ignition	3
Postoperative hemorrhage	3
Subglottic stenosis	3
Cottonoid ignition	2
Subcutaneous emphysema	2
Laryngeal edema	2
Tracheal stenosis	1
Endobronchial explosion	1
Perichondritis	1
Carbon granuloma	1
Pharyngeal burn	1
Total	81

From Fried.[3]

The anesthesiologist and the otolaryngologist must pay special attention to the type and size of the endotracheal tube used, the way it is fixed in place, and the way the cuff is inflated. In many instances, a tube cannot be used, and a Venturi jet ventilation system is needed. The anesthesiologist and the otolaryngologist must work as a team and be prepared for potential complications, such as burns of vital structures, endotracheal tube fire, perforation of the trachea, or bleeding from a tumor into the distal airway.

Complications of Nd:YAG Laser Surgery

Although the Nd:YAG laser has had a remarkably safe record for more than 10 years, it remains the most powerful and perhaps the most dangerous of medical lasers presently available. The power density of the Nd:YAG laser is concentrated below the surface of the tissue as opposed to the surface effect of the carbon dioxide (CO_2) laser, necessitating intermittent exposure settings of 1 second or less at a power setting of less than 50 W (usually 40 to 45 W). Concentration of the laser power density below the tissue surface can cause tissue explosion or the so-called popcorn effect. This complication usually occurs when the laser is used at high powers (greater than 50 W) and long exposure times (several seconds).

Complications of CO_2 Laser Surgery

The CO_2 laser is useful for many procedures in otolaryngology; however, in many instances its use, particularly in the tracheobronchial airway, is difficult because of technical problems associated with delivery systems. It is somewhat awkward to use this laser in the trachea and bronchi because of limitations of the presently available waveguides and bronchoscopic coupler delivery systems (Fig. 6–1). It should not be used in laryngeal surgery when the exposure is suboptimal.

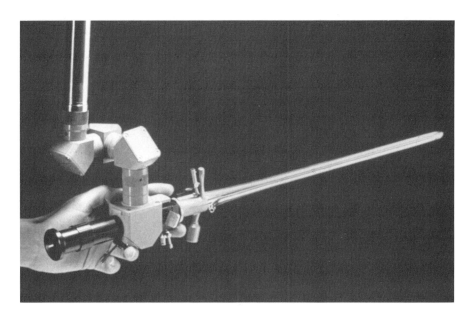

Figure 6–1. Endoscopic CO_2 laser coupler attached to the articulating arm used in bronchoscopy.

The laser should always be tested for proper alignment of the laser beam with the helium-neon aiming beam. Good binocular vision is essential. The operating microscope should be set at $16\times$ power initially and up to $25\times$ for precision microlaryngeal use. With the CO_2 laser, the surgeon should avoid using high energies and continuous exposure. This laser is not an efficient coagulating instrument and must not be used as an electrocautery. The surgeon should always observe the tissue being subjected to the laser beam to avoid drying the mucosa or "cooking" the tissues.

Bleeding may occur because the CO_2 laser does not coagulate vessels larger than 0.5 to 1 mm. This is encountered in large laryngeal and oral mucosal hypervascular lesions, and blood will obscure the view and absorb the laser energy. Occasional application of the electrocautery may be used to stop active bleeding, prevent delayed bleeding, and avoid aspiration of blood into the distal airway.

Fires

In general, the use of endotracheal tubes in bronchoscopic surgery should be avoided because of the risk of combustion, particularly in an oxygen-rich environment. In the laryngeal airway, this complication should never occur when care is taken. A time-honored standard is use of a red rubber endotracheal tube carefully wrapped with self-adherent aluminum tape. The polyvinylchloride tube should never be used because it is rapidly punctured by both the CO_2 and Nd:YAG laser beam, causing combustion and production of toxic fumes as well as a potential blow torch effect (Fig. 6–2). It would be difficult to defend use of this tube should a fire occur. External taping of the endotracheal tube does not protect the internal wall from combustion when the fiber of the Nd:YAG laser is used inside the tube (Figs. 6–3 and 6–4). A fire in an endotracheal tube is a catastrophic complication but fortunately is rare and can be avoided easily. Healy et al[4] reported nine complications in more than 4000 procedures.

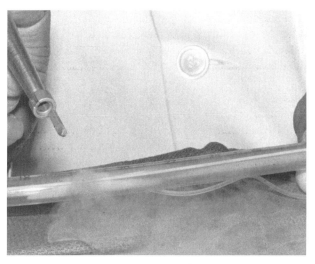

Figure 6–2. Fumes produced by ignition of a polyvinylchloride tube punctured by the CO_2 laser at 5 W continuous mode for 5 seconds with room air filling the tube.

The most common complication was endotracheal tube fire that occurred in six of nine patients. Ossoff and associates[5] reviewed CO_2 laser complications in 204 procedures and encountered no fires involving endotracheal tubes. A survey conducted by Fried[3] revealed the occurrence of endotracheal explosion in 28 of 81 complications, which was the most common complication reported (Table 6–3). Ossoff[1] compared the incendiary characteristics of three endotracheal tubes in various mixtures of oxygen and diluted with either helium or nitrogen. He found that the polyvinylchloride tube should not be used for laser surgery, even when wrapped with reflective metallic tape. The safest anesthetic gas mixture was 30% oxygen in helium; the addition of 2% halothane did not have an adverse effect. Both the Xomed (Jacksonville, Fla) lasershield and Rusch (New York, NY) red rubber endotracheal tubes were found to be safe when used with the laser in the pulsed mode in an atmosphere of 100% oxygen. When the

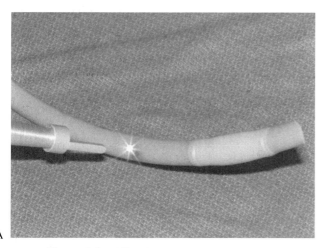

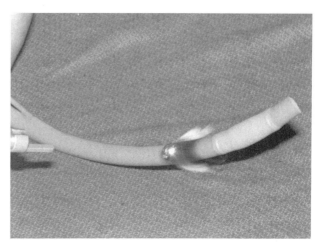

A   B

Figure 6–3. **(A).** Glare produced by aiming the CO_2 laser beam at a nonwrapped Rusch red rubber tube. **(B).** Room air filling the tube followed by rapid ignition.

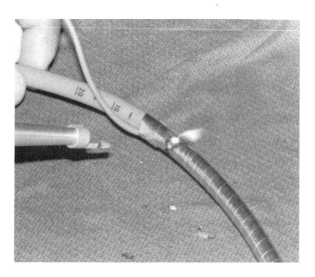

Figure 6–4. Even the perfectly wrapped Risch red rubber tube can be set on fire when subjected to the laser beam long enough.

laser was used in the continuous mode, both tubes ignited in an atmosphere of 30% oxygen in helium. These findings challenged the previously reported levels of safety associated with the use of an unwrapped Xomed tube. Based on the results of this investigation Ossoff[1] concluded that both the Rusch red rubber tube and the Xomed laser-shield tube should be wrapped with reflective metallic tape when used for microlaryngeal surgery with the CO_2 laser.

During Nd:YAG laser bronchoscopy, ignition of the sheath of the flexible bronchoscope can cause a fire. It is crucial to be able to see the laser fiber at all times before activating the laser. The laser fiber must be kept distal to the tip of the bronchoscope (Fig. 6–5). However, combustion of the flexible bronchoscope most often occurs from ignition of charred tumor fragments or flammable material, such as the endotracheal tube. We prefer to use the Nd:YAG laser with a rigid bronchoscope specifically modified for laser fiber application.

Even during rigid bronchoscopy, however, fires may occur. The patients are typically in respiratory distress with poor pulmonary reserve and require high oxygen saturation during anesthesia. Environmental oxygen should be kept at less than 50% when possible. The immediate response to an endobronchial fire is prompt removal of all flammable materials, such as plastic stent devices. If an airway fire occurs during use of the CO_2 laser in the larynx, the oxygen should be disconnected, and the endotracheal tube should be removed immediately. Inspection for tracheobronchial burns should then be carried out to assess the extent of injury, and respiratory support should follow. The patient should be treated with antibiotics and steroids to reduce the inflammatory response and decrease the possibility of subsequent scarring, and close monitoring should be undertaken postoperatively.

Flammable materials within the rigid bronchoscopic system are the laser fiber itself and the plastic suction catheter. The laser fiber should be kept free of debris at all times, and plastic material should be kept proximal to the laser tip when possible (Fig. 6–5).

When a red rubber endotracheal tube is chosen for laser laryngoscopy, the endotracheal tube should be hand wrapped the morning of surgery. The proper wrapping of an endotracheal tube with metallic tape significantly reduces the risk of fire. Care must be taken not to leave any uncovered parts. Wrapping is continuous from distal to proximal so that about 10 cm of the distal tube is covered, and the metallic tape is overlapped so that the thickness of the tape is doubled. The surgeon should inspect the tube before and after its use. In the presence of a tracheotomy tube, the tube is replaced by a wrapped endotracheal tube or, if preferred, a metal tracheotomy tube. The cuff should be inflated with sterile saline solution colored with methylene blue so that, if penetrated by the laser beam, blue-colored liquid is released, which is identified easily. The saline solution also protects against a fire.

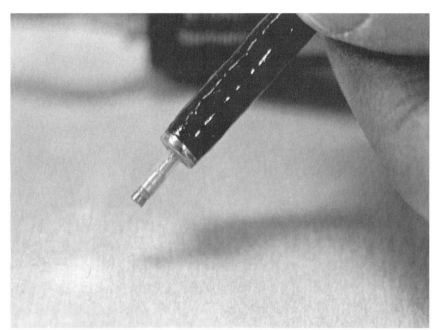

A

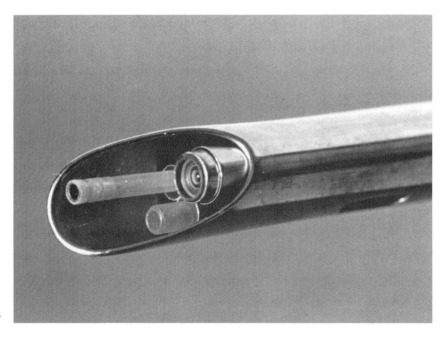

B

Figure 6–5. Ignition of the sheath of the flexible bronchoscope or the plastic suction catheter can cause fire. It is important to be able to see the laser fiber at all times before activating the laser by keeping the laser fiber distal to the tip of the **(A)** flexible bronchoscope and **(B)** rigid telescope.

Burns to Skin and Mucosa

While the laser is being aimed at one vocal cord, the opposite cord should be protected and kept in the lateral position to avoid transmission of heat and possible reflection of the laser beam and indirect injury. To assist in preventing collateral thermal damage to the contralateral vocal cord, we prefer to use an endotracheal tube to keep the vocal cords apart. In addition, a small whistletip suction is used close to the site of laser impact to remove the steam of vaporization before

it has a chance to damage surrounding tissues. The subglottic area and the cuff of the tube should be protected by moist cottonoid pledgets at all times. The laser nurse is instructed to interrupt the procedure every 10 to 15 minutes to moisten the cottonoid pledgets.

Burns to the lips and teeth are particularly possible while excising intraoral lesions.[5] These complications can be avoided easily by covering the face with a moist towel and by aiming the laser beam with precision. Burns to these structures are also possible during laryngeal surgery and are avoided by wrapping the face carefully with moist cotton drapes that are kept moist by a laser nurse during a long procedure.

Burns may be especially serious when the noncontact Nd:YAG laser is used (Fig. 6–6). The effect of the laser cannot be seen on the surface, which does not permit the surgeon to appreciate the depth of damage. The laser must be kept away from reflective surfaces, such as refractors, and the laser should be used in the discontinuous mode. While treating mucosal vascular malformations of the oral cavity, nose, or larynx, the surgeon must be conservative with laser energy because tissue necrosis up to 1 cm below the surface can occur, causing severe swelling and delayed tissue necrosis (Fig. 6–7). Blanching should be the endpoint for these lesions; otherwise, necrosis will be the sequelae.

Injury to operating room personnel is also possible (Table 6–1). The eyes are always protected carefully; however, the face, the clothes, and particularly the hands are at risk, especially when handing instruments to the surgeon and being in the line of fire. A burn to the skin of operating room personnel is usually mild because of reflex withdrawal and, hence, short exposure. With the CO_2 laser, the burn is usually superficial (ie, less than 1 mm deep). The noncontact Nd:YAG laser beam is usually defocused, and even at high power the energy is scattered over a large surface area, causing minimal damage.

Perforation of the Tracheobronchial Tree

The risk of tracheobronchial perforation with the Nd:YAG laser is much greater than with the CO_2 or argon laser. Depth of penetration and scatter are considerably greater with this wavelength, and its soft-tissue interaction is less predictable (Fig. 6–8). The point of maximal power density is not at the surface, as it is with the CO_2 laser, but is a few millimeters below the surface, which cannot be seen readily by the surgeon. Underlying tissue, such as lung, blood vessels, nerves, or muscles, can therefore be damaged, resulting in severe (sometimes fatal) complications.

Cautious intermittent (1 second or less) Nd:YAG laser irradiation using less than 50 W of power is advisable during endoscopy. The Nd:YAG laser fiber should always be used parallel with and never perpendicular to the tracheobronchial wall. The tip of the rigid bronchoscope can be used as a palpating device to help determine the interface of the tumor and the tracheal cartilage. Laser irradiation at continued high power of greater than 40 W with exposure times of greater than 1 second may cause explosive rupture of the tissues—the so-called popcorn effect. The surgeon may see blanching of the surface of the tissue followed by charring before explosion of tissue. Our technique to diminish total laser energy is to use the laser as a no-touch deep coagulating device to diminish the vascularity of the tumor. When the tumor is blanched, the rigid bronchoscope is used to core out the tissue. The laser is then used on the base of the tumor for effective coagulation of the vascular supply to achieve good hemostasis.

Hemorrhage

Hemorrhage from the larynx or oral cavity using the CO_2 laser can be encountered and is usually controlled by defocusing the laser. On occasion, hemorrhage may persist from a slightly large blood vessel and requires control with the electrocautery. Resection of a major vocal cord or excision of a tumor of the oral cavity requires setting up for use of the electrocautery. Once again, it is important to stress that the foot pedals for the laser and electrocautery unit be separated to prevent confusion.

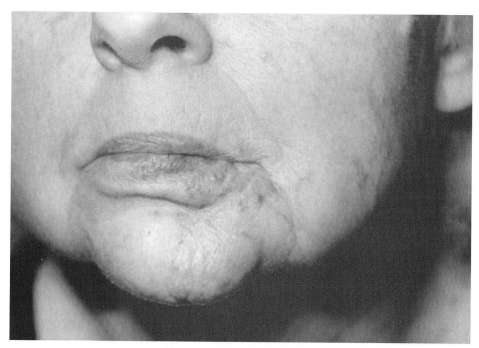

Figure 6–6. Scarring of the skin after Nd:YAG laser coagulation of a venous malformation involving the cutaneous and mucosal surfaces of the lower lip and part of the left commissure.

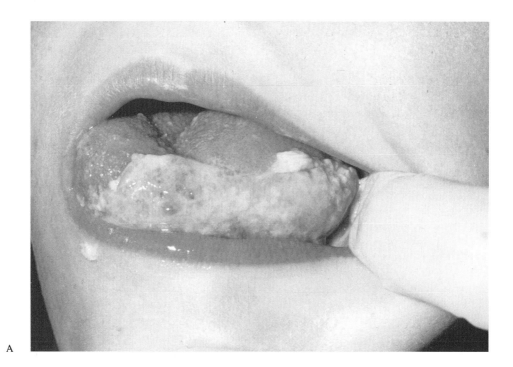

A

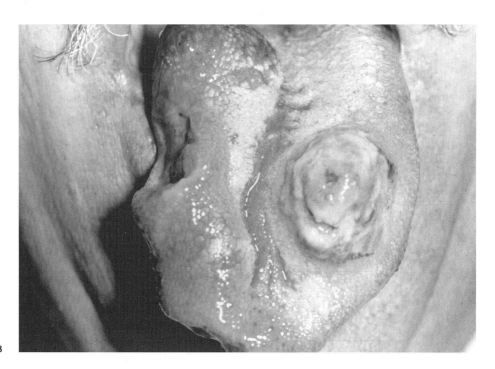

B

Figure 6–7. **(A).** Swelling of the tongue and mucosal sloughing 48 hours after Nd:YAG laser photocoagulation of a lymphangioma in a young boy. **(B).** Delayed partial necrosis of the tongue is the result of excessive laser photocoagulation of a venous malformation in an adult.

The most common hemorrhagic situation is persistent uncontrolled bleeding of the tracheobronchial tree. Massive hemorrhage is usually caused by perforation of a major pulmonary blood vessel and, fortunately, is a rare complication. However, life-threatening hypoxemia may occur from the accumulation of distal tracheobronchial hemorrhagic secretions. Interruption of resection of the tumor and achieving hemostasis are important and are followed by tracheobronchial toilet distal to the site of the tumor. Two semirigid suction catheters passed through the rigid bronchoscope are used to maintain a dry operative field. The laser is applied at a coagulating power of 30 to 40 W, with the fiber about 2 cm from the target tissue. Coagulation should begin circumferentially around the bleeding site and end at the area itself.

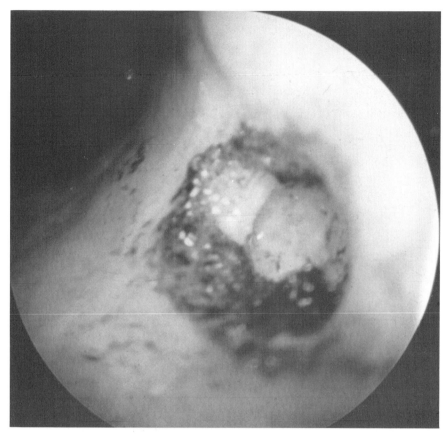

Figure 6–8. Charring may occur during laser treatment, leading to rapid absorption of laser beam and tracheal perforation. This is an experimental tracheal wall perforation in a canine caused by the noncontact Nd:YAG laser.

Massive bronchial hemorrhage necessitates placing the patient in the lateral safety position with the healthy lung above the affected lung. With the patient in this position, the ventilating bronchoscope is used to evacuate blood and secretions and to achieve patency of the airway. Heroic measures should not be taken when hemorrhage secondary to perforation of a pulmonary artery occurs. These patients have poor potential for survival because their carcinoma is not curable, and they usually will not respond to resuscitative measures.

Hypoxemia

The major cause of death during and after tracheobronchial laser resection is hypoxemia. Poor ventilation can be the result of a collection of distal secretions and debris as well as induced respiratory depression caused by anesthetic medications. Uncontrolled hypoxemia leads to cardiovascular complications, such as arrhythmia, bradycardia, myocardial infarction, and subsequent cardiac arrest. Constant monitoring of oxygen saturation using a finger pulse oximeter and frequent monitoring of blood gases are important with high-risk patients. Adequate ventilation and frequent tracheobronchial toilet should be the constant preoccupation of the endoscopist during the laser procedure.

Hypoxemia during laser laryngoscopy can occur in patients with chronic obstructive pulmonary disease if the anesthesiologist is too concerned about the danger of fire with the use of 100% oxygen. It is reasonable to use a helium-oxygen mixture to diminish flammability; however, the overriding consideration is adequate ventilation in these high-risk patients.

Injury to Neural Tissue

When working near nerves, the operator should be careful and predict the extent of thermal scatter around the irradiated field. When hit directly with a CO_2 laser beam, nerve tissue will be injured; however, little indirect thermal damage will result from the CO_2 laser when aiming at adjacent tissue. The Nd:YAG laser, on the other hand, can produce thermal damage up to several millimeters around the target, thus putting surrounding neural tissue at risk. This is important in parotid surgery, neck surgery, or middle ear surgery. The contact Nd:YAG laser would be preferable to noncontact application to limit tissue scatter and deep penetration in a noncontrolled fashion. The contact Nd:YAG laser with the appropriate tip configuration could be used as a precise thermal scalpel.

Several investigators have suggested potential nerve damage during laser surgery. Recently, an animal study by Qadir and Kennedy[6] showed significant thermal damage to the facial nerve during decompression with the holmium:yttrium aluminum garnet (Ho:YAG) laser compared with the drill. Considerable elevation of the temperature and severe nerve degeneration were noted while the mastoid portion of the facial nerve was being decompressed with the Ho:YAG laser. The Ho:YAG laser is a new pulsed laser that limits thermal diffusion. It has good bone interaction and has been used clinically in otolaryngology for endoscopic sinus surgery and endoscopic dacryocystorhinostomy. It should not be used near exposed nerves.

Injury to the Eyes

Because of the extreme care and the safety precautions taken during laser surgery, injury to the eyes has become rare. Unfortunately, experienced laser surgeons tend to become somewhat cavalier and are the most common violators of the safety protocol. Injury to the eyes of experienced workers is actually more common in the laser industry for the same reason.

The site of damage to the eyes differs with different laser wavelengths. With use of visible wavelengths, the laser beam is transmitted through the cornea, lens, and vitreous of the eye to the retina and choroid, where it is transformed to heat, and damage may occur. This is true for the argon wavelength, which is used for coagulation of pigmented lesions and blood vessels on the fundus. In the case of the far infrared invisible CO_2 laser, all the heat is absorbed anteriorly at the cornea or sclera. This risk is eliminated by using appropriate eyewear for each wavelength, which will absorb all the laser light and thus protect the eyes.

The helium-neon light used for aiming the laser beam can emit 1 to 2 mW of power. Although this amount of power is presumed to be safe, direct eye contact with this beam must be avoided. A general rule is never look directly into the source of laser output regardless of the laser and its purported low output.

Inhalation of Laser Plume

Some investigators have suggested that smoke produced from laser vaporization of living tissue may present a hazard to exposed personnel. Garden and associates[7] found intact human papillomavirus DNA in the laser plume of patients being treated for skin warts. Sawchuk et al[8] also demonstrated the presence of live human papillomavirus in the plume of similar patients. Odors detected during laser surgery strongly suggest the presence of noxious gases or particles present in the laser plume and raise questions regarding the efficiency of the smoke evacuators being used. To our knowledge, no known cases of viral contamination from laser plume contents have appeared in the literature. Garden et al,[7] however, showed that particles from the smoke contain live DNA that was inoculated into experimental animals, causing tumors to grow.

In any procedure in which laser smoke occurs, precautions should be taken to remove the smoke efficiently with laser smoke evacuators. Appropriate laser operating room masks should be used. Dual suction should be present—one for mucus, blood, and secretions and the second one for smoke and steam. Constant suctioning in a closed ventilation system is important, and special care must be taken when using a Venturi system not to diminish the fraction of inspired oxygen beyond a safe level. Laser instruments should have built-in suction chambers to evacuate smoke and filters in the suction lines to prevent clogging.

Otology Complications

The CO_2 and argon lasers have been used in otology for middle ear surgery, myringotomy, acoustic neuromas, and glomus tumors. Although the tissue effects of these two lasers are superficial, their use in the ear carries many risks and avoiding complications depends mainly on the expertise of the operator. The laser beam should be focused on the target area to avoid inadvertent damage because the intensity of the beam is greatly reduced away from the focal point.

Heat can build up, especially on dry surfaces, leading to charring of tissue and thermal damage to surrounding structures, such as the saccule and the facial nerve. Injury to the facial nerve is possible as a result of direct exposure of the fallopian canal or because of indirect heat propagation while vaporizing the adjacent footplate. Damage to the inner ear has been reported[9] in animals with the CO_2 and argon lasers. Gantz et al[10] demonstrated perforation of the saccule in three of eight ears of cats.

POSTOPERATIVE COMPLICATIONS

Delayed tissue necrosis can occur up to several days after laser treatment. This is particularly true with the Nd:YAG laser because surrounding tissue damage is considerable, which may lead to delayed necrosis. If this happens to a neighboring blood vessel, massive postoperative hemorrhage may occur. If the tracheal wall undergoes necrosis slowly, delayed tracheal perforation, pneumothorax, and even death may occur.

As with any type of laryngeal surgery, and particularly after CO_2 laser laryngeal surgery, the patient should be watched for delayed laryngeal edema, and perioperative steroids are frequently administered to avoid this complication. This usually occurs as a result of manipulation of the laryngeal mucosa with suction and probes or possibly from thermal insult to the mucosa. It is extremely important to administer cool mist in the immediate postoperative period. It must also be stressed to the patient that humidification must be continued, particularly during the dry winter months, until healing has taken place. Smoking or exposure to smoke after laser surgery on the airway is extremely dangerous because further drying, crusting, and subsequent infection and airway obstruction may take place.

The postoperative period is critical after laser bronchoscopy, and most complications occur from delayed cardiovascular sequelae related to hypoxia. Hypoxia can be the result of a collapsed lung, pneumothorax, hemothorax, or pulmonary edema.

Postoperative septicemia may occur as a result of routine secretions and subsequent atelectasis. When laser resection has been completed, the flexible bronchoscope is used to clear

Table 6–4. Complications of Laser Bronchoscopy
Lahey Clinic Experience

COMPLICATION	OPERATING ROOM	RECOVERY ROOM	AFTER RECOVERY ROOM	TOTAL	DEATHS
Cardiovascular					
Arrhythmias	3	5	10	18	0
Myocardial infarction	0	0	3	3	2
Hemorrhage	1	0	1	2	0
Hypotension	2	1	0	3	0
Pericarditis	0	0	1	1	0
Pulmonary edema	0	1	0	1	0
Respiratory					
Bronchial obstruction	0	0	3	3	0
Hypoxemia	6	2	0	8	0
Pneumothorax	1	0	1	2	1
Bronchospasm	0	1	3	4	0
Respiratory failure	0	3	5	8	1
Other					
Fever	0	0	3	3	0
Laryngospasm	1	0	0	1	0
Total	14	13	30	57	4
Percent	24.6	22.8	52.6	100	7

From Beamis et al.[11]

distal secretions and reexpand segments of the lung that may have been blocked and collapsed during the procedure or may be secondary to the obstructing tumor. Postoperative atelectasis is usually a result of insidious accumulation of distal blood clots.

Fortunately, in more than 400 laser bronchoscopies performed between 1982 and 1993 at the Lahey Clinic,[11] only one death occurred during surgery and that was secondary to tension pneumothorax and pericardial tamponade (Table 6–4). No major hemorrhage, fire, or postoperative septicemia occurred. Two patients with severe coronary artery disease died of myocardial infarction in the postoperative period.

With more than 20 years' experience with laser applications in otolaryngology head and neck surgery, laser safety protocols have been established that should ensure safe use of laser technology in surgery. With each new laser wavelength that is developed for use in clinical practice, new standards and safety guidelines will be established that should be added to the existing protocols, and strict adherence is mandatory. The most important element in safety is attention to details, and the ultimate responsibility lies with the surgeon.

REFERENCES

1. Ossoff RH. Laser safety in otolaryngology—head and neck surgery: Anesthetic and educational considerations for laryngeal surgery. *Laryngoscope.* 1989;99(suppl 48):1–26.
2. Dumon JF, Shapshay S, Bourcereau J, et al. Principles for safety in application of neodymium-YAG laser in bronchology. *Chest.* 1984;86:163–168.
3. Fried MP. A survey of the complications of laser laryngoscopy. *Arch Otolaryngol Head Neck Surg.* 1984;110:31–34.
4. Healy GB, Strong MS, Shapshay S, Vaughan C, Jako G. Complications of CO$_2$ laser surgery of the aerodigestive tract: Experience of 4416 cases. *Otolaryngol Head Neck Surg.* 1984;92:13–18.
5. Ossoff RH, Hotaling AJ, Karlan MS, Sisson GA. CO$_2$ laser in otolaryngology-head and neck surgery: A retrospective analysis of complications. *Laryngoscope.* 1983;93:1287–1289.
6. Qadir R, Kennedy D. Use of the holmium:yttrium aluminum garnet (Ho:YAG) laser for cranial nerve decompression: An in vivo study using the rabbit model. *Laryngoscope.* 1993;103:631–636.
7. Garden JM, O'Banion MK, Sheinitz LS, et al. Papillomavirus in the vapor of carbon dioxide laser-treated verrucae. *JAMA.* 1988;259:1199–1202.
8. Sawchuk WS, Weber PJ, Lowy DR, Dzubow LM. Infectious papillomavirus in the vapor of warts treated with carbon dioxide laser or electrocoagulation: Detection and protection. *J Am Acad Dermatol.* 1989;21:41–49.
9. Wilpizeski C. Experimental labyrinthotomy in monkeys by argon and carbon dioxide lasers. *Otolarygol Head Neck Surg.* 1981;89:197–203.
10. Gantz BJ, Jenkins HA, Kishimoto S, Fisch U. Argon laser stapedotomy. *Ann Otol Rhinol Laryngol.* 1982;91:25–26.
11. Beamis JF Jr, Vergos K, Rebeiz EE, Shapshay SM. Endoscopic laser therapy for obstructing tracheobronchial lesions. *Ann Otol Rhinol Laryngol.* 1991;100:413–419.

7 Complications of Sinonasal Surgery

William R. Wilson, M.D.

PATIENT ASSESSMENT FOR NASAL AND SINUS SURGERY

Surgery for benign disease of the nose and paranasal sinuses should be undertaken with the objective of relieving one or all of the common symptoms of nasal or sinus disease—namely, respiratory obstruction, recurrent or persistent nasal infection, and acute or chronic pain. A highly focused preoperative evaluation is directed toward identifying the etiology of the symptoms so that a realistic surgical plan can be developed that has a high probability of providing the desired result. Most commonly an evaluation includes a thorough history followed by rhinoscopy, nasopharyngoscopy, cultures when indicated, and computerized tomography (CT scans) with coronal and axial views. Most patients are anxious to review CT scans with their doctor and, with some instruction, usually can readily understand the radiographic picture of a septal deviation or an opacified sinus and the pathophysiological mechanism behind their symptoms. The rationale of how the proposed surgical procedures are designed to correct their symptoms can be made apparent using the films, and the potential complications (such as orbital or anterior cranial floor injury) can be discussed in an informative way. Patients who are prepared in this manner more fully comprehend the importance of proposed pre- and postoperative treatment plans and are more cooperative with treatment regimens and precautions, thus improving results. In addition, patients develop a sense of partnership in their care with the surgeon and feel some control over, and shared responsibility for, the final result.

It is incumbent on the surgeon to remember that because an anatomic abnormality exists on an x-ray, correction is not always mandatory. Surgery is for the patient, not to correct an x-ray. An incidentally discovered asymptomatic septal deviation does not need to be fixed, nor does an asymptomatic cyst on the floor of the maxillary sinus. Acute sinusitis most often resolves without sinus surgery, and the x-ray findings will gradually self-correct. Moreover, for patients for whom surgery would be of definite benefit, the expectations should be reasonable. Chronic allergic rhinosinusitis, aspirin triad

syndrome, vasomotor rhinitis, and so on can all benefit symptomatically from skilled surgery. But the underlying disorder is still in place despite surgery, and the patient should understand that surgery is not a cure and the disease will persist. Perhaps it will be completely ameliorated or there may be recurring symptoms at some point in the future. The proper medical and surgical care of patients with nasal and sinus disorders is as much art as science, and with experience the physician will learn the blend best suited to most patients.

A further admonition for the prevention of complications is not to take on the impossible. Surgery is usually harmful in conditions that cause internal scarring of the nose. The most common example is sarcoidosis, and surgery, by introducing further cause for scarring and infection, is in general counterproductive. Wegener's granulomatosis, rhinoscleroma, and tuberculosis also fall into this group.

For patients undergoing nasal and sinus surgery, there are two categories of complications that may be unrelated to surgical technique—namely, those involving coagulopathies and those related to anesthesia, particularly general anesthesia. In preparation for any procedure, such as sinus surgery, which leaves a large raw surface, the surgeon depends on normal clotting to prevent persistent hemorrhage. For this reason it is recommended that the patient take no medication with anticoagulating properties, especially acetylsalicylic acid (ASA), in any form for at least 2 weeks preoperatively. Most patients are unaware of how many proprietary medicines contain ASA and do not realize that a small amount can have a profound effect on platelet aggregation and bleeding time. In addition, within a few days prior to surgery, a prothrombin time (PT), partial thromboplastin time (PTT), and, most importantly, a bleeding time are obtained. Any abnormalities of these tests should automatically trigger a retest, and continued abnormality, however minor, should result in a deferral of surgery and a hematologic evaluation. With these precautions we have essentially eliminated bleeding complications in our patients due to unrecognized coagulopathies and, in the process, identified a substantial number of patients each year with unrecognized bleeding disorders. The most common of these is von Willebrand's disease, which occurs in approximately

1:200 individuals and is readily correctable with appropriate doses of DDAVP (1-desamino-8-D-arginine) and Amicar (aminocaproic acid) in the perioperative period (see Chapter 2). We have identified a smattering of coagulation factor deficiencies as well. One lesson learned is that a positive bleeding history is useful, but a negative history for bleeding, even in patients who have had surgery, is not meaningful.

Another cause for unacceptable hemorrhage during nasal and sinus surgery is a failure on the surgeon's part to avoid interrupting or avulsing major branches of the sphenopalatine artery as it enters the nasal cavity superior to the posterior tip of the inferior turbinate. The posterior lateral branches of this artery ramify from posteriorly to anteriorly over the inferior turbinate and the lateral wall of the nose, anastomosing with the anterior and posterior ethmoidal arteries as they enter superiorly after branching from the ophthalmic artery. In addition, the posterior septal branch of the sphenopalatine artery crosses from the lateral nose to the nasal septum in the soft tissue overlying the anterior face of the sphenoid and should be recognized and controlled. If the surgeon is cognizant of the location of these vessels and interrupts them only if necessary (preferably near the completion of the procedure) and then quickly takes steps to control bleeding permanently with ligation, arterial clips, Bovie or bipolar cautery, or bone wax, bleeding can be reduced. Packing plus Surgicel or Avitene is effective but a less satisfactory method of control.

ANESTHETIC CONSIDERATIONS FOR NASAL AND SINUS SURGERY

Both monitored local anesthesia and general anesthesia are acceptable means of pain control for many types of septal and sinus surgery. Our practice has tended toward increased use of general anesthesia for several reasons. First, most patients prefer to have a general anesthetic. Second, even with good local anesthesia the pain of cautery often cannot be controlled. Third, with general anesthesia, the anesthesia team has full control of the patient's airway, eliminating concerns of intraoperative respiratory suppression and aspiration. The drawbacks are that the side-effects and cross-reactions of inhalational and intravenous anesthetic agents and muscle relaxants become a potential hazard. In addition, there is increased recovery time and cost.

Whether the planned nasal or sinus surgery is to be performed with monitored local anesthesia or general anesthesia, our patients receive oxymetazoline HCl 0.5% nasal spray in the preoperative holding area to ensure good vasoconstriction at the time of nasal prepping and intranasal injections.[1] This drug has essentially no central nervous system or cardiac effects in the doses used at surgery, yet it is intensely vasoconstricting for up to 8 hours. Sharma et al (1992) have shown that spraying a vasoconstricting medication is more effective than packing with soaked pledgets because vasoconstriction is more uniform, there is less preoperative bleeding, and spraying saves time.[2]

Complications in nasal and sinus surgery are avoided by an appropriate operating room routine. Patient positioning is important. First, the patient's head and thorax should be raised 30° to decrease venous bleeding. Second, all nasal and sinus procedures should be positioned in the same way so that anatomic relationships (eg, the relative position of the patient to the surgeon) for every patient are the same. For instance, we place all patients with the dorsum of the nose parallel to the floor, and then the height of the table is adjusted to the surgeon. This puts the cribriform, anterior face of the sphenoid, and palate in relatively similar positions for each patient.

Good intranasal vision is paramount. The vibrissae, no matter how scant, should be trimmed because one's eyes tend to focus there. Next a light that is bright and can be focused down into the depths of the nose is vital. Many of the new fiberoptic lights have such a large, bright spot that the outside of the nose is intensely illuminated, impairing vision inside the nose.

If the procedure is to be done under monitored local anesthesia, then a topical anesthesia is applied. Five milliliters of 4% cocaine solution in well-wrung-out cottonoids may be placed up to the proposed safe limit of 200 mg for a 70-Kg male. Cocaine should not be used with epinephrine because this combination increases the likelihood of cardiac arrhythmias. The mixture of dry cocaine with epinephrine ("cocaine mud") is particularly troublesome in this regard. The onset of effect of cocaine occurs within 1 minute of application and lasts 1 hour. Cocaine, as well as all local anesthetics, rapidly crosses the blood-brain barrier. Early warning signs of impending toxic reaction include euphoria, excitement, agitation, tachycardia, hypertension, shivering, twitching, tremor followed by seizure, and vascular collapse (particularly in a heart sensitized to the effects of cocaine by hypertension, cardiovascular disease, or certain general anesthetics). Every surgeon using local anesthetics must be prepared to treat these complications. First, it is essential to maintain an airway and protect the patient from hypoxia, which may be accomplished with 100% oxygen by mask. Cardiac and cerebral perfusion must be maintained. Ultra-short-acting barbiturates are considered best for interrupting convulsive activity; however, diazepam is also effective.[3]

Lidocaine hydrochloride is one of the most popular local anesthetics for topical use or infiltration. As a plain solution 300 mg is the suggested maximum dose, and when combined with epinephrine the dose may be increased to 500 mg due to the reduction in absorption secondary to the vasoconstrictive effects of epinephrine. Rapid absorption of lidocaine due to a relative overdose from an intravascular injection may cause convulsions, but central nervous system depression is more common. Allergic reactions to local anesthetics are unusual and occur most commonly among health professionals who have had repeated exposures.

For infiltration anesthesia we use approximately 20 cc of lidocaine 0.5% with 1:200,000 epinephrine injected through a 27-gauge needle. A good plan is to inject in the same steps as the planned operation because this ensures that the entire surgical field is well infiltrated. With the less concentrated solution in larger amounts, there is better distribution of the injected material.

Intra- and extranasal injections should be done with a control syringe. There are reports of blindness secondary to submucosal injection of lidocaine with epinephrine. The probable mechanism is the inadvertent injection of a branch of the anterior or posterior ethmoidal artery with retrograde flow through the ophthalmic artery to the retinal artery followed by intense vasospasm and ischemia of the optic nerve and retina[4,5] (Fig. 7–1). Plate and Asboe report an incidence of three cases in an estimated 20,000 rhinosurgical operations.[6]

The rate of infection following nasal surgery is surprisingly low when one considers that the incidence of *Staphylococcus aureus* in the nasal vestibule of the nonhospitalized adult population is roughly 30%,[7] with the reported incidence increasing to 65% for patients with deviated septa or damaged turbinates.[8] Although most surgeons might take increased precautions in diabetics, patients with impaired immunity, those with infections about the face and nose, and those at risk for endocarditis, it has become apparent that the risks associated with antibiotic prophylaxis may well outweigh the risks of infection with septoplasty or rhinoplasty. Eschelman et al, in a prospective, double-blind study, could demonstrate no advantage of penicillin or ampicillin over placebo.[9] Yoder and Weimert report only five minor infections among 1040 patients who received no antibiotics for nasal surgery pre- or postoperatively.[10] No doubt there is a small risk of endocarditis from episodes of staphylococcal bacteremia; however, among 50 patients studied by Coursey, 23 of whom had culture-proven coagulase(+) staphylococcal colonization of the nose, there were no identifiable episodes of bacteremia.[11] Slavin et al, in a similar study of 52 patients undergoing rhinoplasty, had the same result: no bacteremia identified.[12]

Undoubtedly there are more serious infections that occur following septoplasty or rhinoplasty than are reported in the literature; however, case reports describe a death secondary to septic cavernous sinus thrombosis occurring approximately 2 weeks following an uneventful surgery and recovery to that time.[13] Another patient developed meningitis associated with facial swelling secondary to staphylococcal infection on the second postoperative day, with eventual complete recovery.[14] A third patient developed chronic granulomatous meningoencephalitis secondary to histoplasmosis almost 2 weeks following rhinoplasty.[15] Finally, one patient developed staphylococcal osteomyelitis of the lower spine 1 day following septoplasty.[16]

In 1978, Todd et al described toxic shock syndrome in seven children aged 8 to 17 years who presented with marked hypotension (shock), high fever, desquamating scarlatiniform rash, vomiting, diarrhea, hematuria, and delirium.[17] This syndrome has been reported to be caused most often by staphylococcal enterotoxin F and has been noted to be a complication of intravaginal tampon use and postoperative nasal packing[18] and splints.[19,20] The estimated incidence is 16.5 per 100,000 nasal surgeries. Toxic shock usually begins with

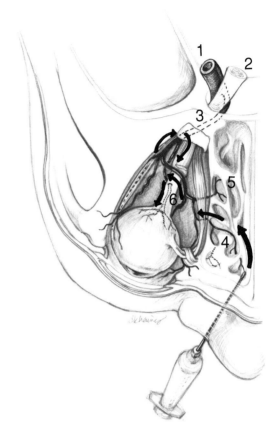

Figure 7–1. Arterial routes whereby intranasal injections of vasoconstrictors or particulate matter may cause blindness. (1) Internal carotid, (2) optic nerve, (3) ophthalmic artery, (4) anterior ethmoid artery, (5) posterior ethmoid arteries, (6) central retinal artery (after Rettinger and Christ[4]).

nausea and vomiting, generally 24 to 48 hours postoperatively. Blood cultures are negative, but nasal cultures are positive for *S. aureus* even though the nose may not appear infected. It is an unusual complication perhaps because 80% of the adult population has sufficient antibody titers against enterotoxin F, leaving 20% of the population susceptible to the disorder.[21]

It is likely that any foreign body associated with enterotoxin-producing *S. aureus* in a warm, moist, bloody environment can lead to toxic shock syndrome. Prevention is probably best achieved by avoiding postoperative nasal packing and splints. In a study of 15 nasal *S. aureus* carriers, preoperative intravenous cefazolin prophylaxis proved ineffective because it failed to eliminate the presence of *S. aureus* in 80% of patients.[22] Treatment is best facilitated by an early recognition of the disorder and aggressive management of this potentially fatal complication. The source of staphylococcal infection should be removed immediately. Treatments include vigorous fluid replacement and vasopressors as needed to improve hemodynamics. Ventilatory support may be required. Intravenous antistaphylococcal antibiotics are not beneficial but prevent recrudescence of the infection. An occasional patient may suffer renal failure and require dialysis.[23] Toxic shock syndrome is an unusual but extremely serious complication of nasal surgery.

COMPLICATIONS OF SEPTAL SURGERY

There are three principal complications of septal surgery: (1) failure to correct the obstructed breathing,(2) septal perforation, and (3) unacceptable cosmetic change.

Much has been written of the relative superiority of septoplasty versus submucous resection, when in truth the experienced surgeon will blend the techniques, providing each patient with the appropriate procedure depending on the problem at hand. The submucous resection is a limited procedure, in general done through a Killian incision placed at a centimeter or more behind the caudal edge of the septal cartilage. This presumes that the anterior caudal centimeter is not deviated and is not obstructing. This operation is reserved for patients with a straight dorsum so that a centimeter or more of dorsal cartilage strip can be left.

The surgical technique is vital. First, make certain that visualization is adequate and injections have been made properly and thoroughly. Next, use instruments which are the appropriate size for the work. Many of the old instruments—such as numbers 8 and 10 Frazer suctions, Ballenger swivel knives, and Jansen-Middleton forceps—are too large for many noses and can cause damage. For suction, number 5 or 7 ear suctions are atraumatic and are usually sufficient.

Either a hemitransfixion or Killian incision is placed on the side of the deviation (ie, side of greatest obstruction). Next, cartilage should be resected under direct vision and the vertical cuts made with an Anderson knife (similar to an ear canal knife), anteriorly and posteriorly, with horizonal cuts made with tenotomy or iris scissors (this prevents inadvertent cuts through the opposing mucoperichondral surfaces and removes only the cartilage which is obstructing). If there are large obstructing spurs along the maxillary crest, the Killian incision can be extended to the floor and an inferior tunnel can be created, permitting sharp dissection of the decussating fibers. On the side opposite the Killian incision, an incision can be made directly in the mucosa of the floor to permit creation of a second inferior tunnel. Bony spurs are best removed with a 4-mm or smaller osteotome or chisel. Deviations in the vomer and, ethmoid plate are generally removed piecemeal with Takihashi forceps. There is little concern about removing too much bone except near the cribriform plate. If at the completion of the submucous resection the mucosal leaves of the septum are intact, as is most often the case, a drainage hole 5 mm in diameter must be placed posteroinferiorly through one side of the mucoperiosteum to provide drainage and to prevent postoperative septal hematoma. Any straight pieces of cartilage or bone may be replaced as desired. The Killian incision is closed with interrupted 4-0 chromic sutures.

For nasal obstructions involving the caudal end of the septal cartilage, either a hemitransfixion incision or transfixion incision is required. The cartilage must be separated from the anterior nasal spine and maxillary crest and, if possible, a "swinging door" technique which leaves one mucosal surface adherent to mucoperichondrium should be employed. Removal and replacement of the caudal strut runs a higher risk of a retracted columellar deformity. Judicious scoring of the cartilage, employment of cartilaginous battons (especially anteriorly between the middle crura), and stiffening sutures and anchoring sutures to the nasal spine all help improve success rates. As with any commonly performed procedure, there are as many techniques as surgeons and thousands of tricks. There is no fixed method that can be applied to every septal deviation surgery.

Several studies have shown that certain surgeons (generally attending surgeons) have encountered few, if any, septal perforations and residual obstructions. Tzadik et al studied 263 septal operations performed by three attending surgeons and seven residents and found an overall complication rate of 6.4% perforated septa, 3.8% unsatisfactory corrections, and one saddle-nose deformity.[24] Peacock reviewed 913 cases of submucous resection at the Royal National Throat, Nose and Ear Hospital in London and found 4.3% perforations and 12.6% deviations still present.[25] Dommerby et al, in a similar study of 161 septoplasty patients examined 2 to 5 years postoperatively, found 2.5% perforated septa and 14% failure to correct the obstructing deviation. Saddle deformity occurred in three cases.The difficulty of long-term correction of anterior dislocations and deflections of the nose was reflected in a higher failure rate in these categories (namely, 16% and 41%, respectively[26]). Miller, in a study which included 650 nasal septal operations, reported an incidence of 0.6% septal perforations during the early postoperative period but did not comment on the number of failures to correct nasal obstruction.[27]

Jessen et al evaluated 35 patients who underwent septoplasty for high nasal resistance at 9 months and 9 years postperatively. By patient evaluation the satisfaction rate was 74% initially and 69%, at the later date. Rhinometric studies showed a small but measurable decrease in nasal airway over time.[28]

There has been a frequently expressed, but rarely documented, opinion concerning a gradual displeasing cosmetic change secondary to supratip depression of the nasal dorsum or columellar retraction following submucous resection. Does this retraction occur following a technically poor operation, or is it an unwanted feature that is an inescapable sequela of a properly performed submucous resection? This question was studied by Phillips with 50 patients who had a full set of preoperative nasal photographs followed by a repeat set at a minimum of 2 years. The surgeries were performed by five experienced nasal surgeons. On comparison of the photos, there was only one patient in whom a change in the nasal appearance could be appreciated. Other complications included a septal perforation and three patients with minor septal-turbinate adhesions.[29]

Upon completion of septal surgery, the question of whether to use packs or splints or not has been examined. Cook et al prospectively studied the benefit of silicone sheeting splints in a group of 100 patients undergoing combined septal and turbinate surgery, 50 of whom had splints placed for 1 week and the remainder none. There was no difference in the septal position or in airway improvement between the splint and nonsplint patients. Total complications, including septal perforation, adhesions, tip cellulitis, and maxillary sinusitis, were significantly higher in the splint patients as well as increased pain, especially at the time of removal.[30]

Nasal packings have been studied as well. The well-known complications of nasal packing include immediate airway obstruction with possible hypoventilation and hypoxemia; dysphagia with potential aspiration; and eustachian tubal obstructive symptoms including otitis media and hearing loss. In addition, nasal and sinus infections and rarely toxic shock may be seen. Later, adhesions may form secondary to the trauma of nasal packing. Watson et al (1989) compared the complications in 106 consecutive patients divided into three groups: one with balloon packing, one with ribbon gauze packing, and one with fingercot packs. The fingercots were the best of the groups because they were the least uncomfortable and were associated with the fewest adhesions.[31] Illum et al (1992) made a similar study comparing fingercot packs to ribbon gauze to Meracel packs with ventilation tubes. The fingercots were again found to be superior because they were the easiest to remove with no adherence to mucosa, caused the least bleeding, and these patients had the least persistence of nasal secretions. At 3 months postsurgery, there was no gross difference in the rhinometric studies between the three groups.[32]

Middle-ear blockage is a common complaint of patients with nasal packing. Johannessen and Poulsen (1984) could find no change in middle-ear pressure in 27 patients with anterior nasal packing.[33] Thompson and Crowther (1991) studied 63 patients who had surgery to correct septal deformities and found on impedance audiometry that 46% developed a reduction of middle-ear pressure of at least 50 daPa. However, only 10% of these ears had eustachian tube dysfunction lasting more than 24 hours after packing removal, and all had resolved within 6 weeks.[34]

Sessions (1984) described lacing the mucoperichondrium and mucoperiosteum of the septal leaves together using a 4-0 chromic suture on an atraumatic straight needle (Fig. 7–2). This "quilting" maneuver has the effect of closing down dead space and holding cross-hatched or replaced cartilage in position. It has the added benefit of eliminating the need for nasal packing in many instances, thus reducing the morbidity of nasal septal surgery.[35] Nunez and Martin (1991) studied 52 patients prospectively. Half the patients were packed with Vaseline gauze and half had Dacron suture quilting of the nasal septum. In this small study, the septal suture was clearly superior.[36] The quilting technique is relatively new, and with experience complications resulting from its use may become evident.

Our policy is to use no packing with septal or septal-turbinate surgery if there is no turbinate bleeding that requires packing and if the septal repair has been accomplished without inferior tunnels. In this event, the septum is laced together with 4-0 chromic suture. When inferior tunnels have been created and the potential for hematoma along the nasal floor is present, then fingercot packs are placed for 3 days.

The proper technique for turbinate surgery has been an area of controversy among nasal surgeons. The turbinates play an

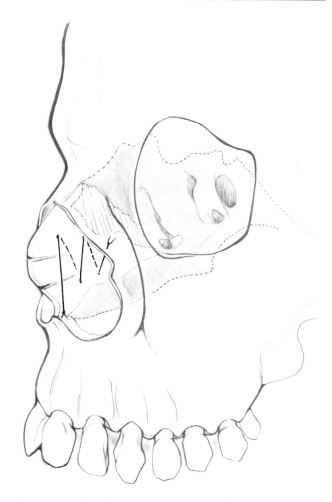

Figure 7–2. "Quilting" technique: one technique for opposing the mucoperichondrial leaves of the septum and stabilizing replaced cartilage.

important role in nasal hygiene and comfort because they are in large part responsible for humidity and temperature regulation as well as for providing a dynamic surface for cilia and the mucous blanket that continuously carries trapped debris to the pharynx to be swallowed. Over 1 liter of fluid carried at a rate of 1 mm/min passes over the nasal mucosal surfaces daily. Nonetheless, turbinates may become obstructing perhaps on a congenital basis, or more likely due to allergy, vasomotor rhinitis, and rhinitis medicamentosa. Commonly there is compensatory hypertrophy on the patent side of the nose in cases of septal deviation. The turbinate requires correction if the septoplasty is to be of benefit. Other causes of hypertrophy are antihypertensive medications, pregnancy, and hypothyroidism.

There have been multiple treatments for turbinate hypertrophy, some more successful than others. Although intraturbinal injection of steroids is not a surgical procedure per se, it is worthy of comment because of the association of this procedure, albeit rarely, with blindness. Simmons (1960) first reported the injection of inferior turbinates using Hydelta TBA (prednisolone) 0.2 cc superficially injected into the topically anesthetized tip of each inferior turbinate and repeated in 3 to 4 days one or two times. In 78% of his 419 patients, this treatment resulted in relief from turbinate hypertrophy for 1 year or more. He reported no complications.[37] Thereafter, increasing numbers of reports of temporary and permanent partial and complete blindness secondary to these injections made it clear that inadvertent intravascular injection could result in embolic obstruction of the retinal artery. Byers (1979) and Evans et al (1980) believe that branches of the external carotid artery of the lip, which are part of the blood supply to the anterior inferior turbinate, anastomose with the anterior ethmoidal artery, which in turn anastomoses with the ophthalmic artery and the retinal artery (Fig. 7–1).[38,39] Mabry (1978, 1981) has looked into this problem in some detail and, despite estimating the incidence of blindness to be very low, warns practitioners that the procedure is not approved by the FDA or manufacturers.[40,41]

Otolaryngologists as a group, recognizing the importance of the turbinates to nasal health, have been cautious in their approach to enlarged nasal turbinates. In addition to steroid injection, some conservative measures include scarification with caustic materials such as silver nitrate or trichloroacetic acid. Although these therapies are relatively harmless, the beneficial effects are small and short lived. Crushing of turbinates is of little benefit, and the technique of forceful lateral displacement of the turbinates by pushing them through the medial wall of the maxillary sinus with a heavy elevator has never gained popularity. Electrical coagulation (whether superficial or submucosal bipolar) is effective, but the beneficial effects (thought to be due to scar formation obstructing or limiting the expansion of the turbinal vascular bed) have a short life—roughly 1 year—before obstructive symptoms reappear. In 1951, Howard House described submucosal resection of the inferior turbinate bone and observed relief of obstruction and no increase in nasal drying and crusting after the procedure. This operation has strong proponents but has not been subjected to a prospective comparative analysis; however, it has withstood the test of time. The main drawback is that it is a somewhat difficult, time-consuming procedure.[42] Ozenberger (1970) first proposed cryosurgery for hypertrophied turbinates. The advantages are that it can be done as an office procedure under local anesthesia, it takes less than 30 minutes, and there is no bleeding at the time of the procedure or 1 week later when sloughed tissue is removed. The turbinates reepithelialize with healthy respiratory tissue.[43] Principato (1979) wrote of his experiences with 350 patients with good to excellent results in 84% of patients and with decreased nasal stuffiness in 86%. There were no complications among this group, and 5-year follow-up biopsy demonstrated normal respiratory tissue. Thirty percent of his patients were followed for 5 years, and of these 17 patients had repeat cryotherapy to the turbinates.[44] Bumsted (1984) also used cryotherapy for chronic rhinitis in 50 patients followed for a minimum of 2 years. He found obstruction to be eliminated in 92% and improved in the remaining 8%. Subjective excessive drainage, or postnasal drip (PND), was relieved in 47% and markedly improved in 41%. There was temporary crusting in three patients, but no permanent rhinitis sicca.[45] From the aforementioned

accounts, this is a safe and effective procedure and is a popular treatment method for hypertrophied turbinates. The drawbacks are that it does not work well for patients in whom the bony choncha is responsible for some of the enlargement, and precise removal of a predetermined amount of turbinate tissue is hard to accomplish.

Courtess et al (1978) reported 88 cases of near total (from his description) inferior turbinate resections in patients undergoing rhinoplasty and stated that following 2 to 37 months there were no untoward effects.[46] This paper led to a reexamination of previously held views of most otolaryngologists that inferior turbinate resection would lead to excessive crusting and chronic infection secondary to rhinitis sicca. There remain many questions in this regard and strongly held opinions. Most surgeons would agree that a partial turbinectomy, consisting of approximately 30% to 50% of turbinal tissue, is effective for relief of airway obstruction and leaves sufficient turbinate to function satisfactorily. Ophir (1985) looked at this question and followed 150 patients who had total inferior turbinectomies with no other nasal surgery for 1 to 7 years. There was a patent nasal airway in 91% and no complaints of crusts, dryness, or foul odor. Because of his method of high resection, he apparently cut a branch of the sphenopalatine artery because seven patients required posterior packing and two patients required transfusion.[47] Martinez (1983) followed 29 patients after total turbinectomy. One case was complicated by excessive dryness (rhinitis sicca), two by mild dryness, and three by excessive secretions.[48] Moore et al (1985) followed 18 patients who underwent total inferior turbinectomy. Of these, 16 complained of a dry nose, 66% had chronic nasal crusting, and another 22% had ozena. These authors conclude that total inferior turbinate resection should not be performed.[49]

Goode (1990), Drumheller (1983), and Mabry (1988) are in agreement that total turbinectomy may serve many patients well; however, they state that inevitably there will be instances of smelly crusting or persistent infection with heavy PND secondary to loss of sufficient respiratory membrane to maintain proper humidity and ciliary flow.[50–52] These patients are very uncomfortable. I have seen these patients, and unfortunately little has been devised to help them.

Our technique for management of hypertrophied turbinates (see Fig. 7–3) has evolved from cryotherapy to partial turbinate resection, principally because the latter takes less time and can be done with increased precision. Because we train residents, it is necessary to provide a guide for the new surgeon regarding how and where to make the turbinate excision. The technique is as follows: The turbinates have been shrunken as far as possible with oxymetazoline 0.5%. They are moved away from the lateral wall of the nose with a Sayer elevator. A DeBakey aorta clamp placed at the level of the junction of the turbinate with the lateral wall of the nose and kept parallel with the floor of the nose is fastened along the entire length of the turbinate. This is left in place for 30 to 60 seconds and it forms a groove, approximately at the junction between the inferior one third and superior two thirds of the turbinate. The groove is then traced both on the medial

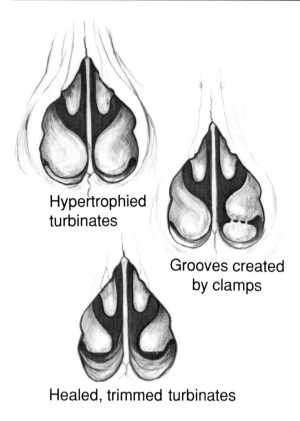

Hypertrophied
turbinates

Grooves created
by clamps

Healed, trimmed turbinates

Figure 7–3. Technique for management of hypertrophied turbinates. Resection of the inferior one third to one half of the inferior turbinate insures a good airway and proper turbinate functioning.

and lateral surfaces using an insulated, long, needle-tipped Bovie at a relatively high coagulation setting. The tissue is coagulated down to the turbinate bone. It is then a simple matter with the Knight turbinate scissors to trim off this lower section of turbinate. Any bleeding is controlled with spot cautery using an insulated cautery suction tip. In general, no packing or splints are required when this technique is used in combination with septal quilting following septal surgery. Elwany and Harrison (1990) compared submucosal resection of the turbinates, cryoturbinectomy, and partial inferior turbinectomy with either scissors or laser and found the best results from partial turbinectomy.[53]

PITUITARY SURGERY

There are two potential sources of complications in transseptal surgery as an approach to the pituitary gland. The first is that the nasal interior must be rapidly and accurately disassembled to provide wide exposure of the sphenoid and sella in a manner such that it can be restored immediately to its original or better condition. Second, the nasal portion of the procedure must provide accurate access to the sella without impinging on the nearby anterior cranial fossa or orbits. The best description of the basic sublabial transseptal approach to the pituitary gland is by Kern and Laws. All modifications of the transseptal operations (such as substitution

of lateral alotomy or open rhinoplasty techniques) contain the elements of this operation.[54] If you are beginning, learn this operation first.

The operation begins with careful positioning of the patient, oxymetazoline 0.5% spray in the nose, and the injection of 20 cc of 0.5% lidocaine with 1:200,000 epinephrine.[55] A moistened vaginal packing is placed around the endotracheal tube in the hypopharynx to prevent the aspiration of blood, mucus, or surgical debris. Special care must be taken with the injections in Cushing's disease patients because the nasal mucosal will be thin and tear easily and these patients are sensitive to the epinephrine. There will be troublesome bleeding due to hypertension if satisfactory injections are not made.

The operation begins with a right hemitransfixion incision that is made down the anterior margin of the cartilaginous septum after the columella has been retracted. In an occasional patient, the medial crura of the lower lateral cartilage will overlap the septal cartilage and this should be recognized to avoid injury. First by sharp dissection and then by blunt dissection, a left mucoperichondrial pocket is made that extends for the full surface of the left cartilaginous and bony septum. Any septal deviations or spurs must be carefully dissected free without tearing the mucoperichondrium. It is important that this dissection be complete from the roof of the nose down to the decussating fibers at the maxillary crest and posteriorly to the face of the sphenoid.   Next, the inferior tunnels are made along the floor of the nose on the right and left sides, with the elevation extending from the maxillary crest to the insertion of the inferior turbinates. Injury to the mucosa can easily occur if the dissection has not been completed so that only the decussating fibers at the maxillary crest remain. These are then sharply divided under direct vision, creating a large, loose sheet of mucosa extending from the uppermost septum to the lateral wall of the nose. The separation of the septal cartilage from the maxillary crest is an easy maneuver, as is the separation of the cartilage from the ethmoid plate and vomer, and is generally done bluntly with the sharp end of a Cottle elevator. The cartilaginous septum with the mucosa still adherent on the right side can be moved laterally against the right lateral wall of the nose after the decussating fibers are cut, again under direct vision. At this point, the decision to use a sublabial incision or a lateral alotomy incision should be made. The sublabial incision is best for small noses and for persons for whom a minor external scar would be objectionable (especially in patients who form hypertrophic scars). The lateral alotomy should be used in patients who wear dentures, older individuals or those who are not as concerned with cosmesis, and especially in individuals with a large nose. The alotomy is carried approximately halfway up the alar crease, which gives enough relaxation to avoid any risk of tearing the edge of the ala.

The sublabial incision is generally made with the cutting cautery to control bleeding, but caution must be taken not to heat the premaxilla with the cautery because injury to the dental roots can occur. As the periosteum is elevated with a Freer elevator, the nasal spine is encountered. A generous covering of soft tissue should be left on this structure and should not be removed or altered in any way, because that unadvised maneuver may result in a dropped nasal tip. The dissection into the nasal tunnels and the transseptal dissection are relatively easy. Next, the pituitary speculum is brought under the lip, pushing the cartilaginous septum to the right and advancing on either side of the ethmoidal plate until the end of the blades touch the face of the sphenoid. The speculum is gently advanced further as the blades are opened. At this point, a large piece of ethmoid plate is removed and will be used to reconstruct the sella following tumor removal. The face of the sphenoid has a characteristic appearance—namely, it looks like the bottom of a sailboat with the vomer forming the keel. If the dissection does not have this appearance, obtain an intraoperative x-ray to check your position. Identification of the sphenoid ostia will confirm location as well. The vomer is grasped with a heavy Takihashi forceps, and with a twisting motion the sphenoid can be opened. The sphenoid face is removed with Kerrison rongeurs and the sphenoid septa with pituitary forceps. Any doubt about the location of the sella can be corrected by placing a metal Frazier suction in the sphenoid and obtaining a lateral x-ray.

The neurosurgical team is concerned with exposure and will often readjust and open the pituitary speculum further. If the transseptal dissection has not been generous enough, the mucosa can be torn, leading to septal perforation.

Following completion of the neurosurgical portion of the procedure, the speculum is removed. Any continued bleeding is handled with electrocautery or bone wax. If there are no mucosal perforations, a drainage hole must be made posteroinferiorly on one side. A 4-0 Vicryl stitch is used to anchor the anterior septum to the soft tissues remaining on the nasal spine, ensuring proper replacement. Upon suturing the wounds, soft packing (such as fingercot packs) is placed in the nose for 3 days.

The potential nasal complications include epistaxis, septal perforation, deviated septum, persistent sinusitis, and a dropped tip if the nasal spine has been removed. The complications occur approximately 1% or less in experienced hands. Numb incisor teeth, usually temporary, are also a sequelae despite what variation of the transseptal approach is used.[56] A "dead" tooth can result from overheating the premaxilla with the electrocautery; cerebrospinal fluid (CSF) leak from cracking of the cribriform plate and accompanying loss of sense of taste and smell are known complications. There are reports of blinding secondary to misplacement of the speculum tips inside the sphenoid sinus, resulting in sphenoid fracture through the optic canals and injury to the optic nerves. Malocclusion from diastasis or fracture of the hard palate can result from overexpansion of the speculum and is another rare complication.[57,58]

SECONDARY PITUITARY SURGERY

Occasionally there will be a need to reexplore the sella following pituitary surgery. Most immediate reexplorations—namely, within 2 months—can be accomplished by opening the old incisions. After this time, the mucoperichondrial leaves of the septum have become firmly adherent and separation can be accomplished only with high risk of septal perforation. For these cases, we employ a transnasal septal displacement technique, which moves the previously dissected septum aside as a unit, thereby eliminating the risk of septal injury.[59]

The procedure begins with a right hemitransfixion incision, which is then extended posteriorly in the nose along the margin of the right maxillary crest and remaining vomer to the posterior septal edge. Next, through the hemitransfixion incision, the anterior septum is dissected away from the nasal spine and a left inferior tunnel is created along the floor of the nose, beginning sharply with iris scissors and then bluntly with a Cottle elevator. The cartilaginous septum is sharply dissected off the maxillary crest; and with care not to cut or rip the left mucosa, the dissection becomes continuous with the left inferior tunnel. This dissection is extended posteroward until the septum swings as a unit, tethered on the left mucosa inferiorly, thereby exposing the face of the sphenoid and the previously made openings. A sublabial incision or right alotomy incision is made to provide room for the pituitary retractor. We have had no complications with approximately 20 of these procedures. Following the neurosurgical portion of the procedure, cartilaginous septum is resutured to the anterior nasal spine and the mucosa is closed along the maxillary crest with absorbable suture as far intranasally as can be reached. Only the left side of the nose requires packing to hold the septum back in the center of the nose. We remove it after 3 days.

THE CALDWELL-LUC OPERATION

George Caldwell, a surgeon at the New Amsterdam Hospital in New York City, described his operation for maxillary sinus disease in 1893. The procedure included a sublabial incision, an opening through the canine fossa, and making a counteropening through the lateral wall of the nose. Henri Luc, a Frenchman, wrote of his experience with essentially the same operation 1897. Although others were writing about maxillary sinus surgery, the appellation *Caldwell-Luc* has been used in the American literature.[60]

The principal complication of Caldwell-Luc surgery is recurrent disease. There are many possible causes for this, such as failure to remove all chronically infected mucosa. However, normal mucosa is best left behind to foster remucosalization of the sinus cavity. Failure to treat adjacent ethmoid sinus disease or dental disease will contribute to the onset of the reinfection. Finally, it is necessary to provide a satisfactory nasal antral opening, either through the natural osteum or below the inferior turbinate. Estimates of continued disease in several larger series range from 2% to 16%.[61,62]

Numbness of the upper lip and gum is a well-known complication due to infraorbital nerve injury. Although symptoms most often are temporary, occasionally they can be protracted. Several suggestions have been made to protect the infraorbital nerve from injury. First, a cheek retractor should never be placed directly on the nerve, but rather should be placed obliquely in the wound, pulling away from the nerve to avoid crushing or stretching it. Second, an atraumatic technique for opening the sinus has been suggested by many authors to avoid an inadvertent fracture of the anterior wall of the sinus into the infraorbital foramen, which may occur when a chisel and mallet are used. Use of a large diamond or cutting bur is the most common recommendation.

Persistent cheek swelling is occasionally troublesome. It has been suggested that a long incision extending above the gingiva posteriorly reduces postoperative swelling.[63] Closure of nasal antral windows is a common problem. In addition to making those located below the inferior turbinate of a generous size in anticipation of partial closure, some authors bring a nasal mucosal flap, developed under the inferior turbinate and based on the nasal floor, through the opening and into the sinus to preclude closure. Too generous a nasal antral opening, particularly posteriorly, invites another complication of this operation—namely, excessive bleeding due to injury to a branch of the sphenopalatine artery. Care (and, if necessary, cautery or judicious packing) should prevent this complication.

Dental root injury is a hazard especially when the roots protrude into the sinus with only a thin covering. A tip-off that the maxillary sinusitis in question is due to a periapical abscess is that the sinus drainage will be malodorous both to the examiner and the patient. The tooth should be repaired or extracted prior to or at the time of the sinus surgery.

Many surgeons, at the completion of the procedure, will pack the sinus with antibiotic-impregnated ribbon gauze or a long Pennose drain and bring it out through the nasal antral window. Our main objective for the packing is to prevent the sinus from filling with blood clot; and when this danger is past, usually in 24 hours, the packing is removed. Some authors bring the packing out through the wound; however, this technique enhances the risk of yet another complication, oral-antral fistula.

Finally, no matter how well performed, the Caldwell-Luc operation has some morbidity and it behooves the surgeon to make certain that the symptoms of the patient are greater than the anticipated sequellae of the surgery. Many postoperative patients, if questioned closely, have one or two numb teeth and also have a tender cheek overlying the antrostomy that may last 6 months. In addition, if the mucosa is stripped from the sinus, the sinus will become contracted, developing a thickened scar covered by regenerated mucosa that may have sufficient ciliary function to provide the patient with an abnormal but hopefully asymptomatic sinus.

PTERYGOMAXILLARY FOSSA SURGERY

The indications for pterygomaxillary fossa surgery have decreased in recent years because many centers have found that sphenopalatine artery epistaxis can be managed by microarteriography and embolization. Vasomotor rhinitis is not well controlled by vidian neurectomy, and nasal neuralgia is in general unaffected by sphenopalatine ganglionectomy. In addition, the pterygomaxillary space is filled with hazards for the unwary surgeon. The foramen rotundum, containing the infraorbital nerve, and the inferior orbital fissure, leading posteromedialward into the posterior orbit, present potential for injury. In addition, the fossa is filled with adipose tissue concealing the third division of the internal maxillary artery and accompanying veins.

To avoid complications during maxillary and sphenopalatine artery ligation, a few precautions are advised. First, a wide anterior maxillary antrostomy is made. Under magnification with an operating microscope and using a diamond bur, the posterior wall of the maxillary sinus is thinned down, cracked, and removed with a stapes curette. The periosteum is cauterized in a cruciate manner and opened with a sickle knife. With a blunt nerve hook, the fat can be moved away to some degree and the maxillary artery located. It should be captured by the hook as far medially as possible and lifted gently forward as an arterial clip is applied. If possible, identify the sphenopaltine artery and apply a clip there as well. There is no need to divide the vessels.

Cooke (1985) reported, in 24 cases of internal maxillary artery ligation, that three patients had permanent facial numbness three had temporary numbness, and one had permanent diplopia.[64]

Postoperative suppurative maxillary sinusitis has been reported, and in most instances a nasal-antral window would be advised. Epiphora has been reported secondary to narrowing of the lacrimal duct near the nasal outlet. However, the most serious complications are ophthalmic. Johnson and Parkin (1976) report a pressure injury to the structures of the superior orbital fissure and contents of the optic canal resulting in blindness secondary to marked swelling of oxidized cellulose gauze, which had been packed in the pterygomaxillary space to control bleeding.[65] Beall et al (1985) report a total ophthalmoplegia following internal maxillary artery ligation.[66]

ETHMOIDECTOMY

The intranasal ethmoidectomy has been long recognized as one of the most difficult to teach and learn of the operations in otolaryngology. The external ethmoidectomy is safer because it provides the surgeon with a better view as well as a better angle of attack to the ethmoid and sphenoid sinuses. Many surgeons make a practice of offering the patient an intranasal ethmoidectomy initially and, should there be recurrent disease, external ethmoidectomy.

The remarks about the importance of screening for clotting dysfunction, a standard position for patients, good vasoconstriction and injections, and posterior pharyngeal packing are especially applicable to ethmoidectomy. Many surgeons type and cross these patients. In a prospective study of 73 patients, Hinton and Buckley (1990) found that the average blood loss from bilateral intranasal ethmoidectomy was 400 mL. In addition, surgeon's estimates of blood loss were usually lower than the actual loss, and even after 6 weeks (the length of the study) many patients had not fully recovered from the blood loss.[67] One tip is that there is less bleeding if the polyps themselves are injected with epinephrine 1:100,000.

A CT scan of the sinuses is helpful with both coronal and axial cuts, if necessary. They give the surgeon a good estimate of the height of the roof of the ethmoid and the relationship of the posterior ethmoid cells to the posterior orbit. The films forewarn the surgeon of any defects in the lamina papyracea and roof of the ethmoid, especially in patients with long-standing polypoid rhinosinusitis who may have had multiple office polypectomies or a previous ethmoid procedure. In addition, the films would demonstrate the rare encephalocele that might be present.

Many surgeons routinely begin a bilateral intranasal ethmoidectomy with a septoplasty to gain working room and improved visualization. Once completed, the major polyps are removed as bloodlessly as possible to identify the middle turbinate and its insertion superiorly on the lateral edge of the cribriform plate. A rule of thumb is that the cribriform plate is no lower than and at roughly the height of the medial canthus. Next, the rostrum of the sphenoid should be identified, and with a blunt probe the natural osteum can usually be found. The upper margin of the osteum is located a few millmeters below the roof of the ethmoid, at a distance of 7 cm and at roughly a 30° angle from the nares. It should be opened with a small Kerrison working downward to remove the lower portion of the anterior face of the sphenoid. The septal branch of the sphenopalatine artery should be cauterized as it crosses the face of the sphenoid. If the natural osteum cannot be identified, the face of the sphenoid should be opened with an osteotome and Kerrison forceps. The roof of the sphenoid is at the same level as the roof of the ethmoid.

After identifying the cribriform plate, the sphenoid, and the level of the roof of the ethmoid in relationship to the sphenoid roof, the ethmoidectomy can begin either from posteriorly to anteriorly or vice versa. It is a good idea to identify the posterior ethmoid cell and work forward because bleeding does not interfere so much with vision working from posteriorly forward. A few general rules are necessary. First, unless there is significant scar formation, polyps are easily avulsed with a gentle tug. Any structure that does not come away easily must be examined carefully before more force is applied. Second, always work lateral to the insertion of the middle turbinate. Third, the operating forceps should be kept as much as possible in a plane parallel to the roof of the ethmoid. Fourth, the lamina papyracea should not be removed and the patient's eyes kept in view throughout the operation. Fifth, to reduce scar formation, take care not to tear out normal mucosa. Sixth, operate on one side until the bleeding interferes with the work, pack with vasoconstrictor-soaked pledgets, and commence work on the other side. If possible, preserve at least the attachment of the middle turbinate for a landmark. Breaking off the middle turbinate at the cribriform plate can cause a CSF leak, and it should be cut away carefully with scissors or forceps.

As the dissection procedes, the scalloped (or reverse cobblestone) appearance of the ethmoid roof will gradually become apparent. As the anterior ethmoids are approached, the osteum to the maxillary sinus can be probed and opened. The nasofrontal duct can be probed, and polypoid tissue lateral and anterior may be removed and the aggar-nasi cells opened. Admittedly this is a hazardous operation, but a thorough understanding of the anatomy and intranasal and external relationships lessens the risk.

A number of authors have reviewed their large series of intranasal ethmoidectomy and report their complications, usually divided into major complications (intracranial—CSF leak, intracranial hemorrhage, meningitis, brain abscess; orbital—blindness, oculomotility defects due to muscle or nerve injury; and hemorrhage—internal carotid or cavernous sinus injury and loss of olfaction) and minor complications (orbital hematoma, persistent low-volume bleeding, aspiration pneummonia, infraorbital neuralgia, nasolacrimal duct obstruction, and recurrent disease).

Freedman and Kern (1979) report a complication rate of 2.8% on 1000 consecutive intranasal ethmoidectomies. They experienced 28 complications in 26 patients. There were 12 hemorrhages, 4 orbital hematomas, but no blindness, no loss of ocular motility, and no excision of brain tissue. They make the point that most of the complications occurred on the right side, which is more difficult to visualize for the right-handed surgeon.[68] Eichel (1982) reported on his 12-year experience of 236 intranasal ethmoidectomies on 123 patients with a 1.7% complication rate. He pointed out that he had an 83% initial success rate in controlling the symptoms of polypoid rhinosinusitis, and following revision surgery a 91% success rate. He reported no deaths, no blindness, and no permanent orbital injury.[69] Taylor et al (1982) reported four major complications in 526 intranasal ethmoidectomies on 284 patients—namely, one retro-orbital hematoma and three fistulae.[70] Friedman et al (1986) had two CSF leaks and two frontal sinus mucoceles in 510 intranasal sphenoethmoidectomies for a major complication rate of under 1%.[71] Lawson reports a 1.1% significant complication rate among 1077 operations with a surgical success rate of 88% in nonasthmatics and 50% among asthmatics. He reports three CSF leaks, two orbital hematomas, three periorbital ecchymoses, two hemorrhages requiring posterior packing, and two instances of epiphora. All three CSF leaks resolved spontaneously. The eight intracranial and orbital complications occurred on the right side. Lawson correctly notes that the factors which promote complications are revision surgery, altered anatomy (especially an absent middle turbinate), obstructed vision from excessive bleeding (which often accompanies chronic infection), and lack of surgical experience.[72]

Other authors have reported on the sinus complications of other physicians that they have called on to treat. Calcaterra (1985) describes the appearance of a CSF leak as the appearance of pulsating, clear fluid into the nose.[73] The defect should be repaired immediately from below, either by turning a septal mucosal flap over the defect or, if this is not available, packing the opening with a pledget of abdominal fat. The repair should be held in position with nasal packing for 7 to 10 days. Appropriate antibiotic coverage is begun. An indwelling lumbar drain should be placed in the operating room (OR). The extent of the defect must be evaluated on CT scan and the patient kept in a sitting position until the leak is considered sealed. If the leak fails to seal, a neurosurgical repair via the bifrontal approach will be required. In addition to increased hospitalization, scarring, and morbidity, this procedure usually results in permanent anosmia. Toselli et al (1991) report on intracranial complications, one a major opening in the roof of the ethmoid leading to right frontal hematoma and meningitis resulting in permanent neurological impairment and a second resulting in recurring meningitis and epidural abscess. They note that if there is a potential for intracranial vascular injury, arteriography must be considered. Two cases of iatrogenic carotid cavernous sinus fistulae have been reported.[74]

Orbital complications following sinus surgery were well reviewed by Dutton (1986). Complications from intranasal ethmoidectomy, among experienced operators, range from 0.5% to 3%, and orbital complications represent 16% to 50% of the total.[75] These include orbital edema, which is the most common orbital injury. It is the consequence of a fracture of the lamina papyracea, which may have been eroded by pressure from polyps. This is usually a self-limited injury that may be accompanied by prolapse of orbital fat. Usually this is of no consequence. However, if the orbital fat is unrecognized by the operator and removed, there may result intraorbital hemorrhage secondary to torn blood vessels and possibly injury to the medial rectus muscle. Early recognition of these introgenic injuries is vital. The immediate consequences may be blindness secondary to optic nerve compression and retinal artery and vein occlusion. Late consequences include enophthalmos and permanent extraocular muscle dysfunction secondary to orbital fibrosis, which most often affects the medial rectus and superior oblique muscles.[76]

The treatment for intraorbital hemorrhage is immediate lateral canthotomy followed by orbital decompression and drainage of the hematoma by widely opening the periorbita medially and, if necessary, inferiorly. Intravenous (IV) steroids and acetazolamide (Diamox) are recommended.

If the injury occurs in the posterior orbit by an unrecognized break through the lateral wall of the posterior ethmoid cell, the optic nerve may be injured directly.

Optic nerve compression may occur in the immediate postoperative period secondary to tight packing or from the use of oxidized cellulose gauze, which swells and forms a firm mass when blood soaked. The packings should be removed immediately and orbital decompression, as described earlier, initiated.[77]

Although many procedures are performed in the presence of serious sinus infections, postsurgical orbital infection or abscess are rare complications. However, to avoid infected packing, it is our practice to remove all packing within 24 hours after it has served its purpose of controlling immediate postsurgical bleeding.

Injury to the lacrimal duct can occur as it enters or traverses its bony canal. The resulting epiphora is usually short lived. If persistent, a cryocystorhinostomy will correct the problem. Despite the location of the lacrimal duct and the risk of frequent injury, epiphora does not seem to be a common complication of ethmoid surgery.

EXTERNAL ETHMOIDECTOMY

External ethmoidectomy is reserved, in general, for reoperations or cases made more difficult by the presence of mucocele or known lamina papyracea injury, or a procedure in which the periorbita requires opening, as in orbital abscess. It also provides good exposure for the repair of CSF leaks from the sphenoid or ethmoid and can be used as an approach for pituitary surgery. In addition, it is used as an approach for ligation of the anterior and posterior ethmoidal arteries for superior nasal epistaxis.

There are several complications that are unique to this procedure due to the surgical approach. The first is scarring. The incision (see Fig. 7–4) should be in the form of a small W-plasty, because the older, conventional circular incision is much more pronounced on the face; and in time, as the scar shortens, it may lift away, forming a web and thereby becoming even more apparent. The W-plasty presents a broken line that the observer's eye does not pick up, and

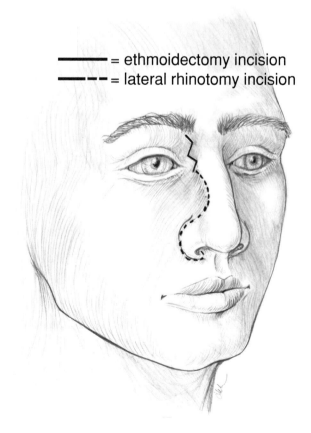

= ethmoidectomy incision
= lateral rhinotomy incision

Figure 7–4. External ethmoidectomy and lateral rhinotomy incisions. If incisions are carefully placed they cause minimal scarring.

because of the multidirectionality of the scar, the normal 25% in length of scar contraction does not lift it away from the nose. Next, care must be used in closing external ethmoidectomy wounds. First, nonabsorbable sutures can form persistent, small fibrous knots below the skin that are tender, particularly for eyeglass wearers. In addition, the periosteum overlying the lateral nose must be repaired carefully because this maneuver returns the medial canthal ligament to its original position. Failure to reattach the medial canthal ligament can result in a pseudohypertelorism.

Exploration (in cases of epistaxis) of the high medial orbit along the frontoethmoid suture line for ligation of the anterior and posterior ethmoidal arteries can result in either transient or permanent superior oblique muscle palsy due to direct trochlear damage from separation of periosteum or localized hematoma formation under the adjoining periosteum. This is probably a more common occurrence than reported.[78,79]

Finally, Maniglia et al have written two papers that contain a series of case reports concerning patients referred after suffering rare, fatal, major complications secondary to nasal and sinus surgery. Because surgeons rarely write of their own complications, Maniglia has provided a useful service of compiling these anonymously presented cases so that all those interested may learn how to avoid the traps and errors that led to these tragic outcomes.[80,81]

LATERAL RHINOTOMY

Bernard et al (1989) report a complication rate of 21% following 162 lateral rhinotomy operations. Of these, 120 or 74% were combined with medial maxillectomy. They report no serious bleeding or CSF leaks. Orbital complications include transient blepharitis and lid edema and lacrimal duct obstruction with associated dacryocystitis. Four patients required a secondary dacryocystorhinostomy. Ten percent of patients had late cosmetic complications, which included unacceptable scars, shift of the bony pyramid with saddle deformity, and vestibular stenosis. In heavily irradiated patients, nasocutaneous fistula may result secondary to poor healing potential.[82]

In summary, most of the reported complications are the result of the placement and design of the incision; the loss of underlying facial, nasal, or orbital bony support; and the mandatory transaction of the lacrimal duct.

The best incision for lateral rhinotomy (see Fig. 7–4) begins under the medial edge of the brow as a W-plasty, with the midpoint of the letter W near the medial canthus and the lower limb extending high onto the nasal bridge until the alar crease is reached. At this point, it follows the crease under the nares and crosses the sill of the nose at the narrowest point. The rationale for making this incision is to provide a broken line that in time becomes invisible, in part because scar contracture is multidirectional and does not lift the scar away from the nose. Below the inferior orbital rim the scar is carried high on the lateral wall of the nose, where the skin is thin and heals well because it is under little tension. The alar crease hides the remainder of the scar. We do not find it necessary to divide the upper lip for this procedure because it can be avoided by extending the sublabial incision both laterally and medially.

The bony removal along the anterior face of the maxilla should be kept as close to the medial wall of the nose as the disease will allow, and the orbital rim is cut just lateral to the lacrimal fossa. Some authors recommend a chisel for these cuts; however, a narrow Kerrison bone forceps gives more control over eggshell fractures. Likewise, the bone of the nasal dorsum is cut, usually along the frontal process of the maxillary bone at the suture line with the nasal bone, again using fine Kerrison forceps and thus preserving as much bony nasal support as possible.[83]

Patients must be forewarned of the potential morbidity of lateral rhinotomy and medial maxillectomy, including areas of temporary and permanent numbness about the cheek, nose, and teeth. All patients will have large nasal mucous crust formations, especially those who have received radiation, and they must learn to deal with these—in general, with saline irrigations.

We have found epiphora and dacryocystitis to be occasional problems. If the lacrimal sac can be easily opened and sutured back, as in a standard dacryocystorhinostomy, it should be done at the time of the medial maxillectomy. If it is unusually difficult or impractical to open the sac at the initial procedure and the lacrimal duct is exposed as it enters the combined maxillary nasal cavity, it is often sufficient to cut the duct on a bias, thus reducing the chance for stenosis by scar contracture. Details of a technique for handling the late complication of persistent epiphora following this operation have been described.[84]

TREPHINATION OF THE FRONTAL SINUSES

When acute sinusitis involving the frontal sinuses fails to resolve after adequate nasal mucosal decongestion and intravenous antibiotic therapy, the sinus should be explored (eg, opened, cultured, cleared of infected material) in an effort to resolve the infection and reduce mucosal swelling and to reestablish the patency of the nasofrontal duct. This is accomplished most often by trephination of the frontal sinus through a medial incision, which exposes the floor of the frontal sinus. The floor is then opened with a cutting bur. At this point, the interior of the sinus can be inspected with sinus scopes, and cultures and biopsies are taken if necessary. A large drain is placed in the sinus and brought out of the wound for irrigation purposes. The complications of this procedure include edema of, and at times bleeding into, the upper lid. Superior trochlear nerve injury with a resulting numbness of a portion of the midforehead occurs commonly. Rarely diplopia secondary to inflammation or injury to the trochlea or superior oblique tendon and sheath may occur.[85] While the irrigating catheter remains in place, it is an irritant to the eye. There is one report of blindness secondary to orbital infection through the trephination site due to a recrudescence of the frontal sinusitis several weeks following therapy.[86] Finally, the scar can be noticeable even with the passage of time.

The osseous trephine is made through the floor of the sinus to take advantage of the fact that the floor is laminar bone and is at less risk for the introduction of osteomyelitis than if the trephine were made through the cancellous bone of the anterior wall.[87] However, the introduction of potent, broad-spectrum antibiotics which have excellent bony penetration have sufficiently reduced the risk of frontal osteomyelitis from trephinations. Our trephinations are now made through an 8-mm skin incision (to admit sinuscopes) placed in a furrow in the brow. A 4-mm drill bit and drill guide are used in a fashion that will allow the drill to penetrate the sinus by a millimeter or two. Then a plastic irrigating catheter is sutured into place. There are multiple advantages to this technique. First, it can always be performed under local anesthesia because there is no concern for the patient or surgeon of potential eye injury due to operating in the superior orbit. There is no lid swelling, no supratrochlear nerve injury, and no risk to the trochlea or superior oblique muscle tendon or sheath. The catheter is in a more comfortable place for the patient, and the irrigations are easily tolerated by the patient because irrigating syringes and solutions do not come near the eye. Finally, the scar is smaller and hidden in a forehead furrow. Our series is small; however, no complications have presented themselves to date, even among the cases of sinusitis associated with AIDS.

OSTEOPLASTIC FRONTAL OSTEOTOMY AND FAT OBLITERATION

Although the operation has been described by others previously, Goodale and Montgomery should be credited with popularization of this operation in the United States.[88] They developed a large experience over the years. In a review of 250 consecutive cases, Hardy and Montgomery found that 93% of postoperative patients had no further frontal sinus symptoms in a 3- to 19-year follow-up period. Six percent of patients had revision surgery for recurrent sinus disease. There were operative or immediate postoperative complications in 47 patients (18%). In the forehead wound there were eight abscesses, with six requiring revision. The abdominal wounds for obtaining the fat for obliteration of the sinus accounted for 11 hematomas and two abscesses. Bone cuts were made outside the confines of the frontal sinus on eight occasions, resulting in dural tears. All were immediately repaired, seven by suturing of the laceration and one required a dural patch. There were five miscellaneous complications, including two scars secondary to tight dressings, one anosmia, one temporary ptosis that lasted for 1 month, and one temporary loss of frontalis muscle function that resolved in 6 months. Thirty-five percent of patients had persistent anesthesia or paresthesia of the forehead. Cosmesis was judged to be excellent in 88%. Adoption of the coronal incision for most patients reduced the incidence of noticeable scars and forehead numbness.[89]

Our techniques for avoiding complications with the osteoplastic frontal operation begin with the incisions. The above-and below-brow incisions are difficult to make so that they are not readily noticeable postsurgery. However, both incisions cut the supratrochlear and supraorbital nerves, leaving the forehead insensate. For this reason, we use the coronal incision whenever possible, or occasionally one placed in a brow furrow for bald patients. The patients are instructed to wash their hair with antiseptic soap preoperatively. We do not shave the hair except for a 1-cm strip from the right to the left temple 1.5 to 2 cm behind the hairline. This strip is sufficient to accommodate the incision and closure. The adjoining hair is braided or combed out of the way. To prevent excessive bleeding from the scalp, neurosurgical hemostatic clips are applied to the scalp margin as the incision is made. To prevent tearing or excessive thinning of the periosteum overlying the frontal bone, sharp dissection must be used to separate the plane between the galea aponeurotic and the periosteum. The dissection is carried to the orbital rims and the nasofrontal suture line. It is at this point that the supraorbital and supratrochlear nerves are at risk. With care, injury can usually be avoided. A sterilized template of the outline of the frontal sinus cut from a standard Caldwell sinus x-ray is temporarily tacked into place with number 18 IV needles. The periosteal cuts are made 1.5 cm beyond the margin of the film, and the periosteum is elevated to the point at which the bone cuts are begun just under the margin of the film.[90] This technique provides a nice rim of periosteum to suture the bone flap back into place. If the bone flap does not stay back in position, marginal 0.5-mm drill holes permit the bone to be sutured in place, assuring the proper placement. We make the bone cuts with fine chisels rather than with a reciprocating saw. The cuts done in this manner are much sharper, there is no loss of bone to sawdust, and the bone flap fits back more precisely when the procedure is completed. In addition, the chisels allow the surgeon to feel when the instrument has passed through bone and entered the sinus, thus minimizing the risk of misdirection and dural tears due to penetration of the posterior wall of the sinus.

Dural tears should be repaired immediately using 5-0 prolene suture on a vascular needle. A rent in the dura can be patched with heavy fascia or pedicled pericranium. Fibrin glue is helpful. Often a lumbar drain is useful to reduce CSF pressure while the dural wounds are sealing. A good choice of antibiotics in this situation, because of their good CSF penetration, is nafcillin and gentamicin.

Recurrent mucoceles are prevented by removing every vestige of mucosa using otic drills.

NEEL-LAKE MODIFICATION OF THE LYNCH PROCEDURE

A drawback to the osteoplastic frontal operation is that it is difficult to combine with simultaneous ethmoid and other sinus surgery; and because frontal sinusitis often occurs in conjunction with other sinus disease, it is important to have a reliable technique available to the surgeon for a combined procedure that corrects the frontal sinus disease as well. The

Lynch technique, described in 1921, lost popularity because of an unacceptably high recurrence rate. The Neel-Lake modification of the Lynch procedure is the result of an analysis of the causes for failure of the operation as originally described—namely, there was too much bone removal about the lateral ethmoid and medial orbit, allowing orbital soft tissues to expand into and reobstruct the newly enlarged nasofrontal duct. In addition, extensive removal of normal ethmoid mucosa and middle turbinates was responsible for reinfection secondary to excessive drying of mucous and crust formation. With attention to these details and the introduction of a nasofrontal duct stent comprised of rolled, soft, thin, Silastic sheeting left in place on average for 3 months, the procedure has gained a high success rate. In a long-term follow-up of 5 to 20 years, the failure rates of the procedure were 7% and 11% in two groups totaling 29 patients.[91] The good candidates for the Neel-Lake procedure include patients in whom previous obliterative or nonobliterative sinus surgery has failed; patients with multiple sinus disease, following fractures through the nasofrontal duct, with and without osteomyelitis; and patients with extensive, ramifying frontal sinuses in whom it would be difficult to remove all remnants of mucosa. The Neel-Lake modification of the Lynch operation is an important operation in the armamentarium of the sinus surgeon.

MAXILLECTOMY

The maxillectomy represents a combination of procedures that are used or not used in combination depending on the extent of the malignancy and the dictates of good resection margins. It may or may not include orbital exenteration and resection of the hard palate, overlying skin of the cheek, pterygoid plates, and contents of the pterygomaxillary space.

These are bloody operations, and it is best that they are done expediciously and with the steps ordered according to increasing risk of blood loss. The incision described earlier for lateral rhinotomy can be employed with or without a lip-splitting incision.

If the lip is to be split, it is best concealed with multiple sharp angles rather than a straight line, which causes a noticeable contracture. To avoid splitting the lip, the sublabial incisions can be extended laterally and medially, as a minimal degloving technique. Liberal use of cautery, bone wax, and temporary packing with oxidized cellulose gauze or epinephrine (1:100,000)-soaked sponges is useful in addition to proceeding through the steps of the operation with timely purpose. The final scissor cut, after the chisel cuts across the pterygoid plates, divides multiple veins of the pterygoid plexus, the internal maxillary artery, and some arterial branches. The internal maxillary artery should be suture ligated. Having the anesthesiologist do a Valsalva test for the patient will reveal many of the hidden pterygoid venous bleeders. Another potential complication is CSF leak, which can occur following orbital exenteration through the optic foramen either immediately or during convalescence, par-

ticularly if there is sloughing in this area secondary to heavy cautery. We have had one CSF leak though the pores in the cancellous bone following a chisel cut across the greater wing of sphenoid. Whether the CSF leaks are an immediate or delayed occurrence, they are treated with placement of a lumbar CSF drain, head elevation, and antibiotic coverage.

If split skin grafting techniques are to be used that require packing for 5 to 10 days, the use of Xeroform gauze packing greatly reduces infection and odor. The graft site is made essentially painfree by the use of Op site which when properly applied and cared for can remain in place for several weeks until reepithelization has taken place. In addition, it can be replaced. Occasional late (> 10 days postoperatively), high postoperative fevers may be the result of graft site infection. It is important to check for cloudy drainage beneath the dressing.

The long-term sequelae are perhaps the worst complications of this procedure. With an open orbital-sinus cavity, the patient still requires weekly postoperative office care until the skin graft and mucosa cover all the internal surfaces. After cleaning, Betadyne swabs are good for keeping the wound clean and odor free. It is essential that the patient becomes an active participant in this wound care.

Our recent techniques include use of the fore-arm free flap for reconstruction of the hard palate, so that the troublesome opening between the mouth and postmaxillectomy space are permanently and solidly closed. In addition to the cavity remaining cleaner, there is no longer a need for an elaborate obturator. A modified denture will suffice, and most patients can chew on both sides of the mouth.

More recently, in selected cases (primarily those with large cheek skin losses) the techniques have included full obliteration of the defect, including the orbit and reconstruction of the hard palate with rectus abdominis or latissimus dorsi free flaps. The disadvantage of this technique is the clear potential for burying disease in some patients. Careful informed consent should be obtained when quality of life has been exchanged for the risk of concealed recurrence.

REFERENCES

1. *AMA Drug Evaluations* Chicago: American Medical Association; 1991.
2. Sharma RK, Paulose KO, al-Khalfa S, Shenoy P. Pre-operative nasal preparation—nasal packing and spraying compared. *J Laryngol Otol.* 1992;106:39–41.
3. Raj PP, Winnie AP. Immediate reactions to local anesthetics. In: Orkin FK, Cooperman LH, eds. *Complications in Anesthesiology.* New York: Lippincott; 1983:51–74.
4. Rettinger G, Christ P. Visual loss following intranasal injection. *Rhinology* 1989;9(suppl):66–72.
5. Cheney ML, Blair PA. Blindness as a complication of rhinoplasty. *Arch Otolryngol Head Neck Surg.* 1987;113:768–769.
6. Plate S, Asboe S. Blindness as a complication of rhinosurgery. *J Laryngol Otol.* 1981;95:371–322.
7. Leedom JM, Kennedy RP, Lepper MH, et al. Observations of the staphylococcal nasal carrier state. *Ann NY Acad Sci.* 1966;128:381–403.
8. Jacobs SI, Williamson GM, Willis AT. Nasal abnormality and the carrier rate of *Staphylococcus aureus.* *J Clin Path.* 1961;14:519–521.

9. Eschelman LT, Schleuning AJ, Brummett RE. Prophylactic antibiotics in otolaryngologic surgery. A double-blind study. *Trans AM Acad Ophthalmol Otolaryngol.* 1971;75:387–394.

10. Yoder MG, Weimert TA. Antibiotics and topical surgical preparation solution in septal surgery. *Otolaryngol Head Neck Surg.* 1992;106:243–244.

11. Coursey DL. Staphylococcal endocarditis following septorhinoplasty. *Arch Otolaryngol.* 1974;99:454–455.

12. Slavin SA, Rees TD, Guy CL, et al. An investigation of bacteremia during rhinoplasty. *Plast Reconstr Surg.* 1983; 71:280–281.

13. Casaubon JN, Dion MA, Larbrisseau A. Septic Cavernous sinus thrombosis after rhinoplasty. *Plast Reconstr Surg* 1977;59: 119–123.

14. Lacy GM, Conway H. Recovery after meningitis with convulsions and paralysis following rhinoplasty; cause for pause. *Plast Reconstr Surg.* 1965;36:254–256.

15. Gilden DH, Miller EM, Johnson WG. Central nervous system histoplasmosis after rhinoplasty. *Neurology* 1974;24:874–877.

16. Cohen BJ, Johnson JD, Raff MJ. Septoplasty complicated by staphylococcal spinal osteomyelitis. *Arch Intern Med.* 1985; 145:556–557.

17. Todd J, Fishaut M, Kapral F, et al. Toxic shock syndrome associated with phage group 1 staphyloccocci. *Lancet* 1978; 2:1116–1118.

18. Thomas SW, Baird IM, Frazier RW. Toxic shock syndrome following submucous resection and rhinoplasty. *JAMA* 1982; 247:2402–2403.

19. Wagner R, Toback JM. Toxic shock syndrome following septoplasty using plastic septal splints. *Laryngoscope.* 1986;96: 609–610.

20. deVries N, van der Baan S. Toxic shock syndrome after nasal surgery: Is prevention possible? *Rhinology.* 1989;27:125–128.

21. Jacobson JA, Kasworm EM. Toxic shock syndrome after nasal surgery. *Arch Otolaryngol.* 1986;112:329–332.

22. Jacobson JA, Stephens MH, Kasworm EM. Evaluation of single-dose cefazolin prophylaxis for toxic shock syndrome. *Arch Otolaryngol Head Neck Surg.* 1988;114:326–327.

23. Jones J, MacRae DL. Toxic shock syndrome. *J Otolaryngol.* 1990;19:211–213.

24. Tzadik A, Gilbert SE, Sade J. Complications of submucous resections of the nasal septum. *Arch Otolaryngol.* 1988;245:74–76.

25. Peacock MR. Sub-mucous resection of the nasal septum. *J Laryngol Otol.* 1981;95:341–356.

26. Dommerby H, Rasmussen OR, Rosborg J. Long-term results of septoplastic operations. *J Orl Relat Spec.* 1985;47:151–157.

27. Miller, T. Immediate postoperative complications of septoplasties and septorhinoplasties. *Trans Pac Coast Otoophthal Soc.* 1976;57:201–205.

28. Jessen M, Ivarsson A, Malm L. Nasal airway resistance and symptoms after functional septoplasty. *Clin Otolaryngol.* 1989;14:231–234.

29. Phillips JJ. The cosmetic effects of submucous resection. *Clin Otolaryngol.* 1991;16:179–181.

30. Cook JA, Murrant NJ, Evans KL, Lavelle RJ. Intranasal splints and their effects on intranasal adhesions and septal stability. *Clin Otolaryngol.* 1992;17:24–27.

31. Watson MG, Campbell JB, Shenoi PM. Nasal surgery: Does the type of packing influence results? *Rhinology.* 1989;27: 105–111.

32. Illum P, Grymer L, Hilberg O. Nasal packing after septoplasty. *Clin Otolaryngol.* 1992;17:158–162.

33. Johannessen J, Poulsen P. The influence of anterior nasal packing on middle ear pressure. *Acta Otolaryngol.* 1984;97:363–364.

34. Thompson AC, Crowther JA. Effect of nasal packing on eustacian tube function. *J Laryngol Otol.* 1991;105:539–540.

35. Sessions RB. Membrane approximation by continuous mattress sutures following septoplasty. *Laryngoscope.* 1984;94:702–703.

36. Nunez DA, Martin FW. An evaluation of post-operative packing in nasal septal surgery. *Clin Otolaryngol.* 1991;16:549–550.

37. Simmons MW. Intranasal injection of corticosteroids. *Calif Med.* 1960;92:155–158.

38. Evans DE, Zahorchak JA, Kennerdell JS. Visual loss as a result of primary optic neuropathy after intranasal corticosteroid injection. *Am J Ophthal.* 1980;90:641–644.

39. Byers, B. Blindness secondary to steroid injections into the nasal turbinates. *Arch Ophthal.* 1979;97:79–80.

40. Mabry RL. Visual loss after intranasal corticosteroid injection. *Arch Otolaryngol.* 1981;107:484–486.

41. Mabry RL. Intraturbinal steroid injection: Indications, results, and complications. *South Med J.* 1978;71:789–791.

42. House HP. Submucous resection of the inferior turbinal bone. *Laryngoscope.* 1951;61:637–648.

43. Ozenberger JM. Cryosurgery in chronic rhinitis. *Laryngoscope.* 1970;80:723–734.

44. Principato JJ. Chronic vasomotor rhinitis: Cryogenic and other surgical modes of treatment. *Laryngoscope.* 1979;89:619–639.

45. Bumsted RM. Cryotherapy for chronic vasomotor rhinitis: Technique and patient selection for improved results. *Laryngoscope.* 1984;84:539–544.

46. Courtess EH, Goldwyn RM, Obrien JJ. Resection of obstructing inferior turbinates. *Plast Reconstr Surg.* 1978;62:249–251.

47. Ophir D, Shapira A, Marshak G. Total interior turbinectomy for nasal airway obstruction. *Arch Otolaryngol.* 1985;111: 93–95.

48. Martinez SA, Nissen AJ, Stock CR, et al. Nasal turbinate resection for relief of nasal obstruction. *Laryngoscope.* 1983;93: 871–875.

49. Moore GF, Freeman TJ, Ogren FP, Yonkers AJ. Extended follow-up of total inferior turbinate resection for relief of chronic nasal obstruction. *Laryngoscope.* 1985;95:1095–1099.

50. Goode RL. Resection of obstructing inferior turbinates. *Plast Reconstr Surg.* 1990;86:1236–1238.

51. Drumheller GH. Nasal turbinate resection for relief of nasal obstruction [Letter]. *Laryngoscope.* 1983;93:1489–1490.

52. Mabry RL. Inferior turbinoplasty: Patient selection, technique, and long term consequences. *Otolaryngol Head Neck Surg.* 1988;98:60–66.

53. Elwany S, Harrison R. Inferior turbinectomy: Comparison of four techniques. *J Laryngol Otol.* 1990;104:206–209.

54. Kern EB, Laws ER Jr. The transseptal approach to the pituitary gland. *Rhinology.* 1978;16:59–78.

55. Campbell JP, Campbell CD, Warren DW, et al. Comparison of the vasoconstrictive and anesthetic effects of intranasally applied cocaine vs. oxylometazoline/lidocaine solution. *Otolaryngol Head Neck Surg.* 1992;107:697.

56. Schoem SR, Khan A, Wilson WR, et al. Minimizing upper lip paresthesias in approaches to transsphenoidal surgery. In press.

57. Black PM, Zervas NT, Candia GL. The incidence and management of complications of transsphenoidal operation for pituitary adenomas. *Neurosurgery.* 1987;20:920–924.

58. Laws ER Jr, Kern EB. Complications of transsphenoidal surgery. *Clin Neurosurg.* 1976;23:401–416.

59. Wilson WR, Laws ER Jr. Transnasal septal displacement approach for secondary transsphenoidal pituitary surgery. *Laryngoscope.* 1992;951–953.

60. MacBeth R. Caldwell-Luc Operation 1952–1966. *Arch Otolaryngol.* 1968;87:630–636.

61. Yarington CT. The Caldwell-Luc operation revisited. *Ann Otol Rhinol Laryngol.* 1984;93:380–384.

62. Murry, JP. Complications after treatment of chronic maxillary sinus disease with Caldwell-Luc procedure. *Laryngoscope.* 1983;93:282–284.

63. Pradhan KA, Baser B. Caldwell-Luc operation without facial swelling. *Auris Nasus Larynx.* 1990;16:223–226.
64. Cooke ETM. An evaluation and clinical study of severe epistaxis treated by arterial ligation. *J Laryngol Otol.* 1985;99:745–749.
65. Johnson DP, Parkin JL. Blindness and total ophthalmoplegia. *Arch Otolaryngol.* 1976;102:501–504.
66. Beall J, Scholl P, Jafek B. Total ophthalmoplegia after internal maxillary artery ligation. *Arch Otolaryngol.* 1985;111:696–698.
67. Hinton AE, Buckley GJ. Blood loss and hematological consequences related to nasal surgery. *Clin Otolaryngol.* 1990;15:253–256.
68. Freedman HM, Kern EB. Complications of intranasal ethmoidectomy: A review of 1000 consecutive operations. *Laryngoscope.* 1979;89:421–434.
69. Eichel BS. The intranasal ethmoidectomy: A 12-year perspective. *Otolaryngol Head Neck Surg.* 1982;90:540–543.
70. Taylor JS, Crocker PV, Keebler JS. Intranasal ethmoidectomy and concurrent procedures. *Laryngoscope.* 1982;92:739–743.
71. Friedman WH, Katsantonis GP, Rosenblum BN, et al. Sphenoethmoidectomy: The case for ethmoid marsupialization. *Laryngoscope.* 1986;96:473–479.
72. Lawson W. The intranasal ethmoidectomy: An experience with 1,077 procedures. *Laryngoscope.* 1991;101:367–371.
73. Calcaterra TC. Diagnosis and management of ethmoid cerebrospinal rhinorrhea. *Otolaryngol Clin North Am.* 1985;18:99–105.
74. Toselli RM, dePapp A, Harbaugh RE, et al. Neurosurgical complications after intranasal ethmoidectomy. *J Neurol Neurosurg Psych.* 1991;54:463–465.
75. Dutton JJ. Orbital complications of paranasal sinus surgery. *Ophthal Plast Reconstr Surg.* 1986;2:119–127.
76. Johnson LP, Parker JL. Blindness and total ophthalmoplegia. *Arch Otolaryngol.* 1976;102:501–504.
77. Giammanco P, Binns PM. Temporary blindness and ophthalmoplegia from nasal packing. *J Laryngol Otol.* 1970;84:631–635.
78. Jacobson DM, Pesicka GA. Transient superior oblique palsy following arterial ligation for epistaxis. *Arch Ophthalmol.* 109:320–321.
79. Cough JM, Somers ME, Gonzalez C. Superior oblique muscle dysfunction following anterior ethmoidal artery ligation for epistaxis *Arch Ophthalmol.* 1990;108:1110–1113.
80. Maniglia AJ, Chandler JR, Goodwin WJ, et al. Rare complications following ethmoidectonies. *Laryngoscope.* 1981;91:1234–1244.
81. Maniglia AJ. Fatal and major complications to nasal and sinus surgery. *Laryngoscope.* 1989;99:276–283.
82. Bernard PJ, Biller HF, Lawson W, et al. Complications following rhinotomy. Review of 148 patients. *Am Otol Rhinol Laryngol.* 1989;98:684–692.
83. Schramm VL, Myers EN. Lateral rhinotomy. *Laryngoscope.* 1978;88:1042–1045.
84. Wilson WR, Grove AS. A method for combined dacryoceptorhinostomy with external ethmoidectomy. *Head Neck Surg.* 1981;4:9–12.
85. Blanchard CL, Young LA. Acquired inflammatory superior oblique tendon sheath (Brown's) syndrome. *Arch Otolaryngol.* 1984;110:120–122.
86. Thompson JN, Niccole MW, Wong E, et al. Blindness following frontal sinus irrigation. *Arch Otolaryngol.* 1980;106:358–360.
87. Montgomery WW. Surgery of the frontal sinuses. *Otolaryngol Clin North Am.* 1971;4:97–126.
88. Goodale RL, Montgomery WW. Experiences with the osteoplastic anterior wall approach to the frontal sinus. *Arch Otolaryngol.* 1958;68:271–283.
89. Hardy JM, Montgomery WW. Osteoplastic frontal sinusotomy: An analysis of 250 operations. *Ann Otol.* 1976;85:523–532.
90. Ward PH, Bauknight S. A serious cosmetic complication of the osteoplastic frontal flap. *Arch Otolaryngol.* 1973;98:389–390.
91. Neel HB III, McDonald TJ, Facer GW. Modified Lynch procedure for chronic frontal sinus diseases: Rationale, technique and long term results. *Laryngoscope.* 1987;97:1274–1279.

8 Complications of Endoscopic Sinus Surgery

Kim R. Jones, M.D., Ph.D.

The use of endoscopic sinus surgery for the management of sinus disease has exploded in the last decade. Messerklinger[1] first popularized the use of endoscopes for the diagnosis and treatment of sinus disease, and descriptions of his techniques were followed by those of Wigand[2] and Kennedy.[3]

Unfortunately, the introduction of endoscopes has done little to contradict Mosher, who stated in 1912 that "intranasal ethmoidectomy is one of the most dangerous. . .of all surgical operations."[4] This is borne out by a computer search of literature between 1985 and 1991, which shows nearly 20 articles dealing with complications of endoscopic sinus surgery.

COMPLICATIONS

Bleeding

Excessive operative bleeding (see Table 8–1) is fortunately more often an inconvenience than a complication. However, it is important to remember that prevention of bleeding complications begins preoperatively. Coagulation tests and, if indicated, a bleeding time should be obtained on all patients. In addition, because many sinus patients suffer from headaches, they should be questioned about their use of nonsteroidals or aspirin, and these medications must be stopped 1 week prior to surgery.

As one proceeds with surgery, there are several areas in which one may encounter troublesome bleeding. The first of these is where the anterior ethmoid artery crosses the ethmoid roof on its way out of the orbit. Occasionally, this artery may hang down 1 to 3 mm from the roof, connected to it by a thin bony septum.[3] If accidentally transected, bleeding from this artery can usually be controlled with packing. However, there is a report[5] of the proximal portion of this artery apparently retracting back into the orbit after cauterization or hemoclip ligation and causing an orbital hematoma.

Other areas in which one may encounter bleeding problems are in the vicinity of the posterior ethmoid artery or from branches of the sphenopalatine artery. However, an arterial "pumper" is rarely encountered; rather, the surgeon suddenly

Table 8–1. Some Complications of Functional Endoscopic Sinus Surgery

Bleeding
  Intraoperative
  Orbital hematoma
  Postoperative
Damage to intraorbital structures
Cerebrospinal fluid leak
Damage to intracranial structures
Epiphora
Restenosis of middle meatus
Death

finds himself or herself in an area where profuse bleeding seems to be coming from everywhere. In these cases, applying gentle pressure to the area with a cotton pledget that is soaked with a vasoconstrictive agent such as xylometazoline or epinephrine 1:10,000 will often control the bleeding. Pressure should not be held too tightly or too long, however, because there is a possibility that blood could be forced through a crack or surgical dehiscence in the lamina papyracea and cause an intraorbital hematoma.

It has been the impression of several authors that bleeding may be somewhat more troublesome when endoscopic sinus surgery is performed under general anesthesia as compared to local.[6,7] However, both of these studies were retrospective, and it is clear that in each series, patients with extensive disease were more likely to be done under general anesthesia rather than local. Thus, it may be that the greater blood loss seen in patients done under general anesthesia was due more to differences in the extent of the disease than in the type of anesthesia used. Obviously, a prospective randomized study would be necessary to answer this question definitively.

One area in which it is hoped that one will never encounter bleeding problems is the internal carotid artery in the lateral wall of the sphenoid. Cadaver studies have indicated that the carotid may cause projection of the sphenoid wall into the lumen of the sphenoid approximately 50% of the time.[8] True dehiscence is exceedingly rare; however, one should always enter the sphenoid as medial as possible. In addition, any patient who presents with a mass in the sphenoid should undergo at least an enhanced computed tomography (CT) scan or even an arteriogram to ensure that the mass is not a carotid aneurysm before undergoing a biopsy. Maniglia[9] has reported two cases using traditional (nonendoscopic) sinus techniques that resulted in inadvertent biopsy of a carotid aneurysm in the sphenoid; both of these resulted in exsanguination and death.

Orbital Hemorrhage

Orbital hemorrhage is of concern because of the possible sequelea of orbital compression and blindness. Because the orbital cavity can be thought of as a closed space, bleeding in this space may result in an elevated intraorbital pressure, which in turn leads to an elevated intraocular pressure. However, the exact nature of how this increase in pressure leads to possible blindness is still unclear. Occlusion of the central retinal artery is the most simplistic explanation, but visual loss secondary to an increase in intraocular pressure has been noted even in patients who have pulsatile central retinal arteries by fundoscopic exam. Studies of patients with retrobulbar hemorrhage following blepharoplasty have indicated that occlusion of the posterior ciliary arteries, which supply the choroid layer of the retina, may instead be the precipitating event. This is based on several observations in patients with retrobulbar hemorrhage that showed extreme pallor of the optic disk but had normal central retinal vessels.[10] In addition, experimental studies on monkeys have indicated that central venous occlusion is not sufficient to cause the symptoms seen in patients with intraorbital hemorrhages.[11]

Orbital hemorrhage can occur in several ways during endoscopic sinus surgery. The first is by retraction of one of the ethmoidal arteries back into the orbit after transaction, where it may continue to bleed. The second, and by far the most common, is violation of the lamina papyracea, with extravasation of blood into the orbit and/or bleeding of small orbital vessels themselves. Two areas in which this may occur are just lateral to the osteomeatal complex, where sometimes there is only a thin layer of ethmoid cells medial to the orbit, and more posteriorly, where the ethmoid cells themselves are more robust but the lamina is eggshell thin.

To understand some of the signs of intraorbital hematoma, some knowledge of orbital anatomy is helpful. The orbit is lined with periosteum that is loosely adherent to its bony walls (periorbita). There is a potential space between this periorbita and the bone (the site of a periorbital abscess), which can fill with extravasated blood if the lamina papyracea is dehiscent or missing but the periorbita is intact.

Deep to the periorbita, the intraorbital space itself is divided into the intraconal (retrobulbar) and extraconal spaces by the intraocular muscles and the intermuscular septae which connect them. Both spaces are filled primarily with orbital fat and connective tissue, with the intraconal space also containing the optic nerve and other associated nerves and vessels. Bleeding in either the retrobulbar or extraconal space may cause an increase in intraorbital pressure which is directly transmitted to the globe itself.

The treatment of intraorbital hemorrhage (see Table 8–2) depends on the severity of the symptoms. Postoperative periorbital ecchymosis (caused by simple extravasation of blood into the periorbital tissues and occurring without attendant proptosis, ophthalmoplegia, or visual changes) can usually be treated with cold packs and elevation. If such ecchymosis occurs in the middle of surgery, however, especially if the patient is under general anesthesia and unable to report any visual changes that may be occurring, it would be prudent to stop surgery, remove any nasal packs, and call for an ophthalmology consultation to measure intraocular pressure. If it is normal and no proptosis has developed, it would probably be safe to continue, although this decision must be based on the risks and benefits inherent in each case.

When proptosis or visual changes occur, prompt action is the key to preventing further complications. As Thompson et al[5] have pointed out, the problem is a simple one: an increase in intraocular pressure due to an increase in the volume of a noncompressible liquid (blood) within a nonexpandable cavity (the orbit). Treatment should thus be aimed at decreasing the intraocular pressure by (1) removing any blood or hematoma, (2) expanding the volume of the orbit, or (3) reducing the pressure by pharmacological means.

One should first request an ophthalmology specialist to help in management and to obtain accurate measures of intraocular pressure. Second, the patient's head should be elevated, any nasal packs removed, and the tarsorrhaphy suture, if present, removed. Acetazolamide (500 mg) and mannitol (0.5 to 1.0 g/kg) may be given intravenously for diuresis and the periorbita, if already exposed, should be incised longitudinally both to allow blood to extravasate and to allow the intraorbital space to expand.

If the orbit does not decompress, lateral canthotomy can be performed to increase orbital volume by allowing the eye to expand 4 to 5 mm anteriorly. The canthotomy is performed by inserting one blade of a pair of scissors on the conjunctival side of the lateral canthus and one on the skin side and then carrying this cut laterally to the marginal tubercles of the zygoma. To cut down on the bleeding that inevitably follows this maneuver, a hemostat can be used to clamp the lateral commissure prior to making the incision. If orbital pressure is not reduced sufficiently by this maneuver, the lateral canthotomy can be extended by turning the scissors

Table 8–2. Treatment of Orbital Hematoma

Obtain ophthalmology consultation
Measure intraocular pressure
Elevate head
Remove nasal packing and tarsorrhaphy, if present
Acetazolamide 500 mg IV
Mannitol 0.5–1.0 g/kg IV
Incise periorbita, if possible
Perform lateral canthotomy and cantholysis
Medial decompression via external ethmoidectomy

90 degrees inferiorly and completely dividing the inferior attachment of the lateral canthal tendon. This incision should continue through the orbital septum to release completely the support provided by the lower lid.

If, after performing these maneuvers, elevated intraocular pressure is still present, an external ethmoidectomy should be performed to medially decompress the orbit. Removal of the lamina papyracea in this manner is much safer than attempting this via an intranasal approach and can be extended to include the lower floor of the orbit as well.

Other Orbital Complications

In addition to orbital hemorrhage, a number of other orbital complications have been described. Maniglia[12] has reported a chilling case in which a patient awoke totally blind following bilateral endoscopic sinus surgery. A postoperative CT scan showed partial to complete transection of both optic nerves. Neuhaus[13] has described three cases of extraocular muscle injury, one of which resulted in permanent diplopia.

Cerebrospinal Fluid Leak

A perioperative or postoperative cerebrospinal fluid (CSF) leak is fortunately a rare occurrence but is one of the more serious complications of endoscopic sinus surgery. The most extensive analysis of the causes and treatment of CSF leaks has been by Stankiewicz.[7,14,15] He reported four perioperative and four postoperative CSF leaks in a series of 800 endoscopic enthmoidectomies. Four of these occurred in the posterior ethmoid/base of skull area, two in the fovea ethmoidalis, and one each in the cribiform plate and sphenoid. No factors that might increase a patient's risk of CSF leak stood out, although Stankiewicz noted that seven out of eight fistulae occurred on the patient's right side. Stammberger and Posawetz[16] noted only three CSF leaks in a total of 4500 cases. Two of these patients had extensive polyposis and had undergone multiple previous sinus surgeries. In both patients there were few landmarks, and both leaks occurred in the medial anterior roof where the anterior ethmoid artery leaves the ethmoids to pass into the olfactory fossa. One leak was noted intraoperatively and the other 3 days postoperatively when the patient sneezed and developed a pneumocephalus.

Maniglia[12] has also reported two cases of CSF penetration during endoscopic sinus surgery; both of these were in the region of the cribiform plate. Lazar et al[17] noted two dural tears in their series of 513 adult patients; the location was not given. Rice,[18] Schaefer et al,[19] Levine,[20] and Matthews et al[21] did not report any CSF complications in their respective series totaling 605 patients.

Fortunately, the treatment of CSF leaks following sinus surgery rarely requires a neurosurgical approach. Both dural tears reported by Lazar et al[17] were patched successfully with temporalis muscle and fascia and a turbinate mucosa free flap. One of the cases reported by Maniglia[12] required an anterior frontal craniectomy for control of an intracerebral hemorrhage, but the other case was repaired using an external

ethmoidectomy approach, a septal flap, and a lumbar drain. Stankiewicz[14] utilized a technique in which a temporalis muscle/fascia graft is "tucked in" through the bony defect to hold the graft in place. If this is not technically possible, the graft is simply laid on the exposed dura and bone to cover the defect. Gelfoam packing is applied and left in place for 5 days. Stankiewicz used no antibiotics, and no meningitis occurred. Lumbar drains were used on only two of his eight patients, and one patient underwent a single lumbar tap. Interestingly, one patient closed his leak spontaneously with bed rest and head elevation.

Epiphora

Epiphora can occur when the nasolacrimal duct is blocked postoperatively by scarring, edema, etc. The location of the blockage is usually just anterior to the maxillary ostium, where the duct travels through its bony canal on its way toward exiting underneath the inferior turbinate. Although this complication is rarely reported in the otolaryngologic literature (the only mention is one case by Davis et al[22] and a 1% incidence of "dacryocystorhinitis" by Lazar et al[17]), almost a dozen cases have been described in the ophthalmology journals. Serdahl et al[23] saw eight cases of epiphora following endoscopic sinus surgery over a single 18-month period. Six of these patients complained of epiphora immediately following the procedure, whereas the other two developed symptoms 1 to 2 weeks later. Seven of the eight patients subsequently underwent dacryocystorhinostomy with resolution of their epiphora.

In addition, a recent paper by Bolger et al[24] suggests that the incidence of occult damage to the nasolacrimal system may occur in as many as 25% of patients. Briefly, Bolger et al injected fluorescein dye into the lacrimal canaliculus in 24 patients immediately following endoscopic sinus surgery. The dye emanated from under the middle meatus rather than the inferior meatus in six patients (25%). Postoperatively, none of these patients developed epiphora or dacryocysfitis. Of the five patients available for follow-up 1 year later, two had persistent drainage of the dye into the middle meatus, whereas in three patients the dye drained from the proper location underneath the inferior turbinate.

Restenosis

Although restenosis of the middle meatus antrostomy may not technically be a complication, its occurrence postoperatively can certainly be discouraging for both the patient and surgeon. In one of the earliest series, Wigand[2] reported a 10% incidence of postoperative closure of the surgical ostium due to recurrent polyps or adhesions forming between the middle turbinate and lateral nasal wall. The patency rates from two recent studies (with follow-up of at least 2 years) are almost identical at 92% and 93%.[18,20]

Davis et al[22] have analyzed the conditions which may affect middle meatus patency rates. Their sample consisted of 178 patients who underwent functional endoscopic sinus surgery and were followed for 3 to 36 months postoperatively. Eighty-seven percent of the antrostomies remained patent throughout the follow-up period. The one factor which was associated with a higher rate of failure was the presence of nasal polyps. Asthma or a history of perennial allergies was not associated with an increased failure rate. Seasonal allergy could not be assessed independently because all patients with seasonal allergy also had polyps. Middle turbinectomy was performed on approximately two thirds of the patients in the study, and these patients had an improved patency rate (96.5%). Additional patients have been added to this study, and further follow-up has been reported by LaMear et al.[25] Patients who presented preoperatively with polyps had an 11% closure rate, whereas only a 3% rate was seen in patients without polyps. Interestingly, although there were fewer stenoses with the addition of a middle turbinectomy in the patients without polyps, this procedure did not statistically improve the patency rate in patients with polyps.

Death

Only two deaths directly attributable to endoscopic sinus surgery have been reported.[12,26] Both of these occurred as the result of laceration of the anterior cerebral artery with resultant intracerebral hemorrhage. In both cases excessive bleeding occurred during the procedure and the procedure was terminated. Details of the diagnostic workup were not given in the one instance, but in the other[26] the severity of the problem was not recognized until the patient became hemiparetic in the recovery room. Both patients underwent emergency craniotomies for evacuation of the hematoma and ligation of the involved vessel but died 2 and 12 days later, respectively.

CONCLUSION

The fact that a very low complication rate has been noted in several large series of endoscopic sinus cases[6,20,21] suggests that this procedure can be done safely and effectively. However, the series of complications reported by Stankiewicz[7,14,15] suggests that a "learning effect" is certainly present. That is, in each successive report by this author, the complication rate was noted to drop significantly. Thus, some of the early concerns about endoscopic sinus surgery were perhaps due to the fact that some surgeons did not initially appreciate the differences between the standard and endoscopic approaches and perhaps did not accord the latter procedure the caution it deserved. However, as the special dangers of the endoscopic technique become better known and as residents are trained in this approach from the beginning of their careers, it is not unreasonable to expect that the nationwide complication rate of this procedure will continue to decline.

REFERENCES

1. Messerklinger W. *Endoscopy of the Nose.* Baltimore: Urban & Schwarzenbert; 1968.
2. Wigand ME. Transnasal ethmoidectomy under endoscopical control. *Rhinology.* 1982; 92:1039–1041.
3. Kennedy DW. Functional endoscopic sinus surgery. Technique. *Arch Otol Head Neck Surg.* 1985;111:643–649.
4. Mosher HP. The applied anatomy and intranasal surgery of the ethmoid labyrinth. *Trans Am Laryngol Assoc.* 1912;94:25–39.
5. Thompson RF, Gluckman JL, Kulwin D, Savoury L. Orbital hemorrhage during ethmoid sinus surgery. *Otolaryngol Head Neck Surg.* 1990;102:45–50.
6. Gittelman, PD, Jacobs JB, Skorina J. Comparisons of functional endoscopic sinus surgery under local and general anesthesia. *Arch Otol Rhinol Laryngol.* 1993;102:289–293.
7. Stankiewicz JA. Complications of endoscopic intranasal ethmoidectomy. *Laryngoscope.* 1987;99:1270–1273.
8. Van Alyea OA. Sphenoid sinus. Anatomic study with consideration of the clinical significance of the structural characteristics of the sphenoid sinus. *Arch Otolaryngol.* 1941;34:225–253.
9. Maniglia AJ. Fatal and major complications secondary to nasal and sinus surgery. *Laryngoscope.* 1989;99:276–283.
10. Heinze JB, Hueston JT. Blindness after blepharoplasty: Mechanism and early reversal. *Plastic Reconstr Surg.* 1978;61:347–354.
11. Hayrehn SS. An experimental study of central retina vein occlusion. *Trans Ophthal Soc UK.* 1964;84:586–595.
12. Maniglia AJ. Fatal and other major complications of endoscopic sinus surgery. *Laryngoscope.* 1991;101:349–354.
13. Neuhaus RW. Orbital complications secondary to endoscopic sinus surgery. *Ophthalmology.* 1990;97:1512–1518.
14. Stankiewicz JA. Complications in endoscopic intranasal ethmoidectomy: An update. *Laryngoscope.* 1989,99:686–690.
15. Stankiewicz JA. Cerebrospinal fluid fistula and endoscopic sinus surgery. *Laryngoscope.* 1991;101:250–256.
16. Stammberger H, Posawetz W. Functional endoscopic sinus surgery. Concept, indication and results of the Messerklinger technique. *Eur Arch Otorhinolaryngol.* 1990;247:63–76.
17. Lazar RH, Younis RT, Long TE. Functional endonasal surgery in adults and children. *Laryngoscope.* 1993;103:1–5.
18. Rice DH. Endoscopic sinus surgery: Results at 2-year follow up. *Otolaryngol Head Neck Surg.* 1989;107:476–479.
19. Schaefer SD, Manning S, Close LG. Endoscopic paranasal sinus surgery: Indications and considerations. *Laryngoscope.* 1989;99:1–5.
20. Levine HL. Functional endoscopic sinus surgery: Evaluation, surgery and followup of 250 patients. *Laryngoscope.* 1990;100:79–84.
21. Matthews BL, Smith LE, Jones R, Miller C, Brookschmidt JK. Endoscopic sinus surgery: Outcome in 155 cases. *Otolaryngol Head Neck Surg.* 1991;104:244–246.
22. Davis WE, Templer JW, Lamear WR, et al. Middle meatus antrostomy: Patency rates and risk factors. *Otolaryngol Head Neck Surg.* 1991;104:467–472.
23. Serdahl CL, Berris CE, Chole RA. Nasolacrimal duct obstruction after endoscopic sinus surgery. *Arch Ophthalmol.* 1990; 108:391–392.
24. Bolger WI, Parson DS, Mair EA, Kuhn FA. Lacrimal drainage system injury in functional endoscopic sinus surgery. Incidence, analysis, and prevention. *Arch Otol Head Neck Surg.* 1992; 118:1179–1184.
25. LaMear WR, Davis WE, Templer JW, McKinsey JP, Del Port H. Partial endoscopic middle turbinectomy augmenting functional endoscopic sinus surgery. *Otolaryngol Head Neck Surg.* 1992;107:382–389.
26. Reinhart DJ, Anderson JS. Fatal outcome during endoscopic sinus surgery: Anesthetic manifestations. *Anesth Anal.* 1993; 77:188–190.

9 Complications of Surgery for Neoplasms of the Oral Cavity, Pharynx, and Cervical Esophagus

Jack L. Gluckman, M.D., F.A.C.S., Markus Gapany, M.D.

The spectrum of surgery for neoplasms of the upper aerodigestive tract ranges from the most simple transoral resection with healing by secondary intention to infinitely more complex resections usually combined with equally complex reconstructive techniques. To understand and appreciate the inevitable sequelae and occasional complications that may arise from these procedures, a fundamental knowledge of the anatomy and function of the oral cavity, oro- and hypopharynx, and cervical esophagus is essential. Of particular importance is an appreciation of the mechanisms involved in swallowing, articulation, and mastication. This information is available in many fine textbooks, and the reader is encouraged to become familiar with them.

SEQUELAE VERSUS COMPLICATIONS

In any given surgical procedure, what constitutes a sequela and what constitutes a complication is debatable. One surgeon's complication is often another surgeon's sequela.

A sequela can be defined as a logical consequence of a particular procedure, whereas a complication constitutes an unexpected, untoward event. Today, with greater understanding and expertise, many sequelae can be avoided and what were once regarded as inevitable decades ago are now regarded as unfortunate complications. Obviously, many factors may predispose to a higher incidence of surgical complications even in the hands of the most experienced surgeon (eg, poor general health, prior radiation, extensive ablation and complex reconstruction). In addition, it stands to reason that the incidence of complications will be less in a more experienced surgeon's hands.

There are obviously multiple operations described for neoplasms of the upper aerodigestive tract, all with their own set of complications. To cover them all in detail would be impossible, but in an attempt to organize this chapter, procedures on the oral cavity and oropharynx have been divided as per Table 9–1 and procedures on the hypopharyx and esophagus as per Table 9–2.

Table 9–1. Surgery for Neoplasms of the Oral Cavity and Oropharynx

Intraoral resection
Mandible-sparing procedures
  Transhyoid pharyngotomy
  Lateral pharyngotomy
  Pull-through procedure
Mandible-splitting procedures
  Lateral mandibulotomy
  Anterior mandibulotomy
Mandible resection procedure
  Jaw-neck (commando operation)
Transpharyngeal approach to the parapharyngeal space

TRANSORAL RESECTION

Indications and General Principles

Transoral resection is usually reserved for benign or low-grade malignant tumors; small superficial exophytic cancers arising anywhere within the oral cavity and oropharynx; and "condemned mucosa," which consists of multicentric areas of early malignancy and premalignancy. The key to successful transoral resection is adequate exposure of the tumor, usually necessitating a variety of mouth gags, cheek retractors, and tongue depressors. The excision may be accomplished using a scalpel, electrocautery, or laser. After resection the defect may be allowed to heal by secondary intention, be closed primarily, or be skin grafted.

Complications

Complications of transoral resection can be divided into those due to obtaining exposure; those due to the resection; and those due to the repair of the defect.

Table 9–2. Surgery for Tumors of the Hypopharynx and Cervical Esophagus

Partial pharyngectomy
Partial pharyngectomy with total laryngectomy
Total laryngopharyngectomy with partial esophagectomy
Total laryngopharyngectomy with total esophagectomy

DUE TO EXPOSURE

Exposure of the anterior oral cavity is usually accomplished easily, but there can be a problem in accessing the posterior oral cavity and oropharynx.

Although a variety of gags exist, the most commonly used is the Crowe-Davis gag, which enables the mouth to be stented open while simultaneously depressing the tongue. In our experience, the most common complication due to this instrument is contusion or even laceration of the posterior pharyngeal wall due to rough or blind insertion of the gag without adequately visualizing the tip of the tongue blade. This can be remedied by carefully selecting the appropriate-length blade and inserting the blade under direct visualization using adequate illumination from a headlight.

Another complication attributable to the gag is prolonged pressure on the tongue during a long procedure. This may affect the lingual nerve, resulting in aberration in taste and sensation which may persist for weeks or even months after the procedure. Knowledge of this potential complication should remind the surgeon to release the pressure periodically during the procedure.

DUE TO RESECTION

Hemorrhage occurs to some degree with any resection but is usually minimal. Excessive and uncontrolled hemorrhage may present either at the time of surgery, in the immediate postoperative period, or after a delay of 7 to 10 days (secondary hemorrhage). Although hemorrhage can occur with any intraoral resection, surgery on the tongue, particularly the tongue base, is prone to hemorrhage because of the extensive vasculature encountered. Although the use of electrocautery and laser tends to minimize this complication, the size of the vessels in the tongue base precludes truly bloodless surgery.

If significant bleeding is encountered intraoperatively, cautery and/or ligation of the offending vessel is usually possible. If, however, the bleeding site cannot be identified because of retraction of the vessel, "blind" clamping or cautery should be avoided. Rather, a deep judiciously placed suture ligature should be used to control the retracted vessel. A similar approach should be utilized for postoperative or secondary hemorrhage. Rarely, if the bleeding cannot be controlled, angiography with embolization or even open exploration of the neck and ligation of the relevant external carotid artery branches may be necessary.

A problem unique to surgery of the tongue is the development of an interstitial hematoma, which may lead to significant swelling and even airway obstruction. This is due to bleeding from retracted blood vessels with the hemorrhage spreading between the muscle fibers. This usually is self-limiting because of the tamponade affect from the hematoma. Characteristically, vessels cannot be identified to ligate and the hematoma cannot be evacuated in a conventional sense. The best treatment, therefore, is to protect the airway with a nasal trumpet or, if absolutely necessary, a tracheotomy, and await spontaneous resolution, which normally occurs in 2 to 3 days.

Obviously, aspiration of blood or secretion can result in secondary pulmonary complications, and therefore a throat pack should always be placed if performing the surgery under general anesthesia.

Damage to the lingual or hypoglossal nerves may rarely occur if "blind" surgery is performed. Inadvertent damage to the submandibular ducts may result in stenosis with resultant submandibular sialadenitis. This can be avoided by dissecting these out, marsupializing the openings, and relocating the ducts to the wound edges. The alternative is to use a CO_2 laser when transacting the ducts, which results in a lower incidence of duct stenosis.

Excision of small superficial lesions does not usually cause any alteration in oropharyngeal function, but significant through-and-through defects of the soft palate will result in velopharyngeal incompetence with hypernasal speech and even reflux of food and liquids through the nose. Secondary eustachian tube dysfunction is also an inevitable sequela of resection of the soft palate musculature. Treatment consists of the placement of an appropriate obturator to fill the defect (Fig. 9-1). Surgical reconstruction with local or regional flaps is not particularly successful and is usually unnecessary. If eustachian tube dysfunction should develop and persist, the placement of ventilation tubes will be needed.

Through-and-through resection of the hard palate, as in an infrastructure maxillectomy, will require closure with an obturator to ensure oral competency.

The use of the CO_2 laser for intraoral resection is gaining in popularity. Extending the indications for this technique (eg, for more advanced lesions requiring more extensive resection) will naturally increase the complication rate. Nonhealing ulcers, fistula formation, and even osteonecrosis of the mandible have been described.[1,2] Animal experiments confirm that wounds created by CO_2 laser have impaired healing compared to those created by a knife.[3] Deep dissection should, therefore, be avoided and the periosteum of the mandible should not be breached, if possible.[4]

DUE TO REPAIR

Most defects created can be allowed to heal by secondary intention with no sequelae or complications. However, if the underlying musculature is damaged, the resultant scarring can cause distortion of the anatomy and may affect function (eg, velopharyngeal incompetence, secondary eustachian tube dysfunction dysphagia, and dysarthria). Rarely, if circumferential dissection has been performed, nasopharyngeal stenosis may result.[1]

To overcome some of these problems, a skin graft may be placed. This is best held in place with a bolster, which is perfectly satisfactory in the anterior oral cavity, but the bulkiness of the bolster in the posterior oral cavity and oropharynx usually necessitates a tracheostomy to protect the airway. The alternative is to "quilt" the graft into place to

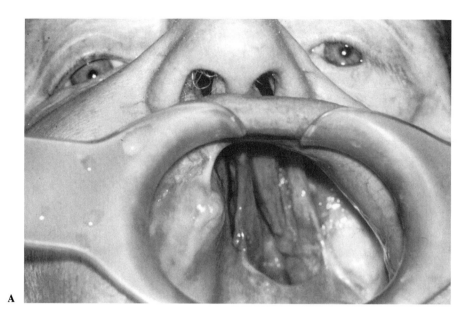

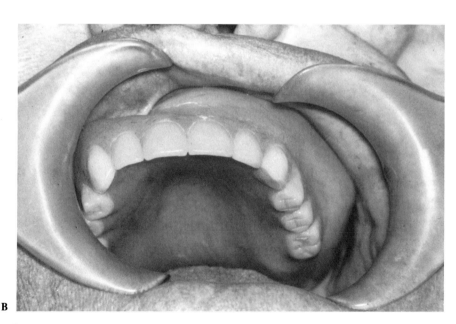

Figure 9–1. **(A).** Defect after palatal resection. **(B).** Defect filled by prosthesis.

obviate the need for the bolster, but this has never proved to be as satisfactory in our experience.

MANDIBLE-SPARING PROCEDURES

These techniques permit exposure to the oral cavity and oropharynx without disrupting the continuity of the mandible.

Lateral Pharyngotomy

INDICATIONS AND GENERAL PRINCIPLES

The lateral pharyngotomy approach has been described for access to tumors of the base of tongue, epiglottis, and

posterior pharyngeal wall. We have not found it particularly satisfactory for base of tongue or epiglottic cancers, but some authors have found it useful in select situations.[5] It can be combined with a neck dissection and extended superiorly by performing a lateral mandibular osteotomy.

COMPLICATIONS

Due to Exposure. Many of these procedures are combined with an ipsilateral neck dissection, and therefore exposure of the lateral pharyngeal wall is usually accomplished easily. However, if a neck dissection is not performed, the internal jugular vein and carotid artery may need to be retracted significantly. This is usually without incident, but if excessively manipulated an atherosclerotic plaque may become dislodged, resulting in a cerebral embolism and, rarely, carotid artery thrombosis.[6] This rare phenomenon has been described secondary to hyperextension of the neck and direct trauma due to overexuberant retraction. The intima is torn by the trauma with the development of a subintimal hematoma and thrombosis. Unfortunately, the condition may not be recognized immediately, with a delay in onset of symptoms from the time of injury varying from a few hours to days.[7,8]

The best treatment is obviously prevention, with the surgeon being cognizant of the potential for this complication and ensuring that the retraction is relaxed at regular intervals. If the patient develops localized neurological symptoms or signs, thrombosis or embolus should be suspected and a head computed tomography (CT) scan and angiography should be performed and vascular consultation sought. Emergency thrombectomy may be indicated.

Damage to the superior laryngeal or hypoglossal nerves either by stretching or disruption may also result from overaggressive exposure. This may result in temporary or permanent damage with aspiration, dysphagia, and dysarthria.

Due to Resection. Obviously the complications that may result from resection are directly dependent on the extent of the resection and size of the resultant defect. The larger the resection, the higher the incidence of complications. Because in our hands this approach is reserved for posterior and lateral pharyngeal wall cancers, hemorrhage and aspiration of blood and secretions are the major concerns. It is hoped that meticulous hemostatic dissection will prevent these problems. Inadvertent nerve damage may have serious consequences.

Due to Repair. After resection, the defect can be closed by primary repair, skin graft, or regional flap reconstruction. The most serious complication common to all three types of repair is the development of a pharyngocutaneous fistula. Athough many local and systemic factors may predispose to wound disruption and fistula formation, probably the most important is poor technique in closing the wound with too much tension on the anastomosis. The most common scenario for fistula formation is therefore an ill-conceived closure. The consequences of a fistula may vary from minor inconvenience to the disastrous, and therefore every attempt should be made to prevent this complication and to treat it energetically if it should develop.

Prevention consists of careful planning of the reconstruction and meticulous attention to the anastomosis. If primary closure is considered too risky, a skin graft should be placed. If this is used, ensure that not only the mucosal edges of the defect are sutured to the skin graft, but that (particularly in posterior pharyngeal wall defects) the graft is also sutured to the prevertebral musculature to ensure that the closure is stable and waterproof. Likewise, the skin graft should be quilted to the prevertebral musculature. If the defect is larger, a regional flap can be used. A pectoralis major myocutaneous flap may be too bulky and, therefore, either a deltopectoral flap with a de-epithelialized pedicle, a temporalis muscle flap, or even a free flap may be a better choice.

Treatment of the fistula itself consists of early identification and, if indirect (ie, undermining the flaps), conversion to a direct fistula by incising directly over the tract and diverting the saliva away from the great vessels and ensuring that the neck flaps are not elevated (Fig. 9–2). In most cases, the fistula will heal spontaneously. Only if it fails to close over a prolonged period of time should surgical closure be considered.

Prophylactic carotid artery protection is probably always advisable if a neck dissection and lateral pharyngotomy are performed. In our institution this consists of a dermal skin graft, although the pedicle of a myocutaneous flap will suffice. Perioperative antibiotics may aid in diminishing the incidence of fistula formation,[9,10] with a 24-hour regimen probably being as effective as a 5- to 7-day course.[11]

Although the use of a skin graft or flap ensures a tension-free anastomosis, a major disadvantage is the denervated, adynamic tissue, which interferes significantly with deglutition and results in loss of coordinated peristalsis and fixation of the larynx with resultant dysphagia and aspiration. This is compounded if there is associated injury to the superior laryngeal or hypoglossal nerves. There is no ready remedy for this problem other than to use as thin and pliable a flap as possible and to subject the patient to agressive swallowing therapy in the postoperative period. Removal of the tracheostomy tube before commencing swallowing is important because the tracheostomy may compound the laryngeal fixation. The routine prophylactic use of a cricopharyngeal myotomy to improve swallowing has been advocated but has not proven to be of value in our hands and is only used at a later stage if cricopharyngeal spasm appears to be the definitive cause of the dysphagia.

Transhyoid Pharyngotomy

INDICATIONS AND GENERAL PRINCIPLES

The transhyoid pharyngotomy is a little used but valuable approach to the oropharynx. Although its use has been advocated for cancer of the epiglottis, base of tongue, and posterior pharyngeal wall,[12,13] in our hands it has proved most useful for moderately sized cancers of the lower posterior pharyngeal wall. It is our impression that the blind entry into the vallecula, with a concern for violating tumor margins, precludes its use for base of tongue cancers.[14]

The hyoid bone may be left intact, with the entire dissection being performed in the suprahyoid area, or the hyoid may be excised (completely or partially), which permits a better exposure.

COMPLICATIONS

Due to Exposure. Inadvertent stretching or severing the hypoglossal and superior laryngeal nerves represents the most serious complications.[12] If the greater horn of the hyoid is left undissected and only the body is removed, the chance of nerve damage is diminished significantly. The resultant dysarthria, dysphagia, and aspiration from this nerve damage may be severe.

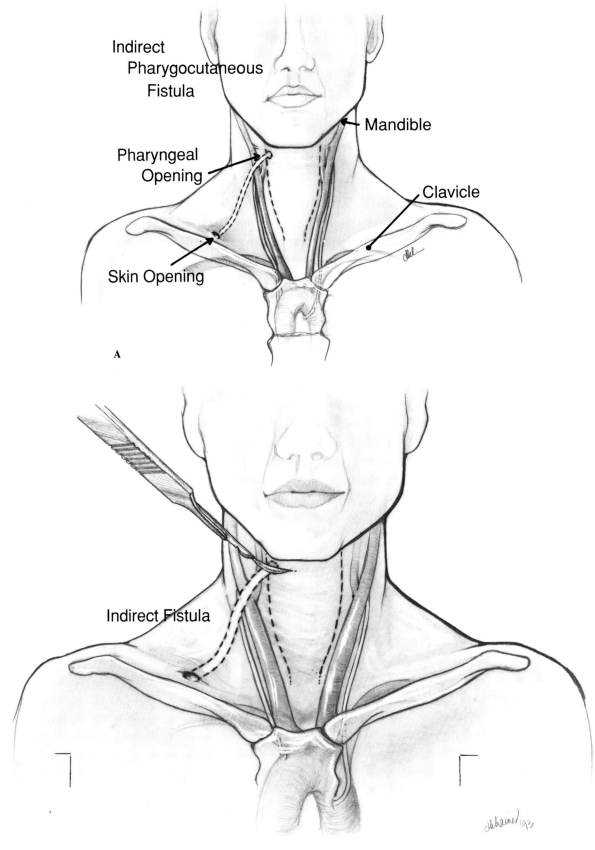

Figure 9–2.   Conversion of indirect fistula to direct fistula. **(A).** Indirect pharyngocutaneous fistula undermining flaps. **(B).** Conversion of indirect fistula to direct by incising skin overlying defect in pharynx.

Due to Resection. Because in our hands this technique is limited to resection of cancers of the posterior pharyngeal wall, the complications are similar to those encountered with lateral pharyngotomy. In the hands of those authors who use it for base of tongue cancers apparently minimal complications have been encountered.[12]

Due to Repair. The site of resection will require repair, using the same principles as described for lateral pharyngotomy. Fistula formation, aspiration, dysphagia, and so on are all potential sequelae or complications, and management is as already described. The advantage of this technique is that the approach per se is relatively atraumatic and primary closure results in no functional or anatomic impairment. Wound dehiscence and fistula formation at the site of incision are rare. A prophylactic tracheotomy should probably be performed in case of edema or hemorrhage, although in some cases this may not be necessary.

Pull-Through Procedures

INDICATIONS AND GENERAL PRINCPLES

This approach is used for resection of advanced tumors of the anterior oral cavity without overt involvement of the mandible, and it is usually combined with unilateral or bilateral neck dissections. It may be combined with a mandibular shave to ensure wide resection of the tumor without compromising the integrity of the mandible. It offers poor exposure to the posterior oral cavity and oropharynx, and these areas are best approached via a mandibulotomy.

COMPLICATIONS

Due to Exposure. There are three potential approaches to performing a pull-through procedure: lip splitting, intraoral release, and via a visor flap. The first two approaches protect the mental nerves, whereas the last compromises these nerves, leading to anesthesia and paraesthesia of the lips and mental area. For this reason, the visor flap approach is rarely used.

Due to Resection. A significant aspect of the pull-through procedure is the mandibular shave, which permits removal of the inner table or alveolar ridge. Although this is usually performed easily without sequelae or complication, the mandible may be fractured inadvertantly. The key to avoiding this disastrous complication is to perform the bone cuts with a saw, avoiding the more cumbersome hammer and chisel. If a fracture does occur, it should be plated immediately using compression plates.

Other complications include hemorrhage and aspiration, which have been described already.

Due to Repair. The sequelae that result obviously depend on the size of the defect and particularly the amount of tongue removed. Significant functional deficits may result, particu-

larly related to speech, swallowing, and mastication. Appropriate reconstruction may go a long way toward minimizing these sequelae. Complications, however, may also result from an inappropriate reconstructive technique, with wound breakdown, infection, and fistula formation. Careful selection of a suitable reconstructive technique and meticulous attention to detail in suturing the flap are therefore essential. Skin graft, various myocutaneous flaps, and even free flaps have been used to reconstruct, all of which have their proponents and detractors.

MANDIBLE-SPLITTING PROCEDURES

Lateral Mandibulotomy

INDICATIONS AND GENERAL PRINCIPLES

The lateral mandibulotomy (Fig. 9–3) was originally described by Trotter[15] and is particularly useful when superior extension of the lateral pharyngotomy is required to obtain access to larger lesions of the oropharynx and posterior oral cavity. The actual site of the osteotomy is dictated by the site of the tumor and whether the patient is dentulous or edentulous. It is usually performed with an ipsilateral neck dissection.

COMPLICATIONS

Due to Exposure. The complications described in the section on lateral pharyngotomy may all occur with this procedure along with those due to the osteotomy. Because of the site of the lateral osteotomy, the inferior alveolar nerve and vascular bundle will be severed, with resultant numbness of the ipsilateral teeth, alveolar ridge, and mental skin and even possible subsequent devitalization of the teeth. Although it has been suggested that this anesthesia will recover in a year,[16] this has not been our experience. These sequelae are a significant disadvantage of this technique.

Performing the osteotomy may result in damage to the neighboring teeth, and therefore it is best to extract a tooth at the site of the osteotomy rather than risk damage to two viable adjacent teeth.

Temporomandibular joint dysfunction as a result of too vigorous retraction of the posterior mandible segment is a common sequela which is usually temporary, but it can be more problematic if care is not taken to avoid excessive retraction. Intra-articular injection of steroids can offer symptomatic control.

Due to Resection. Tumors that necessitate this approach are by definition larger and, therefore, require wider resection. The incidence of hemorrhage, fistula formation, wound infections, and so on is, therefore, likely to be greater.

Due to Repair. Complications due to repair include all those related to closure of the mucosal defect (ie, dehiscence, fistula formation, and infection) but also those uniquely due to the

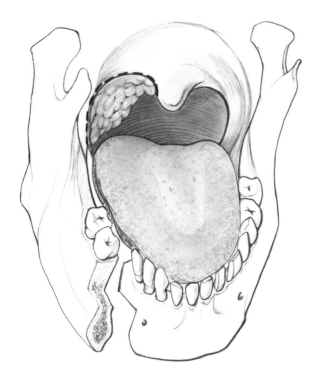

Figure 9–3. Lateral osteotomy. Note that site of osteotomy is posterior to the mental foramen.

repair of the osteotomy. Malunion or nonunion is likely, particularly if the area has undergone preoperative radiation or if postoperative radiation is to be used.[14,17] In this scenario this technique should not be used, but rather an anterior osteotomy outside the radiation field should be performed. Other steps to minimize this complication include designing the osteotomy to ensure maximal stability (eg, a stair-step osteotomy). Likewise, careful attention to fixation of the osteotomy will decrease the incidence of malunion. The older technique of wiring the segments with or without intermaxillary fixation was less than satisfactory and led to a high incidence of malunion, with occasional infection of the hardware and osteomyelitis.[17] The use of modern plating techniques permits more rigid fixation and has decreased the incidence of this problem and obviates the need for intermaxillary fixation.[16]

Malunion is frequently associated with osteomyelitis, which may lead to infection around the plates or wires with a discharging sinus tract or even fistula formation. Damage from the saw or inadequate soft-tissue coverage may also predispose to osteomyelitis. Once the diagnosis has been made clinically and radiographically, intravenous antibiotics and hyperbaric oxygen should be commenced. If this fails to improve the situation, the hardware should be removed and the osteomyelitic bone debrided. The mandible should then be stablized by external splints, and when the infection has become quiescent, a bone graft should be plated into position. The usual donor site is the iliac crest. If the osteomyelitis is too extensive or the malunion proves refractory to grafting, the posterior mandible segment should be removed and the soft tissue allowed to collapse in.

Finally, a poorly repaired mandibulotomy will result in dental malocclusion, with impaired mastication and secondary temporomandibular joint dysfunction. The key to the management of this problem is prevention, with accurate positioning of the screw holes prior to performing the osteotomy to ensure exact reapproximation of the fragments.

Anterior Mandibulotomy
INDICATIONS AND GENERAL PRINCPLES

In our hands, the anterior osteotomy (Fig. 9–4) is the procedure of choice when splitting of the mandible is indicated to obtain access to the oral cavity and oropharynx. Its major advantage over the lateral osteotomy is that it will lie outside the radiation field if delivered pre- or postoperatively and thus damage to the inferior alveolar nerve can be avoided.

The osteotomy can either be performed in the symphyseal[18] or parasymphyseal[19] sites, but the key is always to perform the osteotomy anterior to the mental foramen.

Once the osteotomy has been performed, the mandible is swung laterally by performing a release incision along the floor of the mouth (mandibular swing) or through the midline of the tongue (median labiomandibular glossotomy). This latter technique is for practical purposes only and is used for benign or low-grade malignancies of the base of the tongue.[14,20,21]

COMPLICATIONS

Due to Exposure. The osteotomy is usually accomplished via a lip-splitting incision.[19] The design of the osteotomy is

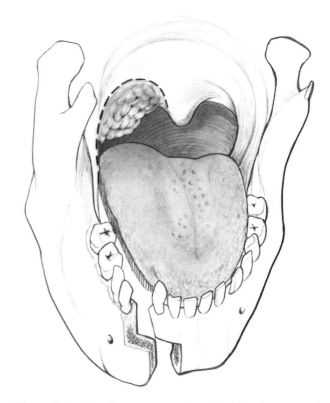

Figure 9–4. Anterior osteotomy. Note that site of osteotomy is anterior to the mental foramen.

intended to maximize stability and minimize any dental trauma. The stair-step osteotomy is the most common configuration used. The best technique to avoid dental damage is to remove a tooth at the site of the osteotomy and avoid thermal damage by using copious irrigation. Some advocate making a straight cut between the teeth without extraction and claim no increased dental trauma.[19]

As the mandible is swung laterally to obtain exposure, temporomandibular joint disruption may result if this is performed too vigorously.

Due to Resection. Cancers necessitating this approach will usually be large and will require more extensive resection and elaborate reconstruction. Wound dehiscence, hemorrhage, infection, and fistula formation will inevitably, therefore, occur in a significant percentage of cases[18] and will require appropriate management.

Due to Closure. A common but easily preventable complication of this approach is the development of an orocutaneous fistula due to disruption of the floor of mouth mucosal closure. The key to prevention of this complicaton is to ensure that an adequate cuff of mucosa is left on the alveolar ridge when making the incision, which will permit a satisfactory closure. Once the fistula has developed, it should be managed like any other fistula.

Malunion or nonunion related to instability of the reconstituted mandible, along with osteomyelitis or infection around the hardware used to stablize the fragments, are all difficult problems. A stair-stepped osteotomy using meticulous technique, mini-plates, eccentric compression plates, and lag-screw osteosynthesis have resulted in superior stabilization, obviating the need for mandibular splints and intermaxillary fixation.[21,22]

If osteomyelitis is suspected either clinically or radiographically, the mandible should be immobilized by means of external fixation and the patient should be placed on antibiotics and hyperbaric oxygen. If this fails to resolve the problem, the plate should be removed, the area of osteomyelitis debrided, and at a later stage the segment replaced with a bone graft from hip or rib.

Jaw-Neck Procedure

INDICATIONS AND GENERAL PRINCIPLES

The jaw-neck procedure, which consists of an in-continuity neck dissection, segmental mandibulectomy, and resection of the mucosal cancer, remains the cornerstone of surgical treatment for advanced cancer of the oral cavity and oropharynx, particularly if the tumor involves the mandible.

The sequelae associated with this procedure in the past were primarily related to the large defects created and ill-advised attempts at primary closure. The resultant contracture and distortion led to significant problems with speech, mastication, deglutition, and cosmesis. In the modern era, with excellent techniques available for reconstruction of both soft tissue and bone, these sequelae are no longer acceptable and function, cosmesis, and the complication rate have declined significantly, although satisfactory reconstruction remains a challenge.

COMPLICATIONS

Due to Exposure. Unlike many of the previously described procedures, there are few complications associated with the exposure per se because the performance of the neck dissection and mandibulectomy permits a wide field of exposure. Because these resections are usually performed for advanced cancer, the surgeon should be cognizant that the tumor may have extended significantly into the floor of mouth and submandibular triangle. The contents of the submandibular triangle are therefore best resected with the primary tumor as opposed to the neck dissection to avoid compromising the oncologic resection.

Due to Resection. Hemorrhage is the most common complication relating to the resection. Intraoperative bleeding may be secondary to damage to any of the branches of the external carotid system. The internal maxillary artery may be transected when performing the posterior osteotomy and may require removal of the posterior mandible segment to gain control of the vessel. Oozing from the pterygoid plexus of veins can also be troublesome but usually responds to meticulous cautery or intraoperative packing.

In the early postoperative period, hemorrhage may manifest as increased drainage from the hemovac drains or as an accumulation under the skin flaps if the hemorrhage is significant or the drains become plugged. Because flap necrosis and wound infection are significant consequences of hematoma formation,[23] the wound should be explored immediately, the hematoma evacuated, and bleeding areas isolated and controlled and fresh drains inserted. Inadequate evacuation of the hematoma or premature removal of the drains can result in seroma formation, which at the least will require repeated aspiration with a 15-gauge needle and the application of a pressure dressing. Occasionally incision and drainage is indicated. A seroma should not be drained through the neck incision itself because the local trauma and secondary infection may result in the wound becoming "unzipped."

Other complications due to resection are directly dependent on the extent of the ablative procedure. Nerve damage (eg, hypoglossal or superior laryngeal and glossopharyngeal nerves) and extensive pharyngeal and tongue resection all will severely compromise normal function.

Excision of a portion of the mandible has its own set of sequelae and complications. Following posterior mandibulectomy, the free edge of the remaining mandible segment may protrude through the skin or even into the oral cavity. This can be prevented intraoperatively by rounding off any sharp edges with a rongeur or rasp. If this does become a problem in the postoperative period, open exploration and amputation of any protruding segment should be performed. Osteomyelitis of the mandible stump has also been reported.[24] Treatment consists of wide debridement.

Due to Repair. Resection of the posterior segment of the mandible without reconstruction will result in varying degrees of scarring and collapse of the lateral wall of the oropharynx, with impairment of function depending on the extent of the resection. If only a small portion of the body is removed, the consequences are minimal, but if a hemimandible is removed particularly beyond the midpoint, the support of the tongue is lost and respiratory obstruction, sleep apnea, and other functional problems may result. Resection of the anterior body of the mandible leads to even more significant functional and cosmetic deformity ("Andy Gump deformity"), rendering the quality of life often unacceptable.

Until fairly recently, most defects after posterior mandibulectomy were closed primarily with significant distortion of the pharynx, leading to malocclusion and problems with mastication, dysphagia, and dysarthria. In addition, the cosmetic deformity following this resection was significant. These deformities were accepted as the norm. Today, the almost routine use of skin grafts, regional cutaneous and myocutaneous flaps, and more recently free flaps have greatly diminished the distortion and impaired function and decreased the incidence of complications. In spite of this, the incidence of pharyngocutaeous fistula may be as high as 10% to 30%.[25] The vast majority will heal with conservative therapy (ie, converting the indirect to a direct fistula, packing, and routine wound care), but a small percentage will require surgical closure if this therapy fails. The consequences of a poorly managed fistula range from a prolonged hospital stay to flap necrosis, wound infection, and carotid rupture, which is potentially life threatening. It is our routine, therefore, to protect prophylactically the exposed great vessels with a dermal graft or muscle pedicle to guard against such an eventuality.[26]

To minimize the cosmetic deformity and dysfunction, a case can be made for routine posterior mandible reconstruction together with a flap reconstruction of the mucosal defect. Various techniques, including plate reconstruction,[27] autogenous free graft, osteomyocutaneous flaps, and free flaps all have their advocates. Even the simplest procedure (ie, plate reconstruction) can, however, result in intraoral exposure, nonhealing wounds, and loosening of the plates,[27] although these complications can be minimized by using myocutaneous flaps concomitantly. The debate therefore continues whether the advantages of mandible reconstruction outweigh the disadvantages.

Although it is our experience that there is some advantage to posterior mandible reconstruction in select situations,[28-30] others have demonstrated little advantage over the use of a simple myocutaneous flap for soft-tissue coverage.[31] In expert hands, microvascular mandibular reconstruction and endosteal implants of dentures have demonstrated superior functional results without any increase in complications as compared to other reconstructive procedures.[32]

Reconstruction of the mandible after anterior mandibulectomy, on the other hand, is essential to maintain the functional integrity of the oral cavity. As can be expected, this is an extremely difficult reconstructive task that taxes the imagination and the skill of the reconstructive surgeon.

Whichever technique is utilized (eg, free autografts with plates, plates alone, or free revascularized grafts using radius, fibula, scapula, or iliac crest), the most important complication encountered is graft failure. Our experience with plates alone has been unsatisfactory, and these plates should be combined with bone and myocutaneous flaps to achieve any chance of success. If these procedures fail, the graft should be removed immediately and the remaining mandible segments held in position with external splints.

Even if these techniques are successful, the function of the reconstructed mandible is usually less than satisfactory and only rarely will permit the insertion of dental implants. In any event, every attempt should be made to restore the integrity of the mandible.

TRANSPHARYNGEAL APPROACH TO PARAPHARYNGEAL SPACE TUMORS

This approach is included only for completeness because it is the opinion of the authors that this approach should be mentioned only to be condemned. The limited and blind nature of the approach results in a great risk for neural and vascular damage,[33-35] inadequate tumor resection,[36] and tumor spillage. Unfortunately, the literature is replete with reports of successful resections performed by this route.[36-38] Although in the hands of an experienced surgeon, with careful case selection, this may occasionally be feasible, this approach should be discouraged and the external approach should be advised for all cases.

SURGERY FOR TUMORS OF THE HYPOPHARYNX AND CERVICAL ESOPHAGUS

These procedures are categorized as per Table 9–2 and are designed for resection of cancer in this area.

Partial Pharyngectomy (with or without Total Laryngectomy)
INDICATIONS AND GENERAL PRINCIPLES

Partial pharyngectomy alone is used in select situations for cancer of the superior pyriform sinus and posterolateral pharyngeal wall. It is, however, more frequently combined with total laryngectomy for pyriform sinus cancers, with the extent of the pharyngectomy depending on the size of the hypopharyngeal cancer. The complications of the procedure when combined with total laryngectomy are discussed in the section on laryngeal surgery.

COMPLICATIONS

The complications associated with partial hypopharyngectomy are identical to those described in the section on lateral pharyngotomy for oropharyngeal tumors.

Due to Exposure. If a concomitant neck dissection has been performed, the exposure to the lateral pharynx is easy; but if not, excessive retraction of the great vessels may lead to thrombosus or embolism. Damage to the hypoglossal, superior laryngeal, and recurrent laryngeal nerves should be avoided because it will result in dysphagia.

Due to Resection. Complications of partial pharyngectomy alone include hemorrhage, aspiration of blood, and edema, and therefore a temporary tracheostomy is usually performed.

Due to Repair. The most important complication of the repair is wound breakdown with fistula formation. To prevent this, flap reconstruction should be used to minimize the tension on the anastomosis. Flaps, however, have their own set of problems. A large, bulky flap potentially predisposes to airway obstruction, and therefore a thin, pliable flap (eg, deltopectoral flap with a de-epithelialized pedicle or a free cutaneous flap) is preferable. Chronic aspiration because of the presence of a denervated flap may be a problem and may necessitate a tracheostomy. On the other hand, an inappropriate primary closure may result in stenosis and obstructive dysphagia.

Total Laryngopharyngectomy with Partial or Total Esophagectomy
INDICATIONS AND GENERAL PRINCIPLES

Total laryngopharyngectomy is indicated for advanced-stage hypopharyngeal cancers with circumferential or near-circumferential involvement and cervical esophageal cancers. Partial esophagectomy is usually necessary to obtain adequate inferior margins, but if there is significant inferior extension or there is a second cancer in the distal esophagus, or gastric pull-up is the reconstruction of choice, total esophagectomy will be required. Unilateral or bilateral neck dissections and occasionally a superior mediastinal dissection may need to be performed.

COMPLICATIONS

Due to Exposure. Although it is an extremely radical operation, total laryngopharyngectomy is technically easy to perform and is associated with complications similar to the other procedures already described. If a total esophagectomy is to be performed, however, the complications of the laparotomy and the thoracotomy need to be considered. Most patients do not require a formal thoracotomy; however, the superior mediastinum frequently will need to be dissected.

Due to Resection. Any resection of this magnitude will inevitably be associated with complications. These include hemorrhage, either primary or secondary; hematoma; chyle leak; wound sepsis; and subsequent flap necrosis.[39] These complications can have catastrophic consequences in patients in whom a mediastinal dissection has been performed or a free revascularized graft has been used. Major vessel rupture or thrombosis of the vascular anastomoses with graft necrosis

are possible. Therefore, if hematoma or seroma should develop, these should be evacuated immediately and drains should be kept in prophylactically a little longer than usual.

Total thryoidectomy is frequently performed, and although every effort should be made to preserve at least one functioning parathyroid, the serum calcium should be monitored carefully postoperatively and treated accordingly. Disproportionate hypocalcemia has been described when a gastric pull-up is used for reconstruction,[40] with the impaired calcium metabolism not only secondary to the parathyroid resection but compounded by altered gastrointestinal function, resulting in impaired calcium absorption.[41] The surgeon should be aware of this phenomenon.

Due to Repair. Complications associated with reconstruction of the pharyngoesophageal conduit after total laryngopharyngectomy depend on the technique utilized. Older methods, such as split-thickness skin grafts and regional and distant skin flaps, were associated with an unacceptably high rate of stricture and fistula formation. The pectoralis major myocutaneous flap, with its excellent blood supply, decreased significantly the rate of fistulae but continued to result in significant dysphagia because of its bulk, stricture formation, and the adynamic conduit formed.

Two techniques most commonly utilized today to reconstruct the pharynx and cervical esophagus are the free jejunal graft and gastric pull-up. Although these are highly successful techniques, both can be associated with formidable complications.

Complications associated with jejunal free grafts may be related to harvesting of the jejunum and the placement of the bowel in the recipient site.[41-43]

In general, the laparotomy, harvesting of the graft, bowel anastomosis, and placement of the gastrostomy result in minimal morbidity. In poorly nourished and debilitated patients, impaired wound healing can be a problem and abdominal wound dehiscence may occur. Other possible complications include intestinal obstruction due to adhesions, leak from the bowel anastomosis, and wound sepsis.[41]

Of the complications encountered in the neck, graft necrosis is the most serious, with potentially catastrophic consequences. These include a high incidence of major vessel rupture, with life-threatening hemorrhage and the possibility of cerebrovascular accident.[42] The most important aspect in the management of graft necrosis is prevention. This is one of the few free flaps that are completely covered with skin flaps, and therefore the viability is difficult to assess. Graft viability and competence of the microvascular anastomosis should therefore be reassessed before concluding the operation. If any problem exists, revision of the microvascular anastomosis should be performed at that time. If revision surgery fails to provide vascular patency, an alternate means of reconstruction should be performed.

In the postoperative period, the graft needs to be monitored in some fashion because early diagnosis of graft necrosis is vital. If the diagnosis is established within a few hours, the neck can be explored and the necrosed graft replaced with

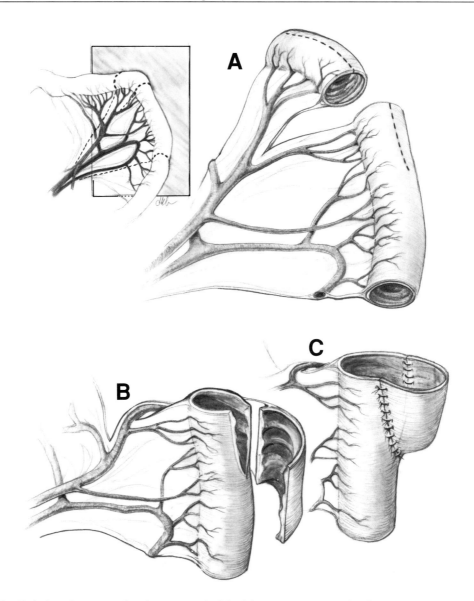

Figure 9–5. Technique for augmenting the upper end of the jejunum to overcome the discrepancy in lumen between the jejunum and pharyngeal remnant.

another free jejunal graft, with no serious sequelae. However, when the diagnosis is delayed for a few days, this is not possible and usually a temporary pharyngostoma and esophagostoma need to be created and definitive alternative reconstruction performed at a later stage.

Clinical evidence of graft necrosis is surprisingly undramatic, and thus it is important to maintain a high index of suspicion. Systemic features of graft failure, such as pyrexia and elevated white blood count, are not found consistently. Edema of the overlying skin flap is suggestive of graft necrosis, but not diagnostic. The appearance of an early pharyngocutaneous fistula is suspicious.

The best method of determining the status of the graft is direct visualization, either through the mouth (if the pharyngeal anastomosis is performed high enough) or a fiberoptic scope (which is more difficult because of the accumulation of secretions). A highly satisfactory alternate technique is to exteriorize a redundant segment of jejunum

and directly monitor this and amputate it on the fifth postoperative day.

Great vessel rupture is usually associated with late-diagnosed graft failure with secondary thrombosis and infection. If just the arterial anastomosis has ruptured, this can usually be oversewn and the lumen of the carotid artery preserved intact, but if the carotid itself has ruptured, this will need to be oversewn and resected with acceptance of the possible consequences. A ruptured jugular vein requires ligation and resection. Cerebrovascular sequelae may result from retrograde extension of the thrombosis from the anastomosis to the internal carotid artery or as a result of vessel rupture.

The incidence of pharyngocutaneous fistulae is relatively infrequent considering the radical nature of the surgery. Most occur at the superior jejunal-pharyngeal anastomosis due to the discrepancy in size between the pharynx and jejunum and the great difficulty in performing this anastomosis. Most pharyngocutaneous fistulae will heal spontaneously with conservative management, but it is essential to divert the fistula away from the vascular anastomosis.

Although most patients will have some degree of initial dysphagia, due to edema of the jejunal graft, this subsides within the first few months. Stenosis of the inferior anastomosis rarely occurs but responds well to dilatation. Stenosis of the upper anastomosis is invariable because of the discrepancy in size between the lumen of the jejunum and pharynx, making the anastomosis difficult. This can be overcome by filleting the jejunum on its antimesenteric border to widen the lumen or, better yet, fashioning a redundant segment of jejunum to augment the size of the upper lumen[42] (Fig. 9–5). A redundant bowel syndrome can result if the free jejunal graft is too long, causing pooling of secretions and food at the lower end, resulting in dysphagia. Functional dysphagia due to neuromuscular incoordination can be prevented by performing a myotomy in the jejunal musculature.

Gastric pull-up is an extensive surgical procedure associated with significant postoperative morbidity and even mortality. Patients selected to have this reconstruction must be relatively healthy and able to withstand the surgery.

The complications of gastric pull-up can be categorized as due to the laparotomy, thoracic dissection, the cervical anastomosis, and malfunction of the transposed stomach.[44] Among the most common pulmonary and mediastinal complications are pneumothorax, pleural effusion, atelectasis, and pulmonary infiltrates. These complications are usually minor enough and usually do not result in significant morbidity. Other more ominous but rarely encountered chest complications include postoperative intrathoracic hemorrhage, chylothorax, mediastinitis, sternal dehiscence, and gastropleural fistula, resulting in mediastinal empyema.[44-47] The abdominal complications include prolonged postoperative ileus, abdominal wound dehiscence, gastrointestinal bleeding, pancreatitis, and mechanical small bowel obstruction due to volvulus.[44-47]

Anastomotic breakdown due to distal ischemia of the stomach with pharyngocutaneous fistula is a serious complication with potentially life-threatening consequences, including mediastinitis and major vessel rupture both in the chest and neck.[44] Even if rupture does not occur, stenosis at the anastomosis may result. The key to prevention is to ensure a tension-free anastomosis by adequate mobilization of the stomach and even removal of the clavicular heads to decrease any pressure on the stomach.

If a fistula develops, open exploration and diversion of the fistula away from the major vessels should be performed. If, however, effective diversion is not feasible, a controlled pharyngostoma and gastric-cutaneous fistula should be created and closed at a later phase with a myocutaneous flap.

A more common problem is delayed gastric emptying, with regurgitation of gastric contents into the oral cavity while leaning forward or lying down shortly after a meal. This problem is managed by decreased meal size and head elevation. Minor episodes of postprandial diarrhea can occasionally occur but respond well to conservative management.

CONCLUSION

As is apparent, surgery on the upper aerodigestive tract is fraught with serious sequelae and complications and should only be undertaken by experienced surgeons with a clear appreciation of the sequelae and complications and with the expertise to manage these complications if they occur.

REFERENCES

1. Nagorsky MJ, Session DG. Laser resection or early oral cavity cancer—results and complications. *Ann Otol Rhinol Laryngol.* 1987;96:556–560.
2. Guerry RL, Silverman S, Dedo HH. Carbon dioxide laser resection of superficial oral carcinoma. *Ann Otol Laryngol.* 1986;95:547–555.
3. Fisher SE, Frame JW, Browne RM, et al. A comparative histological study of wound healing following CO_2 laser and conventional surgical excision of canine buccal mucosa. *Arch Oral Biol.* 1983;28:287–291.
4. Fisher SE, Frame JW. The effects of carbon dioxide surgical laser on oral tissues. *Br J Oral Maxillofac Surg.* 1984;22:414–425.
5. Moore DM, Calcaterra TC. Cancer of the tongue base treated by a transpharyngeal approach. *Ann Otol Rhinol Laryngol.* 1990;99:300–303.
6. Miller DR, Bergstrom L. Vascular complications of head and neck surgery. *Arch Otolaryngol.* 1974;100:136–140.
7. Fleming JF, Petrie D. Traumatic thrombosis of the internal carotid artery with delayed hemiplegia. *Canad J Surg.* 1968;11:166–172.
8. Pitner SE. Carotid thrombosis due to intraoral trauma. *N Engl J Med.* 1966;274:764–767.
9. Robbins KT, Byers RM, Fainstein V, et al. Wound prophylaxis with metronidazole in head and neck surgical oncology. *Laryngoscope.* 1988;98:803–806.
10. Becker GD, Parell GJ. Cefazolin prophylaxis in head and neck cancer surgery. *Ann Otol Rhinol Laryngol.* 1979;88:183–186.
11. Johnson JT, Schuller DE, Silver F, et al. Antibiotic prophylaxis in high-risk head and neck surgery: One-day vs. five-day therapy. *Otolaryngol Head Neck Surg.* 1986;95:554–557.
12. Zeitels SM, Vaughn CW, Ruh S. Suprahyoid pharyngotomy for oropharynx cancer including the tongue base. *Arch Otolaryngol Head Neck Surg.* 1991;117:757–760.
13. Zeitels SM, Vaughn SW, Toomey JM. A precision technique for suprahyoid pharyngotomy. *Laryngoscope.* 1991;101:565–566.
14. Gluckman JL, Thompson R. Cancer of the oropharynx. In: Suen JW, Meyers EM, eds., *Cancer of the Head and Neck.* New York: Churchill Livingstone; 1989.
15. Trotter W. Operation for malignant disease of the pharynx. *Br J Surg.* 1929;16:485–495.
16. Pinsolle J, Siberchicot F, Emparanza A, Caix P, Michelet FX. Approach to the pterygomaxillary space and posterior part of the tongue by lateral stair-step mandibulotomy. *Arch Otolaryngol Head Neck Surg.* 1989;115:313–315.
17. Desanto LW, Whicker JH, Devine KD. Mandibular osteotomy and lingual flaps. *Arch Otolaryngol.* 1975;101:652–655.
18. Spiro GR, Gerold FP, Shah JP, Sessions RB, Strong EW. Mandibulotomy approach to oropharyngeal tumors. *Am J Surg.* 1985;150:466–469.
19. McGregor IA, MacDonald DG. Mandibular osteotomy in the surgical approach to the oral cavity. *Head Neck Surg.* 1983;5:457–462.

20. Martin H, Tollefsen HR, Gerold FP. Median labiomandibular glossotomy. *Am J Surg.* 1971;102:753–759.

21. Tollefsen HR, Spiro RH. Median labiomandibular glossotomy. *Annals Surg.* 1971;173:415–420.

22. Dawson DE, Gapany M, LaVelle WE. Titanium lag-screw osteosynthesis for the restoration of mandibular continuity in mandibular "swing" procedures. *Laryngoscope.* 1990;100: 1241–1244.

23. McGuirt WF, McCabe BF, Krause CJ. Complications of radical neck dissection: A survey of 788 patients. *Head Neck Surg.* 1979;1:481–487.

24. LaFerriere KA, Sessions DG, Thawley SE, Wood BG, Ogura JH. Composite resection and reconstruction for oral cavity and oropharynx cancer. *Arch Otolaryngol.* 1980;106:103–110.

25. Conley JJ. Oropharyngeal fistula. In: Conley JJ, ed. *Complications of Head and Neck Surgery.* Philadelphia: WB Saunders; 1979.

26. Shumrick DA. Carotid artery rupture. *Laryngoscope.* 1973; 83:1051–1061.

27. Chow JM, Hill JH. Primary mandibular reconstruction using the AO reconstruction plate. *Laryngoscope.* 1986;96:768–773.

28. Logemann JA, Bytell DE. Swallowing disorders in three types of head and neck surgical patients. *Cancer.* 1979;44:1095–1105.

29. McConnel FMS, Teichenberg JF, Adler RK. A comparison of three methods of oral reconstruction. *Arch Otolaryngol Head Neck Surg.* 1987;113:496–500.

30. Teichenberg J, Bowman J, Geopfert H. New tests series for the functional evaluation of oral cavity cancer. *Head Neck Surg.* 1985;8:9–20.

31. Komisar A. The functional results of mandibular reconstruction. *Laryngoscope.* 1990;100:364–374.

32. Urken ML, Buchbinder D, Weinberg H, et al. Functional evaluation following microvascular oromandibular reconstruction of the oral cancer patient: A comparative study of reconstructed and nonreconstructed patients. *Laryngoscope.* 1991;101: 935–950.

33. Som PM, Biller HF, Lawson W. Tumors of the parapharyngeal space. Preoperative evaluation, diagnosis and surgical approaches. *Ann Otol Rhinol Laryngol.* 1981;90(suppl 80):3–15.

34. Baker DC, Conley J. Treatment of massive deep lobe parotid tumors. *Am J Surg.* 1979;138:572–575.

35. Carrau RL, Myers EN, Johnson JT. Management of tumors arising in the parapharyngeal space. *Laryngoscope.* 1990;100: 583–589.

36. Goodwin WJ, Chandler JR. Transoral excision of lateral pharyngeal space tumors presenting intraorally. *Laryngoscope.* 1988;98:266–269.

37. Havens FZ, Betler LC. Mixed tumors of the posterior pharyngeal wall. *Ann Otol Rhinol Laryngol.* 1955;64:457–465.

38. McIlrath DC, Remine WH, Devine KD, Dockerty MB. Tumors of the parapharyngeal region. *Surg Gynecol Obstet.* 1963;116: 88–94.

39. Gluckman JL, McCafferty GJ, Black RJ, et al. Complications associated with free jejunal graft reconstruction of the pharyngoesophagus—a multiinstitutional experience with 52 cases. *Head Neck Surg.* 1985;7:200–205.

40. Krespi YP, Wurster CF, Wang TD, Stone DM. Hypoparathyroidism following total laryngpharyngectomy and gastric pull-up. *Laryngoscope.* 1985;95:1184–1187.

41. Price JC, Ridley MB. Hypocalcemia following pharyngoesophageal ablation and gastric pull-up reconstruction: Pathophysiology and management. *Ann Otol Rhinol Laryngol.* 1988;97: 521–526.

42. Gluckman JL, McDonough JJ. Free jejunal grafts. In: Baker S, ed. *Microsurgical Reconstruction of the Head and Neck.* New York: Churchhill Livingstone; 1989:229–254.

43. Gluckman JL, McDonough JJ, Donegan JO. The role of the free jejunal graft in reconstruction of the pharynx and cervical esophagus. *Head Neck Surg.* 1982;4:360–369.

44. Ujiki GT, Pearl GJ, Poticha S, Sisson GA, Shields TW. Mortality and morbidity of gastric pull-up for replacement of the pharyngoesophagus. *Arch Surg.* 1987;122:644–647.

45. Griffin SM, Woods SDS, Chang A, Chung PCS, Li AKS. Early and late surgical complications of subtotal oesophagectomy for squamous carcinoma of the oesophagus. *J Res Coll Surg Edinb.* 1991;36:170–173.

46. Shah JP, Shemen L, Spiro Rh, Strong EW. Selecting variants in pharyngeal reconstruction. *Ann Otol Rhinol Laryngol.* 1984;93:318–321.

47. de Vries EJ, Stein DW, Johnson JT, et al. Hypopharyngeal reconstruction: A comparison of two alternatives. *Laryngoscope.* 1989;99:614–617.

10 Complications of Laryngeal Surgery

Carl E. Silver, M.D., David H. Henick, M.D.

Surgical procedures performed for extirpation of laryngeal carcinoma range from massive soft-tissue resections for control of advanced disease to the precise limited-field dissections required for removal of relatively early stage lesions with preservation of the essential functions of the larynx. Naturally the complications experienced with these distinct types of surgical procedure, as well as their management, will differ considerably. An entire volume would be required to review the complications unique to each surgical procedure. In addition, the complications related to radical dissection of the neck and the use of particular reconstructive methods involving free or pedicled transfer of tissue from remote sites are many and are not unique to surgery of the larynx. This discussion will focus on the major types of complications specific to extirpation of the larynx itself which will be considered according to whether they are associated with procedures requiring total laryngectomy or with the various conservation operations. In addition, the discussion will focus mainly on intermediate and long-term complications and exclude discussion of events in the immediate postoperative period that are common to all major operative procedures in the head and neck or in general.

COMPLICATIONS ASSOCIATED WITH TOTAL LARYNGECTOMY
Infection, Fistula, and Necrosis

Pharyngocutaneous fistula is a major problem in radical surgery of the pharynx and larynx. Fistulization occurs when the pharyngeal closure does not heal completely, leading to leakage of pharyngeal secretions beneath the skin flaps, infection, and external drainage through the cervical wound. The extent and severity of a fistula depend on the amount of associated tissue necrosis. Thus fistulae may range from narrow tracts surrounded by relatively healthy tissue to massive open wounds with wide exposure of the hypopharynx and, often, the carotid artery (Fig. 10–1A). All fistulae will delay onset of oral feeding and increase length of hospitalization, and the more severe varieties can set the stage for carotid artery rupture. Pharyngocutaneous fistulae are often respon-

sible for significant metabolic depletion and, by delaying the administration of postoperative radiotherapy, may contribute to recurrence of cancer.

PREDISPOSING FACTORS

Numerous contributing factors have been implicated in fistula formation, but actual study of experience by various authors has produced somewhat conflicting conclusions. Many surgeons have believed that previous radiation therapy is a major predisposing factor. Stell and Cooney[1] and Lundgren and Olofsson[2] found that radiation therapy markedly increased the rate of fistula formation, whereas Bresson et al[3] concluded that radiotherapy determined the severity of the fistulae. Cummings et al[4] and Weingrad and Spiro[5] also reported that although radiotherapy did not increase the absolute number of fistulae in their experience, fistulae in previously irradiated patients were more severe and required more time to heal. Johansen et al[6] showed a pronounced increase of fistulae and late complications after high-dose radiotherapy and large field sizes. Prophylactic metronidazole resulted in a significant decrease in the frequency of postoperative fistulae from 60% to 13% for patients receiving 6800 cGy of irradiation and laryngectomy for salvage. On the other hand, Gall et al,[7] in a multifactorial analysis, related the incidence of fistulae to tumor site (hypopharynx more than larynx) and to positive margins, as opposed to radiation or stage of disease.

Other factors play a role in fistula formation. Lavelle and Maw[8] associated preoperative tracheostomy, radical neck dissection, and low postoperative hemoglobin level with an increased rate of fistula formation. Myers[9] and Cantrell[10] stressed wound tension as an important etiologic factor. Shemen and Spiro[11] demonstrated only preoperative weight loss and microscopic margins as significant factors influencing the fistula rate. Mendelsohn and Bridger[12] reported that in addition to preoperative radiation therapy in doses exceeding 5000 cGy, postoperative anemia (hemoglobin below 12.0 mg/dL), the presence of a pyriform sinus tumor, and large tumor burden were contributing factors. Previous

107

radiotherapy as well as the site of the fistula opening had the greatest influence on the ease or difficulty of fistula management.

Many reports have shown a strong correlation between fistula formation and the extent of pharyngeal resection as well as the type of repair employed. Weingrad and Spiro[5] found a major complication rate of 27% and a fistula rate of 4% in those patients who had a conventional total laryngectomy performed for endolaryngeal tumors, whereas the complication rate was 77% and the fistula rate was 37% in those patients with laryngopharyngectomies performed for tumors involving the hypopharynx. Most of the latter group of patients included in the aforementioned report required planned temporary pharyngostomies and staged reconstruction with cutaneous flaps to close the large hypopharyngeal defects. These staged repairs often involved prolonged hospitalizations, multiple surgical procedures, and extensive intervals before institution of oral feeding. The advent of the myocutaneous flap produced a marked reduction in postoperative morbidity, permitting single-stage closure of extensive hypopharyngeal defects and thus minimizing the effect of size of the surgical defect in pharyngeal mucosa upon the incidence of postoperative fistula and morbidity, as demonstrated in a subsequent study at the same institution by Shemen and Spiro.[11]

MANAGEMENT

Simple wound infections unassociated with necrosis, skin loss, or fistula can be managed by opening the wound to provide adequate drainage. Salivary fistulae are usually manifested by purulent drainage beneath intact skin flaps. If necessary, confirmation of a pharyngeal defect can be ascertained after the oral administration of methylene blue. When there is minimal loss of tissue, the fistula may be treated adequately by establishing continuous drainage with sump wound catheters, which are changed frequently. Oral feedings should be stopped and oral suctioning of saliva is recommended to prevent further soilage of the wound. As the fistula drains freely through the catheters, the surrounding tissue granulates and the fistulous tract contracts progressively. The catheters are removed when the tract has contracted sufficiently and contains healthy granulation tissue, and when clear saliva rather than purulent drainage issues from the fistula.

Larger fistulae require surgical closure. Such closure requires two epithelial surfaces: one to line the pharynx and one to resurface the cervical skin. Stell and Cooney[1] classified fistulae according to the method required for repair:

Type I: Both surfaces may be developed locally.
Type II: One surface may be developed locally, and one from a distance.
Type III: Both surfaces must be provided by distant flaps.

Closure of a Type I fistula must await complete epithelialization of skin to mucosa circumferentially around the defect. The mucosal defect is then closed by development of crescentic or "trap door" flaps based on the mucocutaneous junc-

tion and turned inward, whereas the external defect can be resurfaced by an advancement or rotation flap of adjacent skin and subcutaneous tissue. The mucosal defect of a Type II fistula may be repaired similarly by direct approximation of tissue or by turning in of local flaps, but it will require transfer of a pedicled or revascularized flap from the chest or other site to resurface the cervical skin. Closure of Type III fistulae is usually accomplished by transfer of free or myocutaneous flaps, with islands of skin employed to replace the mucosal defect as well as the external surface.

Disruption of the pharyngeal closure and leakage of pharyngeal contents beneath the skin flaps is often associated with necrosis of the overlying skin and loss of coverage of the neck wound, producing the simultaneous occurrence of fistula, necrosis, and infection. Such wounds require debridement and control of infection as well as surgical closure. The timing of surgery will often depend on whether the carotid artery is exposed in the wound and hence in danger of rupture. If the carotid has been covered successfully with a muscle flap or dermal graft, the surgeon may opt for a period of wound debridement, antibiotic therapy, and hyperalimentation prior to surgically closing the wound. If the carotid artery is exposed, however, it must be covered immediately with healthy skin, muscle, or a myocutaneous flap.

We have employed a "sandwich" pectoralis myocutaneous flap for coverage of large necrotic cervical defects associated with pharyngeal fistula, infection, and carotid exposure. Successful results with seven patients treated in this manner were reported by Goldstein et al.[13] The technique is demonstrated in Figure 10–1. In departure from the previously standard procedure, we do not wait for clean granulation tissue to develop at the recipient site, but we debride the wound in the operating room and immediately apply the myocutaneous flap to the freshly debrided cervical tissue. The skin paddle is turned inward to close the defect in pharyngeal mucosa, whereas a meshed skin graft is applied to the external aspect of pectoralis muscle to resurface the skin defect. Use of the skin graft avoids sacrifice of unnecessarily large amounts of pectoral skin for repair of the complex wound.

Tracheal Stomal Stenosis

A well-functioning postlaryngectomy tracheostoma should provide normal laminar airflow without the need for stenting to maintain an adequate airway, facilitate normal clearing of tracheobronchial secretions, and provide a wide enough lumen to allow the insertion of a tracheoesophageal speech prosthesis. Tracheal stomal stenosis may be considered extant when any of these functions are not met. There is considerable variation in the reported incidence ranging from 4%[14] to 42%.[15] Stenosis of the tracheostoma after laryngectomy compromises optimal air exchange, the efficacy of the mucociliary transport system, and the ability of the patient to clear tracheobronchial secretions.[16] Recurrent pulmonary infections may result. The functional effect of tracheostomal stenosis varies. Whereas a patient with normal pulmonary function will maintain normal exercise tolerance with up to

75% reduction in luminal surface area, a patient with chronic obstructive pulmonary disease will manifest respiratory insufficiency.[17]

PREDISPOSING FACTORS

Certain factors seem to predispose to tracheal stomal stenosis. Black individuals have a higher incidence of keloid and hypertrophic scar formation. Females have a narrower tracheal circumference and softer tracheal cartilage, which is affected more easily by extrinsic pressure. Short neck, prominent thyroid gland, prominent muscles, and, rarely, congenital absence of tracheal rings are also predisposing factors. The question of whether radiation therapy is a predisposing factor remains controversial.

PREVENTIONS OF STOMAL STENOSIS

In the immediate postoperative period, obstruction of the trachea or the laryngectomy tube with clotted blood is of primary concern. A short double-cannula number 10 or 12 laryngectomy tube should always replace the single-cannula anesthesia endotracheal tube at the termination of the procedure. If ventilatory assistance is required postoperatively, a number 8 or 10 cuffed plastic tracheostomy tube can be used alternatively.

Prevention of tracheal stomal stenosis can be accomplished by providing a tension-free anastomosis, displacing prolapsing tissues, and lengthening and interrupting the tracheal circumference. The tracheostoma may be created by incorporating the tracheal stump directly into the transverse cervical incision, or it may be placed in the inferior flap, either through a separate incision or a vertical extension from the junction of flaps. A short tracheal stump is best managed by exteriorization into the inferior flap and employment of tension-releasing sutures of 0 or 00 silk or nylon.[18] If the tracheal stump is substernal or fails to reach the level of the suprasternal notch without excessive tension, a manubriectomy with mediastinal tracheostomy may be necessary.[19] Advancement of a cutaneous or myocutaneous flap funneled to the trachea may be employed as an alternative to manubriectomy with thoracotracheostomy.

Montgomery[20] classified tracheal stenosis into three types: concentric (60%), vertical shelf (30%), and inferior shelf stenosis (10%). Concentric stenosis is caused by circumferential scar contracture or keloid formation. Resection of excessive cutaneous and subcutaneous adipose tissue, proper trimming of protruding tracheal cartilaginous rings, and exact mucocutaneous approximation will allow primary healing and help prevent this type of stenosis. Lengthening and interrupting the circumference of the tracheal stoma will help prevent circumferential stenosis secondary to benign scar contracture. Bevelling the tracheal stump at a 45° angle in an anteroposterior direction changes the configuration of the opening from a circle to an ellipse and increases the circumference of the stoma. Other techniques to lengthen and stagger the mucocutaneous suture line, often employed for

correction of established tracheostomal stenosis, may be used at the time of initial surgery to prevent stenosis.

Vertical shelf stenosis results from the lateral restriction exerted by the sternocleidomastoid muscle or the remaining thyroid lobe. Transection of the clavicular insertion of the sternomastoid muscle or partial resection of the bulky thyroid lobes will prevent this form of stenosis. Inferior shelf stenosis is caused by redundant skin folds, and it accounted for fewer than 10% of the cases reported by Montgomery.[20] It is best prevented by excising the redundant tissue prior to creation of the stoma.

MANAGEMENT OF TRACHEAL STOMAL STENOSIS

A variety of nonsurgical techniques may be employed for initial management or for mild cases. These include dilatation with placement of progressively larger tracheostomy tubes or stoma buttons. Occasionally, after prolonged dilatation, the stoma may remain adequately patent, but more often stenosis recurs after removal of the stent.

A simple method of surgical correction was described by Montgomery[20] and later by Callins and Applebaum.[21] This

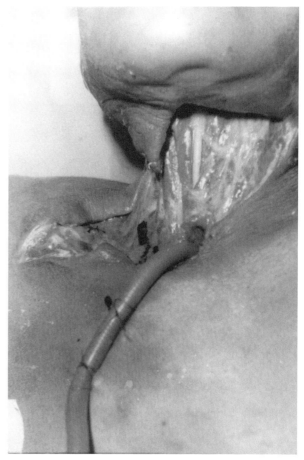

A

Figure 10–1. "Sandwich" pectoralis major myocutaneous flap for immediate coverage of a necrotic cervical wound with gaping pharyngeal fistula. **(A).** Massive cervical wound with open pharynx and exposed carotid artery.

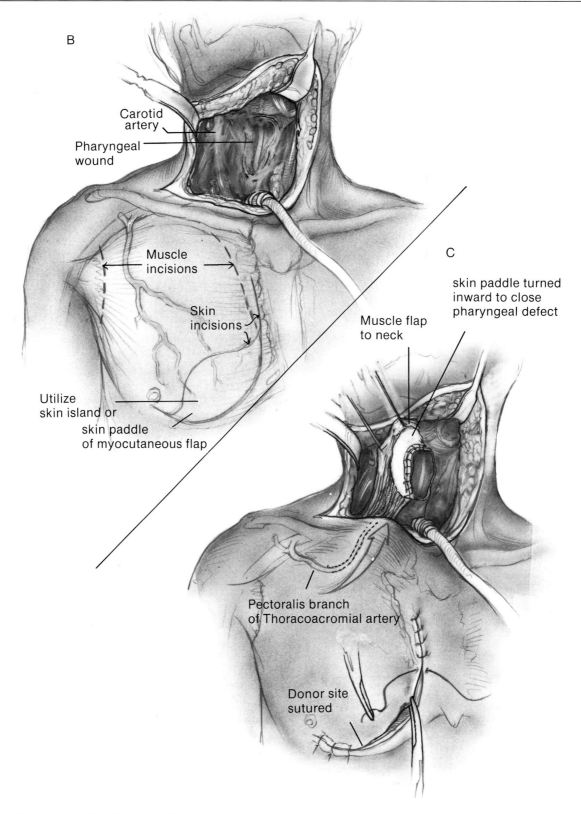

Figure 10–1 (continued).   (B). Pectoralis major flap designed for coverage of wound. **(C).** Myocutaneous flap transferred to the cervical wound. The skin paddle is turned inward and sutured to the edges of the pharyngeal defect.

consists of multiple radial incisions made with electrocautery through the mucosa, skin, and fibrous bands of the stenotic area, followed by insertion of a number 10 laryngectomy tube, which is left in place for 1 month.

More formal techniques of correction of tracheostomal stenosis combine excision of all cutaneous and cartilaginous scar tissue and mobilization of adjacent normal tissues, with Z-plasties and/or relaxing incisions to create an irregular

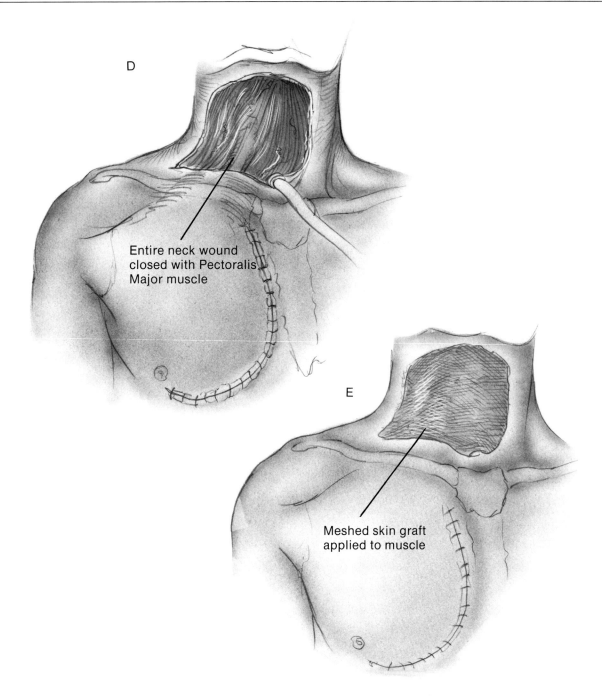

D

Entire neck wound
closed with Pectoralis
Major muscle

E

Meshed skin graft
applied to muscle

Figure 10–1 (continued). **(D).** The pectoralis major muscle covers the entire cervical defect and carotid artery. **(E).** A meshed skin graft is applied over the muscle to resurface the neck.

stomal perimeter and redistribute the forces of scar formation to prevent concentric stenosis. Single Z-plasties[22,23] are usually placed in the posterior membranous tracheal wall, allowing for the transposition of both skin and mucosal triangles (Figs. 10–2A–F). Dual Z-plasties are usually created in the anterior and posterior portions of the stoma. Relaxing incisions in the trachea are created by simple perpendicular transections of the trachea with advancement of a superiorly based triangular skin flap.[24,25] Double relaxing incisions, followed by interdigitation of triangular cutaneous advancement and rotation flaps (Figs. 10–2G–I) create a characteristic "bow tie" appearance of the stoma. Placement of the relaxing

incisions on the lateral aspects of the trachea as shown will avoid interference with a subsequently inserted prosthetic device.[26] Other procedures employed include transposition of cervical skin flaps sutured to the lateral tracheal walls and transfer of fenestrated deltopectoral or myocutaneous flaps in patients with severe skin compromise secondary to radiation therapy.

Hypopharyngeal Stenosis

Varying degrees of hypopharyngeal stenosis occur after total laryngectomy with some frequency. After laryngectomy for

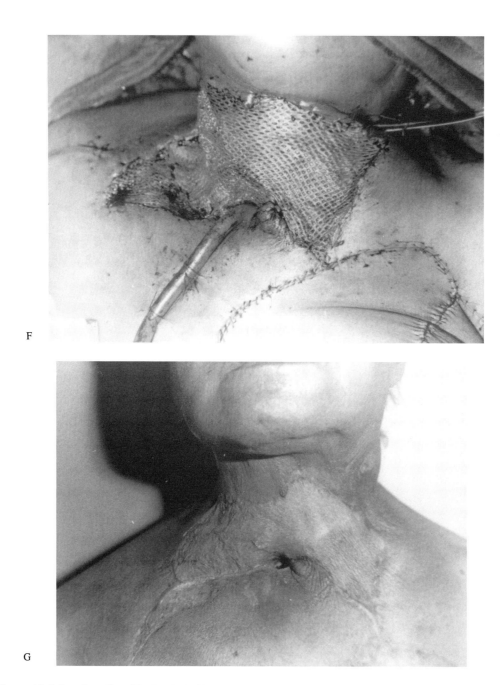

Figure 10–1 (continued).   (F). Meshed skin graft covering the neck wound. **(G).** The completely healed wound.

endolaryngeal carcinoma, most patients can swallow without much difficulty, but when mucosal resection is extended to include portions of the hypopharynx, the incidence of postoperative stenosis, particularly when primary closure has been attempted, is high. Kaplan et al[27] reported some degree of stenosis in 73% of patients after laryngectomy for pyriform sinus carcinoma, whereas Gates and Hearne[28] found that only 8% of their patients acquired esophageal speech after surgery for pyriform sinus lesions, most likely due to the high incidence of hypopharyngeal stenosis.

Most surgeons recognize that tight closure of hypopharyngeal mucosa around a nasogastric tube is not desirable. Stell[29] determined that in laryngectomy for pyriform sinus car-

cinoma, primary closure of the pharynx with less than 3 cm of hypopharyngeal mucosa will lead to a significant risk of stenosis. Hypopharyngeal stenosis is best prevented by the same techniques employed to prevent fistula when insufficient mucosa remains for adequate primary closure: transfer of myocutaneous flaps or free transfer of revascularized jejunal or fasciocutaneous flaps. Staged reconstructions with pedicled cutaneous flaps associated with temporary pharyngostoma are older methods of reconstruction beset with the disadvantages enumerated previously in this discussion.

Initial management of postoperative stenosis is by diet restriction to soft or pureed foods and progressive pharyngoesophageal dilation. Many patients will respond to conservative

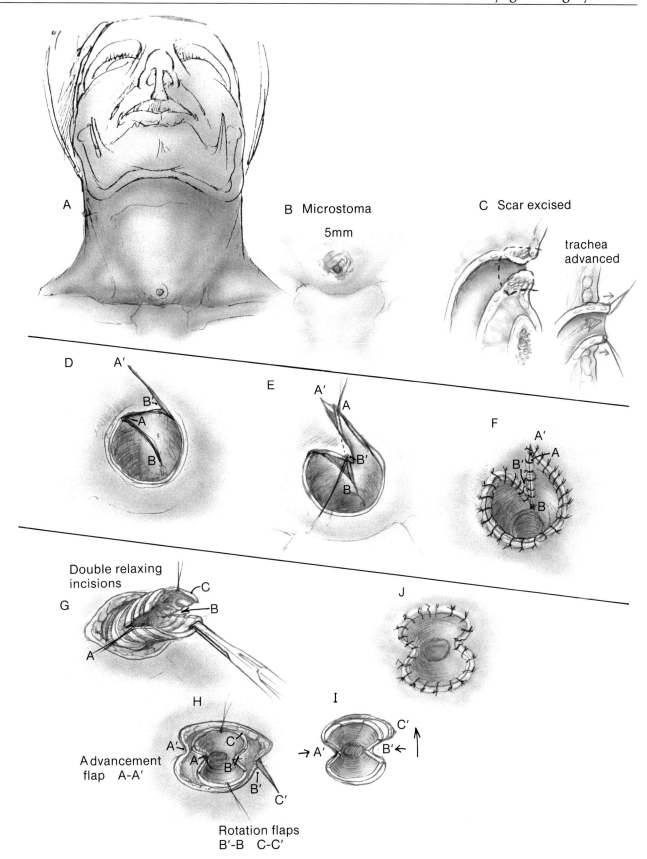

Figure 10–2. Correction of tracheal stomal stenosis. **(A).** A microstoma surrounded by a ring of scar. **(B).** Sagittal view of the distal end of trachea contracted by scar tissue. **(C).** The scar at the mucocutaneous junction has been excised. Normal trachea is mobilized and brought to skin level. **(D).** Z-plasty technique for recreating mucocutaneous junction; incisions are planned on the posterior tracheal wall (a-b) and skin (a′-b′). **(E, F).** Flaps are interposed and sutured. **(G).** Double laterally placed relaxing incisions are made in the trachea. **(H, I).** On the right side the skin is advanced into the tracheal incision (a′ to a); on the left side a small rotation flap (b′-c′) is rotated into the other tracheal incision. **(J).** The completed stoma has a characteristic bow-tie appearance.

management in the initial postoperative period, and others may be maintained successfully with periodic dilatations, often self-administered with a mercury-filled rubber bougie.

More severe cases require surgical correction. Depending on the exact nature of the obstruction, short segments of stenosis may be corrected by release of scar tissue, cricopharyngeal myotomy, or Z-plasty for narrow-band strictures. Patients with long segments of stenosis may require replacement or bypass of the stenotic segment. The tubed pectoralis major myocutaneous flap has been employed successfully for this purpose.[30,31] Various forms of visceral replacement have been employed, including gastric transposition, free jejunal autografts, esophagocoloplasty, and reversed gastric tube esophagoplasty. Revascularized free fasciocutaneous flaps used in the reconstruction of the hypopharyngeal defect include lateral thigh, radial forearm, and scapular and parascapular grafts.

The aforementioned procedures have been employed more frequently in dealing with primary replacement of circumferential pharyngoesophageal defects after resection for cancer. Choice of operation and complications inherent with these individual procedures are beyond the scope of this discussion.

Alterations in Esophageal Motility

In addition to mechanical obstruction due to hypopharyngeal stenosis, postlaryngectomy patients may experience varying degrees of dysphagia due to alterations in esophageal motility. Dysmotility may be due to several factors, including interruption of the upper digestive tube, interruption of the pharyngeal branches of the vagus nerve, anterior fixation of tracheal structures due to surgically induced cicatrix, loss of the negative pressure generated by the pharyngoesophageal segment,[32] and inefficient peristalsis of the pharyngoesophageal musculature. During normal swallowing, laryngeal elevation aids in the opening of the pharyngoesophageal segment. This segment develops negative pressure that is important for bolus passage. The total laryngectomy patient is unable to develop negative pressure in the pharyngoesophageal segment, without which there is less of a pressure gradient to drive bolus flow. This is reflected in increased pharyngeal transit time and decreased pharyngeal bolus velocity. In addition, interruption of the laryngeal constrictors (especially the cricopharyngeus) will tend to obliterate the high-pressure pharyngeal segment zone and impair upper esophageal sphincter relaxation because such relaxation requires an adequate pharyngeal pressure stimulus.

Lund[33] has suggested that pharyngeal branches of the vagus nerve probably contribute to the maintenance of resting tone, relaxation, and contraction of the upper esophageal sphincter. Interruption of these branches as well as bilateral division of the superior laryngeal nerves may interfere with sphincteric motor function.[34]

Alterations in Nasal Physiology

The mucous blanket that covers the nasal mucosa is produced continuously by the mucoserous nasal glands and intraepithelial goblet cells. This mucous film has two layers: an inner serous layer, called the sol phase, in which cilia beat; and an outer more viscous layer, the gel phase, which is transported by the ciliary beat. In normal individuals, inspired air causes drying of the sol part of the mucous layer and consequently some destruction of cilia in the anterior part of the nose. After completion of total laryngectomy, the lower respiratory tract becomes completely disconnected from the nose, mouth, and pharynx. Respiratory airflow takes place directly through the end tracheostoma. Light microscopy studies by Dixon et al[35] have demonstrated a change toward a more densely ciliated nasal epithelium in laryngectomized subjects; this has also been demonstrated by scanning electron micrographs. Nasal mucociliary function tests demonstrate a functional improvement in mucociliary transport in laryngectomy patients. This functional improvement seems to correlate with the structural change toward a more densely ciliated mucosa with an increase in mucous secretion.

Henkin et al[36] suggested that smell via the olfactory epithelium and olfactory nerve was completely abolished by laryngectomy, and any residual sensitivity to a vapor stimulus was mediated by "accessory areas of olfaction" present in the lateral nasal wall and the oropharynx and larynx and supplied by cranial nerves V, IX, and X. They postulated that surgical interference with sensory nerves in the larynx at the time of laryngectomy altered olfactory acuity by some complex feedback mechanism, and they suggested that anatomic connections between the laryngeal nerves and the olfactory cortex may exist. The authors concluded that anosmia was an inevitable consequence of laryngectomy.

Hypothyroidism

Hypothyroidism has been a well-recognized complication of treatment for head and neck cancer. Its incidence has ranged from 3.5%[37] to 29.1%.[38] In most total laryngectomies, one lobe of the thyroid gland and its adjacent parathyroid tissue are preserved, thus preserving normal thyroid and parathyroid function. However, infarction of either thyroid or parathyroid tissue may occur, resulting in endocrine deficiencies.

Thus insidious hypothyroidism may develop slowly during the first few postoperative weeks. This, in turn, may exert a profound effect on wound healing as well as the entire postoperative course. Kranz et al[39] proved that thyroid hormone influences DNA-synthesizing connective tissue cells, release of tropocollagen by fibroblasts, and tensile strength of wounds in rats with varying levels of thyroid activity. Wound healing was delayed an average of 2 days in hypothyroid rats compared to a control group.

Talmi[40] reported four patients who had undergone combined treatment for squamous cell carcinoma of the larynx and who developed hypothyroidism with treatment-resistant pharyngeal fistulae. All patients demonstrated marked rapid improvement in their general condition and wound healing ability after initiation of thyroid hormone therapy. Several mechanisms have been implicated: protein and nucleic acid synthesis, mitochondrial oxidative phosphorylation, the Krebs cycle enzyme system,[37,39,41] and the rate of release of tropocollagen.[39] Alexander et al[42] described three patients who, after receiving surgery and radiation to the head and neck region, developed pharyngocutaneous fistulae and hypothyroidism which responded to levothyroxine sodium. These authors proposed that wound healing, which can be delayed in the hypothyroid state, can be accelerated with appropriate replacement therapy.

Thus patients undergoing surgical treatment, particularly total laryngectomy, with or without irradiation for head and neck cancer should be evaluated preoperatively and postoperatively for thyroid function. Suspicion is warranted because symptoms and signs may be minimal or absent. Prompt diagnosis and treatment can be the key to an uninterrupted postoperative course.

Hypoparathyroidism

Postoperative hypoparathyroidism is not a common sequel of traditional operations on the pharynx, larynx, cervical esophagus, and neck. With intentional resection of the thyroid gland for subglottic, hypopharyngeal, and postcricoid carcinomas, however, hypoparathyroidism is particularly prone to occur. An increased incidence of hypoparathyroidism has been documented when the cervical esophagus is resected along with the larynx and hypopharynx.

Sisson and Vandar Aarde[43] noted that 10 of 14 patients experienced significant hypocalcemia with radical ablative procedures of the head and neck. Krespi et al[44] retrospectively reviewed three groups of head and neck surgery patients to assess the incidence of hypoparathyroidism. In patients with conventional total laryngectomy with thyroid preservation, the incidence of hypoparathyroidism was 12%. There was a 50% incidence of hypoparathyroidism among patients after total laryngectomy with mediastinal dissection, whereas 75% of patients developed hypoparathyroidism after total pharyngolaryngo-esophagectomy and gastric transposition. These authors noted that management of severe hypocalcemia and vitamin D hypovitaminosis seemed more difficult in patients undergoing gastric transposition than in patients undergoing the same operation reconstructed with other methods, and they concluded that the difficulties were related to diminished calcium absorption secondary to truncal vagotomy and decreased gut transit time. Similar observations were reported by Price and Ridley,[45] who found that the magnitude of difficulty of calcium management was reduced substantially once the jejunostomy tube feedings had been discontinued and oral feedings commenced. Jejunostomy tube feedings bypass the duodenum and proximal jejunum, where most calcium absorption takes place.

Price and Ridley[45] made the following recommendations for the management of hypoparathyroidism after total thyroparathyroidectomy performed with total pharyngolaryngoesophagectomy:

1. Parathyroid autotransplantation, confirmed by frozen section, should be done when it is oncologically feasible.

2. Postoperative hypocalcemia should be treated with intravenous calcium to an adjusted serum calcium of 7.6 to 8.0 mg/dL.
3. Water-soluble preparations of calcium (gluconate, glubionate, lactate) should be given during the administration of jejunostomy feedings.
4. Vitamin D therapy should be started immediately in the form of either 1,25[OH]2D (calcitriol, Rocaltrol) or dihydrotachysterol (DHT).
5. Exogenous thyroid should not be administered during the early postoperative course because it inhibits intestinal uptake of calcium, and clinically significant hypothyroidism does not occur for at least 2 to 3 weeks.

Medical Complications of Total Laryngectomy

The extraparietal nature of head and neck surgery tends to preclude the fluid compartment shifts, pain, and disturbance of basic physiological functions associated with intraabdominal and intrathoracic major surgical procedures. Patients resume ambulation promptly and only rarely experience altered genitourinary and gastrointestinal function.[46] Separation of the respiratory and digestive tracts by total laryngectomy can relieve airway obstruction, improve pulmonary toilet, and resolve life-threatening aspiration. Total laryngectomy patients experience primarily cardiovascular, neurological, and pulmonary complications rather than general medical complications, such as sepsis and renal failure.

Arriaga et al[47] evaluated preanesthetic risk factors retrospectively and correlated these with the incidence and significance of postoperative complications in 414 patients undergoing total laryngectomy. The mortality rate was 1.2%. Major, nonfatal medical complications occurred in 6.3%. There were seven instances of stroke, three myocardial infarctions, and two cases of pulmonary embolus. Twelve patients incurred respiratory failure requiring mechanical ventilation. Patients over age 65 experienced medical complications more frequently than did younger patients; however, major medical complications of respiratory failure, myocardial infarction, pulmonary embolus, and stroke were not significantly more frequent in the elderly. Thus advanced age in itself could not be considered a contraindication to total laryngectomy. Specific risk factor assessment revealed postoperative mortality to be associated with history of stroke or presence of a significant cardiac murmur. Strokes were associated with history of diabetes mellitus, and respiratory failure was associated with history of severe chronic obstructive pulmonary disease.

COMPLICATIONS ASSOCIATED WITH CONSERVATION SURGERY

The larynx serves three basic functions in its anatomic situation at the junction of the digestive and respiratory systems. The first is as a sphincteric mechanism for the protection of the respiratory tract against aspiration of food and liquids during deglutition; the second is to maintain a patent airway for respiration; and the third is as an organ for production of voice. Radical or conservative surgery modifies these basic functions to varying degrees. The objective of conservation laryngeal surgery may be stated as eradication of tumor while maintaining or restoring the sphincteric, respiratory, and sound-producing structures to as functional a level as possible.[48] Inability to reconstruct a functioning larynx is the main limiting factor to the extent of surgical resection.[49]

Long-term functional disability after partial laryngectomy may be termed *glottic insufficiency*, which occurs either as glottic incompetence with aspiration, inability to cough or strain, and weak voice; or as stenosis with stridor and respiratory obstruction. Respiratory impairment is somewhat more prevalent than aspiration after vertical hemilaryngectomy, whereas after supraglottic laryngectomy aspiration of food is the most common problem and airway obstruction occurs infrequently.[50]

Selection of Patients

The pioneers of conservation surgery learned that patients over the age of 65 tended to fare poorly after conservation operations on the larynx. A certain amount of neuromuscular coordination is required to overcome the anatomic and neurological disruptions resulting from removal of major portions of the larynx, and elderly patients tend to be less capable of such adaptation than are younger individuals. Nevertheless, recent improvements in reconstruction have helped minimize problems experienced by older patients. Tucker[51] reported results of conservation surgery in 27 patients over the age of 65. The overall complication rate was 11.1% with no mortality; this compares favorably with results in younger patients. On the other hand, Alajmo et al[52] compared results of conservation surgery in 171 patients over 65 with a control group of 287 younger patients. The authors concluded that although the complication rates were similar in both groups after vertical hemilaryngectomy, the incidence of bronchopneumonia and serious complications with high risk of mortality was significantly higher in the older group of patients. Supraglottic laryngectomy was recommended only if neck dissection was not required, pulmonary function was over 50% of predicted normal, and the patient accepted the increased risk. The risk presented by more extensive procedures such as partial pharyngolaryngectomy or subtotal laryngectomy were felt to be prohibitive.

Patients suffering from chronic debilitating illnesses are not good candidates for conservation surgery. Chronic pulmonary disease is a greater deterrent to successful conservation surgery than any other factor. Glottic narrowing and altered tussic function contribute to pulmonary insufficiency, poor deglutition, and pulmonary sepsis. Previous radiation therapy is not a contraindication to conservation surgery, but patients must be selected judiciously. Complications such as perichondritis and necrosis with subsequent stenosis and fistula formation occur more frequently in irradiated patients. Lesions unsuitable for conservation surgery prior to irradiation should

not be treated with partial laryngectomy, even if tumor size appears to have been reduced to within suitable limits.

Glottic Incompetence (Aspiration)

A review of 61 complications reported in several large combined series of subtotal supraglottic laryngectomy revealed 25 (41%) instances of aspiration and 8 (13%) instances of pneumonia.[53] Flores et a[54] determined that relatively normal swallowing could be expected in only 85% to 90% of patients after supraglottic laryngectomy. Approximately half the remaining patients can swallow and cough well enough to prevent pneumonia but are unable to ingest sufficient food to maintain adequate nutrition and require either gastrostomy or completion laryngectomy. The remaining 5% to 7% develop persistent pulmonary infection and require completion laryngectomy. In many instances, chronic pulmonary sepsis is more subtle and tenacious than is readily apparent. A retrospective study of patients after supraglottic laryngectomy by Murray[55] noted that respiratory infections and deaths from pneumonia occurred more often than generally realized.

CAUSES AND PREVENTION

Supraglottic subtotal laryngectomy, extended supraglottic laryngectomy, and partial laryngopharyngectomy involve resection of the epiglottis, false vocal cords, and, occasionally, portions of the base of the tongue. Loss of the supraglottic structures not only removes the anatomic protection of the laryngeal introitus but also interrupts the sequential sensory input of the swallowing mechanism. This sensory derangement is the most important factor in loss of adequate deglutition after supraglottic resections.[56] Ablation of the internal branch of the superior laryngeal nerve is inherent in the surgical procedure of supraglottic laryngectomy. This deficiency in sensory reception can be compensated for by the residual structures as long as damage to the external branch of the superior laryngeal nerve as well as the recurrent laryngeal nerve is avoided.[48] The external branch is situated posterior and lateral to the thyroid cartilage and is vulnerable to injury by the horizontal cut across the thyroid cartilage during the course of supraglottic laryngectomy. Injury to this nerve on one or both sides of the already surgically injured larynx will reduce sensation and sphincteric function to a degree for which the healing larynx may or may not be able to compensate. In extensive resections for larger tumors (which may include arytenoid resection and tongue base excision), injury to these nerves as well as erratic healing, edema, and scarring may combine to further reduce sphincteric function.

In addition to sensory loss, failure to achieve adequate glottic closure is the major cause of glottic incompetence. Following horizontal partial laryngectomy or partial laryngopharyngectomy, closure of the glottis upon deglutition is essential for adequate deglutition. At the time of resection, every effort should be made to ensure adequate glottic closure. Biller et al[57] attributed failure to either partial or total arytenoid removal, partial resection of the true cord to obtain a tumor-free inferior margin, or inadvertent injury of the recurrent laryngeal nerve during cricopharyngeal myotomy. The authors found the first circumstance (namely, partial arytenoid resection with exposure of the residual cartilage) to be the most common cause, leading frequently to arytenoid fixation in the abducted position. Som[58] reported postoperative fixation of the ipsilateral vocal cord in 4 of 93 cases, which he attributed to incision into the arytenoid during resection with resultant fixation by scar.

Biller et al[57] suggested that coverage of the exposed cartilage with a mucosal flap may avoid chondritis and, ultimately, fixation of the cord. The authors noted that resection of the superior aspect of the arytenoid to the level of the vocal process will lead to fixation in most cases, even with mucosal coverage, and they advised fastening the vocal cord in the posterior midline with a nonabsorbable submucosal suture extending from the vocal process to the perichondrium of the cricoid cartilage. Following complete arytenoid resection, however, the authors advised against simply suturing the vocal process to the cricoid because this maneuver tends to result in a posterior glottic defect. A free or pedicled cartilage graft, interposed between the vocal process and the cricoid, was employed to augment the posterior glottis. Occasional failure was attributed to lateral placement of the graft or infection with resorption of the cartilage graft.

Cricopharyngeal myotomy at the time of initial resection and preservation of the hyoid bone have been employed as means of minimizing postoperative aspiration. A retrospective analysis by Flores et al[54] of 51 patients operated at the Cleveland Clinic indicated that preservation of the hyoid bone facilitated closure but improved deglutition only if both superior laryngeal nerves were preserved along with the hyoid, which is not feasible in most resections. Cricopharyngeal myotomy could not be shown to affect ultimate swallowing success but seemed to facilitate more rapid return of deglutition.

Glottic incompetence after vertical hemilaryngectomy occurs mainly when the arytenoid has been resected and is due to loss of the structure of the posterior laryngeal vestibule, creating a troughlike effect in which food and saliva in the hypopharynx may spill into the glottis, as well as to inadequate glottic closure due to lack of bulk of the pseudocord. Approximately 50% of patients will experience significant aspiration unless adequate reconstructive measures are employed.[57] Various methods have been employed to provide bulk and/or replace the posterior vestibule. Single and bipedicled muscle flaps,[59,60] and free grafts of fat,[61] muscle,[62] and cartilage[50] have been employed for this purpose, but all tend to atrophy over time, producing loss of glottic competence. Use of a flap of thyroid cartilage pedicled on the inferior constrictor muscle, as described by Blaugrund and Kurland,[63] has proven more effective in maintaining vestibular integrity and glottic bulk. Various modifications of this flap have been employed for extended resections for lesions with subglottic extension or bilateral involvement.[64]

MANAGEMENT OF GLOTTIC INCOMPETENCE

Various nonsurgical techniques may be helpful in minimizing postoperative aspiration or hastening the return of adequate deglutition. Decannulation of the tracheotomy and removal of the nasogastric feeding tube prior to offering the patient semisolid food appear to help with deglutition in the immediate postoperative period. A "three-swallow" technique has been described by Tucker.[56] The patient, while holding a deep breath, takes a small bolus of semisolid material, swallows twice, and then coughs and swallows a third time. Leaning to the unoperated side may help some patients. It is generally easier to swallow semisolid material than free liquids, and the latter should be withheld until adequate deglutition has been restored. Some patients will always find certain food easy and other foods difficult to swallow and must learn to adjust their diet accordingly.

Teflon injection has been used since 1962 for vocal cord augmentation to correct dysphonia following vocal cord paralysis[65] and has been applied to correction of glottic insufficiency after laryngeal surgery. Its use for this purpose has been generally ineffective for several reasons. Scarification of the laryngeal sphincter, lack of potential space in the pseudocord for augmentation, as well as the high viscosity of Teflon prevent dispersal of the material to where augmentation may be required. In addition, a marked inflammatory reaction may be elicited by the injected Teflon. Injectable collagen has been shown to be useful for vocal and laryngeal rehabilitation and appears to be more useful for correction of glottic incompetence after partial laryngectomy.[66,67] Gax collagen is a purified, soluble bovine collagen which has excellent properties, including the ability to be integrated by host tissues, low viscosity, and minimal cellular and immunologic response. Remacle et al[67] reported improvement in all eight patients treated by them with Gax collagen for aspiration problems after subtotal laryngectomy. The authors note that the material is useful only when aspiration is due to anatomic rather than neurological factors.

Biller et al[57] have used a cartilage implant to correct posterior glottic incompetence after supraglottic laryngectomy with arytenoid resection. Unlike other techniques which employ an anterior thyrotomy approach for insertion of the implant and are suitable for anterior glottic defects, the authors utilize a posterior approach similar to a Woodman type of external arytenoidectomy. After disarticulation of the inferior cricoarytenoid joint, the posterior cricoid is exposed submucosally, and the implant is inserted and fixed with a wire into the bed of the previously resected arytenoid. Good results were reported in four of six patients followed for a minimum of 18 months.

Biller and Urken[68] have applied a technique of hemicricoid collapse for patients who have undergone extended supraglottic laryngectomy that included resection of the arytenoid and in whom reconstruction had failed (Fig. 10-3). After exposing and reflecting the pyriform sinus mucosa superiorly, vertical cuts are made in the cricoid from the superior to the inferior border with an oscillating saw, leaving the laryngeal mucosa intact. These vertical cuts begin

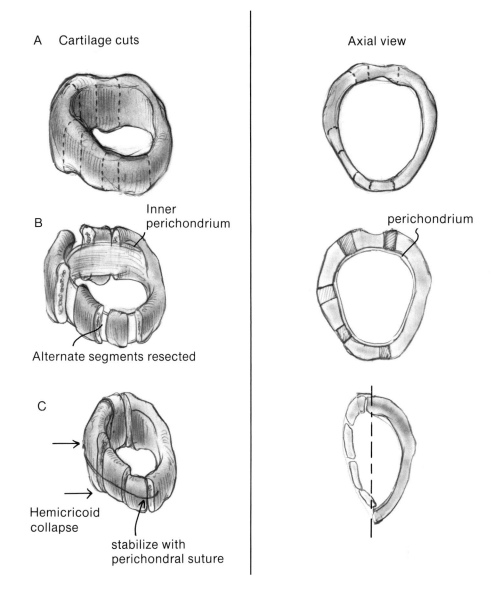

A   Cartilage cuts

Axial view

B

Inner
perichondrium

perichondrium

Alternate segments resected

C

Hemicricoid
collapse

stabilize with
perichondral suture

Figure 10–3.   Cricoid collapse technique (modified from Biller and Urken[68]). **(A).** Dotted lines indicate cartilage cuts. **(B).** Alternate cartilage segments resected. **(C).** Hemicricoid collapsed to midline and segments stabilized by perichondrial suture.

at the posterior midline and are placed every 2 to 3 mm until the anterior midline is reached. Alternate sections of the cartilage are removed, with hemicricoid collapse toward the midline while maintaining the integrity of the inner perichondrium. The authors reported good results in three of four patients, who regained ability to swallow without aspiration after the procedure. Postoperative examination revealed the normal vocal cord abutting a midline mucosal band during phonation.

Airway Obstruction
GRANULOMA AND REDUNDANT MUCOSA

In performing supraglottic laryngectomy, the line of resection should traverse the ventricles bilaterally, even if not necessary to secure an adequate resection margin. Portions

of false vocal cord left in situ tend to become edematous and may produce postoperative airway obstruction. Similarly, in vertical hemilaryngectomy, the portion of aryepiglottic fold used for reconstruction should be thinned of remnants of corniculate and cuneiform cartilages as well as the thickened aryepiglottic ligament. This not only creates a more pliant mucosal flap for advancement into the hypopharynx but also removes tissue that otherwise tends to become edematous postoperatively and to prolapse into the glottis, producing obstruction. In either case, obstructing masses of redundant or edematous supraglottic mucosa may be removed endoscopically. The CO_2 laser is of particular use for this purpose.

Excessive granulation tissue or intralaryngeal granuloma may form, most often after vertical resection, producing postoperative airway obstruction, hoarseness, and glottic insufficiency. Diabetes, radiation, nonabsorbable suture material, infection, and inadequate reconstruction may all contribute to granuloma formation, most commonly at the anterior commissure and anterior third of the neocord.[69] Most granulomas develop a few months after surgery and will regress spontaneously. Endoscopic biopsy to rule out tumor recurrence and removal with the laser should be done for granulomas that persist beyond a reasonable follow-up period. Treatment with topical or systemic steroids may be employed briefly in the conservative management of granuloma or in an effort to prevent subsequent scarring.

GLOTTIC STENOSIS

Krespi and Khetarpal,[69] in a literature review, quantified the incidence of persistent laryngeal edema and stenosis, with delayed decannulation or late recannulation, as varying from 2% to 15% after horizontal partial laryngectomy and from 1% to 20% after vertical partial laryngectomy, with or without irradiation. Infection with cartilage necrosis and loss of mucosa is the most frequent precursor of stenosis, which may be due to web formation, intraluminal scarring, or inadequate residual laryngeal framework. Preservation of cricoid cartilage, meticulous reconstruction, and immediate treatment of postoperative infection are the most effective means of preventing postoperative glottic stenosis. Planned radiation therapy is associated with a lower incidence of postoperative complications than when surgery is performed for salvage of radiation failure.[70]

Stenosis due to web and synechia formation is best prevented by adequate resurfacing of the endolarynx or by compartmentalization of the larynx by a stent or keel. If mucosa can be preserved on most of one side of the larynx, then stenting is unnecessary. If resection will leave bare one side of the glottis and more than one third of the opposite side, then resurfacing with external skin, stented grafts, or a midline partition such as a silastic "keel" will be required.[71] Once an anterior web has formed, if confined mainly to the glottic level it may be treated by endoscopic division (using a laser, if desired) and insertion of a midline partition, such as the keel described by McNaught.[72]

More extensive stenosis, involving necrosis and loss of laryngeal framework or due to excessive resection, must be dealt with by various reconstructive methods, including staged reconstruction with skin flaps, laryngotracheal reconstruction with stented cartilage grafts, or resection of supraglottic obstructive rings or bands. Often such reconstruction cannot be accomplished without loss of glottic competence, and many patients may simply continue tracheotomy cannulation, with preservation of voice and deglutition, rather than risk loss of swallowing function.

Voice after Partial Laryngectomy

Lack of standardized criteria for comparing voice results in the literature makes the true incidence of phonatory problems difficult to define. The incidence of poor voice has been reported as low as 3.3% after partial laryngectomy or cordectomy.[73] At the other extreme, Moore[74] stated that almost all cases of vertical partial laryngectomy and supraglottic laryngectomy had suboptimal postoperative voice.

The ability of a patient to generate an adequate voice depends on ability to develop adequate subglottic pressure, resonate the vocal cords, and develop adequate sphincteric activity of the supraglottic strictures. After cordectomy, compensatory hyperkinesia of the supraglottis may result in supraglottic hypertrophy or constriction. Krespi[69] concluded that in an attempt to preserve the vibratory mechanism in the glottic area, the supraglottic sphincter may act as a generator of noise, thus distorting the phonatory effect. After supraglottic laryngectomy, the loss of adjunctive phonatory function of the supraglottic structures results in suboptimal voice, even in the presence of a normal glottis. Supraglottic webbing or constriction at the tongue base anastomosis may exacerbate voice quality even further. Avoidance of tight wound closure could obviate this possible complication. The development of postoperative granulation tissue, scar formation, glottic incompetence, and paralysis of laryngeal nerves will adversely affect ultimate voice quality.

Prevention and treatment of voice difficulties are accomplished by the same procedures employed to prevent or treat aspiration, by providing bulk to enhance glottic closure. During the past decade, interest in the original work of Isshiki[75,76] has led to rising popularity of laryngeal framework surgery for functional voice problems.[77-80] Procedures for altering the framework to improve voice may be categorized according to the functional alteration of the vocal folds as follows: Type I, medial displacement; Type II, lateral displacement; Type III, shortening or relaxation; and Type IV, elongation or tensioning.[81] Medialization of the neocord, vocal fold tightening, and implantation of cartilage grafts or silastic prostheses have proven an effective means of vocal improvement for various problems and may be employed in selected cases after conservative laryngeal surgery.

CONCLUSIONS

Radical and conservation surgical procedures on the larynx carry with them various complications, some unique to the individual procedures and some common to all extirpative operations on the head and neck. Severe medical complications do not occur as frequently after laryngectomy as with many other types of surgery, but careful selection of patients is necessary for conservation surgery. Necrosis, fistula, tracheal stomal stenosis, swallowing difficulties, and endocrine disturbances are the major problems occurring after total laryngectomy. The chief complications of conservation surgery are glottic incompetence with related problems of aspiration pneumonia and inability to ingest food orally, glottic stenosis, and poor voice.

Considerable progress both in prevention and management of complications has enhanced the ability of the surgeon to perform safely increasingly extensive radical and conservation operations for various laryngeal and hypopharyngeal cancers.

REFERENCES

1. Stell PM, Cooney TC. Management of fistulae of the head and neck after radical surgery. *J Laryngol Otol.* 74;88:819.

2. Lundgren J, Olofsson J. Pharyngocutaneous fistulae following total laryngectomy. *Arch Otolaryngol.* 1979;4:13–23.

3. Bresson K, Rasmussen H, Rasmussen PA. Pharyngocutaneous fistulae after totally laryngectomized patients. *J Laryngol Otol.* 1972;88:835–842.

4. Cummings CW, Johnson JT, Chung CK, Sagerman R. Complications of laryngectomy and neck dissection following planned preoperative radiotherapy. *Ann Otol.* 1977;86:745–750.

5. Weingrad DN, Spiro RH. Complications after laryngectomy. *Am J Surg.* 1983;146:517–520.

6. Johansen LV, Overgaard J, Elbrond O. Pharyngo-cutaneous fistulae after laryngectomy. Influence of previous radiotherapy and prophylactic metronidazole. *Cancer.* 1988;61:673–678.

7. Gall AM, Sessions DG, Ogura JH. Complications following surgery for cancer of the larynx and hypopharynx. *Cancer.* 1977;39:624–631.

8. Lavelle RJ, Maw AR. The etiology of post-laryngectomy pharyngo-cutaneous fistulae. *J Laryngol Otol.* 1972;86:785.

9. Myers EN. The management of pharyngocutaneous fistula. *Arch Otolaryngol.* 1972;95:10–17.

10. Cantrell RW. Pharyngeal fistula: Prevention and treatment. *Laryngoscope.* 1978;88:1204–1208.

11. Shemen LJ, Spiro RH. Complications following laryngectomy. *Head Neck Surg.* 1986;8:185–191.

12. Mendelsohn MS, Bridger GP. Pharyngocutaneous fistulae following laryngectomy. *Aust NZ J Surg.* 1985;55:177–179.

13. Goldstein RD, Komisar A, Silver CE, Strauch B. Management of necrotic neck wounds with a "sandwich" pectoralis myocutaneous flap. *Head Neck Surg.* 1988;10:246–251.

14. Loewy A, Larker HI. Tracheal stoma problems. *Arch Otolaryngol.* 1968;87:477–481.

15. Yonkers AJ, Mercurio GA Jr. Tracheostomal stenosis following total laryngectomy. *Otolaryngol Clin North Am.* 1983;16:391–405.

16. Myers EN, Gallia LJ. Tracheostomal stenosis following total laryngectomy. *Ann Otol Rhinol Laryngol.* 1982;91:450–453.

17. Bain J. Late complications of tracheostomy and prolonged endotracheal intubation. *Int Anesthesiol Clin.* 1972;10:25–44.

18. Clairmont AA. Tracheostoma construction during laryngectomy: Techniques to prevent stenosis. *J Laryngol Otol.* 1978;92:75–78.

19. Grillo HC. Terminal or mural tracheostomy in the anterior mediastinum. *J Thorac Cardiovasc Surg.* 1966;51:422–427.

20. Montgomery W. Stenosis of tracheostoma. *Arch Otolaryngol.* 1962;75:76–79.

21. Callins WP, Applebaum EL. Correction of laryngectomy stomal stenosis. *Laryngoscope.* 1980;90:159–161.

22. Trail ML, Chambers R, Leonard JR. Z-Plasty of tracheal stoma at laryngectomy. *Arch Otolaryngol.* 1968;88:84–86.

23. Chandler JR. Construction and reconstruction of the laryngeal stoma. *Int Surg.* 1967;48:233–239.

24. Hartwell SW, Dykes ER. Construction and care of the end tracheostomy. *Am J Surg.* 1967;113:498.

25. Carleton JS. Revision of the tracheal stoma. *Laryngoscope.* 1980;80:260–266.

26. Panje WR, Kitt VV. Tracheal stoma reconstruction. *Arch Otolaryngol.* 1985;111:190–192.

27. Kaplan JN, Dobie RA, Cummings CW. The incidence of hypopharyngeal stenosis after surgery for laryngeal cancer. *Otolaryngol Head Neck Surg.* 1981;89:956–959.

28. Gates GA, Hearne EM III. Predicting esophageal speech. *Ann Otol Rhinol Laryngol.* 1982;91:454–457.

29. Stell PM. Total laryngectomy. In: Silver CE, ed. *Laryngeal Cancer.* New York: Thieme; 1991:212–223.

30. Cusumano RJ, Silver CE, Brauer RJ, Strauch B. Pectoralis myocutaneous flap for replacement of cervical esophagus. *Head Neck.* 1989;11:450–456.

31. Silver CE, Cusumano RJ, Fell SC, Strauch B. Replacement of upper esophagus: Results with myocutaneous flap and with gastric transposition. *Laryngoscope.* 1989;99:819–821.

32. McConnel FM, Cerenko D, Mendelsohn MS. Dysphagia after total laryngectomy. *Otolaryngol Clin North Am.* 1988;21:721–726.

33. Lund WS. A study of the cricopharyngeal sphincter in man and in the dog. *Ann R Coll Surg Engl.* 1965;37:225.

34. Duranceau A, Jamieson G, Hurwitz AL, Jones RS, Postlethwait RW. Alteration in esophageal motility after laryngectomy. *Am J Surg.* 1976;131:30–35.

35. Dixon FW, Hoerr NL, McCall JW. The nasal mucosa in the laryngectomized patient. *Ann Otol Rhinol Laryngol.* 1949;58:535–547.

36. Henkin RI Hoye RC, Ketcham AS, et al. Hyposmia following laryngectomy. *Lancet.* 1968;2:479–481.

37. Zohar Y, Ben Tovim R, Laurian N, Laurian L. Thyroid function following radiation and surgical therapy in head and neck malignancy. *Head Neck Surg.* 1984;6:948–952.

38. Vrabec DP, Heffron TJ. Hypothyroidism following treatment for head and neck cancer. *Ann Otol Rhinol Laryngol.* 1981;90:449–453.

39. Kranz D, Hecht A, Fuhrmann J. The influence of hyperthyroidism and hypothyroidism on the wound healing of experimental myocardial infarction in the rat. *Exp Pathol.* 1976;12:129–136.

40. Talmi YP, Finkelstein Y, Zohar Y. Pharyngeal fistulas in postoperative hypothyroid patients. *Ann Otol Rhinol Laryngol.* 1989;98:267–268.

41. Sterling K. Thyroid hormone action at the cell level. *N Engl J Med.* 1979;300:117–123.

42. Alexander MV, Zajtchuk JT, Henderson RL. Hypothyroidism and wound healing. *Arch Otolaryngol.* 1982;108:289–291.

43. Sisson GA, Vandar Aarde SB. Control of hypoparathyroidism. *Arch Otolaryngol.* 1971;93:249.

44. Krespi YP, Wurster CF, Wang TD, Stone DM. Hypoparathyroidism following total laryngopharyngectomy and gastric pull-up. *Laryngoscope.* 1985;95:1184–1187.

45. Price JC, Ridley MB. Hypocalcemia following pharyngoesophageal ablation and gastric pull-up reconstruction: Pathophysiology and management. *Ann Otol Rhinol Laryngol.* 1988;97:521–526.

46. Jun M, Strong E, Salzman E, Gerold F. Head and neck cancer in the elderly. *Head Neck Surg.* 1983;4:376–382.

47. Arriaga MA, Kanel KT, Johnson JT, Myers EN. Medical complications in total laryngectomy: Incidence and risk factors. *Ann Otol Rhinol Laryngol.* 1990;99:611–615.

48. Ward PH. The second Joseph H. Ogura memorial lecture. Compilations of laryngeal surgery: Etiology and prevention. *Laryngoscope.* 1988;98:54–57.

49. Biller HF. Conservation surgery past, present and future. *Laryngoscope.* 1987;97:38–41.

50. Sessions DG, Ogura JH, Ciralsky RH. Late glottic insufficiency. *Laryngoscope.* 1975;85:950.

51. Tucker HM. Conservation laryngeal surgery in the elderly patient. *Laryngoscope.* 1977;87:1995–1999.

52. Alajmo E, Fini-Storchi O, Agostini V, Polti G. Conservation surgery for cancer of the larynx in the elderly. *Laryngoscope.* 1985;95:203–205.

53. Silver CE. *Surgery for Cancer of the Larynx.* New York: Churchill Livingstone; 1981:140.

54. Flores TC, Wood BG, Levine HL, et al. Factors in successful deglutition following supraglottic laryngeal surgery. *Ann Otol Rhinol Laryngol.* 1982;91:579.

55. Murray GM. Pulmonary complications following supraglottic laryngectomy. *Clin Otolaryngol.* 1976;1:71.

56. Tucker H. Deglutition following partial laryngectomy. In: Silver CE, ed. *Laryngeal Cancer.* New York: Thieme; 1991:197–200.

57. Biller HF, Lawson W, Sacks S. Correction of posterior glottic incompetence following partial laryngectomy. *Ann Otol Rhinol Laryngol.* 1982;91:448–449.

58. Som ML. Conservation surgery for carcinoma of the supraglottis. *J Laryngol Otol.* 1970;84:655.

59. Ogura JH, Biller H. Glottic reconstruction following extended frontolateral laryngectomy. *Laryngoscope.* 1969;79:2181.

60. Bailey BJ. Glottic reconstruction after hemilaryngectomy: Bipedicled muscle flap laryngoplasty. *Laryngoscope.* 1975;85:960–977.

61. Dedo HH. A technique for vertical hemilaryngectomy to prevent stenosis and aspiration. *Laryngoscope.* 1975;85:978.

62. Quinn HJ. Free muscle transplant method of glottic reconstruction after hemilaryngectomy. *Laryngoscope.* 1975;85:985–986.

63. Blaugrund S, Kurland S. Replacement of the arytenoid following vertical hemilaryngectomy. *Laryngoscope.* 1975;85:935–941.

64. Biller HF, Lucente FE. Reconstruction of the larynx following vertical partial laryngectomy. *Otolaryngol Clin North Am.* 1979;12:761–766.

65. Arnold G. Vocal rehabilitation of paralytic dysphonia. IX. Techniques of intracordal injection. *Arch Otolaryngol.* 1962;76:358–368.

66. Ford CN, Bless DN. Clinical experience with injectable collagen for vocal fold augmentation. *Laryngoscope.* 1986;96:863–869.

67. Remacle M, Hamoir M, Marbaix E. Gax-collagen injection to correct aspiration problems after subtotal laryngectomy. *Layrngoscope.* 1990;100:663–669.

68. Biller HF, Urken M. Cricoid collapse, a new technique for management of glottic incompetence. *Arch Otolaryn.* 1985;111:740–741.

69. Krespi YP, Khetarpal U. *Laryng Surg.* 215–231.

70. Thawley SE. Complications of combined radiation therapy and surgery for carcinoma of the larynx and inferior hypopharynx. *Laryngoscope.* 1981;91:677–700.

71. Som ML, Silver CE. The anterior commissure technique of partial laryngectomy. *Arch Otolaryngol.* 1968;87:42.

72. McNaught RC. Surgical correction of anterior web of the larynx. *Laryngoscope.* 1950;60:262.

73. Neel BH, Devine KD, Desanto LW. Laryngofissure and cordectomy for early cordal carcinoma: Outcome in 182 patients. *Otolaryngol Head Neck Surg.* 1980;88:79–84.

74. Moore GP. Voice problems following limited surgical excision. *Laryngoscope.* 1975;85:619.

75. Isshiki N, Okamura H, Ishikawa T. Thyroplasty Type I (lateral compression) for dysphonia due to vocal cord paralysis or atrophy. *Acta Otolaryngol.* 1975;80:465–473.

76. Isshiki N, Tanabe M, Sawada M. Arytenoid adduction for unilateral vocal cord paralysis. *Arch Otolaryngol.* 1978;104:555.

77. Tucker HM. Anterior commissure laryngoplasty for adjustment of vocal fold tension. *Ann Otol Rhinol Laryngol.* 1985;94:547–549.

78. Koufman JA. Laryngoplasty for vocal cord medialization: An alternative to Teflon. *Laryngoscope.* 1986;96:726–731.

79. Maves MD, McCabe BF, Gray S. Phonosurgery: Indications and pitfalls. *Ann Otol Rhinol Laryngol.* 1989;98:577.

80. Tucker HM, Wanamaker J, Trott M, Hicks D. Complications of laryngeal framework surgery (phonosurgery). *Laryngoscope.* 1993;103:525–527.

81. Isshiki N, Taira T, Kajima H, Shoji K. Recent modifications in thyroplasty type I. *Ann Otol Rhinol Laryngol.* 1989;98:777.

11 Complications of Neck Surgery

William W. Shockley, M.D., Chapman T. McQueen, M.D., Gregory N. Postma, M.D.

Complications of neck surgery occur in every surgeon's practice. The types of problems and their severity range widely and vary with the procedure involved, patient factors, and the clinical judgment and technical expertise of the surgeon. As the use of modified neck dissection techniques become more popular, the profile of associated complications will undoubtedly change. In general, one would expect fewer complications (with carotid exposure and potential blow-out) as muscular coverage becomes more routine. Interestingly, venous sequelae, however, may become more likely because the dissected internal jugular vein is now exposed to infections and fistulae, should they occur.

This chapter will deal with complications that may arise during surgery of the neck as well as those that occur postoperatively. Because radical neck dissection and its modifications encompass the contents of the neck, emphasis will be on complications associated with these procedures.

Complications of neck surgery are related to a multitude of predisposing factors. However, proper surgical technique and patient selection are the foremost determinants of a satisfactory surgical outcome. Certainly, one of the most profound predictors is simply whether the surgery involves entry into the oral cavity, larynx, or pharynx. Although prophylactic antibiotics have had a dramatic effect on diminishing the incidence of infection in this setting, it is unlikely that postoperative infections and wound problems will ever be eliminated.

Patient factors play a major role in the tolerance of surgical intervention and in wound healing. The majority of patients cared for by the head and neck surgeon are chronic smokers with a history of moderate to heavy alcohol use. These patients present with varying degrees of pulmonary, cardiac, liver, and vascular disease. Many are malnourished related to their lifestyles as well as to the tumor that has affected their swallowing and mastication. The ischemic changes in the tissues of a smoker should not be underestimated. A complete medical history and a thorough general physical examination are mandatory before major surgical decisions are made. A history of bleeding disorders must be searched for because familial bleeding diathesis, liver dysfunction, and

anticoagulant medication may set the stage for hemorrhage and hematoma. Many patients take over-the-counter aspirin, aspirin-containing products, or nonsteroidal anti-inflammatory agents that prolong the bleeding time by their adverse effect on platelet aggregation.

The surgery itself inherently affects the complications. In tumor surgery, more advanced neck disease is associated with an increased likelihood of vascular or neural complications as the scope and extent of the surgery become more complex. Those having modified neck dissection would be expected to experience a lesser chance of sequelae.

The impact of irradiation on cervical tissues has been explored by many investigators. It is generally agreed that tissues which have been exposed to 4500 cGy or more of irradiation will be less tolerant of surgical manipulation. Higher rates of wound infection, breakdown, hematoma, and fistula formation are linked to surgery performed on patients with prior radiotherapy.

The following sections will explore the various complications encountered in neck surgery. When possible, the subject will be reviewed by discussing the incidence, recognition, pathophysiology, management, and preventive measures. Because it would be difficult to cover each surgery and its inherent risks, the discussion concentrates on individual complications and their treatment.

GENERAL COMMENTS

Prior to the proposed procedure, the surgeon must be cognizant of the patient's medical condition and history. This allows the surgeon to anticipate and plan for potential difficulties associated with the anesthetic risks, cardiopulmonary system, healing, alcohol withdrawal, and other relevant issues. In particular, any prior neck surgery for benign or malignant disease will require careful thought as to the optimal incision to ensure adequate exposure, flap viability, and carotid protection. If an open biopsy was performed for a malignancy, then the scar should be excised and left attached to the neck specimen.

Surgical Technique

Standard surgical principles cannot be violated without an attendant increase in morbidity and possible mortality. These include use of natural tissue planes for dissection, gentle tissue manipulation, maintenance of tissue moistness, proper hemostasis, relaxed tissue closures, proper antibiotic prophylaxis, irrigation of contaminated wounds, and appropriate drainage techniques. Careful management of the patient's fluid and nutritional status in the perioperative period is also crucial for a successful surgical outcome.

In general, the risk of complications in an isolated neck dissection is low. The incidence of complications increases significantly if the dissection is performed in continuity with resection of a primary tumor in the upper aerodigestive tract due to the bacterial contamination.[1-8]

Radiation

The effects of radiation therapy (RT) on the incidence and severity of complications in patients undergoing a neck dissection is an area of significant disagreement. Cummings et al have shown that there is no statistically significant increase in complications after preoperative radiation.[9] This has been corroborated by others.[3,10-12] However, a number of other reviews have shown an increase in both the incidence and severity of complications, particularly when the neck dissection was combined with resection of a primary lesion in the pharynx or larynx.[1,2,7,13-23] Johnson and others strike a middle ground with a similar incidence of wound complications, whereas those in radiated patients are of a more serious nature.[24,25]

Experimental work involving rats has shown that irradiated wounds are unable to tolerate bacterial contamination to the same extent that normal tissue can, and this is dose related.[26] In addition, intravenous antibiotic levels are decreased in irradiated tissue.[27] Further research has shown decreased vascularity in irradiated flaps, but this did not always correlate with decreased flap survival.[28]

In general, it appears that the procedure is technically more difficult in an irradiated field with increased bleeding and difficulty in following tissue planes secondary to fibrosis. Healing is compromised, leading to an increase in the incidence and severity of complications.

Nutrition

The nutritional state of the head and neck cancer patient is of vital importance. Pain, obstruction by tumor, alcohol abuse, and substances produced by the tumor (such as tumor necrosis factor) can lead to a cachectic state. This results in 40% of head and neck oncology patients presenting in a malnourished condition.[29-31] Alcoholism also contributes to malnutrition and leads to vitamin deficiencies, resulting in a macrocytic anemia.

The increased catabolic response to the surgery itself magnifies the premorbid nutritional deficits. This may result in delays in healing, an increased infection rate, and a general overall increase in complications, which can be diminished by preoperative nutritional repletion.[3,32-37] These difficulties are usually not seen until a 20% loss in body weight occurs. Goodwin and Torres have developed a prognostic nutritional index in which nearly all of the head and neck cancer patients classified as markedly malnourished suffered major wound complications and 85% of these patients were dead in 6 months.[38]

Nutritional intervention would appear to be of great potential benefit to patients. Although no conclusive study has shown improved survival rates due to intensive nutritional therapy, improved tolerance to radiation and chemotherapy and a decreased complication rate in severely malnourished patients has been demonstrated.[39-43]

Recent studies have shown an improvement in wound healing response due to short-term food intake without seeing a concomitant improvement in the subject's overall nutritional status.[44] This suggests that a short period of nutritional support prior to surgery could be of significant benefit. The duration of preoperative nutritional support that is both medically and economically effective is not known. Recommendations range from 7 to 14 days with a goal of 40 kcal/kg/d.[45] If the gastrointestinal tract is functional, then enteral feedings are the most advantageous. In patients in which the resumption of oral intake is doubtful, a percutaneous endoscopic gastrostomy should be performed in the preoperative or preradiation period.

Tobacco Use

Smoking continues to be a major health problem and is considered the major cause of preventable deaths in the United States. The head and neck surgeon sees the carcinogenic effect of tobacco abuse but may be unaware of its deleterious effects on blood flow and therefore wound healing.

Studies performed in a rat model have shown that random flaps are less viable in rats that have been exposed to tobacco smoke.[46,47] The reasons for this appear to be multifactorial. The best-known mechanism is vasoconstriction caused by nicotine-induced epinephrine release from the sympathetic nervous system. This has also been shown in dogs in which nicotine infusions decreased flow in small arteries by 72%.[48]

The inhalation of carbon monoxide is also a factor. Carbon monoxide comprises 3% to 6% of tobacco smoke and binds to hemoglobin, causing a decrease in the oxygen-carrying capacity of blood. This coupled with underlying lung disease hinders tissue oxygenation, leading to ischemia with its adverse effect on wound healing.

Finally, nicotine may also induce a hypercoagulable state which may compromise healing and skin flap viability.[49] This has been shown in vitro and is believed to also be mediated by catecholamines. A decrease in fibrinolytic activity has also been shown.[50]

Mosely has performed a clinical study on patients undergoing hand surgery in which decreased digital blood flow and poor healing was observed in smokers.[51] A single cigarette can cause a dramatic decrease in digital blood flow, suggesting that nicotine is clinically a potent vasoconstrictor in humans.[53]

Observations in facial plastic surgery patients and in head and neck cancer patients appear to corroborate this finding. For these reasons, it is recommended that all patients decrease or cease smoking prior to any procedure. A decrease in pulmonary complications has also been seen if smoking is stopped for even a few days preoperatively.[53]

Incisions

The type of incision to be used in the performance of a given procedure should not be arbitrary but rather should take into account a number of issues. The head and neck surgeon must be familiar with a variety of different incisions so that the most advantageous cervical flap for a given patient and situation can be used. A poorly planned incision may lead to flap ischemia and possible infection, most notably in the diabetic or irradiated patient. Wound dehiscence and carotid artery exposure could result as well.

The type of neck dissection contemplated, the primary to be addressed, and whether any skin is to be resected are major concerns. The incision chosen must provide adequate exposure for the extirpation and must protect the carotid artery. Concerns about flap necrosis due to radiation therapy, atherosclerosis, or severe diabetes must be considered in incision planning. Flaps elevated in a subplatysmal plane enhance their viability. Finally, cosmesis should be a concern but is secondary to the issues of oncologic principles, exposure, and wound healing.

A prior biopsy scar requires excision of the scar in conjunction with the specimen and may influence the type of incision used. Likewise, skin involvement by tumor requires resection of involved skin with an adequate margin of normal skin, sometimes necessitating a regional flap for closure of the cutaneous defect.

Incisions for lesser procedures such as cervical biopsies should be given the same degree of careful consideration regarding exposure, appearance, and possible incorporation into a future neck dissection. The more limited exposure with such incisions makes inadvertent nerve and vessel injury more likely.

When feasible, incisions should be made in skin creases or in the relaxed skin tension lines for both cosmesis and greater wound strength.[54] If separate limbs are needed, these must meet at right angles to avoid ischemia at the corners and the trifurcation point should be placed well away from the carotid artery, avoiding possible exposure of the artery. Vertical limbs should be made in a gentle curve to avoid scar contracture.

The MacFee incision, with its bipedicled blood supply, or a broad-based apron flap are excellent choices in the patient who has undergone radiation therapy in that the carotid artery is well protected, with minimal risk for wound breakdown and exposure.[55,56] Preferred incisions (Fig. 11–1) take into account exposure, carotid coverage, and flap survival.

WOUND PROBLEMS
Wound Healing

Wound healing results from a complex interplay between the coagulation cascade, secreted factors, and blood-borne cellular elements. A brief review will be provided. Detailed discussions on the subject are available in appropriate review articles.[57,58]

Soon after a wound is created, an inflammatory response begins and a fibrin clot is formed which serves as a matrix for cellular elements drawn to it by various chemotactic factors. Platelets are critical at this juncture, both for their role in clot formation and as a source of chemotactic, vasoactive, and growth factors.

Polymorphonuclear leukocytes arrive first, followed soon by macrophages. These engulf and destroy bacteria as well as any necrotic tissue. Macrophages are also believed to release factors which promote angiogenesis and attract fibroblasts. These, in turn, begin to form granulation tissue.

Granulation tissue consists of inflammatory cells, fibroblasts, and an extensive system of new capillaries enmeshed in fibrin and collagen.

Wound contracture begins approximately 5 to 6 days after injury and is a function of myofibroblasts derived from fibroblasts. In addition to contracting the wound, the myofibroblast produces collagen (the key structural unit in wound healing), which will begin crosslinking and gaining strength over a period of weeks.

Reepitheliazation begins during the first 24 hours and is a result of migration and growth of epithelial cells from the free wound edges and from any remaining adnexal structures. This proceeds at a rate of 0.25 to 0.50 mm per day and is enhanced in a moist environment.

Wound Infection

Wound infection continues to be a major cause of morbidity and prolonged hospitalization. The incidence is variable, with a range of 5% to 25%, but several general comments can be made.[10,12,59-61] Wound infections add significant morbidity to the surgical patient. A 1985 study of patients undergoing major head and neck surgery estimated that hospitalization increased by 2 weeks and that hospital charges increased more than $10,000 in patients who developed a postoperative wound infection.[11]

Contamination from the oral cavity or pharynx is the greatest single factor. The performance of a neck dissection without entry into the aerodigestive tract carries little infectious morbidity. In fact, it is likely that prophylactic antibiotics are of little benefit in the performance of isolated neck dissections.[3,25,62] However, once entry into the pharynx occurs, the possibility of wound infection increases dramatically. A small pilot study using topical oral clindamycin showed a significant decrease in oral aerobes and anaerobes for at least 4 hours, suggesting that preoperative dental and oral hygiene may play a role in diminishing wound infections.[63] Radiation therapy is associated with a higher rate of infection, as noted by the reviews mentioned earlier.[10,12,59-61]

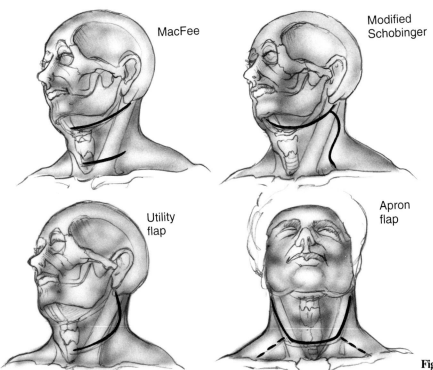

MacFee

Modified Schobinger

Utility flap

Apron flap

Figure 11–1. Preferred incisions for neck surgery.

Early recognition of wound infections leads to early treatment, which decreases further morbidity. Detailed inspection and palpation of the wound and examination of the amount and character of the drainage are mandatory. Any localized swelling under a flap must be expressed from the wound or aspirated to determine whether it is purulent, bloody, or serous. This is diagnostic as well as therapeutic, allowing the flap to make contact with the deep cervical tissues and heal appropriately. Wound infection may manifest as a collection of purulent material under the cervical flaps, coming out of the wound, or in the suction drains. Tenderness, erythema, warmth, mild induration, low-grade fever, and leukocytosis are insufficient findings because they are routinely seen in the postoperative period in nearly all patients. The legion of factors which can predispose or cause wound infection have been alluded to. These include contamination, prior RT, malnutrition, and hematoma or seroma formation.

Drainage is the key to managing infections. Purulent material should be directed away from the carotid artery and the tracheostoma or tracheotomy site. Drainage allows cervical flaps to contact the deep neck tissues and heal, avoiding possible carotid artery erosion.

Prophylactic Antibiotics

The vast majority of infections are polymicrobial in nature. These consist primarily of aerobic gram-positive cocci and anaerobes, with anaerobes predominating. Gram-negative organisms appear to colonize the infected wounds but are usually not the causative organism.[64,65]

Prophylactic antibiotics have been shown in a number of studies to decrease dramatically the incidence of infection in those patients in whom the oral cavity or pharynx has been entered.[3,62,66-69] However, no consensus has been reached on the optimal agent or on the duration of its use, although 24 hours of prophylaxis appear to be sufficient.[4,62,69,70] Antibiotics must be given prior to the procedure to be efficacious.[4,71] Some surgeons continue antibiotic prophylaxis until the drains are removed. Although many head and neck surgeons routinely use antibiotics for 3 to 5 days postoperatively, the additional benefit has not been borne out in controlled studies. Aside from the added expense, this practice may lead to the development of resistant organisms and side-effects, such as pseudomembranous colitis.

Surgical Preparation

Once in the operating room, proper skin preparation is important. Hair removal, when required, should be done with clippers or a depilatory. Shaving with a razor has been shown to increase infection rates when compared to clippers or depilatories.[72,73] The skin should then be scrubbed and prepped with an antibacterial agent such as povidine iodine (Betadine) or a chlorhexidene solution. A 1-minute alcohol cleansing followed by application of an iodophor antimicrobial adhesive film has an equivalent bactericidal effect as the classic 5-minute iodophor soap scrub and Betadine painting.[74]

Preparation and draping should include areas potentially needed as skin graft sites or potential regional or free flap sites.

Wound Closure

Prior to skin closure, a water-tight closure of the oral cavity and pharynx is necessary. This is obtained by gentle handling of the tissues, inversion of the mucosa, and avoidance of tension on the suture lines. Reinforcement of mucosal closures with local tissue is advisable as long as it is also tension free and does not lead to a narrowing of the gullet.

Irrigation with saline at body temperature should be performed vigorously after closure of the pharynx and prior to skin closure. This removes clot as well as other debris, dilutes the concentration of bacteria in the wound, and allows improved visualization of lymphatic vessels and small bleeding points. The use of an antibiotic in the irrigant may be intuitively beneficial, but its efficacy has never been proven.

Closure of the cervical flaps should include only healthy tissue closed without any tension. If there is any question about the viability of the periphery of a skin flap, a small portion of the edge should be excised. The closure includes the platysma incorporated into the dermal closure or as a separate layer.

The type and size of suture material used during the procedure are less important than proper technique. All suture material acts as a foreign body to some degree, and therefore the fewest number of sutures required to do the job correctly should be used. In addition, tissues should be brought only into apposition, not strangulated. Strangulation leads to ischemia and necrosis, with an increase in the opportunity for infection and fistula formation.

Wound Drainage

Appropriate placement and care of suction drains is critical in the care of these patients. When used in the proper fashion, suction drains keep the skin flaps coapted with the underlying tissue, eliminating dead space and reducing the incidence of hematoma and seroma formation.

Drains should be inserted via a separate stab incision and placed in dependent portions of the wound to facilitate drainage. If needed, an absorbable suture is placed in the wound and is wrapped loosely around the drain to keep it from coming into direct contact with major vascular structures, nerves, or an anastomosis. Suction drains should not be placed over the line of closure. We have never seen a patient suffer from overdrainage but have seen serious complications due to the lack of drains or hasty removal of them.

Numerous methods of affixing the drains to the patient have been devised. The particular method used is unimportant as long as it meets four criteria: (1) The drain must be fixed to the patient in such a way that accidental removal is unlikely; (2) the method of attachment should not damage the skin; (3) there should be no air leakage at the drain site; and (4) the drain should be easily removable when it is no longer needed.

At the conclusion of the procedure, the closure of the cervical flaps must be airtight if the drains are to function properly. A persistent air leak may be due to a communication with the tracheotomy site or with the oral cavity or pharyngeal closure or due to inadequate cutaneous closure. This must be investigated and repaired prior to awakening the patient. This is particularly crucial if an opening into the aerodigestive tract exists because air and bacteria-laden secretions may be aspirated under the flaps, leading to infection and fistula formation. Some surgeons favor a vertical incision for the tracheotomy versus a horizontal, attempting to maintain a separation between the neck dissection and the tracheotomy site. Any connection must be closed by suturing the subcutaneous tissue or platysma to the deeper neck tissues.

Drain failure is usually due to inadequate care of the drain but also occurs when a hematoma blocks the drain. A poorly functioning drain may be remedied by aspiration with a syringe using a sterile technique. A small amount of sterile saline may also be injected in an attempt to clear the drain. If this cannot be accomplished, then the drain should be cut off beyond the skin exit wound and converted into a passive drain. A compression dressing should then be applied if the flaps are not at significant risk for ischemia and if compression is not contraindicated by an underlying vascular pedicle flap.

Postoperative care of closed suction drains is simple but if ignored can lead to major wound complications. Some surgeons urge that the drains be it "milked" or "stripped" frequently in the early period after surgery to avoid possible clot formation or debris obstructing the drain. The drainage must also be measured and recorded accurately so that decisions regarding the removal of the drains be made appropriately.

A suction drain should be removed when it is no longer needed. A number of rules have been promulgated to determine when this point has been reached. These range from removing a drain when it drains 10 cc to 40 cc per 24 hours. Some surgeons leave drains in for a minimum of 4 days regardless of the output. The most important principle is not to remove a drain too early. The authors recommend erring on the side of conservatism and retaining a drain for at least 48 hours (major neck procedures) or until the drainage is less than 30 cc (per drain) per 24 hours.

SEROMA

Seromas may occur in any location involving the formation of a potential space or development of a skin flap, both of which are integral to a neck dissection. This has been reported to occur in approximately 10% of radical neck dissections, although in the authors' experience this problem rarely occurs following radical neck dissection.[75,76] Formation of a seroma has been proven to lead to an increase in the incidence of flap necrosis and infection in mastectomy patients.[77] It seems likely to be associated with adverse effects in the neck as well.

A seroma usually presents as an enlarging mildly tender mass under a cervical flap with overlying induration and erythema. Incorrect drain placement, drain failure, or early removal of a drain may all lead to a seroma. Drainage via the suture line or needle aspiration followed by a compression dressing will normally alleviate the problem. Attention given to meticulous hemostasis and placement of closed suction drains should preclude the development of a seroma. A rat model producing seromas has been developed which has shown that the use of intraoperative topical fibrin glue decreased the incidence of seromas.[78]

HEMATOMA

Hematoma formation occurs in about 1% of radical neck dissections and 2.3% to 4.2% of all major head and neck surgical cases.[79,80] It is critical to recognize this complication as early as possible by careful inspection of the neck and watching the character and amount of drainage. Pressure from the hematoma can cause necrosis of a portion of the flap, disrupt suture lines, and cause airway obstruction. If a myocutaneous or free flap has been used, it can compress the vascular pedicle and compromise its viability as well. Infection rates also increase in the presence of a hematoma secondary to tissue ischemia and secondary to iron serving as a bacterial nutrient.[81]

Numerous factors, including preoperative medications, may influence the likelihood of hematoma formation. Salicylates exert their antiplatelet effect for 2 weeks, and surgery should be delayed until this time has passed. For the same reasons, patients should also be instructed to avoid nonsteroidal anti-inflammatory drugs prior to surgery. Hypertension at the conclusion of the case or in the postoperative period may also contribute to excessive bleeding and result in a hematoma.[82] Hepatic dysfunction related to alcohol abuse results in potential coagulation difficulties as well.

The findings of cervical swelling, flap elevation, discolorization, or significant bloody drainage should raise the suspicion of postoperative hematoma. Suction drains may become occluded due to clot, causing further accumulation of blood. Bleeding around the drain site may also signal problems. After evacuation of the clot, major bleeders are rarely seen, but finding a diffuse oozing is common.[60] The hematocrit should be followed but will rarely be of benefit in making a decision about whether to explore the neck.

The key to avoiding hematoma formation lies in identifying any coagulation disorders prior to surgery and ensuring meticulous hemostasis at the close of the case. The wound should be irrigated repeatedly, and each aspect of the wound should be inspected for bleeding, taking care to visualize the undersurface and base of all cervical flaps. Placement of suction drains in dependent areas is important but does not substitute for good hemostasis.

FISTULA

The incidence of postoperative fistula depends on a variety of factors. This incidence has been reported as high as 10% to 30% of cases, depending on many etiologic factors including technical, physiological, and biological parameters.[83-86] Performing these operations following radiation therapy appears to increase these rates, although some authors have not found a statistically significant difference.[1,17,24,85,87]

As saliva passes into the neck, an inflammatory response occurs resulting in a swollen, indurated, and erythematous flap. This collection rapidly becomes purulent. Saliva or purulent debris may be seen collecting in the drains or passing through the suture line into the tracheotomy site or stoma.

The multiple entities which can contribute to the development of a fistula have been discussed earlier. Risk factors for poor wound healing include diabetes, vascular disease, prior radiotherapy, and malnourishment. Special attention must be given to the oral cavity or pharyngeal closure, ensuring that the tissues are handled gently and closed in an inverted fashion without tension. Vascularized tissue should be used in the closure of irradiated patients if there is any question about the adequacy of the closure.

It should not be forgotten that head and neck patients who have undergone combined modality treatment or radiation therapy alone are at risk for hypothyroidism. This is a well-recognized problem which can lead to a significant delay in wound healing with resultant fistula. Thyroid replacement results in rapid improvement.[88-90]

Conservative care and patience on the part of the surgeon will lead to closure of the majority of pharyngocutaneous fistulas. The nutritional state of the patient should be optimized to enhance the patient's ability to heal. Broad-spectrum antibiotics should be started as well. The fistulous tract should be opened via the suture line if possible and an attempt made to direct drainage away from the carotid artery and tracheostoma. Creation of this so-called direct fistula helps protect the carotid artery from possible infection and erosion leading to a vascular catastrophe (Fig. 11–2). Standard wound care consists of gently packing the wound open so that it closes from inside out. If saliva is draining through a suction drain, some authors recommend continued closed drainage on low suction. Other authors recommend using it only as a passive drain because they believe that the suction serves to promote the fistulous tract. After 7 to 10 days it can be taken off suction, used as a passive drain, and withdrawn slowly.

Fistulas that do not heal after a long period of conservative wound care require closure using local flaps or regional flaps. Surgery should not be performed until the fistula has matured and shows no signs of infection or granulation tissue. This could entail the use of a regional myocutaneous flap or a microvascular free flap. One should avoid the temptation of using local flaps of irradiated tissue in the hope of sparing the patient a larger procedure because this is nearly always doomed to failure.

CHYLE LEAK

Chyle leaks are an uncommon but potentially disastrous complication first reported by Cheevers in 1875.[91,92] They occur after 1% to 2% of radical neck dissections, with the majority (75% to 92%) being on the left side.[8,12,93,94] An appreciation of the anatomic variations of the thoracic duct and the right lymphatic duct is one of the keys in the prevention of a chyle fistula.

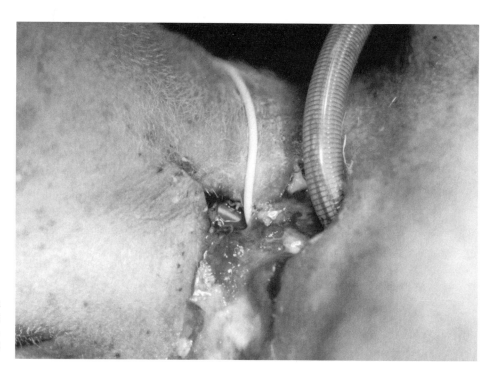

Figure 11–2. Postoperative fistula and wound breakdown following laryngectomy in an irradiated field. Endotracheal tube in stoma; feeding tube in esophagus.

Anatomy

The thoracic duct, only 2 to 4 mm in diameter, usually enters the cervical region on the left side behind the internal jugular vein, anterior to the phrenic nerve, crossing the transverse cervical artery and thyrocervical trunk. Up to 4.5% of patients may have a right-sided thoracic duct.[95] As it courses 3 to 5 cm above the clavicle, it passes from medial to lateral, posterior to both the common carotid artery and the internal jugular vein, and empties into the internal jugular vein at its junction with the subclavian vein. Occasionally, the duct may pass anterior to the common carotid artery and internal jugular vein.[96] A study of more than 1000 cadavers by Van Pernis found all ducts ending within 1 cm of the internal jugular-subclavian junction.[97] In contrast, other studies have shown more variability, with the thoracic duct terminating in the subclavian, innominate, or external jugular veins.[98] In addition, there are often multiple terminal branches occurring in up to 45% of patients.[99,100] The thoracic duct often receives numerous tributaries prior to its termination. This may lead to leakage of chyle despite ligation of the main duct[101] (Fig. 11–3). The right lymphatic duct drains the right cervical region, right arm, right lung, right heart, and the convex surface of the liver. It terminates at the junction of the right subclavian and internal jugular veins usually as a confluence of three trunks, (jugular, subclavian, and bronchomediastinal), or they may all drain separately.[102]

Physiology

Chyle consists of 70% ingested fat and is composed of emulsified fat and lymph, with triglycerides representing the major lipid component.[95] In addition, it has a high protein content (2% to 4%) and between 2000 and 20,000 white blood cells (WBC)/mm.[102] The total volume of chyle produced over 24 hours can vary between 1.5 and 4 L.[93,103] The loss of such a protein-, electrolyte-, and lymphocyte-rich fluid can readily lead to significant metabolic and immunologic disorders, such as dehydration, hypochloremia, hyponatremia, and hypoproteinemia if severe or prolonged. In addition, it may lead to secondary infection under cervical skin flaps with possible flap necrosis.

Intraoperative Chyle Leak

Intraoperative recognition of this complication usually occurs well after the injury to the lymphatic vessels has occurred. It typically manifests as a collection of oily, watery, or milky fluid mixed with blood in the supraclavicular area which persistently reaccumulates during the case, or a greasy residue may be noted on the surgeon's gloves. The tearing or avulsion of the thoracic or right lymphatic duct usually occurs when the lymphatic tissues adjacent to the carotid sheath in the inferior aspect of the neck are being swept superiorly. Enlarged, thin-walled lymphatic channels can often be seen during this point of dissection. Avoidance of chyle leaks comes from consideration of the lymphatics when dissecting in the supraclavicular regions and ligation of lymphatic channels when they are noted.

The treatment of an intraoperative chyle leak begins with finding the leak. If the vessel is identified, it may be ligated with nonabsorbable suture. Any branches noted should be ligated as well. If it cannot be found, the surgeon should have the anesthesiologist apply positive pressure to increase the chylous leak. Placing the patient in the Trendelenberg position can also assist in locating a small chylous leak. Thawley has advocated the use of an operating microscope in difficult cases.[93]

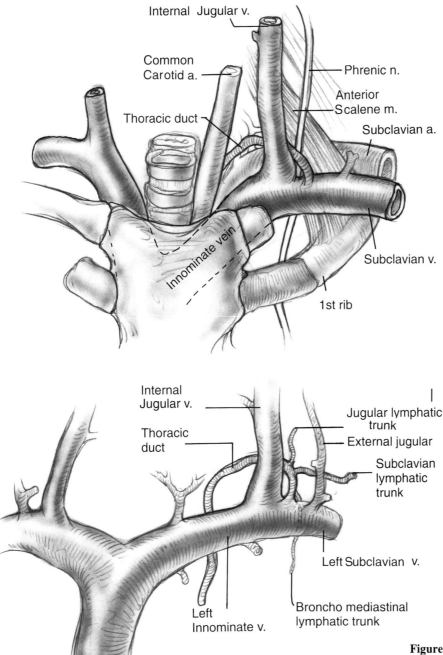

Internal Jugular v.

Common
Carotid a.

Thoracic duct

Phrenic n.

Anterior
Scalene m.

Subclavian a.

Innominate vein

Subclavian v.

1st rib

Internal
Jugular v.

Thoracic
duct

Jugular lymphatic
trunk

External jugular

Subclavian
lymphatic
trunk

Left Subclavian v.

Left
Innominate v.

Broncho mediastinal
lymphatic trunk

Figure 11–3. Anatomy of the
thoracic duct.

If no discrete lymphatic vessels are seen, figure-of-eight ligatures can be used in the area of leakage. Surgicel may also be applied. As an adjunct to this, tetracycline has been used as a sclerosing agent by applying 500 mg of powder on Surgicel and packing this over the area of the leak.[104] Coverage with a local muscle or fascial flap may also be performed.[105] When the surgeon is satisfied with the repair, the patient should be placed in the Trendelenberg position and have positive pressure applied once again as the area is reinspected. Closed-suction drainage is instituted and a pressure dressing is applied in addition to the usual postoperative head elevation. After an intraoperative chyle leak is detected and treated, the possibility of a chylothorax should be considered and chest x-rays obtained for 2 days after enteral feedings are initiated. The authors recommend feedings consisting of medium-chain triglycerides (MCTs). Mallen and Kudryk first advocated the use of an enteral diet consisting of MCTs as a method of supplying adequate nutrition and decreasing chyle formation by bypassing the intestinal lymphatics. MCTs are absorbed directly into the portal venous circulation and are not carried by the gut lymphatics.[106] Total parenteral nutrition has also been shown to be effective but is more expensive and is associated with greater morbidity.[96,103]

Postoperative Chyle Leak

In the postoperative period, after 2 to 5 days a milky effluent may be seen in the suction drains which increases when enteral feeding is begun. A fullness (chyloma) in the supraclavicular region may also appear under a skin flap, causing overlying erythema and induration usually more severe than that of a seroma or early fistula (Fig. 11-4).

The drainage can be analyzed for triglycerides. A chyle fistula will have a triglyceride level > 100 mg/dL and should be greater than the level found in the serum. The presence of chylomicrons in the drainage is not diagnostic and may be due simply to fat breakdown in the wound.[107]

If a chyle fistula or chyloma occurs, a trial of conservative management is begun. This consists of head elevation with continued suction drainage or repeated needle aspiration. A pressure dressing may be of some benefit, and MCT tube feedings should also be used as discussed earlier.

Loss of fluid can reach levels of up to 4 L/d and should be replaced on a cc-per-cc basis. In addition, electrolytes should be followed closely and deficits corrected promptly.

Timing of neck exploration is a subject of controversy. Kassel et al recommend a week of conservative treatment and exploration if the output exceeds 500 cc per day with no decreasing trend noted. Serious complications would necessitate earlier intervention.[104,108] Crumley and others would concur but recommend waiting only 4 to 5 days.[92,93] In a review of 823 neck dissections with 14 chyle fistulas, Spiro et al found that patients with chyle outputs of greater than 600 cc per 24 hours will likely fail conservative treatment. They recommend early reoperation in these individuals to lessen the overall morbidity and hospital stay[94] (Fig. 11-5).

Cream is given by tube or by mouth preoperatively for improved visualization of the chyle during the exploration. The operative techniques useful in these cases have been reviewed in the preceding section. Tetracycline has also been injected percutaneously under flaps or instilled retrograde through suction drains in a manner analogous to the treatment of recurrent pleural effusions or pneumothoraces.[109,110] This could be attempted prior to reexploration, particularly in those patients with significant concurrent medical problems who would represent a major surgical risk. Fibrin glue has also been used for this purpose; however, the authors have no personal experience with this technique.[111]

Prevention of postoperative chyle leaks requires a knowledge of the cervical lymphatic anatomy, as mentioned earlier, and meticulous ligation of all lymphatics during the procedure. A number of postoperative chyle leaks occur after an intraoperative chyle leak was identified and repaired.[92] This makes it imperative that the surgeon do everything possible to control the leak during the initial procedure.

Chylothorax

Unilateral or bilateral chylothorax associated with neck dissection is an extraordinarily rare complication. A patient may complain of dyspnea and chest pain or be entirely asymptomatic. A chest x-ray (CXR) will demonstrate the effusion.

The pathophysiology behind the development of a chylothorax is unproven. Chylothorax has not been reported in conjunction with a pneumothorax; therefore, it is not due to an intraoperative pleural laceration.[112] The most accepted explanation is that chyle under pressure in the neck tracks along fascial planes into the mediastinum. Tissue maceration along with an intense local inflammatory response results in spontaneous rupture of the mediastinal pleura, releasing chyle into the pleural space(s).[112,113] Patients with a chylothorax as the initial manifestation of a chyle leak with minimal or no chyle in cervical suction drains have been reported. The pathophysiological basis for this is believed to be an increase in hydrostatic pressure in the thoracic duct after its ligation in the neck. This overwhelms the posterior mediastinal collaterals, leading to an atraumatic extravasation of chyle into the mediastinum and then into the pleural space.[113,114] The dangers of this are twofold. The metabolic derangements as noted earlier may occur, but in addition cardiopulmonary compromise may develop due to mechanical compression of the lungs and eventual shifting of the mediastinum.

Thoracocentesis as a diagnostic and therapeutic maneuver is performed and repeated if the effusion recurs and the patient is symptomatic. If the patient is asymptomatic, the effusion can be followed by serial chest films and will generally resorb rapidly.[115] Tube thoracostomy or pleurodesis is rarely required[104,116] (Fig. 11-6).

CAROTID ARTERY COMPLICATIONS

Carotid rupture or "blowout" is one of the most feared complications of radical neck dissection. The incidence of rupture or near rupture has been reported from 3% to 7%.[117-122] Most ruptures occur when the neck dissection is accompanied with resection of oral, pharyngeal, or laryngeal structures.[118] Mortality rates with spontaneous postop rupture can reach 18% to 50%. In his study of 574 operative neck procedures, Ketcham[118] found 19 cases of spontaneous carotid artery hemorrhage. The time of rupture ranged from 6 to 81 days, with a median time of 16 days postoperatively in 13 patients. In three other patients hemorrhage occurred at 64, 94, and 264 days after postoperative radiation therapy. Three had repeat blowouts near the previous site. The most common site of rupture was the common carotid followed by the internal carotid and carotid bulb.

The pathophysiology of carotid rupture has been studied in detail. The most common etiologic factors contributing to rupture are en bloc resection of tumor coupled with tumoricidal doses of preoperative irradiation to overlying tissues and to the artery. Radiation doses of 3000 rad have been shown to reduce blood flow to the vasa vasorum as much as 50%, and doses up to 9000 rad decrease flow as much as 70%.[123] Massive tumor invasion into the wall of the artery is uncommon and in one series was noted in only 5.5%

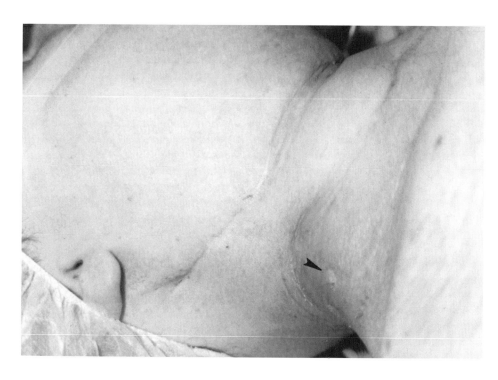

A

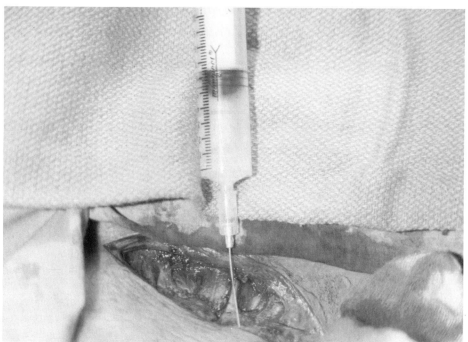

B

Figure 11–4. **(A).** Postoperative chyloma (arrow) right neck. **(B).** Aspiration of chyloma at the time of neck exploration. Note cream-colored fluid in syringe.

of the cases studied.[124] On the other hand, tumor growing around the carotid is a much more likely occurrence. Tumor invasion weakens the arterial wall and predisposes to rupture.

Radiation imposes significant risk. Maran et al reported 17 (4.3%) carotid ruptures in 394 operations.[125] The mean age of this group was 60.1 years. Fifteen (88.2%) of these ruptures had wound breakdown compared with 10.3% of those without carotid rupture. Fourteen (82.4%) of the 17

who had breakdown had had preoperative radiation therapy, whereas only 8.4% of the 167 previously irradiated patients without breakdown developed rupture. Only 1.1% of nonirradiated patients developed rupture.

Wound breakdown and necrosis of overlying tissue and flaps are other major contributors to this problem. Infection, fistula formation, and wound dehiscence resulting in carotid exposure have all been implicated as causative factors predisposing to carotid blowout.

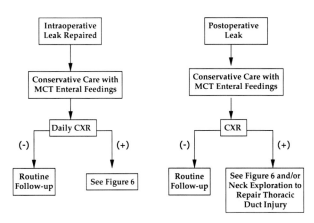

Figure 11-5.   Treatment of chyle leak. MCT = medium chain triglycerides.

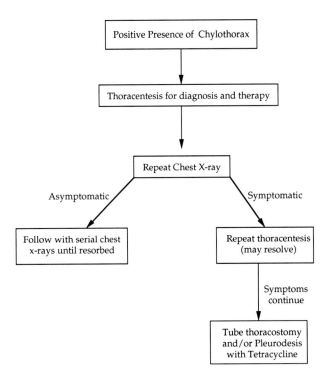

Figure 11-6.   Treatment of chylothorax.

Surgical technique itself also plays a role in ruptures. In the dissection of the carotid, improper manipulation of the vessel can damage the adventitia and lead to compromise of the vascular wall. The adventitia contains the vasa vasorum, which is the major blood supply to the vessel wall. Of the three layers, the adventitia is the most sensitive to dessication and infection.[126] Without a blood supply to the vessel wall, weakening of the tissue may lead to blowout. In addition, atherosclerotic disease may affect both the vasa vasorum and the strength of the arterial wall.[126,127]

The experienced head and neck surgeon will be able to recognize the signs of impending rupture. The clinical setting will generally include those patients who have previously been irradiated and recently undergone major head and neck surgery. Patients at increased risk are those who have

developed a postoperative wound complication which is not responding to conservative measures. Patients who have failed primary treatment with radiation and proceed to surgical salvage are at particular risk. A "sentinel bleed" is the classic warning sign of impending rupture. This bleed will not be as dramatic as an actual blowout and in fact may appear as only minor bleeding. However, if wound breakdown has occurred in a patient with prior radiation, it is incumbent on the responsible surgeon to suspect impending blowout and to take the necessary measures.

Carotid rupture is a surgical emergency. If bleeding is not stopped immediately, mortality approaches 50%. If a sentinel bleed is encountered, surgical exploration is indicated. If the rupture occurs spontaneously without warning, immediate pressure should be applied to slow the bleeding. Large-bore intravenous (IV) lines should be established and support with adequate replacement of fluid and blood products should be initiated immediately to maintain hemodynamic stability. Albumin and type O blood should be used if blood cannot be matched in a timely fashion. Attempts to clamp or ligate the arterial bleeding without being able to visualize the source is to be condemned and resulted in at least one death in the series reported by Ketcham.[118] One of the keys to avoiding cerebrovascular complications is to maintain the patient hemodynamically before formal exploration is undertaken. Once the bleeding is stopped at the bedside, the same physician holding pressure should ideally continue to do so until the operating room is prepared.

There are many considerations affecting surgical intervention. Ligation and excision of the ruptured area should be performed to prevent subsequent bleeds. Most authors agree that elective ligation of the carotid is the treatment of choice if rupture is imminent.[117,128] The postoperative morbidity and mortality is lower for elective surgery. Moore et al showed that cerebral vascular accident following elective ligation was 23% versus 50% in emergent situations.[128]

Emergent ligation should be approached with an appreciation that the area which has eroded is likely infected, ischemic, or involved with tumor.

Therefore, control of the eroded vascular area should be achieved well above and below the site which is likely to be involved. Suturing or repair of the involved arterial segment is usually fruitless and in fact is probably dangerous. Some authors advocate separate incisions to further avoid contaminating the field and decrease the risk of rebleeding.[129] Careful attention during this step may prevent further bleeding. Ligature of the stump closest to the heart should be especially secure because this stump will be exposed to the most intravascular pressure. Once the stumps have been ligated, they should be buried beneath an adjacent muscle or covered by a vascularized flap.

Sanders et al proposed the use of intrarterial balloon embolization catheters for the management of prerupture lesions.[122] Although balloon embolization is used extensively for other head and neck cases, further studies need to be conducted in regard to long-term prevention of bleeding in carotid rupture situations.[130]

Preventive measures should decrease the incidence of carotid rupture. Meticulous surgical technique minimizes damage to the adventitia. Some authors advocate covering the carotid with free dermal grafts.[131,132] The senior author has found dermal grafting in the high-risk patient to be a worthwhile procedure if performed at the time of the primary surgery. These grafts have little value, however, once wound breakdown has taken place and carotid exposure occurs. The treatment for either carotid rupture or impending rupture should include coverage with a myocutaneous flap, bringing in a fresh blood supply from outside the irradiated field.

Other measures to prevent rupture include continuous, diligent cleaning of the wound and diverting secretions away from the wound. Packing with moist gauze or petroleum gauze helps prevent drying of the vessel wall. Antibiotics will help in the treatment of associated infection and cellulitis. Because modified neck dissection has gained popularity, more patients are left with the natural protection of the sterno-cleidomastoid muscle, further minimizing the incidence of rupture.

CAROTID SINUS SENSITIVITY

Intraoperative manipulation of the carotid artery can bring about a quick response from the anesthesiologist. The carotid is a special vascular structure which contains receptors located in the outer muscular layer of the bifurcation which function as a feedback mechanism for blood pressure control. These receptors sense chemical and pressure changes and convey messages to the higher autonomic centers. For the head and neck surgeon, these baroreceptors become very important. Pressure changes in the region of the carotid bulb, whether iatrogenic or native, are transmitted to the medulla via the carotid sinus nerve.[133] These nerves are supplied primarily by the glossopharyngeal nerve.[134] Increased arterial pressure and/or compression during surgery causes a reflex increase in vagal output and a decrease in sympathetic output. This reflex causes a decrease in cardiac stroke volume, contractility, and a lower peripheral resistance (Fig. 11–7).

Surgical manipulation of the carotid baroreceptors will also cause autonomic reflexes. Compression or torquing of the carotid may be interpreted as an increase in blood pressure causing a sudden reflex drop in systemic blood pressure. This could have serious deleterious effects on a patient who is already hemodynamically unstable. Cerebral and visceral perfusion pressures may fall to a dangerous level, resulting in irreversible ischemic damage. Bradycardia, bradyarrhythmias, and hypotension are usually the initial signs.

Patients who have sensitive carotid baroreceptors may benefit from local injection of 1% lidocaine without epinephrine. This solution injected into the subadventitial tissue with a 25- or 27-gauge needle will usually temporarily block the reflex. Atropine is useful for the treatment of extreme bradycardia. Robinul, a newer anticholinergic (antimuscarinic) agent, like atropine can be used to counteract the bradycardia associated with carotid sensitivity. If any of

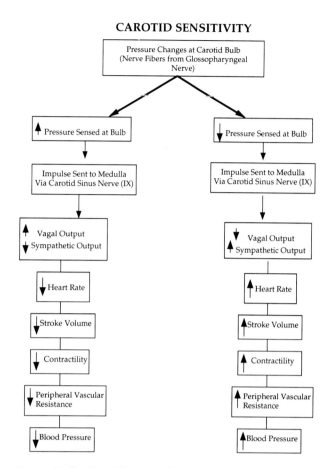

Figure 11–7. Carotid sinus refluxes.

the aforementioned signs appear during the operation, dissection should stop immediately until the problem has been identified and remedied.

AIR EMBOLISM

Air embolism has an unknown incidence because there are many events which go unreported. In one series, air embolism accounted for 1 in 108 operating room deaths.[135] In a surgical setting in which the patient's head is above his or her heart and venous structures are in the operative field, the risk of air embolism is increased. The reverse Trendelenburg position is common for head and neck procedures because it decreases the amount of bleeding secondary to decreased orthostatic pressure. With the head slightly elevated, the pressures within the venous structures of the head and neck are greater than the pressures in the right heart. In most neck dissections the internal jugular vein is exposed, manipulated, and/or sacrificed. Sacrifice of the vein requires ligature and division. With higher pressures within the vein and a point of entry of air into the venous system, air embolization will likely occur. Adams et al discuss the pathophysiology of venous air embolism in detail.[136] They emphasize that two factors must be present if embolization is to occur: (1) The venous system must be breached to allow entry of air, and (2) a pressure gradient between the opened vein and the right side of the heart must be present. The pressure gradient which develops is directly proportional to the height of the opening in relation to the heart and is inversely proportional to the central venous pressure. As a result, the gradient increases with inspiration. Therefore, most of the air introduced enters during inspiration.[137]

After air enters the vein, it travels via the anatomic pathway to reach the heart. Once in the heart, the air has three major pathways available (Fig. 11–5). The first is to continue through the heart, pass through the pulmonary artery, and end up in the lung. If the amount of air is small, it may diffuse into the alveoli and be expired or it may cause platelet aggregation in the small capillaries. This can result in microthrombi and inflammatory mediator release.[138] Ultimately, vasoconstriction, increased pulmonary resistance, and decreased compliance may follow.[139] If a large amount of air enters the system and proceeds to the lung, then an intense pulmonary artery vasoconstriction with resulting cor pulmonale and edema will likely result.[140] Air bolus and cor pulmonale may also initiate cardiac dysrhythmias and obstruct the right ventricular outflow tract.

The second alternative is for the air to remain in the heart. Air which passes into the heart may initially become lodged within the right atrium. Experimental evidence shows that air embolization may cause acute dilation of the right atrium.[141] Dilatation of the right atrium may lead to arrhythmias. If the air enters the right ventricle an airlock phenomenon appears. This airlock prevents proper venous return and reduces cardiac output. Subsequently, hemodynamic instability ensues and cardiovascular failure follows.

Approximately 20% of the normal population has a patent foramen ovale.[142] When right atrial pressure exceeds left atrial pressure, it is possible for the embolized air to pass through this patent foramen and enter the arterial circulation. Once into the arterial side, embolization can occur. This is also known as paradoxical embolization because the air originated on the right side of the heart. Embolization to the cerebral and other vital arterial circulation routes may have significant sequelae. Air emboli of as little as 100 mL of air have proven lethal in humans (Fig. 11–8).[143]

Recognition of air embolism may be difficult in the anesthetized patient. If a major vein is torn or a ligature becomes dislodged and a sucking noise is heard, embolization should be suspected. Auscultation may elicit a mill-wheeling cardiac murmur indicative of air mixing with blood in the heart. Sudden cardiorespiratory collapse in this setting should also alert the team of possible embolization. A sudden rise in central venous pressure and/or a decrease in end-tidal carbon dioxide should also draw the attention of the anesthesiologist. Tachycardia, arrhythmias, cyanosis, and hypotension are associated classic signs and symptoms.[139] Early detection of air embolus is important for treatment. An intraoperative Swan-Ganz catheter can relay changes in pulmonary artery pressures and central venous pressures which may signify the embolus.[142] A transthoracic ultrasonic Doppler device can detect intracardiac air, which will also help in diagnosis.[144]

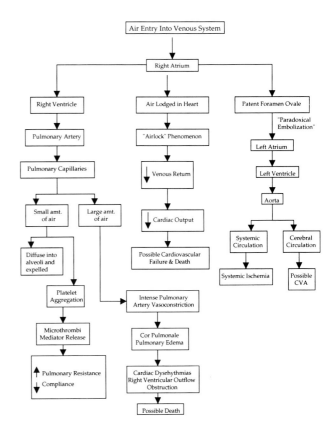

Figure 11–8. Pathophysiology of air embolism.

Treatment of air embolization begins with placing the patient in the left lateral decubitus position and Trendelenburg. This reduces the risk of a paradoxical embolus through a patent foramen ovale and has the ability to shift the embolus out of the right ventricular outflow tract into the apex of the right ventricle and allow antegrade blood flow. Occlusion of the torn vein with either direct pressure or repair will prevent further air entry (Table 11–1.)

If a central venous catheter has been previously placed and has a port within the right atrium, right ventricle, and pulmonary artery (as seen in most Swan-Ganz catheters), then immediate aspiration of the air can resolve the embolus. If nitrous oxide is being used for anesthesia, it should be discontinued immediately and replaced with 100% oxygen because nitrous oxide may increase and sustain the air bubble.[145] Because speed of treatment is so important, closed-chest cardiac massage has been suggested as an alternative treatment of choice. Ericsson et al reported a series of seven neurosurgery patients who sustained an air embolus during

Table 11–1.   Treatment for Air Embolism

1. Place patient in left lateral decubitus position.
2. Stop nitrous oxide—start oxygen at 100%.
3. If pulmonary artery catheter is in place, may use to aspirate air.
4. Closed chest cardiac massage.
5. Transcardiac aspiration from right ventricle—last resort.
6. If paradoxical air embolus to brain occurs, hyperbaric oxygen therapy may help reduce sequelae.

a neurosurgical procedure. Five of these patients were resuscitated successfully using closed-chest cardiac massage.[146] As a last resort, transcardiac aspiration of air may be attempted by placing a needle into the right ventricle to aspirate the air. Finally, central nervous systems (CNS) sequelae of paradoxical air embolus into the arterial circulation may respond to hyperbaric oxygen therapy.[147]

Prevention of embolus is best achieved by careful dissection of the jugular vein, being careful to look for hidden tributaries and following the proper plane of dissection. Preoperative placement of pulmonary artery catheters is helpful in recognition and treatment of air embolus but is not advocated for routine use in surgery of the neck.

INTERNAL JUGULAR VEIN COMPLICATIONS
Jugular Vein Thrombosis

All types of neck dissection and multiple other procedures in the cervical region place the internal jugular vein at some risk. In a radical neck dissection, at least one vein is sacrificed. The opposite internal jugular is left intact. Modified or selective neck dissections are now used more frequently in the treatment of head and neck cancer. Patency rates of internal jugular veins following selective neck dissection have been studied by Fisher et al.[148] In a study of 13 patients with contrast-enhanced computed tomography (CT) scans from 2 to 4 weeks postoperatively, 10 of the 13 patients had patent internal jugular veins with comparable diameters to preoperation. One vein was narrowed but patent, and two were occluded. This represents a patency rate of 85% (11 of 13).

Several factors have been proposed to cause thrombosis of the vein during surgery.[146] Handling of the vessel may cause damage to the endothelial lining, propagating clot formation. Dissection of the soft tissues from the surface of the vein may damage the adventitia, resulting in a transmural injury to the vessel. If attention is not paid to keep the vein moist throughout the procedure, drying may result and vessel wall damage can occur.

During ligation and coagulation of the branches of the vein, thermal injury may be sustained. Occasionally, branches are not ligated close enough to the internal jugular and stumps are left behind. Clot formation can occur in these stumps and propagate into the main vessel. Ligatures placed too close to the trunk may pinch and narrow the vein and impede flow, thereby initiating clot formation. Central venous catheter placement is also a risk factor for clot formation.[149]

Symptoms of unilateral internal jugular thrombosis have been described by several authors.[62,147,150] A tender, ill-defined, nonspecific neck mass on the side of the thrombosis is the most common symptom. Fever, leukocytosis, and a palpable cord may also be present. Pulmonary embolus (5% of cases), septic emboli, and septicemia are the most serious complications of internal jugular thrombosis.[147] Thrombosis can also lead to laryngeal edema, intracranial thromboses, seizures, visual changes, cervicofacial swelling, and

headaches.[151] It is assumed that many cases of thrombosis escape detection and result in no sequelae.

Diagnosis can be made with radionuclide scan, attempted needle aspiration, biopsy, ultrasound, magnetic resonance imaging (MRI), and CT scan. The definitive diagnosis traditionally has been the venogram. Enhanced CT scanning, however is the least invasive study providing maximum information (Fig. 11–9).

Treatment of internal jugular thrombosis begins with removal of the agent which caused the clot (namely, the indwelling catheter). Anticoagulants and fibrinolytics can also be used if the clot appears to be propagating. If these agents do not help, thrombectomy or removal of the vein (if it is not the only remaining vein) may be necessary if septic thrombosis is present. Expectant care may be all that is necessary if there is no sign of sepsis.

Prevention is best achieved by avoiding placement of central venous catheters in the internal jugular vein, especially if it is the only remaining vein. Surgical technique should include careful dissection around the vein and proper placement of ligatures and cautery.

Central Venous Catheter Complications

Long surgical procedures which have a significant risk of blood loss often require the placement of a central venous catheter. The catheters used, and their introduction, are not innocuous. Complications as high as 22% have been reported in some studies.[152] Bernard and Stahl found that the experience of the physician performing the procedure was an important factor. In 202 central catheter placements, no complications were reported for the operator who had performed more than 50 procedures versus a complication rate of 8.1% for operators who had performed fewer than 50.[153]

The injuries caused by central catheters or their placement are wide ranging. Pneumothorax, hemothorax, dysrhythmias, and even cardiac arrest are among the potential cardiothoracic injuries. Vascular tears with resultant hematomas, fistula formation, and aberrant placement also occur. Injury to the thoracic duct or other lymphatic channel can lead to chylothorax or chyle accumulation within the tissues. Thrombosis and infections represent more common complications. Neurological injury to the brachial plexus, phrenic nerve, or other cranial nerves has been described. McGurk and Camilleri independently reported aberrant migration or placement of central venous catheters into the internal jugular vein at the time of surgery.[154,155] Both articles describe the presence of the central venous catheter in the internal jugular vein which had been introduced via the antecubital fossa vein approach. In both instances, at the time of operation the surgeons were unaware that the catheter had found its way into the internal jugular vein. The catheter tip was sectioned in both cases and ended up in the pathologic specimen.

Treatment for catheter placement sequelae is directed toward the identified problem. Prevention of injuries during central line placement is probably best achieved through an understanding of the regional anatomy and technical

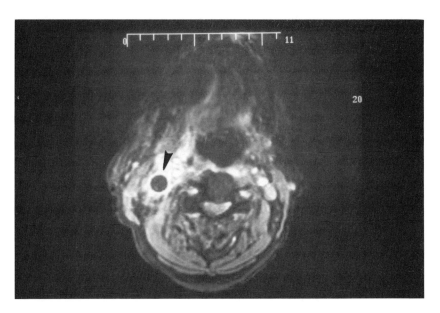

Figure 11–9. Right internal jugular vein thrombosis (arrow) on CT scan.

experience. Chest x-rays should be obtained after the procedure to assess placement and possible cardiothoracic injury. Placement of the catheter on the opposite side of the dissection and avoidance of manipulation of the catheter or the arm (if a long-arm central venous catheter is used) can prevent dislodgment of the catheter and aberrant migration. Palpation of the internal jugular vein prior to ligation or sectioning will notify the surgeon that the catheter lies in the vein.

PNEUMOTHORAX

Pneumothorax associated with neck surgery can be a life-threatening event. Probably the most common cause of pneumothorax is from the tracheostomy which often accompanies head and neck cases. The incidence of this complication following tracheostomy ranges from 0% to 5%.[156–158] Dissections in the posterior triangle of the neck which proceed into the supraclavicular region may also result in pneumothorax. The pleura overlying the apex of the lung, or cupola, may be entered at this point, leading to pneumothorax. Another iatrogenic cause of this problem in the perioperative period is the placement of central venous catheters.

Recognition of a pneumothorax may save the patient's life. Decreased breath sounds and hyperresonation on chest percussion should alert the physician to this possibility. If this is suspected, a chest x-ray should be obtained to check for an air space between the visceral and parietal pleura as well as possible mediastinal shift. If the pneumothorax is small (less than 20% of the lung volume by CXR) and the patient is asymptomatic, then conservative management with serial chest x-rays is appropriate. If the pnuemothorax is larger (greater than 20%), then tube thoracostomy should be performed.

If a tension pneumothorax is present with a shift of the mediastinum, emergent decompression is indicated. This is performed by introducing a large-bore angiocath into the second intercostal space in the midclavicular line (Fig. 11–10). If a rush of air is encountered, then the plastic catheter is left in place until a chest tube can be placed.

Careful dissection and avoidance of a high positive-pressure ventilation are the best prevention for pneumothorax. In performing a tracheostomy, it has been shown that closure of the incision around the trach or tightly packing the incision may predispose the patient to pneumothorax. Presumably these measures prevent egress of air from around the trach tube and the escape of air into the wound is diverted, tracking into the chest and causing pneumothorax or pneumomediastinum.

CRANIAL NERVE COMPLICATIONS
Trigeminal Nerve

Surgical procedures involving the submandibular triangle are at risk for jeopardizing the lingual nerve, a branch of the mandibular division of the trigeminal nerve. Dissection in the submandibular region can also damage the mylohyoid nerve, a branch of the inferior alveolar nerve, a division of the mandibular nerve. The lingual nerve runs medial to the gland and is tethered inferiorly by the submandibular ganglion (Fig. 11–11). Because of this tethering, the nerve is sometimes injured or transected when the submandibular contents are removed. Loss of the lingual nerve on one side causes decreased taste sensation to the anterior two thirds of the tongue and decreased special visceral afferent fiber sensation from the same anterior two thirds. In a study by Milton et al, permanent injury to the lingual nerve occurred during excision of submandibular glands in 3% of patients.[159]

Adjei et al report damage to the mylohyoid nerve during excision of a submandibular gland.[160] The inferior alveolar nerve gives off the mylohyoid nerve as it enters the mandibular canal. From this point, the nerve turns inferiorly and runs in the mylohyoid groove on the medial surface of the

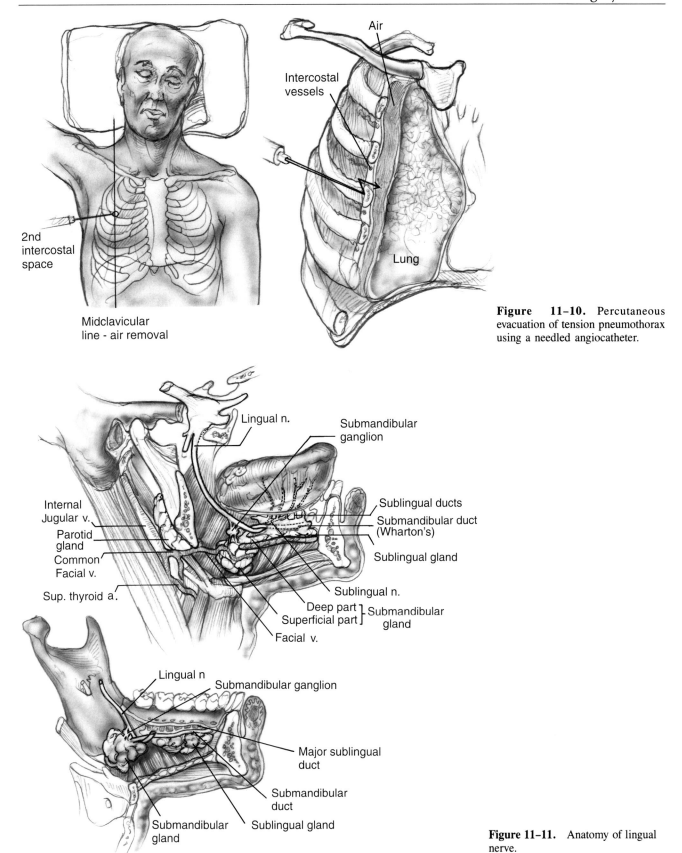

Midclavicular
line - air removal

2nd
intercostal
space

Air

Intercostal
vessels

Lung

Figure 11-10. Percutaneous evacuation of tension pneumothorax using a needled angiocatheter.

Lingual n.

Submandibular
ganglion

Internal
Jugular v.

Parotid
gland

Common
Facial v.

Sup. thyroid a.

Sublingual ducts

Submandibular duct
(Wharton's)

Sublingual gland

Sublingual n.

Deep part ⎱ Submandibular
Superficial part ⎰ gland

Facial v.

Lingual n

Submandibular ganglion

Major sublingual
duct

Submandibular
duct

Submandibular
gland

Sublingual gland

Figure 11-11. Anatomy of lingual nerve.

mandible. The nerve leaves the groove inferiorly to innervate the mylohyoid muscle and the anterior belly of the digastric. Sensory fibers continue forward to supply sensory innervation to the anterior surface of the mental prominence.[158] Damage to the nerve within the submandibular triangle may cause a minor sensory deficit around the chin.

Denervation of the mylohyoid and anterior belly of the digastric would likely go unnoticed.

Direct neurorrhaphy of the lingual nerve or cable grafting may provide resolution of some symptoms. Repair of the mylohyoid nerve is not warranted.

Prevention of damage is related to careful dissection and knowledge of anatomy. Isolation of the lingual nerve medial to the gland and sectioning of the tether to the submandibular ganglion will allow the nerve to retract superiorly. The authors do not hesitate, however, to transect the mylohyoid or lingual nerve when necessary to accomplish proper excision of the gland in cancer surgery.

Gustatory sweating following radical neck dissection has been described by Myers et al.[161] This phenomenon is most likely the result of injury to the secretomotor fibers innervating the parotid, which become misdirected to the skin and sweat glands. Myers reported six patients who presented with gustatory sweating involving the neck and face following radical neck dissection. Treatment varies from supportive care to topical antiperspirants. Surgical intervention is rarely required and is reserved for only the most symptomatic patients.

Facial Nerve

Neck dissections and other upper cervical procedures may involve the tail of the parotid, which swings below the angle of the mandible as it overlies the sternocleidomastoid muscle. As the facial nerve leaves the stylomastoid foramen, the nerve passes lateral to the styloid process before it enters the parotid gland (Fig. 11–12).[162] Surgery around the posterior belly of the digastric or removal of nodes in this region places the nerve at some risk. The marginal mandibular branch as well as the cervical branch may be injured within the parotid tissue or more distally. More anteriorly, the marginal mandibular branch swings inferiorly and laterally to run across the lateral surface of the submandibular gland. Damage to the cervical branch denervates the platysma muscle, whereas marginal nerve injury affects the orbicularis oris muscle, the depressor anguli oris, the mentalis, and the depressor labii inferioris (Fig. 11–12).[163] Loss of function of the platysma may result in loss of tone in the involved neck (usually clinically insignificant), whereas damage of the marginal mandibular branch causes elevation of the ipsilateral oral commissure and facial asymmetry at rest as well as with spontaneous and volitional facial motion.

Repair of the cervical branch is seldom necessary because the platysma is usually considered a vestigial muscle. Repair of facial nerve transaction is best achieved with end-to-end neurorrhaphy, if possible. If a portion of the nerve has been removed and the ends will not approximate without tension, then cable grafting with sural or greater auricular nerve is indicated.

Prevention of facial nerve injury is best achieved by identification and preservation of the nervous structures and avoidance of cutting through the parotid unless oncologically necessary. A nerve stimulator, nerve monitors, and non-paralytic anesthetic agents should be used to help identify the nerve. Because the marginal mandibular branch runs just beneath the platysma and lateral to the submandibular gland, it is generally preferred to identify the nerve so that it can elevated safely out of the operative field.

Vagus Nerve

The vagus nerve exits the jugular foramen and runs in the carotid sheath with the major vascular structures in the neck. In the neck it lies between the common carotid and the internal jugular vein.[164] The first branch off of the vagus is the superior laryngeal nerve. The superior laryngeal nerve has two branches: (1) the internal branch-special visceral afferent from the supraglottic larynx and (2) the external branch-innervation to the cricothyroid muscle. In the lower part of the neck, the vagus has small branches, the superior and inferior cardiac branches, which pass behind the subclavian artery and join the cardiac plexus. In the base of the neck, the recurrent laryngeal nerves arise. The right recurrent nerve loops behind the subclavian artery (from anterior to posterior) and then runs medially and superiorly in the tracheoesophageal groove to reach the larynx. The left recurrent runs below and behind the arch of the aorta and then follows a similar path to the larynx (Fig. 11–13). The recurrent nerves innervate all of the intrinsic muscles of the larynx except the cricothyroid muscle, which is innervated by the extrinsic branch of the superior laryngeal nerve. They also supply innervation to the pharyngeal constrictors. Finally, the recurrent nerves supply special visceral afferent sensation to the glottis and infraglottic larynx.

The superior laryngeal nerve runs in close proximity to the superior thyroid artery and may be damaged by dissection in this region (Fig. 11–13). During thyroidectomy, dissection of the superior pole and superior vascular pedicle places the external branch of the superior laryngeal nerve at particular risk. If injury to this nerve occurs, the cricothyroid muscle is unable to lengthen the vocal cord, resulting in problems with vocal pitch and easy tiring of the voice.[165] The singing range is particulary affected whereas the normal speaking voice may show little change.

Loss of sensation to the supraglottic larynx in the event of superior laryngeal nerve (Fig. 11–13) damage increases the risk of aspiration. Injury to the recurrent nerve results in unilateral vocal cord paralysis and decreased glottic sensation. This would cause hoarseness, slightly increased risk of aspiration, a breathy voice, difficulty with valsalva techniques, and decreased exercise tolerance due to the inability to sustain a breath. Some patients also notice generalized fatigue due to air wastage, using many more breaths than necessary for both speaking and normal respiration.

Recurrent Laryngeal Nerve

Thyroidectomy is the procedure most often associated with recurrent laryngeal nerve injury. Transection of the recurrent nerve and its repair have been studied extensively, and

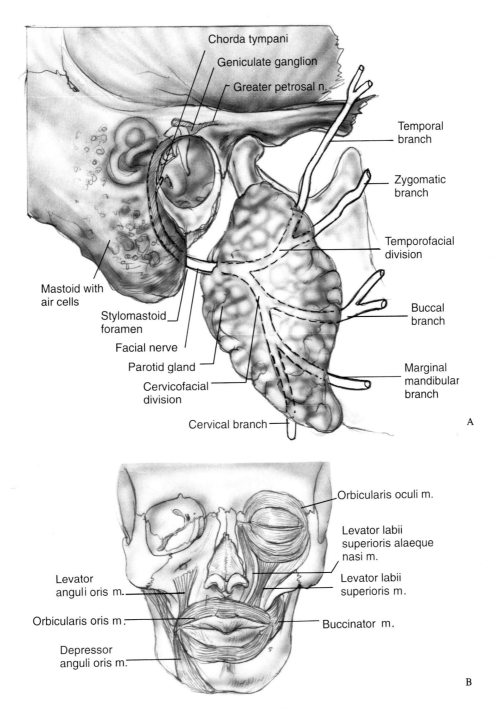

Chorda tympani

Geniculate ganglion

Greater petrosal n.

Temporal branch

Zygomatic branch

Temporofacial division

Buccal branch

Marginal mandibular branch

Mastoid with air cells

Stylomastoid foramen

Facial nerve

Parotid gland

Cervicofacial division

Cervical branch

A

Orbicularis oculi m.

Levator labii superioris alaeque nasi m.

Levator labii superioris m.

Levator anguli oris m.

Orbicularis oris m.

Depressor anguli oris m.

Buccinator m.

B

Figure 11–12. **(A).** Anatomy of the facial nerve. **(B).** Muscles of facial expression.

much controversy continues to make it difficult to make a definitive recommendation about repair in this circumstance. Functional results with neurorrhaphy are variable. Sato et al showed that nerve repair may prevent atrophy of the paralyzed muscles, thus maintaining the tone of the involved vocal cord.[166]

Maniglia et al described a new technique of laryngeal reinnervation by using a superior laryngeal-cricothyroid muscle pedicle flap to reinnervate the posterior cricoarytenoid muscle.[167] Using a canine model, the study looked at reinnervation in an iatrogenically paralyzed vocal cord. At 6 months

postoperatively, the reinnervated side had approximately half the mobility of the unoperated side and did not require tracheotomy in any case.

Doyle et al reported the effects of selective reinnervation of the posterior cricoarytenoid muscle by implantation of the sectioned proximal end of the recurrent laryngeal nerve.[168] Crumley looked at an ansa hypoglossi neuromuscular pedicle in another dog study in attempts to reinnervate the posterior cricoarytenoid muscle and found vocal cord abduction during hyperpnea from airway obstruction in the operated dogs. This abduction was alleviated by transaction of the

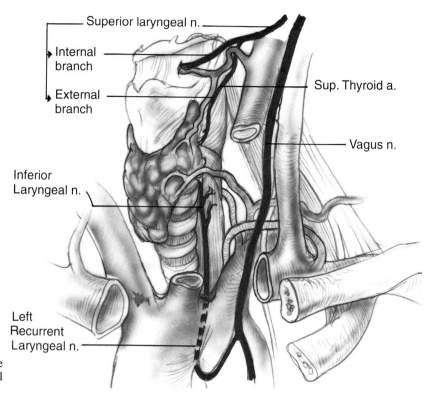

Figure 11–13. Anatomy of the recurrent and superior laryngeal nerves.

superior laryngeal nerve or detachment of the sternothyroid muscle, suggesting that the pedicled neuromuscular flap may not be causing the abduction.[169] Fink described accessory "abduction" during laryngeal inspiratory descent produced by lateral movement of the arytenoid cartilage, thyroid lamina, and vocal cord.[170] The experiments by Crumley suggested that the ansi hypoglossi neuromuscular pedicle may increase glottic patency but does not do so by reinnervation of the posterior cricoarytenoid.[169]

In 1982, Rice described reinnervation of the paralyzed larynx by using the phrenic nerve anastomosed to the abductor branch of the recurrent laryngeal nerve.[171] He reported good movement of the vocal fold during inspiration. He also anastomosed the motor branch of the superior laryngeal nerve to the adductor branch of the recurrent laryngeal nerve (RLN) to improve adduction of the vocal fold. Other authors, however, point out that if significant synkinesis occurs, the vocal quality may be further comprised.

In the event that a recurrent nerve is injured and immediately recognized, intervention may be indicated. Some authors advocate neurorrhaphy, accepting possible synkinesis in return for improved tone. Others prefer medialization techniques such as thyroplasty, which may be permanent but is potentially reversible. Of course, prior to the recent popularization of thyroplasty, Teflon or Gelfoam injection stood as standard treatment for unilateral RLN paralysis.

The best prevention is careful dissection and knowledge of the regional anatomy. Nerve stimulators may be useful in identifying these nerves.

Spinal Accessory Nerve

Since Crile in 1906 described radical neck dissection, injury to and sacrifice of the spinal accessory nerve has caused much morbidity to head and neck patients.[172] The spinal accessory nerve exits the jugular foramen with the IXth and Xth nerves as well as the jugular vein (Fig. 11–14). Soo's study showed that the nerve travels on the lateral aspect of the internal jugular vein in 56% of the specimens and medial in the remaining 44%.[172] It then runs posteriorly and downward to enter the deep surface of the sternocleidomastoid muscle (SCM). The nerve usually runs through the muscle but occasionally runs deep to the muscle. After supplying the SCM, the nerve turns inferiorly and laterally, running through the posterior triangle and deep to the trapezius, which it innervates.[173] The spinal accessory nerve may receive branches from the cervical plexus, which help in supplying the aforementioned muscles. In an article by Soo et al, 29 of 32 cadaveric specimens had contributions from the cervical plexus, with an average of 1.6 branches.[174] Most contributions were from C-2, C2-3, or C-3. Usually the branches joined the accessory nerve deep to the SCM and not in the posterior triangle. It is still unclear whether the cervical plexus contributions carry motor or sensory fibers into the accessory nerve.

During a radical neck dissection, the accessory nerve is sacrificed high in the neck as it exits the jugular foramen. Dissections in the posterior triangle may also injure the nerve. In the posterior triangle, the nerve can be located best by three

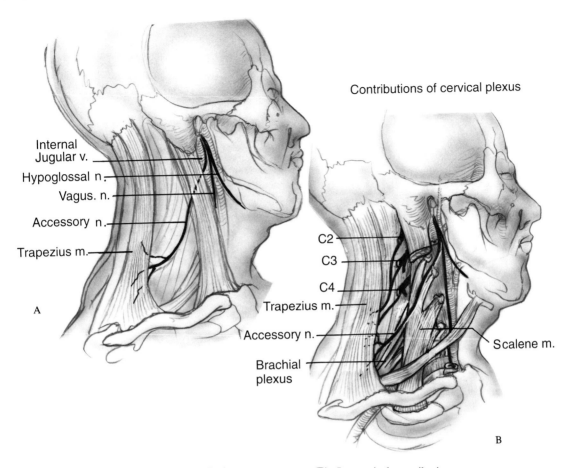

Contributions of cervical plexus

Internal Jugular v.
Hypoglossal n.
Vagus. n.
Accessory n.
Trapezius m.
A

C2
C3
C4
Trapezius m.
Accessory n.
Brachial plexus
Scalene m.
B

Figure 11–14. **(A).** Anatomy of the spinal accessory nerve. **(B).** Its cervical contributions.

landmarks: (1) The distance between the clavicle and the point, where the nerve passes under or pierces the trapezius muscle is generally 2 to 4 cm; (2) the greater auricular nerve is easily located during neck surgery and is found emerging on the posterior border of the SCM and then curving forward across the muscle, and the accessory nerve is found approximately 2 cm above the exit point of the greater auricular nerve; and (3) the nerve can nearly always be found along the top half of the posterior border of the SCM.[174] Selective or modified radical neck surgery has been developed in part to preserve the spinal accessory nerve. The presence of tumor or metastatic nodal involvement around the nerve or in the posterior triangle determines the extent of the dissection.

Patients who suffer from damage to the accessory nerve often are afflicted with the classic "shoulder syndrome." This syndrome consists of pain in the shoulder, limited abduction of the shoulder, a full passive range of motion, anatomic deformity (including scapular flaring, droop, and protraction), and an abnormal electromyogram of the trapezius.[175] Many authors have looked at symptoms and disability of patients following sacrifice of the nerve. These studies include subjective questionnaires, objective strength testing, and electromyography to assess function following surgery.

Fialka et al investigated shoulder function after radical neck dissection and looked at 43 patients who had sacrifice of the accessory nerve.[176] In these patients, 11 to 15 cm of

accessory nerve was removed at the time of surgery. Fialka et al found that 34 of 43 had strong (11), severe (22) or intolerable (1) pain, and 23 of 43 had moderate (13) to marked (10) muscular atrophy. The atrophy also correlated with decreased physical activity. Approximately 83% had damage detectable by electromyography (EMG) which was found to be predominantly in the descending portion of the trapezius. EMG values were only slightly decreased from the ascending portion. These results could represent dual innervation.

Remmler et al compared groups of patients who had undergone radical and modified radical neck dissections.[177] As might be expected, at 6 and 12 months postoperatively, the nerve sparing group showed no change in trapezius muscle strength testing from preoperative evaluations as opposed to the nerve sacrifice group, which had a marked decrease in trapezius muscle strength. No difference was found in range of shoulder motion between the two groups.

Electrodiagnostic testing of the trapezius muscle postoperatively at 12 months showed that 92% of the nerve-sparing group had normal innervation, whereas in the nerve sacrifice group nearly all had complete denervation. Interestingly, 22% of the nerve sacrifice group had denervation preoperatively, suggesting possible metastatic disease or biopsy related injury.

Sobol et al looked at another group of patients and performed an objective comparison of physical dysfunction following neck dissection.[178] They looked at 35 patients who underwent 44 neck dissections. These dissections were either radical neck dissections (RND), modified radical neck dissections (MRND), or supraomohyoid neck dissections (SND). They found that those who underwent radical neck dissection had the greatest reduction in shoulder movement and severely abnormal EMGs. The modified radical neck dissection group suffered less loss of shoulder function than the radical neck dissection group, but not to a significant degree at 16 weeks. However, the EMG studies of the modified radical neck dissection group were significantly better than the radical neck dissection group, suggesting that these patients may improve with time, which was the case when they were reexamined after 1 year. Those patients who underwent SND had only minimal loss of shoulder function at 16 weeks and essentially normal EMGs. All of the aforementioned articles[175-178] suggest that in patients who have a low probability of nodal involvement or tumor invasion of the nerve or surrounding lymphatics, sparing of the nerve results in better shoulder function postoperatively and less morbidity to the patient. The authors feel that the degree to which the nerve is dissected free from the surrounding tissues is also a determinant of postoperative function.

Treatment of patients who have transection of the accessory nerve is twofold. Immediate treatment options consist of preservation of the cervical plexus to preserve any existing alternative muscular innervation as long as this appears to be oncologically feasible. Primary reanastomosis of the severed nerve endings or cable grafting have also been proposed. Weisberger et al describe cable grafting of the accessory nerve to improve shoulder function after radical neck dissection.[179] Nine patients had immediate cable grafting of the accessory nerve after partial removal during radical neck dissection. The ipsilateral or contralateral greater auricular nerve was used as the graft. Using a subjective questionnaire, objective strength testing of the trapezius muscle, and postoperative EMG of the trapezius, comparisons were made with six patients who had undergone radical neck dissection without cable grafting and 10 patients who had undergone modified radical neck dissection with preservation of the accessory nerve. Weisberger et al found that cable grafting of the accessory nerve allowed adequate excision of the metastatic neoplasm and lessened the morbidity. Cable grafting restored some function of the trapezius muscle through reinnervation. Although this appears reasonable, it is seldom performed by most head and neck surgeons. The functional results for grafting were superior to radical neck dissection without cable grafting but less satisfactory than modified radical neck dissection in which the nerve was spared.

The decision to spare the nerve is based on tumor staging. Much evidence has been published on equivalent control of disease in the N_0 or N_1 neck with modified radical neck dissection as opposed to radical neck dissection.[180-184] However, Schuller showed that in the N_2 or N_3 neck, the proximity of the tumor to the nerve prevents preservation of the nerve.[185] Others have pointed out that metastatic nodes greater than 3 cm will often break through the nodal capsule and invade surrounding structures such as the accessory nerve.[186] When the nerve cannot be spared, the cable grafting technique may be useful.

Other treatment modalities have been proposed. Orthopedic reconstruction of the shoulder girdle may release some of the stress on the trapezius and levator scapulae to alleviate some of the symptoms. However, such reconstruction may cause damage to compensatory musculature, such as the serratus anterior, and further destabilize the scapula. Aggressive physical therapy following surgery has been shown to be useful in strengthening supporting musculature (serratus anterior, deltoid, levator scapulae, and rhomboids) as well as maintaining trapezius function in modified or grafting techniques.[177]

Preventing injury to the accessory nerve can be accomplished in several ways. As discussed earlier, avoiding the posterior triangle during neck surgery, if oncologically acceptable, may prevent damage to the nerve. If the posterior triangle is to be entered and nerve preservation is planned, the course of the nerve should be identified as the surgery proceeds. The nerve stimulator may be a helpful adjunct. Finally, if biopsies are to be taken from the posterior triangle, then the accessory nerve should be anticipated during the dissection. Lymph node biopsies in this region are notorious for inadvertent injury to the eleventh nerve.

Hypoglossal Nerve

The hypoglossal nerve is a purely motor nerve containing no afferent fibers. It arises from the medulla and exits the skull via the hypoglossal foramen. Just as it exits the skull, it receives a branch from the upper cervical nerves that helps form the ansa cervicalis.[187] Once the nerve leaves the foramen, it runs downward and forward lateral to the internal carotid, external carotid, and occipital arteries.[188] After the nerve passes the arteries, it runs medial to the posterior belly of the digastric and the stylohyoid muscles. In this region it courses just above the greater cornu of the hyoid bone. The nerve then crosses lateral to the hyoglossus muscle, which it innervates, and begins to branch as it runs deep to the sublingual gland.[189] The distal branches then supply all of the intrinsic muscles of the tongue on the ipsilateral side. The cervical plexus contribution mentioned earlier leaves the hypoglossal just as the nerve crosses lateral to the carotid. This small branch innervates the thyrohyoid muscle.

Surgery in and around the carotid artery (namely, carotid endarterectomy) places the hypoglossal nerve in jeopardy. Because the nerve passes lateral to the carotid, damage to the nerve is not uncommon (Fig. 11–15). Some studies report an incidence of 5.8% to 17.5% of hypoglossal dysfunction following carotid surgery.[190-196] With surgery around the hyoid bone, such as laryngectomy, the hypoglossal nerve must be identified and preserved, if possible (Fig. 11–15). Neoplasms and infections in the floor of mouth, sublingual, and submandibular regions may also involve the nerve. Care should be taken to identify the nerve even though tissues may be distorted secondary to the disease process. Excisions of bronchial cleft cysts high in the neck may take the head and

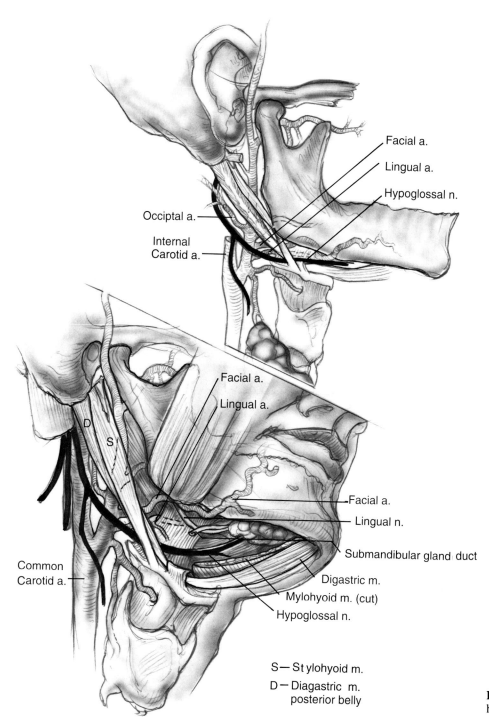

Facial a.

Lingual a.

Hypoglossal n.

Occiptal a.

Internal
Carotid a.

Facial a.

Lingual a.

Facial a.

Lingual n.

Submandibular gland duct

Common
Carotid a.

Digastric m.

Mylohyoid m. (cut)

Hypoglossal n.

S— Stylohyoid m.
D— Diagastric m.
posterior belly

Figure 11–15. Anatomy of the hypoglossal nerve.

neck surgeon near the nerve. Again, careful dissection and identification are essential.

Injury to the nerve during surgery or involvement of the nerve by tumor or infection is recognized easily. Ipsilateral tongue weakness, deviation of the tongue with protrusion to the affected side, speech difficulty, and difficulty swallowing may all be signs and symptoms of hypoglossal nerve paralysis.

If the nerve is transected accidentally or if a portion must be sacrificed secondary to tumor involvement, primary anastomosis or cable grafting seems justified, although results are not predictable. Unilateral tongue paralysis is generally well tolerated, with only minor changes in speech and mastication resulting.

Prevention of injury is best accomplished by a detailed knowledge of the anatomy. A nerve stimulator may aid in identification.

SYMPATHETIC NERVE INJURY

The sympathetic trunk lies deep in the neck posterior and medial to the carotid artery, between the prevertebral fascia and the carotid sheath. The sympathetic trunk passes upward superficial to the longus coli and longus capitis muscles behind the common carotid artery.[197] In some instances, the superior cervical ganglion lies deep to the prevertebral fascia.[198] The fascial layers and their relationship to the sympathetic chain are shown in Fig. 11-16.[197] Tumor resection in or around the sheath may disturb the sympathetic innervation of the head and neck.

When tumors invade this region, the surgeon is forced to follow the tumor extent to achieve clear margins; if resection of the trunk is necessary, it should be undertaken. However, care must be taken not to transect or remove the superior cervical ganglion inadvertently because it can resemble a lymph node at the level of C-1 to C-3. Traction on neck dissection contents may cause rotation of the carotid whereby the sympathetic chain is encountered and must be recognized to avoid injury.

Recognition of this injury postoperatively is characterized by several different signs and symptoms related to the classic Horner's syndrome. Physical findings resulting from loss of sympathetic innervation include meiosis (pupillary constriction), ptosis (eyelid drooping secondary to paralysis of Mueller's muscle), transient blushing, anhydrosis, and nasal congestion. If the lesion is below the stellate ganglion, no Horner's syndrome will occur. If the sympathetic flow is interrupted higher (ie, on the intracranial carotid or within the cavernous sinus), a partial Horner's without anhydrosis may result because sweat fibers leave the oculopupillary fibers after synapsing in the superior cervical ganglion. Likewise, a transaction of the sympathetic chain below the first thoracic ganglion may cause only anhydrosis.[198]

Treatment of Horner's syndrome is generally supportive care. Prevention of stretching or inadvertent transaction by following the aforementioned anatomic guidelines can help avoid these sequelae.

PHRENIC NERVE INJURY

The phrenic nerve originates from the cervical roots C3-5. The nerve descends in the neck on the anterior surface of the anterior scalene muscle beneath the fascia (Fig. 11-17).[199] As the nerve roots leave the cervical foramina, they may join to form the phrenic nerve or they may remain separated on the anterior scalene for some distance. Therefore, it may appear that two phrenic nerves are running beneath the fascia. In this instance, the lower of the two branches is usually referred to as the accessory phrenic nerve. The incidence of an accessory phrenic nerve has been reported from 5% to 54.5%.[200,201] Kelley proposed that the accessory nerve may carry motor fibers because sectioning or crushing of the phrenic nerve in some patients did not produce complete paralysis of the diaphragm.[202] These two branches usually join low in the neck or even in the thorax. From the neck the phrenic nerve enters the thorax by running behind the subclavian vein and in front of the subclavian artery. Occasionally the nerve will pass anterior to the vein.

Injury to the phrenic nerve may occur during neck dissection or any surgery in this region. Dejong and Manni discussed phrenic nerve paralysis following neck dissection and found several complicating factors. These factors include fibrosis or edema in the area of the anterior scalene muscle, tumor infiltration in or near the phrenic nerve, and diffuse bleeding or ligature of the blood vessels near the phrenic nerve.[203]

The phrenic nerve carries motor innervation to the diaphragm as well as somatic afferent fibers (ie, pain fibers) from the pericardium, the mediastinum, the diaphragmatic portions of the parietal pleura, and the parietal peritoneum on the inferior surface of the diaphragm.[203] Patients who suffer injury to the phrenic nerve may suffer the following signs and symptoms: cough, dyspnea, chest pain, cyanosis,

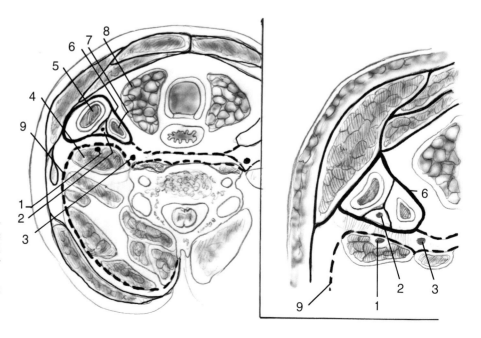

Figure 11-16. Anatomy of the cervical sympathetic trunk. (1) phrenic nerve, (2) vagus nerve, (3) cervical sympathetic trunk, (4) anterior scalene m., (5) internal jugular v., (6) carotid sheath, (7) common carotid artery, (8) thyroid gland, (9) prevertebral fascia.

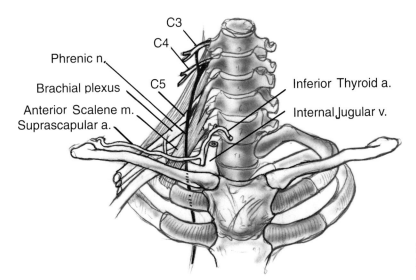

Figure 11-17. Anatomy of the phrenic nerve and the brachial plexus.

palpitations, tachycardia, dyspepsia, abdominal discomfort, nausea, vomiting, excessive belching, paralysis, and/or elevation of the ipsilateral diaphragm and mediastinal shift. The four classical signs according to deJong are (1) elevated hemidiaphragm, (2) absent or paradoxical diaphragm movement, (3) mediastinal shift, and (4) positive Hitzenberger sign (paradoxical movement of the diaphragm when sniffing).[203]

Although symptoms are rarely noted by the patient, the surgeon should be aware of the increased incidence of atelectasis on the involved side and take precautions to prevent postoperative pneumonia. If the nerve is sectioned, immediate neurorrhaphy or cable grafting is indicated. Diaphragmatic electronic pacers are available but are usually not necessary with unilateral phrenic nerve paralysis.

To prevent injury to the phrenic nerve, careful dissection in the area of the scalene fat pad during surgery will minimize the risk. Identifying the nerve as it lies on the anterior surface of the anterior scalene, running in an inferolateral direction, will also help prevent damage. As the dissection in this region proceeds, the fascia over the nerve should be left intact, thus minimizing the possibility of injury. Likewise, when sacrificing the cervical sensory branches in a neck dissection, care must be taken not to stretch the adjacent phrenic nerve or transect these branches too close to the phrenic itself.

BRACHIAL PLEXUS INJURY

Injury to the brachial plexus is rare during neck surgery. This plexus is formed from the nerve roots C5-8 and the first thoracic root. In the neck, the fifth and sixth cervical nerves with any contribution from C-4 will emerge between the anterior and middle scalene muscles and join on the anterolateral surface of the middle scalene to form the superior trunk of the plexus (Fig. 11-17).[204] The middle trunk runs downward and laterally on the middle scalene. The inferior trunk is usually behind the anterior scalene or lateral to it. All of these areas of the brachial plexus are located low in the floor of the neck beneath the deep cervical fascia, which allows the surgeon to develop a plane above the fascia, thus

preserving the nerves. Gacek, however, describes an anatomic variation which endangers this plexus.[205] The primary division of the brachial plexus composed of nerve fibers primarily from C-5 and C-6 nerve roots makes up the most cephalad portion of the brachial plexus. Occasionally this upper division takes a redundant course over the supraclavicular fat pad in the floor of the neck. This portion of the nerve can be unknowingly elevated and dissected, thus injuring the plexus.

Because the upper trunk is most often damaged, the muscles affected would include the biceps, triceps, supraspinatus, and infraspinatus because all receive contributions from the C5-6 roots. Weakness in these muscle groups would manifest the injury. Should the nerve be severed during surgery, primary neurrhoraphy or cable grafting is indicated.

Because of the relationship between the scalene muscles, the deep cervical fascia, and the brachial plexus, blunt dissection is usually achieved easily. However, as Gacek points out, if this plane of dissection is not separated easily, extreme caution should be used to prevent damage to the most cephalad aspect of the brachial plexus. If this cleavage plane is not identifiable easily, then the brachial plexus divisions should be identified and preserved. A nerve stimulator may be helpful in this identification.

CERVICAL NERVE NEUROMAS

The transaction of the cervical plexus can occasionally lead to the formation of neuromas. These are usually seen after a radical neck dissection and involve the sensory nerves located at the C-2 or C-3 level. These may present as painful subcutaneous masses and may be a source of significant discomfort to the patient. Classically these manifest themselves as a firm, tender, subcutaneous nodule less than 1 cm in size. The pain elicited by tapping on the neuroma will often be described as shocklike or tingling in nature. If the surgeon is unsure of the nature of the mass, it is important that it be differentiated from recurrent cancer.

All transected nerves form a bud or neuroma, but few are painful. The pathophysiology of painful neuroma formation is incompletely understood. Clinical and experimental work on peripheral neuromas, primarily involving the hand, has been enlightening. Mackinnon has shown in a primate model that transacted sensory nerves implanted in muscle had significantly less scar tissue and minimal neuroma formation. Histologically these nerve ends were contained by muscle and had no myofibroblasts, as seen in classic neuromas.[206] These myofibroblasts have been described as the source of painful neuromas in humans.[207,208] The authors speculate that injured skin in the area of a transacted nerve may attract regenerating neural fibers toward the skin, forming a painful neuroma. This is apparently blocked by inserting the nerve stump into muscle. Nerve implantation into muscle has been fairly successful clinically in orthopedic and hand surgery patients.

The factors causing painful neuroma formation are not known but would appear to include decreased soft-tissue coverage between the transacted nerve and the overlying skin.

Usually the presentation is so typical that no further diagnostic studies are necessary. If the patient desires or if recurrent malignancy is in question, then the nodule should be excised. Management strategies have included excision and ligation followed by muscle implantation, injection of steroids, or implanting the nerve stump into unscarred subcutaneous tissue.[209,210] Simply coagulating or ligating the nerve stump is also done. The authors recommend excision, ligation, and muscle implantation. The injection of a steroid or a local anesthetic into the neuroma followed by ethanol, if a good response is obtained, is a less invasive alternative.[139] The preventive measure practiced at many institutions is simply ligation of all cervical sensory nerves with silk. This practice is based on dogma, not science, but is rapid and results in few severely symptomatic neuromas. It would appear that implantation of the nerve stump into muscle after ligation is the most accepted form of treatment and would potentially have the lowest recurrence rate.

OPHTHALMIC COMPLICATIONS
Corneal Injury

Corneal injury during any surgical procedure can be a very uncomfortable postoperative problem and can lead to severe eye injury. During long operative procedures, if improper eye protection occurs, drying and/or scratching of the corneal surface is possible. Damage is directly related to time of exposure.

Treatment of corneal abrasion should include an antibiotic ointment such as gentamicin ophthalmic ointment, a temporary patch or special contact lens to cover the cornea, and serial exams by an ophthalmologist. Topical anesthetics may be used for temporary relief. Most corneal abrasions heal within 24 to 48 hours.

Prevention of corneal injury is accomplished by assuring adequate closure of the eyelid during surgery, using a temporary tarsorrhaphy suture, or placing a protective patch or "bubble" over the eye. Lubricants should be instilled into the eye to prevent excessive dryness.

Blindness

Blindness occurring after bilateral neck dissection is a rare but devastating complication, particularly in a patient with the loss of other cranial nerves and possibly requiring care of a stoma or tracheoesophageal fistula. Fewer than a dozen cases have been reported.[211-217]

The literature suggests a variety of contributing factors, of which intraoperative or postoperative hypotension appears to be the most significant (Fig. 11–18). The decreased perfusion creates ischemia and eventual infarction of the optic nerve or ganglion cells of the retina.[218] Obstructed venous and lymphatic outflow leads to impaired drainage from the ophthalmic veins, leading to a further drop in perfusion pressure via the ophthalmic arteries. Increasing facial edema contributes to this. Hypotension can also lead to visual changes due to damage of the primary optic cortex from occipital lobe infarction.[219] Emboli released during manipulation of the internal carotid artery during the course of the dissection could also lead to visual loss. Increased intracranial pressure can bring about both perioperative and delayed ocular changes as well.[3,220] Weiss et al described finding intracranial pressure changes associated with bilateral radical neck dissection. For patients undergoing bilateral radical neck dissections who would be in danger from an intracranial pressure greater than 40 mm Hg, they recommend intraoperative monitoring with central venous catheters and subarachnoid intracranial pressure (ICP) bolts.[221] Intervention for elevated pressures may help prevent complications including blindness.

Management of this problem involves correcting the underlying hypotension and taking steps to decrease intraocular pressure. Proper treatment demands immediate evaluation by an ophthalmologist. Standard measures include the use of mannitol, acetazolamide, and timolol ophthalmologic drops. A lateral canthotomy with inferior cantholysis should also be performed. The use of steroids or even continuous lumbar drainage may be of benefit, but this has not been proven.[2,4]

Prevention of postoperative blindness in these patients may relate to maintaining a stable blood pressure while avoiding fluid overload, which further increases postoperative orbital and facial edema. It must be remembered that many of these patients will develop a mild degree of "antidiuresis" due to increased antidiuretic hormone (ADH) secretion. If not recognized, the patient will receive an inappropriately large amount of intravenous fluids, further aggravating the situation.[222]

Avoidance of occlusive operative eye dressings has also been recommended by Wilson et al to avoid increasing intraocular pressure.[212] A prophylactic decrease in intraocular pressures in patients with glaucoma undergoing bilateral radical neck dissections should be considered.[2] All such patients with underlying ocular disease should be examined in the immediate postoperative period by an ophthalmologist.

Another neuro-ophthalmologic complication of bilateral radical neck dissection is pseudotumor cerebri. This occurs

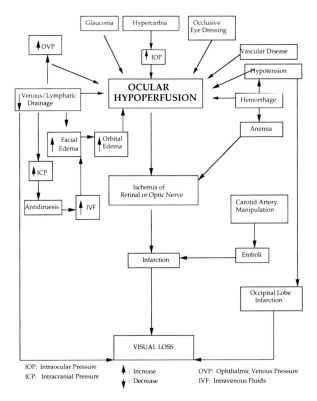

IOP: Intraocular Pressure   ↑ : Increase   OVP: Ophthalmic Venous Pressure
ICP: Intracranial Pressure   ↓ : Decrease   IVF: Intravenous Fluids

Figure 11–18. Blindness following neck surgery.

within a few weeks of surgery and is manifested by headache and diplopia, with papilledema and paralysis of either or both the trochlear and abducens nerves.[223,224] An intracranial lesion or cerebral vascular accident should be ruled out. This condition will normally resolve in 1.5 to 3 months. This has also been reported after unilateral radical neck dissection, presumably when the dominant (usually right) internal jugular vein is ligated.

LYMPHEDEMA

Lymphedema is seen commonly after both unilateral and bilateral neck dissections. Its incidence and severity are directly related to the extent of the surgery—bilateral versus unilateral, radical versus modified—as well as whether the area was irradiated. A preoperative neck biopsy also increases the resultant edema due to further disruption of the lymphatics and venules.

Fisch has shown that the number and size of the cervical lymph nodes decreases and that the majority of the lymphatic tributaries are destroyed over a period of 5 weeks to 1.5 years after radiation treatment.[225] Superficial venous and lymphatic collaterals in the contralateral neck, submental area, oral cavity, and pharynx are available as long as these areas have not been irradiated or the drainage path has not been traversed by an incision. Long-standing edema will eventually give way to fibrosis and atrophy, which will eliminate any further collateral development.[8]

Elevation of the platysma with the skin flap preserves the dermal lymphatics in the flap as long as they have not been

irradiated, and this will allow resolution of edema in a more rapid fashion.

Regional nonirradiated flaps can also be used to advantage in this situation, particularly if bilateral neck dissections are performed.

RECURRENT OR PERSISTENT CANCER

Conley considers recurrent or persistent disease to be the most serious of all complications occurring after neck surgery.[8] Neck recurrence is primarily related to the stage of the neck at the time of initial treatment and whether extracapsular spread (ECS) has occurred. Neck recurrence rates range from 4% to 40% at 3 years in different series, with an average of 15%.[8,12,13,226]

If the cervical nodes are pathologically negative, the incidence is 3% to 7%.[227,228] This increases markedly if positive nodes are found at multiple nodal levels or if ECS is present.[229-231]

A high clinical suspicion for recurrent disease is vital when following head and neck cancer patients. Conley has stressed five warning signs for recurrent tumors:

1. A mass is the most obvious sign, especially if there is a history of rapid tumor growth. Any such lesion should be evaluated with an immediate fine-needle aspiration (FNA) and CT if indicated.
2. Granulation tissue is commonly seen in wounds in which infection or a fistula has developed. Lack of resolution should lead to a suspicion of persistent or recurrent disease. Tissue adjacent to the fistula should be biopsied in this circumstance.
3. Persistent or recurrent edema is also of great concern because it suggests dermal lymphatic involvement with a dismal prognosis.
4. Neuromas which are not classic in presentation should also be evaluated with FNA or excisional biopsy.
5. The final warning sign is an ulcer that does not respond to antibiotics and local care.

Although the tumor biology or the intrinsic aggressiveness of a particular patient's cancer may be the cause of persistent or recurrent disease, there are technical factors that the surgeon can modify to increase the chances of a successful surgical result.

The surgeon must assure that he or she is performing a complete resection of the primary without cutting through tumor as well as execution of an appropriate neck dissection. This refers not only to performing the correct type of dissection but completing it in the correct manner.

Failure to perform a complete neck dissection could leave tumor behind as well as confuse the issue of postoperative radiation therapy. The surgeon must never forget that his or her first concern is to remove the malignancy, followed by restoration of function and preservation of cosmesis. An overly conservative surgeon hoping to prevent disability or disfigurement at the expense of leaving tumor is of no benefit to the patient.

Being prepared to alter one's plans during the case is also important. The surgeon must be prepared to take additional structures, such as the vagus or hypoglossal nerves, if indicated as well as always consider the need for a myocutaneous flap for closure of the pharynx or carotid protection.

The concern with treatment of recurrent neck disease is whether further treatment is likely to alter the course of disease or improve the patient's level of comfort. The initial desire to do something to cure the patient must be tempered with a detailed evaluation of the extent of the cancer, its potential for cure or effective palliation with acceptable risk, and the patient's wishes.

To select the optimal therapy for these challenging patients, it is recommended that all such cases be evaluated by a multidisciplinary tumor board. At our institution this consists of representatives from the Departments of Otolaryngology and Head and Neck Surgery, Radiation Oncology, Medical Oncology, Oral Medicine, and Diagnostic Radiology. A social worker is a crucial member of the team. For advanced-staged tumors, the treatment will involve combination therapy.

If disease recurs in a partially dissected neck, a complete evaluation of the local disease with a CT and/or MRI should be performed as well as a complete work-up for metastatic disease. If surgery appears to be a viable option then the surgeon must be aggressive and attempt to remove all disease, including any potentially involved skin. If not already performed, postoperative radiation therapy is advisable in this setting as well.

Recurrence on the side of a prior radical neck dissection requires the same investigation into locoregional and distant spread, as noted earlier. In these cases the distorted tissue planes give the tumor easy access to the skull base as well as to the carotid and subclavian arteries.

In spite of an extended radical neck dissection or subadventitial dissection of tumor off of the carotid artery, margins may be very close or tumor may be left behind on the carotid, skull base, or other structures. The use of radioactive implants (brachytherapy), which are able to deliver high doses to residual tumor without a large dose to adjacent normal tissue, has a definite role in such individuals. The need for combined therapy is demonstrated by the 7% survival seen in patients with residual disease on the carotid and the <30% survival for patients with N_3 disease.[232] I^{125} seeds or sutures as well as Ir^{192} after loading catheters have been used for this purpose and have resulted in improved survival, good local control, and effective palliation with a low complication rate, even if prior radiation therapy has been given.[233]

The logistically difficult intraoperative radiation therapy (IORT) may also play a role in selected patients.[234] A review of these two modalities has recently been published.[235] Individuals with unresectable malignancies may also be treated with the addition of concomitant chemotherapy to hyperfractionated radiation therapy, which has been shown to improve short-term survival in these unfortunate patients.[236]

Surgical palliation may take many forms, such as pain control, maintaining nutritional intake via a gastrostomy, airway control with a tracheotomy, laser treatment of an endobronchial tumor, or even laryngectomy for obstruction and aspiration.

Accurate preoperative evaluation of the extent of the disease is critical. Radiographic imaging to determine prevertebral muscle and skull base invasion, as well as carotid artery encasement or invasion, is invaluable. Careful panendoscopy performed by an experienced surgeon is also a necessity. In borderline resectable cases, radiation and/or induction chemotherapy may be a viable option prior to surgical resection. The key element is good clinical judgment to prevent the surgeon from having to back out or cut through tumor at the time of initial surgery.

Intraoperatively only complete radical, modified, or selective neck dissections should be performed. Anything less than a radical neck dissection must only be performed when clear indications for the lesser procedure exist. If there is a question as to resectability, then the surgeon must be prepared to perform an extended radical neck dissection or insert radioactive seeds or sutures at the time of initial surgery. The first goal during such a case must be to establish operability with a minimum of morbidity. The pharynx must be clearly separable from the prevertebral fascia and the carotid(s) examined prior to committing to a resection.

To decrease theoretically the risk of tumor cell implantation at the time of surgery, gloves and instruments are changed after tumor extirpation is done. Irrigation with sterile water is also performed to lyse remaining tumor cells osmotically.

BILATERAL RADICAL NECK DISSECTION

Despite the appropriate enthusiasm for modified and selective neck dissections over the past decade, the head and neck surgeon will be confronted with a small number of patients who will require bilateral radical neck dissections (RND). The question of whether to perform a simultaneous bilateral radical neck dissection or proceed with another alternative (due to the presumed excessive risk of the former procedure) has not been answered in any prospective manner. The options available include staged radical neck dissection, radical neck dissection with preservation of the external jugular vein, or modified radical neck dissection with sparing of the internal jugular vein on the least involved side. A number of authors may be quoted to lend credence to any of the viewpoints.[222,237-243]

The concept of a staged radical neck dissection refers to the delay in performing the second neck dissection to allow the development of collateral venous and lymphatic drainage to occur. The length of time these collaterals take to develop is controversial and ranges from 3 weeks to many months. The authors generally wait 4 to 6 weeks when staging a radical neck dissection.[238,239,243,244] Radiation therapy causes a fibrosis of lymphatic channels and would significantly delay the development of collaterals.[1,225]

Those areas involved in collateral venous drainage include the vertebral plexus, pharyngoesophageal plexus, ophthalmic veins, occipital veins, emissary veins, pterygoid plexus, and posterior jugular veins. Of these, the first three have the most clinical significance.[245-247] The classic work by Batson has shown that the vertebral plexus has a cross-sectional area which actually exceeds that of the internal jugular system.[248]

The most common complication of bilateral radical neck dissection is facial and neck edema resulting from the ligation of the internal jugular veins as well as the destruction of small venules and lymphatic vessels serving the head and neck. It is seen in 15% to 63% of patients and is associated with poor wound healing.[76,238,239,249] Its incidence and severity are greatly increased if the patient has received preoperative radiation or if a significant amount of the pharynx has been resected.[1,10] In fact, this edema can lead to upper airway obstruction due to supraglottic swelling even after staged radical neck dissection. Therefore, tracheotomy should be considered in these patients.

The prevention and treatment of this begins with keeping the patient's head elevated with the patient in the reverse Trendelenberg position throughout the perioperative period. In addition, careful attention to the overall fluid status of the patient, avoidance of any constricting ties or dressings around the neck, not turning the neck more that 30 degrees, and not placing pads behind the patient's neck or shoulders are important.[125] Such pads could serve to obstruct the external vertebral plexus, shown by Batson to be the primary collateral system.[133]

The intraoperative use of a Mayfield headrest would not impair venous drainage from the post neck or scalp and would therefore be of benefit. The patient's head must be moved at regular intervals to avoid ischemia at the contact points between the patient's head and the horseshoe-shaped headrest.[250]

We favor the use of perioperative steroids when performing bilateral neck dissections because they may be helpful in decreasing both facial and cerebral edema.[222]

If a simultaneous bilateral radical neck dissection is deemed necessary by the surgeon, then the possibility of jugular venous reconstruction or bypass may be considered, especially if the patient has been irradiated. A vein conduit can be fashioned using autogenous saphenous vein wrapped and sewn around a chest tube. This has been successful in avoiding severe facial edema.[251-253] One study suggests that jugular vein stump pressures of less than 30 mm Hg indicate that no jugular reconstruction is needed and the patient will not develop disfiguring edema or elevated intracranial pressure postoperatively.[251]

It should always be remembered that edema occurring well after surgery or recurring after initial resolution should be or great concern because it may indicate tumor infiltration into the dermal lymphatic.[1]

Visual loss after neck dissection is usually seen after bilateral procedures rather than unilateral neck dissection. Its etiology, treatment, and prevention have been reviewed.

Increased intracranial pressure (ICP) can be seen after bilateral radical neck dissection, as mentioned previously. ICP elevation occurs due to impaired cerebrospinal fluid absorp-

tion after internal jugular vein ligation and leads to cerebral edema. Although usually asymptomatic and of brief duration, it can become problematic. Symptoms may include headache, nausea, visual changes, lethargy, seizures, and eventual coma.[220,,222,254] Sensorineural hearing losses of 10 to 15 dB secondary to increased ICP have also been reported.[255]

A review of the various series concerning bilateral radical neck dissection does not allow direct comparison of complication rates due to different types of neck dissection, different staging intervals, and differences in radiation therapy. The data suggest that there is no significant difference in surgical complications between simultaneous or staged bilateral radical neck dissection and that the morbidity and mortality rates are acceptable. The authors agree that bilateral radical neck dissections can be performed safely when the patients are managed carefully in the perioperative period. The senior author has performed bilateral radical neck dissection on numerous patients without serious sequela, but the risks must be weighed in this decision. However, whenever it is oncologically sound, an attempt is made to spare a single internal jugular vein.

COMPLICATIONS OF TRACHEOTOMY

In the most general sense, complications can be divided into those occurring intraoperatively, during the early postoperative period, and during the late postoperative period. During the operation, damage can be done to the great vessels or party wall between the trachea and esophagus. The cupula of the lung enters the low neck and can be damaged, resulting in pneumothorax or pneumomedistinum, and for this reason postoperative orders after any tracheotomy should include a chest x-ray.

Early postoperative complications include tube obstruction, usually from mucous plugging; tube displacement, seen more frequently in children because of the more pliable neck tissue and the soft, malleable tubes commonly used; postobstructive pulmonary edema, seen commonly in those who have labored for some time with a partially obstructed airway; and infection. Obstruction from dried mucus can be largely prevented by meticulous tracheostomy care. A humidifier should be used postoperatively and the tube should be suctioned frequently after the installation of 1 to 2 cc of sterile saline. Guide sutures can assist with reinsertion of a displaced tracheostomy in the child. Postobstructive pulmonary edema should be treated with mechanical ventilation with positive-end expiratory pressure (PEEP) and possibly diuretics.

Late complications include tracheal stenosis, which can occur at the level of the tracheostoma, at the level of the tracheostomy tube cuff, and at the level of the tube tip. These have become much less common since the introduction of large-volume, low-pressure cuffs. Cuffs should be inflated only to the minimally occlusive volume. Cuff pressure should be checked regularly and kept below 25 cm H_2O, the pressure at which submucosal capillaries are occluded. In children, for whom cuffed tubes are generally not used, a slight air leak around the tube is desirable. A properly sized and fitted tracheostomy tube can decrease the incidence of damage from the tube tip. Some patients with severely distorted neck anatomy may require the use of special tracheostomy tubes, such as the Rusch tube, which is essentially a soft endoracheal tube that can be advanced variably through the neck plate to accommodate a variety of anatomic situations. Stenosis at the level of the tracheastoma usually occurs at the upper anterior border, where the anterior tracheal wall becomes softened and displaced into the tracheal lumen. Granulation tissue forms commonly at the level of the tracheastoma and can occur more distally from too vigorous tracheal suctioning.

One of the most feared complications of tracheotomy is tracheo-innominate artery fistula. This commonly occurs at the level of the tip of the tracheostomy tube and has been ascribed to a too low tracheotomy (below the level of the third tracheal ring), erosion from a high-pressure cuff, tube torsion and movement from a ventilator, and local infection. Sixty percent occur within 2 weeks of the tracheotomy and the complication carries a 73% mortality rate. It may be heralded by some minor sentinel bleeding. It is best treated by initially attempting to control the hemorrhage by overinflating the tracheostomy tube cuff or inserting an endotracheal tube below the level of the bleeding while attempting to compress the innominate artery anteriorly against the sternum with a finger inserted through the tracheotomy wound anterior to the trachea. Definitive treatment involves dividing and suture ligating the two ends of the innominate artery.[256]

The incidence of complications in pediatric tracheotomy is generally considered to be higher than that in adults. Gianoli et al reported a 3.3% incidence of intraoperative complications, a 13% incidence of early postoperative complications, and a 38.3% incidence of late complications in children less than 1 year of age. Tube obstruction was the most common early postoperative complication, and granulation tissue was the most common late complication.[257] The mortality rate for the procedure itself was 1.6%, but the overall mortality in the group of patients was 42%, reflecting the degree of underlying illness. Duration of tracheostomy was the most important factor influencing the rate of late complications. Higher complication rates were seen in preterm infants as opposed to full-term infants, and infants undergoing tracheotomy for upper airway obstruction suffered more complications than those undergoing tracheotomy for ventilator dependency. This correlation, however, seemed to be explained by the longer survival of patients undergoing tracheotomy for upper airway obstruction than those undergoing the procedure for ventilator dependency, with the subsequently greater period of time over which complications had a chance to develop (Table 11-2).

MEDICAL COMPLICATIONS

Hypertension following Radical Neck Dissection

The incidence of postoperative hypertension in patients undergoing major head and neck surgery may be as high as

Table 11–2. Complications of Tracheostomy

Intraoperative	Damage to great vessels
	Damage to tracheoesophageal common wall
	Pneumothorax
	Pneumomediastinum
Early postoperative	Tracheostomy tube obstruction
	Tracheostomy tube displacement
	Pulmonary edema
	Infection
Late	Tracheal stenosis
	Granulation tissue
	Tracheo-innominate artery fistula

10%.[238] In the study by McGuirt et al, 94 patients were reviewed retrospectively for the occurrence of intraoperative and postoperative hypertension.[238] Nine patients (9.6%) had postoperative blood pressures of 200/100 or higher or more than 40 mm Hg systolic and 20 mm Hg diastolic above preoperative blood pressure. Ten (10.6%) had systolic blood pressures greater than 40 mm Hg or diastolic pressures 20 mm Hg above preoperative. These observations were made in the first 2 postoperative hours and lasted an average of 9 hours. Of these 19 patients, four had hypertension preoperatively. Hypertension and hypotension following carotid endarterectomy have also been described.[258] Postoperative hypertension reported in these patients was mostly transient. Long-term hypertension occurred only in those who were hypertensive preoperatively. No CNS sequelae were sustained in this study, but two of the patients developed postoperative hematoma likely secondary to hemorrhage from increased blood pressure.

The pathophysiology of this process is not completely understood. Scher describes the carotid reflexes based on the pressure reflex model.[133] Baroreceptors in the carotid bifurcation transmit changes in pressure to the medullary vasomotor center via the carotid sinus nerve. Stimulation of this nerve due to an increase in blood pressure causes a reflex inhibition of sympathetic output and an increase in vagal activity, resulting in a decrease in blood pressure and heart rate. If this area of the carotid were denervated, as sometimes occurs in a neck dissection, the opposite or increase in blood pressure and heart rate would occur. Hypertension after carotid sinus denervation has been associated with a 10% incidence of fixed neurological deficit and an increased risk of intracranial hemorrhage.[258]

In McGuirt's study, all patients underwent opening of the carotid sheath, dissection of the XIIth cranial nerve in the area of the carotid bulb and bifurcation, and resection of soft tissues in these areas. Although eight of the 94 patients required stripping of tumor from the carotid, only three developed postoperative hypertension.

Another possible explanation for the appearance of hypertension in the postoperative period is that some patients develop hypertension as a reflex to the decreasing vasodilatory effects of general anesthesia. Regardless, prevention of injury to the carotid bulb/bifurcation region and surrounding soft tissues is extremely important.

Treatment of this hypertension is imperative to prevent the aforementioned complications. Vasodilating agents such as nitrates or sodium nitroprusside can be used for immediate control in those patients whose pressures reach 200/100 or elevations above preoperative of 40 mm Hg systolic or 20 mm Hg diastolic. At our institution, patients are usually treated with nitroprusside, nitrates, or other antihypertensives to reduce blood pressure to preoperative levels. Those who continue to show signs of chronic hypertension following surgery should receive long-term therapy.

SIADH

The syndrome of inappropriate secretion of antidiuretic hormone (SIADH) is rarely thought of as a complication of neck dissection but may be fairly common. Six of 17 patients in a series by Wenig and Heller developed various degrees of SIADH after such surgery.[259] SIADH is defined as hyponatremia with low serum osmolarity associated with urine osmolality greater than the serum. It has been reported after both unilateral and bilateral neck dissections but is believed to be more common in the latter.[222]

A patient with SIADH may complain of weakness, headache, lethargy, and mental confusion. This may ultimately progress to cardiac arrhythmias, seizures, and coma. SIADH should be suspected in hyponatremic patients with urine that is hypertonic to plasma.[260]

The mechanism through which this occurs is believed to be related to an increase in intracranial pressure after jugular vein ligation.[254] This pressure has been shown to lead to SIADH.[222] Previous radiation therapy or contralateral neck dissection would further increase the venous and lymphatic obstruction, putting the individual at greater risk for SIADH.

The treatment of this disorder involves fluid restriction to 1 L per day. However, this may not be possible in some surgical patients. If the situation is severe or life threatening, then 200 to 300 cc of 5% sodium chloride is given slowly IV until the patient's symptoms improve, but the treatment is not without its own potential complications.[261]

Avoidance of SIADH involves judicious fluid management in the operative and postoperative periods to avoid fluid overload. This is particularly important in patients who have had previous radiation therapy or a prior neck dissection because these patients will be at higher risk for developing increased intracranial pressure and therefore possibly developing SIADH.[251]

Drug Fevers

Fever associated with drug therapy usually occurs 7 to 10 days following initial administration and persists for the duration of drug use. Temperature usually returns to normal soon after discontinuing the drug; however, the fever will return if the drug is restarted. Initially, the fever may be low grade. In patients felt to have drug-induced temperature elevation, the fever may be spiking in nature and exhibit a normal diurnal rhythm.

Drug-induced fevers may result from several mechanisms, although most are thought to be due to a hypersensitivity reaction. In these instances, the fever cannot be explained by a known pharmacological effect of the drug, is unrelated to dose, and is associated with signs and symptoms that suggest an immunologic etiology. Therefore, it is unusual for fever to be the sole indicator of an allergic drug reaction because patients may experience arthralgias, urticaria, myalgias, gastrointestinal (GI) discomfort, and rashes. Fever may be the first sign of an impending severe drug reaction. Certain patients with autoimmune disorders such as systemic lupus erythematosus (SLE) appear to have a predisposition to developing allergic drug reactions. Other factors include genetic factors, increased age of the patient, duration of therapy, and route and dose of drug administration.

In addition to hypersensitivity reactions, other possible causes of drug-induced fever include the following mechanisms: (1) administration of drugs contaminated with pyrogens in the intravenous solutions (eg, amphotericin B); (2) infuson-related phlebitis (eg, cephalosporins and vancomycin); (3) direct pharmacological action of drug (eg, release of endogenous pyrogens from injured malignant cells as a result of chemotherapy); (4) interference with normal thermoregulatory mechanisms (eg, synthroid and antihistamines in large doses); and (5) idiosyncratic drug reactions (eg, oxidizing agents in patients with G6PD deficiency).

Diagnosis of drug-induced fever is often a diagnosis of exclusion; however, a high clinical index of suspicion may lead to the appropriate diagnosis prior to obtaining an expensive evaluation for a fever of unknown origin. Knowledge of the most common drugs associated with fever is helpful. In addition, the presence of associated allergic symptoms would be further evidence of a drug reaction. Definitive diagnosis is made once complete defervescence occurs after discontinuation of the drug and reappearance of fever with reinstitution of therapy. Rechallenge with the suspected agent should be carefully considered, however, because severe allergic reaction may occur, resulting in serious morbidity.

The list of drugs associated with fever is long and varied, although some are implicated more commonly. Of the drugs cited most frequently, antibiotics that have been administered perioperatively are most suspect for a postoperative fever. Allergic reactions with associated fever are not as common today, presumably due to the increased purity of the antibiotic preparations. Other drugs commonly associated with drug fever include quinidine, procainamide, antituberculars, methyldopa, and phenytoin. Unless first instituted perioperatively, these drugs would be rare causes of a postoperative fever.

UNUSUAL COMPLICATIONS
Arteriovenous Malformation

Arteriovenous (AV) malformations have been reported in the literature following radical neck dissection (RND).[262] The mechanism is thought to be a hematoma which occurs within the adventitia of the involved vessel, causing damage to the vasa vasorum. Out-budding of vascular endothelial cells occurs as part of the reparative process. These initial buds are considered by some to be the initial elements of the communications between the artery and the vein. A shunt phenomenon develops and vascular proliferation ensues, eventually leading to an AV malformation.

Diagnosis of these AV malformations can be made based on the history and physical examination. A history of neck surgery or penetrating neck trauma coupled with the clinical findings suggests an AV malformation. These findings include palpation of a thrill or auscultation of a bruit in the neck and/or history of pulsatile tinnitus or a whooshing sound. Continuous wave Doppler with spectrum analysis can identify flow abnormalities within the vasculature consistent with AV malformations. Arteriography is the gold standard for definitive diagnosis.

Surgical correction of AV malformations is the treatment of choice. Preoperative embolization by invasive vascular radiological technique may prevent unnecessary intraoperative bleeding, although for the easily accessible, well-localized AV malformation this may be unnecessary. Recurrence and reformation after repair of AV malformations have been reported.

Meticulous dissection and gentle handling of vascular structures should help prevent AV malformations. Care must be taken not to traumatize the vasa vasorum of major vessels. It has been recommended that even small arteries and veins be ligated separately to minimize this risk further. All vessels which have been ligated should also be divided to prevent possible AV malformation.

Clavicle Disorders

Clavicular pseudotumor after radical neck dissection without radiation therapy has been reported to occur with an incidence of 0.4% to 0.5%.[263-265] This complication usually presents within the first 6 months after surgery as a round, hard mass over the medial aspect of the clavicle which may measure 4 to 6 cm in size. It is often painless. Fine-needle aspiration or formal biopsy is usually not required, assuming that there are no associated abnormalities. Spontaneous clavicular fracture may also occur.

The proposed mechanism involves neither trauma nor metastatic disease but results from a distortion of the normal force vectors working on the shoulder girdle region. Loss of the spinal accessory nerve leads to a lowering of the shoulder in the absence of a functioning trapezius muscle, resulting in a relative increase in the weight of the upper limb. Resection of the sternocleidomastoid muscle then allows its antagonists, the pectoralis major and subclavius muscles, to act unimpeded on the clavicle. These forces stress the sternoclavicular joint and can lead to fracture or subluxation. Hypertrophic changes may also be seen.[266] No treatment beyond reassurance of the patient is required, and the fracture will heal or form a psuedoarthrosis.

Osteoradionecrosis

Osteoradionecrosis (ORN) has also been reported within the clavicle after radiation treatment. ORN and pathologic fracture have been reported as high as 4% to 22% in irradiated patients with head and neck cancer.[267,268] The incidence of ORN is proportional to radiation dosages delivered and inversely proportional to the number of fractions and total days of treatment.[269] Clinically, ORN may present with intractable pain, pathologic fracture, infection, and sometimes fistulization. Stofman et al reported a clavicular tracheal fistula following ORN of the head of the clavicle and sternum.[269] Treatment for ORN attempts to relieve pain and maintain appearance and function. Hyperbaric oxygen may be effective in treating ORN of the clavicle. Surgical debridement may be required if infection or intractable pain persists. Flap coverage may be necessary in recalcitrant cases.

Subcutaneous Emphysema

Subcutaneous emphysema following neck surgery is a relatively uncommon occurrence. Soft-tissue swelling and crepitus in the neck, face, and/or anterior chest wall are usually apparent. Respiratory compromise may also occur.[270] The pathophysiology of this process stems from several possible problems.

Tracheostomy can be associated with this complication. Escape of air into the surrounding tissues from the trach site may be the inciting event. If the wound is closed too tightly, air can track up the fascial planes instead of into the evacuation drains or through the skin incisions. If the trach tube becomes blocked or displaced, subcutaneous emphysema may occur. In the article by John et al, improper use of a vacuum drainage system caused inadvertent expulsion of air into the neck while attempting to empty or reset the drainage bulb.[270]

Treatment of subcutaneous emphysema may consist of observation if the air pockets are not enlarging or causing airway compromise. If the emphysema is expanding, decompression can be undertaken by opening the main incision. This will allow for escape of the air. If the patient develops pneumomediastinum, antibiotic coverage is warranted because the air tracking down from the trach site is likely contaminated.

Prevention can be achieved by assuring proper trach care and by making a separate incision for tracheostomy placement to maintain a tissue barrier between the primary neck incision and the air escape from the trach. Proper training of supportive staff in drain care can prevent accidental injection of air into the neck.

REFERENCES

1. Arian S. *Rad Neck Dissection Surg Clin North Am.* 1986; 66:133–147.
2. Beahrs OH. Complications of surgery for cancer of the head and neck. In: Artz CP, Hardy JD, eds. *Management of Surgical Complications.* Philadelphia: WB Saunders; 1975;277.
3. Robbins KT, Favrot S, Hanna D, Cole R. Risk of wound infection in patients with head and neck cancer. *Head Neck.* 1990;143–148.
4. Johnson JT, Myers E, Sigler B, Thearle P, Schramm V. Antimicrobial prophylaxis for contaminated head and neck surgery. *Laryngoscope.* 1984;94:46–51.
5. Dor P, Klastersky J. Prophylactic antibiotics in oral pharyngeal, and laryngeal surgery for cancer: A double-blind study. *Laryngoscope.* 1973;83:1992–1998.
6. Becker GD. Identification and management of the patients at risk for wound infection. *Head Neck.* 1986;8:205–210.
7. Yoder MG, Krause J, Kwyer TA. Infectious and noninfectious complications in head and neck surgery. *Otolaryngol Head Neck Surg.* 1979;87:797–806.
8. Conley JJ. Operative complications. In: Conley JJ, ed. *Complications of Head and Neck Surgery.* Philadelphia: WB Saunders; 1979;25–39.
9. Cummings CW, Johnson J, Chung CK, Sagerman R. Complications of laryngectomy and neck dissection following planned preoperative radiotherapy. *Ann Otol Rhinol Laryngol.* 1977;86:745–750.
10. Mendenhall WM, Million RR, Cassisi NJ. Squamous cell carcinoma of the head and neck treated with radiation therapy: The role of neck dissection for clinically positive neck nodes. *Int J Radiat Oncol Biol Phys.* 1986;12:1005–1011.
11. Brown BM, Johnson JT, Wagner RL. Etiologic factors in head and neck infections. *Laryngoscope.* 1987;97:587–590.
12. Khafif RA, Gelbfish GA, Attie JN, Tepper P, Zingale R. Thirty-year experience with 457 radical neck dissections in cancer of the mouth, pharynx, and larynx. *Am J Surg.* 1989;158:303–308.
13. Olofsson J, Tytor M. Complications in neck dissection. *Otol Rhinol Laryngol.* 1985;47:123–130.
14. Yarington CT, Yonkers AJ, Beddoe GM. Radical neck dissection. Mortality and morbidity. *Arch Otolar.* 1973;97:306–308.
15. Krause LG, Moreno-Torres A, Campos R. Radical neck dissection. Evaluation of 230 consecutive cases. *Arch Otolar.* 1971;94:153–157.
16. Taylor JMG, Mendenhall WM, Parsons JT, Lavey RS. The influence of dose and time on wound complications following post-radiation neck dissection. *Int J Radiation Oncol. Biol Phys.* 1992;23:41–46.
17. Joseph DI, Shumrick DL. Risks of head and neck surgery in previously irradiated patients. *Arch Otolaryngol Head Neck Surg.* 1973;97:381–384.
18. Yarington CT, Yonkers AJ, Beddoe GM. Avoiding complications in radical neck dissection. *Laryngoscope.* 1976;86:325–330.
19. McGuirt WF, McCabe BF, Krause CJ. Complications of radical neck dissection: A survey of 788 patients. *Head Neck Surg.* 1979;1:481–487.
20. Mantravadi RVP, Skolnik EM, Applebaum EL. Complications of postoperative and preoperative radiation therapy in head and neck cancers. *Arch Otolaryngol.* 1981;107:690–693.
21. Marchetta FC, Sako K, Maxwell W. Complications after radical head and neck surgery performed through previously irradiated tissues. *Am J Surg.* 1967;114:835–838.
22. Nichols RT, Greenfield LJ. Experience with radical neck dissection in the management of 426 patients with malignant tumors of the head and neck. *Ann Surg.* 1968;167:23–24.
23. Harris AE, Cassone RD. Surgery of the neck. In: Johns ME, ed. *Complications in Otolaryngology—Head and Neck Surgery.* Philadelphia: BC Decker; 1986.
24. Johnson JT, Bloomer WD. Effect of prior radiotherapy on postsurgical wound infection. *Head Neck.* 1989;132–136.
25. Carrau RL, Byzakis J, Wagner RL, Johnson JT. Role of prophylactic antibiotics in uncontaminated neck dissections. *Arch Otol Head Neck Surg.* 1991;117:194–195.
26. Arian S, Marfuggi RA, Harder G, Goodie MM. An experimental model to determine the effect of adjuvant therapy on the incidence of postoperative wound infection. I. Evaluating preoperative radiation therapy. *Plast Reconstr Surg.* 1980;65:328–337.
27. Cruz NI, Ariyan S, Miniter P, Andriole VT. An experimental model to determine the level of systemically administered antibiotics in radiated tissue. *Plast Reconstr Surg.* 1984;73:811–817.
28. Clarke HM, Howard CR, Pynn BR. Delayed neovascularization in free skin flap transfer to irradiated beds in rats. *Plast Reconstr Surg.* 1985;75:560–564.
29. Bassett MR, Dobie RA. Patterns of nutritional deficiency in head and neck cancer. *Otolaryngol Head Neck Surg.* 1983;91:119–125.
30. Brookes GB. Nutritional status in head and neck cancer. *Otolaryngol Head Neck Surg.* 1985;93:69–74.
31. Hever D, Byerley LO, Chi J, et al. Pathophysiology of nutrition in the adult cancer patient. *Cancer.* 1986;58:1867–1873.
32. Chandra S, Chandra RK. Nutrition, immune response, and outcome. *Prog Food Nutr Sci.* 1986;10:1–65.
33. Hussain M, Dish JA, Crane L, et al. The role of infection in the morbidity and mortality of patients with head and neck cancer undergoing multimodality therapy. *Cancer.* 1921;67:716–721.
34. Hooley R, Levine H, Flous TC, Wheeler T, Steiger E. Predicting postoperative head and neck complications using nutritional assessment. The Prognostic Nutritional Index. *Arch Otolaryngol.* 1983;109:83–85.
35. Hill GL. Malnutrition and surgical risk: guidelines for nutritional therapy. *Ann Royal Coll Surg Engl.* 1987;69:263–265.
36. Warnold I, Lundholm K. Clinical significance of preoperative nutritional status in 215 non-cancer patients. *Ann Surg.* 1984;199:299–305.
37. Muller JM, Brenner U, Dienst C, Pichlmaier H. Preoperative parenteral feeding in patients with gastrointestinal carcinoma. *Lancet.* 1982;1:68–71.
38. Goodwin WJ, Torres J. The value of the prognostic nutritional index in the management of patients with advanced carcinoma of the head and neck. *Head Neck Surg.* 1984;6:932–937.
39. Daly JM, Hearne B, Dunaj J, et al. Nutritional rehabilitation in patients with advanced head and neck cancer receiving radiation therapy. *Am J Surg.* 1984;148:514–520.
40. Pexner RD, Archambeau JO, Lipsett JA, Kokal WA, Thayer W, Hill LR. Tube feeding enteral nutritional support in patients receiving radiation therapy for advanced head and neck cancer. *Int J Radiat Oncol Biol Phys.* 1987;13:935–939.
41. Chencharick JD, Mossman KL. Nutritional consequences of the radiotherapy of head and neck cancer. *Cancer.* 1983;51:811–815.
42. Fietkau R, Iro H, Sailer D, Sauer R. Percutaneous endoscopically guided gastrostomy in patients with head and neck cancer. *Recent Results Cancer Res.* 1991;121:269–282.
43. Copeland EM, Duby JM, Dudrick JJ. Nutritional concepts in the treatment of head and neck malignancies. *Head Neck Surg.* 1979;1:350–363.
44. Windsor JA, Knight GS, Hill GL. Wound healing response in surgical patients: Recent food intake is more important than nutritional status. *Br J Surg.* 1988;75:135–137.

45. Johnson JT. Postoperative infection. In: Eisele DW, ed. *Complications in Head and Neck Surgery.* St. Louis, MO: Mosby-Year Book Inc; 1993;39–45.

46. Kaufman T, Eichenlaub EH, Levin M, Hurwitz DJ, Klain M. Tobacco smoking: Impairment of experimental flap survival. *Ann Plast Surg.* 1984;13:468–472.

47. Lawrence WT, Murphy MC, Heggers JP. The detrimental effect of cigarette smoking on flap survival: An experimental study in the rat. *Br J Plast Surg.* 1984;37:216–219.

48. Rao VK, Morrison WA, O'Brien B McC. Effect of nicotine on blood flow and patency of experimental microvascular anastomosis. *Ann Plast Surg.* 1983;11:206–209.

49. Engelberg H, Futterman M. Cigarette smoking and thrombotic coagulation of human blood. *Arch Environ Health.* 1967;14:266–270.

50. Meade TW, Chakrabarti R, Haines AP, North WR, Stirling Y. Characteristics affecting fibrinolytic activity and plasma fibrinogen concentrations. *Br Med J.* 1979;1:153–156.

51. Mosely LH, Finseth F. Cigarette smoking: Impairment of digital blood flow and wound healing in the hand. *Hand.* 1977;9:97–101.

52. Sarin LC, Austin JC, Nickel WO. Effects of smoking on digital blood flow velocity. *JAMA.* 1974;229:1327–1328.

53. Tish GM. Preoperative identification and evaluation of the patient with lung disease. *Med Clin North Am.* 1987;71:399–411.

54. Bernstein L. Incisions and excisions in elective facial surgery. *Arch Otolaryngol.* 1973;97:238–243.

55. MacFee WF. Transverse incisions for neck dissection. Ann Surg. 1960;151:279–284.

56. Deniell CH, Fee WE Jr. MacFee incisions: Dispelling the myth of cervical flap vascular inadequacy. *Head Neck Surg.* 1987;9:167–171.

57. Madden JW, Arem AR. Wound healing: Biologic and clinical features. In: Sabiston DC, ed. *Textbook of Surgery,* 13th ed. Philadelphia: WB Saunders; 1986;193–213.

58. Angel MF. Wound healing and its complications. In: Eisele DW, ed. *Complications in Head and Neck Surgery.* St. Louis, MO: Mosby-Year Book Inc; 1993;34–38.

59. Krizek TJ, Ariyan S. Infection. In: Conley JJ, ed. *Complications in Head and Neck Surgery.* Philadelphia, WB Saunders; 1979:99–123.

60. Johnson JT, Myers EN. Management of complications of therapeutic intervention. In: Myers EN, Suen JY, eds. *Cancer of the Head and Neck,* 2nd ed. New York; Churchill Livingstone; 1989;953–978.

61. Johnson JT, Schuller DE, Silver FS et al. Antibiotic prophylaxis in high-risk head and neck surgery: One-day vs. five-day therapy. *Otolaryngol Head Neck Surg.* 1986;95:554–557.

62. Johnson JT, Wagner RL. Infection following uncontaminated head and neck surgery. *Arch Otolaryngol Head Neck Surg.* 1987;113:368–369.

63. Kirchner JC, Edberg SC, Sasaki CT. The use of topical oral antibiotics in head and neck prophylaxis: Is it justified? *Laryngoscope.* 1988;98:26–29.

64. Rubin J, Johnson JT, Wagner RL, Yu VL. Bacteriologic analysis of wound infection following major head and neck surgery. *Arch Otolaryngol Head Neck Surg.* 1988;114:969–972.

65. Johnson JT, Yu V, Myers EN, Wagner RL. An assessment of the need for gram-negative coverage in antibiotic prophylaxis for oncological head and neck surgery. *J Infect Dis.* 1987;115:331–333.

66. Seagle MG, Duberstein LE, Gross CW. Efficacy of Cefazolin as a prophylactic antibiotic in head and neck surgery. *Otolaryngology.* 1987;86:568–572.

67. Becker GD, Parrel GJ. Cefazolin prophylaxis in head and neck cancer surgery. *Ann Otol Rhinol Laryngol.* 1979;88:183–186.

68. Fee WE, Glenn M, Handen C, Hopp ML. One day vs two days of prophylactic antibiotics in patients undergoing major head and neck surgery. *Laryngoscope.* 1984;94:612–614.

69. Brand B, Johnson JT, Myers EN, Thearle B, Sigler B. Prophylactic perioperative antibiotics in contaminated head and neck surgery. *Otolaryngol Head Neck Surg.* 1982;90:315–318.

70. Piccart M, Dor P, Klastersky J. Antimicrobial prophylaxis of infections in head and neck cancer surgery. *Scand J Infect Dis Suppl.* 1983;39:92–96.

71. Burke JF. The effective period of preventive antibiotic action in experimental incisions and dermal lesions. *Surgery.* 1961;50:161–168.

72. Seropian R, Reynolds BM. Wound infections after preoperative depilatory versus razor preparation. *Am J Surg.* 1971;121:251–254.

73. Cruse PJE. Prospective study of 20,105 surgical wounds with emphasis on the use of topical antibiotics and prophylactic antibiotics. Presented at the Fourth Symposium on Control of Surgical Infection; November 10, 1972; Washington, DC.

74. Geelhoed GW, Sharpe K, Simon GL. A comparative study of surgical skin preparation methods. *Surg Gyn Obs.* 1983;157:265–268.

75. Shaw JHF, Rumball EM. Complications and local recurrence following lymphadenectomy. *Br J Surg.* 1990;77:760–764.

76. Summers GW. Physiologic problems following ablative surgery of the head and neck: Symposium on revision surgery in otorhinolaryngology. *Otolaryngol Clin North Am.* 1974;7:217–250.

77. Budd DC, Cochran RC, Sturtz DL, Fouty WJ. Surgical morbidity after mastectomy operations. *Am J Surg.* 1978;135:218–220.

78. Lindsey WH, Masterson TM, Llaneras M, Spotnitz WD, Wanebo HJ, Morgan RF. Seroma prevention using fibrin glue during modified radical neck dissection in a rat model. *Am J Surg.* 156:310–313.

79. Gall AM, Sessions DG, Ogura JH. Complications following surgery for cancer of the larynx and hypopharynx. *Cancer.* 1977;39:624–631.

80. Johnson JT, Cummings CW. Hematoma after head and neck surgery—a major complication? *Trans Am Acad Ophthalmol Otolaryngol.* 1978;86:171.

81. Krizek TJ, Davis JH. The role of the red cell in subcutaneous infection. *J Trauma.* 1965;5:85–95.

82. McGuirt MD, May, John S. Postoperative hypertension associated with radical neck dissection. *Arch Otolaryngol Head Neck Surg.* 1987;113.

83. Conley JJ. Oropharyngocutaneous fistula. In: Conley JJ, ed. *Complications of Head and Neck Surgery.* Philadelphia: WB Saunders; 1979;92–98.

84. Robbins RE, Budden MK, MacDougall JA. Analysis of mortality and morbidity in 100 composite resections for oral carcinoma. *Am J Surg.* 1975;130:178–181.

85. Dedo DD, Alonso WA, Ogura JH. Incidence, predisposing factors and outcome of pharyngocutaneous fistulas complicating head and neck cancer surgery. *Ann Otol Rhinol Laryngol.* 1975;84:833–840.

86. Lavelle RJ, Maw RA. The aetiology of postlaryngectomy pharyngocutaneous fistulae. *J Laryngol Otol.* 1972;86:785–793.

87. Weingrad DN, Spiro RH. Complications after laryngectomy. *Am J Surg.* 1983;146:517–520.

88. Talmi YP, Finkelstein Y, Zohar Y. Pharyngeal fistulas in postoperative hypothyroid patients. *Ann Otol Rhinol Laryngol.* 1989;98:267–268.

89. Alexander MV, Zajuchuk JT, Henderson RL. Hypothyroidism and wound healing: Occurrence after head and neck radiation and surgery. *Arch Otolaryngol.* 1982;108:289–291.

90. Palmer BV, Gaggar N, Shaw HJ. Thyroid function after radiotherapy and laryngectomy for carcinoma of the larynx. *Head Neck Surg.* 1981;4:13–15.

91. Allen DP, Griggs CE. Wounds of the thoracic duct occurring in the neck: Report of two cases. Resume of 17 cases. *Am Med* 1901:401–404.

92. Crumley RL, Smith JD. Postoperative chylous fistula prevention and management. *Laryngoscope.* 1976;86:804–813.

93. Thawley SE. Chylous fistula prevention and management. *Laryngoscope.* 1980;90:522–525.

94. Spiro JD, Spiro RH, Strong EW. The management of chyle fistula. *Laryngoscope.* 1990;100:771–774.

95. Younus M, Chang RWS. Chyle fistula, treatment with total parenteral nutrition. *J Laryngol Otol.* 1988;102:384.

96. Greenfield J, Gottlieb MI. Variations in the terminal portion of the thoracic duct. *Arch Surg.* 1956;73:955–959.

97. Van Pernis PA. Variations of the thoracic duct. *Surgery.* 1949;26:806–809.

98. Gray H, Goss CM, ed. *Gray's Anatomy of the Human Body,* 36th ed. Philadelphia: WB Saunders; 1980;784–786.

99. Kinnaer TD. Anatomical variation of the cervical part of the thoracic duct in man. *J Anatomy.* 1973;115:45–52.

100. Parsons FG, Sargent PWG. On the termination of the thoracic duct. *Lancet.* 1909;1:1173–1176.

101. Hollinshead WH. *Textbook of Anatomy,* 3rd ed. Hagerstown, MD: Harper & Row; 1974:784–785.

102. Bozetti F, Arullani A, Baticci F, et al. Management of lymphatic fistulas by total parenteral nutrition. *J Parent Nutr.* 1982;6:526–527.

103. Ng RS, Kerbavaz RJ, Hilsinger RL. Bilateral chylothorax from radical neck dissection. *Otolaryngol Head Neck Surg.* 1985;93:814–817.

104. Kassel RN, Havas TE, Gullane PJ. The use of topical tetracycline in the management of persistent chylous fistulae. *J Otolaryngol.* 1987;16:174–178.

105. Lucente FE, Diktaban T, Lawson W, Biller HF. Chyle fistula management. *Otolaryngol Head Neck Surg.* 1981;89:575–578.

106. Mallen RW, Kudryk WH. Chylous fistula following right radical neck dissection. *J Otolaryngol.* 1975;4:177,–179.

107. Rodgers GK, Johnson JT, Petruzzelli GJ, Warty VS, Wagner RL. Lipid and volume analysis of neck drainage in patients undergoing neck dissection. *Am J Otolaryngol.* 1992;13:306–309.

108. Coleman JJ III. Complications in head and neck surgery. *Surg Clin North Am.* 1986;66:149–167.

109. Metson R, Alessi D, Calcaterra TC. Tetracycline sclerotherapy for chylous fistula following neck dissection. *Arch Otolaryngol Head Neck Surg.* 1986;112:651–653.

110. Austin EH, Flye MW. The treatment of recurrent malignant pleural effusion. *Ann Thorac Surg.* 1979;28:190–203.

111. Fitz-Hugh GS, Cowgill R. Chylous fistula. *Arch Otolaryngol.* 1970;91:543–547.

112. Frazell EL, Harrold CC, Rasmussen L. Bilateral chylothorax: An unusual complication of radical neck dissection with recovery. *Ann Surg.* 1951;134:135–137.

113. Cavallo CA, Hirata RM, Jaques DA. Chylothorax complication radical neck dissection. *Am Surg.* 1975;41:266–268.

114. Har-el G, Segal K, Sidi J. Bilateral chylothorax complicating radical neck dissection: Report of a case with no concurrent external chylous leakage. *Head Neck Surg.* 1985;7:225–230.

115. Pace-Balzan A, Moriarty B. Bilateral chylothorax following left radical neck dissection. *J Laryngol Otol.* 1988;102:288–290.

116. Kurtz TW, Hsu CH. Resolution of chylothorax after positive end-expiratory pressure ventilation. *Arch Surg.* 1980;115:73–75.

117. Shumrick DA: Carotid artery rupture. *Laryngoscope.* 1973;83:1051–1060.

118. Ketcham AS, Hoye RC. Spontaneous carotid artery hemorrhage after head and neck surgery. *Am J Surg.* 1965;110:649–655.

119. Leikensohn J, Milko D, Cotton R. Carotid artery rupture: Management and prevention of delayed neurological sequelae with low dose heparin. *Arch Otolaryngol.* 1978;104:307–310.

120. Dibbel DG, Gowen GF, Shedd DP, et al. Observations on postoperative carotid hemorrhage. *Am J Surg.* 1965;109:765–770.

121. Heller KS, Strong E. Carotid artery hemorrhage after radical head and neck surgery. *Am Med Surg.* 1979;138:607–610.

122. Sanders EM, Davis KR, Whelan CS, et al. Threatened carotid artery rupture: A complication of radical neck surgery. *J Surg Oncol.* 1986;33:190–193.

123. Smith DJ. Effects of gamma radiation on isolated surviving arteries and their vasa vasorum. *Am J Physiol.* 1961;201:901–904.

124. Kennedy JT, Krause CJ, Loevy S. The importance of tumor attachment to the carotid artery. *Arch Otolaryngol.* 1977;103:70–73.

125. Maran AGD, Amin M, Wilson JA. Radical neck dissection: A 19-year experience. *J Laryngol. Otol.* 1989;103:760–764.

126. Swain RE, Biller HF, Ogura JH, Harvey HE. An experimental analysis of causative factors and protective methods in carotid artery rupture. *Arch Otolaryngol.* 1974;99:235.

127. Huvos AG, Leaming RH, Moore OS. Clinicopathologic study of the resected carotid; analysis of sixty-four cases. *Am J Surg.* 1973;126:570.

128. Moore OS, Karlan M, Sigler L. Factors influencing the safety of carotid ligation. *Am J Surg.* 1969;118:666–668m.

129. Porto DP, Adams GL, Foster C. Emergency management of carotid artery rupture. *Am J Otolaryngol.* 1986;7:213–217.

130. Khoo CT, Molyneux AJ, Rayment R, et al. The control of carotid arterial hemorrhage in head and neck surgery by balloon catheter tamponade and detachable balloon embolization. *Br J Plast Surg.* 1986;39:72–75.

131. Smithdeal CD, Corso PF, Strong EW. Dermis graft for carotid artery protection; Yes or no? *Am J Surg.* 1974;128:484.

132. Moore OS, Papaionnou AN. Use of muscle flap for reconstruction after head and neck surgery for cancer. *Am J Surg.* 1965;110:514.

133. Scher AM. Carotid and aortic regulation of arterial blood pressure. *Circulation.* 1977;56:521–527.

134. Hollinshead WH, Rosse C. *Textbook of Anatomy.* 4th ed. 1985;835.

135. Dornette WH, Orth OS. Death in the operating room. *Anesth Analg.* 1956;35:545–569.

136. Adams VI, Hirsch CS. Venous air embolism from head and neck wounds. *Arch Pathol Lab Med.* 1989;113:498–502.

137. O'Quin RJ, Lakshminarayan S. Venus air embolism. *Arch Intern Med.* 1982;142:2173–2176.

138. Butler BD. Biophysical aspects of gas bubbles in blood. *Med Instrum.* 1985;19:59–62.

139. Koch WM. Complications of surgery of the neck. In: Eisele DW, ed. *Complications in Head and Neck Surgery.* St Louis, MO: Mosby-Year Book, Inc. 1993;393–413.

140. Munson ES, Paul WC, Perry JC, et al. Early detection of venous air embolism using a Swan-Ganz catheter. *Anesthesiology.* 1975;42:223–226.

141. Durant TM, Long J, Oppenheimer M. Pulmonary (venous) air embolism. *Am Heart J.* 1947;33:269–281.

142. Everts EC. Surgical complication. In: Cummings, CW, Fredrickson JM, Harker LA, et al, eds. *Otolaryngology—Head and Neck Surgery.* 1992;1673–1690.

143. Yeakel AE. Lethal air embolism from plastic blood storage container. *JAMA.* 1968;204:267–269.

144. Maroon JC, Edmonds-Seal J, Campbell RL. An ultrasonic method for detectng air embolism. *J Neurosurg.* 1969;31:196–201.

145. Marshall WK, Bedford RF. Use of pulmonary-artery catheter for detection and treatment of venous air embolism: A prospective study in man. *Anesthesiology.* 1980;52:131–134.

146. Ericsson JA, Gottlieb JD, Sweet RB. Closed-chest cardiac massage in the treatment of venous air embolism. *N Engl J Med.* 1964;270:1353–1354.

147. Dunbar EM, Fox R, Watson B, et al. Successful late treatment of venous air embolism with hyperbaric oxygen. *Postgrad Med J.* 1990;66:469–470.

148. Fisher CB, Mattox DE, Zinfeich JS. Patency of the internal jugular vein after functional neck dissection. *Laryngoscope.* 1988;98:923–927.

149. McNeill R. Internal jugular vein thrombosis. *Head Neck.* 1981;3:247–250.

150. Albertyn LE, Alcock MK. Diagnosis of internal jugular vein thrombosis. *Radiology.* 1987;162:505–508.

151. Storper ES, Calcaterra TC. Laryngeal edema induced by neck dissection and catheter thrombosis. *Am J Otolaryngol.* 1992;13:101–104.

152. Kaye WE, Dublin HG. Vascular cannulation. *Critical Care.* 1988;211–225.

153. Bernard RW, Stahl WM. Subclavian vein catheterizations: A prospective study. *Ann Surg.* 173:184.

154. McGurk M, Thomson PJ. A central venous catheter complicating head and neck surgery. *Br J Oral Maxillofac Surg.* 1991;29:388–391.

155. Camilleri AE, Davies FW. Aberrant central venous catheter complicating radical neck dissection. *J Laryngol Otol.* 1991;105:491–492.

156. Meade JW. Tracheotomy; its complications and their management: A study of 212 cases. *N Engl J Med.* 1961;265:519.

157. Skaggs JA, Cogbill CL. Tracheotomy: Management, mortality, complications. *Am Surg.* 1969;35:393.

158. Chew JV, Cantrell RW. Tracheotomy: Complications and their management. *Arch Otolaryngol.* 1972;96:538.

159. Milton CM, Thomas BM, Bickerton RC. Morbidity study of submandibular gland excisions. *Ann Coll Surg Engl.* 1986;68:148.

160. Adjei SS, Hammersley N. Mylohyoid nerve damage due to excision of the submandibular salivary gland. *Br J Oral Maxillofac Surg.* 1989;27:209–211.

161. Myers EN, Conley J. Gustatory sweating after radical neck dissection. *Arch Otolaryngol.* 1970;91:534–542.

162. Everts EC. *Surgical Complications.* Cummings. p. 1682.

163. Hollinshead WH. *Textbook of Anatomy,* 4th ed. Hagerstown, MD: Harper & Row; 878.

164. Hollinshead WH. *Textbook of Anatomy.* 3rd ed. Hagerstown, MD: Harper & Row; 1974:831–833.

165. Hollinshead WH. *Textbook of Anatomy,* 3rd ed. Hagerstown, MD: Harper & Row; 1974:1005.

166. Sato F, Ogura J. Neurorrhaphy of the recurrent laryngeal nerve. *Laryngoscope.* 1978;88:1034–1041.

167. Maniglia AJ, Dodds B, Sorensen K, Kumar N, Katirji MB. Newer techniques of laryngeal reinnervation. *Ann Otol Rhinol Laryngol.* 1989;98:8–14.

168. Doyle PF, Brummett RE, Everts EC. Results of surgical section and repair of the recurrent laryngeal nerve. *Laryngoscope.* 1967;77:1245–1254.

169. Crumley RL. Experiments in laryngeal reinnervation. *Laryngoscope.* 1982;92(suppl 30).

170. Fink FN. Folding mechanism of the human larynx. *Acta Otolaryngol.* 1974;78:124–128.

171. Rice DH. Laryngeal reinnervation. *Laryngoscope.* 1982;92:1049–1059.

172. Crile G, Cleveland NO. Excision of cancer of the head and neck with special reference to the plan of dissection based on one hundred and thirty-two operations. *JAMA.* 1906;47:1780–1783.

173. Hollinshead WH. *Textbook of Anatomy,* 3rd ed. Hagerstown, MD: Harper & Row; 1974;829.

174. Soo KC, Hamlyn PJ, Pegington J, Westbury G. Anatomy of the accessory nerve and its cervical contributions in the neck. *Head Neck Surg.* 1986;9:111–115.

175. Nahum AM, Mullally W, Marmor L. A syndrome resulting from radical neck dissection. *Arch Otolaryngol.* 1961;74:424–428.

176. Fialka V, Vinzenz K. Investigations into shoulder function after radical neck dissection. *J Cranio-Max-Fac Surg.* 1988;16:143–147.

177. Remmler D, Byers R, Scheetz J, et al. A prospective study of shoulder disability resulting from radical and modified neck dissections. *Head Neck Surg.* 1986;8:280–286.

178. Sobol S, Jensen C, Sawyer W, Costiloe P, Thong N. Objective comparison of physical dysfunction after neck dissection. *Am J Surg.* 1985;150:503–509.

179. Weisberger EC, Lingeman RE. Cable grafting of the spinal accessory nerve for rehabilitation of shoulder function after radical neck dissection. *Laryngoscope.* 1987;97:915–918.

180. Bocca E, Pignataro O. A conservation technique in radical neck dissection. *Ann Otol Rhinol Laryngol.* 1957;76:975–987.

181. Lingeman RE, et al. Neck dissection: Radical or conservative. *Ann Otol Rhinol Laryngol.* 1977;86:737–744.

182. Skolnik EM, Deutsch EC. Conservative neck dissection. *Laryngoscope.* 1985;95:561–565.

183. Jesse RM, Ballantyne AJ, Larson D. Radical or modified neck dissection: A therapeutic dilemma. *Am J Surg.* 1978;136:516–519.

184. Brandenburg J. Eleventh nerve in radical neck surgery. *Laryngoscope.* 1981;91:1851–1859.

185. Schuller DE. Spinal accessory lymph nodes: A prospective study of metastatic involvement. *Laryngoscope.* 1978;88:439–450.

186. Zoller M, Goodman ML, Cummings CW. Guidelines for prognosis in head and neck cancer with nodal metastasis. *Laryngoscope.* 1978;88:135.

187. Hollinshead WH. *Textbook of Anatomy.* 3rd ed. Hagerstown, MD: Harper & Row; 1974;937.

188. Hollinshead WH. *Textbook of Anatomy,* 3rd ed. Hagerstown, MD: Harper & Row, 1974;835.

189. Hollinshead WH. *Textbook of Anatomy,* 3rd ed. Hagerstown, MD: Harper & Row, 1974:906.

190. Tucker JA, Gee W, Nicholas GG, et al. Accessory nerve injury during carotid endarterectomy. *J Vasc Surg.* 1987;5:440–444.

191. Evans WE, Mendelowitz DS, Liapis C, et al. Motor speech deficit following carotid endarterectomy. *Ann Surg.* 1982;196:461–469.

192. Rosenbloom M, Friedman SC, Lamparello PJ, et al. Glossophoryngeal nerve injury complicating carotid endarterectomy. *J Vasc Surg.* 1987;5:469–471.

193. Hertzer NR, Felman BJ, Beven EG, et al. A prospective study of the incidence of injury to the cranial nerves during carotid endarterectomy. *Surg Gynecol Obstet.* 1980;151:781–784.

194. Deweese JA, Robb CG, Satran R, et al. Results of carotid endarterectomy for transient ischemic attacks—five years later. *Ann Surg.* 1973;178:258–264.

195. Hertzer NR. Postoperative management and complications following extracranial carotid reconstruction. In: Rutherford RB, ed. *Vascular Surgery,* 2nd ed. Philadelphia: WB Saunders; 1984;1300.

196. Verta MJ, Applebaum EL, McCluskey DA, et al. Cranial nerve injury during carotid endarterectomy. *Ann Surg.* 1977;185:192–195.

197. Hollinshead WH. *Textbook of Anatomy,* 3rd ed. Hagerstown, MD: Harper & Row; 1974;826.

198. Collins SL. Cervical sympathetic nerves in surgery of the neck. *Otolaryngol Head Neck Surg.* 1991;105:544–555.

199. Hollinshead WH. *Textbook of Anatomy.* 3rd ed. Hagerstown, MD: Harper & Row; 1974;566, 838.

200. Caliot P. Variations anatomiques de l'origine du nerf phrenique. *Rev Laryngol Rhinol Otol.* 1982;103:239–244.

201. Kikuchi T. A contribution to the morphology of the ansa cervicalis and the phrenic nerve. *Acta Anat Nippon.* 1970;45: 242–282.

202. Kelley WO. Phrenic nerve paralysis. Special consideration of the accessory phrenic nerve. *J Thorac Surg.* 1950;19:923–928.

203. deJong AA, Manni JJ. Phrenic nerve paralysis following neck dissection. *Eur Arch Otorhinolaryngol.* 1991;248:132–134.

204. Hollinshead WH. *Textbook of Anatomy,* 3rd ed. Hagerstown, MD: Harper & Row; 1974:842.

205. Gacek RR. Neck dissection injury of a brachial plexus anatomical variant. *Arch Otolaryngol Head Neck Surg.* 1990; 116:356–358.

206. Mackinnon SE, Dellon AL, Hudson AR, Hunter DA. Alteration of neuroma formation by manipulation of its microenvironment. *Plast Reconstr Surg.* 1985;76:345–353.

207. Badalamente MA, Hurst LC, Ellstein J, McDevit CA. The pathobiology of human neuroma: An electron microscopic biochemical study. *J Hand Surg.* 1985;10B:49–53.

208. Rudolph R, Utley JR, Woodward M. Contractile fibroblasts (myofibroblasts) in a painful pacemaker pocket. *Ann Thorac Surg.* 1981;31:373–376.

209. Graham WP III. Cervical neuromas following extensive maxillofacial surgery. *J Surg Oncol.* 1973:485–489.

210. Dellon AL, Mackinnon SE. Treatment of the painful neuroma by neuroma resection and muscle implantation. *Plast Reconstr Surg.* 1986;77:427–438.

211. Nawa Y, Jaques JD, Miller NR, Palermo RA, Green WR. Bilateral posterior optic neuropathy after bilateral radical neck dissection and hypotension. *Graefe's Arch Clin Exp Ophthalmol.* 1992;230:301–308.

212. Wilson JF, Freeman SB, Breene DP. Anterior ischemica optic neuropathy causing blindness in the head and neck surgery patient. *Arch Otol Head Neck Surg.* 1991;117:1304–1306.

213. Kiers L, King JO. Increased intracranial pressure following bilateral neck dissection and radiotherapy. *Aust NZ J Surg.* 1991;61:459–461.

214. Balm AJM, Brown DH, De Vries WAEJ, Snow GB. Blindness: A potential complication of bilateral neck dissection. *J Laryngol Otol.* 1990;104:154–156.

215. Marks SC, Jaques DA, Hirata RM, Saunders JR Jr. Blindness following bilateral radical neck dissection. *Head Neck* 1990;12:342–345.

216. Milner GAW. A case of blindness after bilateral neck dissection. *J Laryngol.* 1960;74:880–885.

217. Torti RA, Ballantyne AJ, Berkeley RG. Sudden blindness after simultaneous radical neck dissection. *Arch Surg.* 1964;88: 271–274.

218. Chutkow JG, Sharbrough FW, Riley FC. Blindness following simultaneous bilateral neck dissection. *Mayo Clin Proc.* 1973;48:713–717.

219. Aldrich MS, Alessi AG, Beck RW, Gilman S. Cortical blindness. *Ann Neurol.* 1987;21:149–158.

220. De Vries WAEJ, Balm AJM, Tiwari RM. Intracranial hypertension following neck dissection. *J Laryngol Otol.* 1986;100:1427–1431.

221. Weiss KL, Wax MK, Hayden RC, Kaufman HH, Hurst MK. Intracranial pressure changes during bilateral radical neck dissections. *Head Neck.* 1993;546–552.

222. McQuarrie DG, Mayberg M, Ferguson M, Shons AR. A physiologic approach to the problems of simultaneous bilateral neck dissection. *Am J Surg.* 1977;134:455–460.

223. Walsh FB, Hoyt WF. *Clinical neuro-ophthalmology,* 3rd ed, vol. 2. Baltimore: Williams & Wilkins; 1969;1899.

224. Marr WG, Chambers RG. Pseudotumor cerebri syndrome. *Am J Ophthalmol.* 1961;51:605–611.

225. Fisch U. *Lymphography of the Cervical Lymphatic System.* Philadelphia: WB Saunders; 1968.

226. Calearo CV, Teatini G. Functional neck dissection. Anatomical grounds, surgical technique, clinical observations. *Ann Otol Rhinol Laryngol.* 1983;92:215–222.

227. Leemans CR, Tiwari R, van der Wall I, Karim ABMF, Nauta JJP, Snow GB. The efficacy of comprehensive neck dissection with or without postoperative radiotherapy in nodal metastases of squamous cell carcinoma of the upper respiratory and digestive tracts. *Laryngoscope.* 1990;100:1194.

228. DeSanto LW, Beahrs OH, Holt JJ, O'Fallon WM. Neck dissection and combined therapy. *Arch Otolaryngol.* 1985;111:366.

229. Johnson JT, Barnes EL, Myers EN, Schramm VL, Borochovitz D, Sigler BA. The extracapsular spread of tumor in cervical node metastasis. *Arch Otolaryngol.* 1981;107:725–729.

230. Carter RL, Barr LC, O'Brien CJ, Soo K, Shaw HJ. Transcapsular spread of metastatic squamous cell carcinoma from cervical lymph nodes. *Am J Surg.* 1985;150:495–499.

231. Strong EW. Preoperative radiation and neck dissection. *Surg Clin North Am.* 1969;49:271–276.

232. Vikram B, Hilaris BS, Anderson L, Strong EW. Permanent iodine-125 implants in head and neck cancer. *Cancer.* 1983;51:1310–1314.

233. Stafford N, Dearnaley D. Treatment of "inoperable" neck nodes using surgical clearance and postoperative interstitial irradiation. *Br J Surg.* 1988;75:62–64.

234. Freeman SB, Hamaker RC, Singer MI, et al. Intraoperative radiotherapy of head and neck cancer. *Arch Otolaryngol Head Neck Surg.* 1990;116:165–168.

235. Close LF, Morrish TN, Nguyen P. Intraoperative versus interstitial radiotherapy: A comparison of morbidity in the head and neck. *Laryngoscope.* 1993;103:231–246.

236. Weissler MC, Melin S, Sailer SL, Qaqish BF, Rosenman JG, Pillsbury HC III. Simultaneous chemoradiation in the treatment of advanced head and neck cancer. *Arch Otolaryngol Head Neck Surg.* 1992;118:806–810.

237. Ahn C, Sindelar WF. Bilateral radical neck dissection: Report of results in 55 patients. *J Surg Oncol.* 1989;40:252–255.

238. McGuirt WF, McCabe BF. Bilateral radical neck dissections. *Arch Otolaryngol.* 1980;106:427–429.

239. Razack MS, Baffi R, Sako K. Bilateral radical neck dissection. *Cancer.* 1981;47:197–199.

240. Medina JE, Rigual NR. Neck dissection. In: Bailey BJ, ed. *Head and Neck Surgery—Otolaryngology,* vol 2. Philadelphia: JB Lippincott Co; 1993:1192–1220.

241. Weingarten CZ. Simultaneous bilateral radical neck dissection. Preservation of the external jugular vein. *Arch Otolaryngol.* 1973;97:309–311.

242. Moore OS, Frazell EL. Simultaneous bilateral neck dissection. *Am J Surg.* 1964;107:565–568.

243. Frazell EL, Moore OS. Bilateral radical neck dissection performed in stages. *Am J Surg.* 1961;102:809–814.

244. Brown AMS, Millar BG. Acute upper airway obstruction following "staged" bilateral radical neck dissections in previously irradiated patients. *Br J Oral Maxillofac Surg.* 1990;28:272–274.

245. Balm AJM, Brown DH, De Vries WAEJ, Snow GB. Blindness: A potential complication of bilateral neck dissection. *J Laryngol Otol.* 1990;104:154–156.

246. Gius JA, Grier DH. Venous adaptation following bilateral radical neck dissection with excision of the jugular veins. *Surgery.* 1950;28:305–321.

247. Fitz-Hugh GS, Robins RB, Craddock WD. Increased intracranial pressure complicating unilateral neck dissection. *Laryngoscope.* 1966;76:893–906.

248. Batson OV. Anatomical problems concerned in the study of cerebral blood flow. *Fed Proc.* 1944;3:139–144.

249. Moore OS. Bilateral neck dissection. *Surg Clin North Am.* 1969;49:277–283.

250. Wengen DF, Donald PJ. Complications of radical neck dissection. In Shockley WW, Pillsbury HC, eds. *The Neck: Diagnosis and Surgery.* Chicago: Mosby-Year Book, Inc.; 1994;483–509.

251. Comerota AJ, Harwick RD, White JV. Jugular venous reconstruction: A technique to minimize morbidity of bilateral radical neck dissection. *J Vasc Surg.* 1986;3:322–329.

252. Citrin P, Dasmahapatra KS. Interposition spiral saphenous vein graft bypass in bilateral simultaneous radical neck dissection. *Surg Gyn Ob.* 1988;167:79–80.

253. Leafstedt SW, Rubenstein RB, Pallanch JF, Wilder WH. Spiral saphenous vein graft for replacement of internal jugular vein: A series of case reports. *Angiology.* 1985;827–831.

254. Sugarbaker ED, Wiley HM: Intracranial pressure studies incident to resection of the internal jugular veins. *Cancer.* 1951;4:242–250.

255. Gamble JE, Peterson E. The effect of increased venous pressure on hearing. *South Med J* 1968;61:580–584.

256. Yang YY, Criado E, Schwartz JA , et al. Trachea-innominate artery fistula: retrospective comparison of treatment methods. *South Med J.* 1988;81:701–706.

257. Gianoli GJ, Miller RH, Guarisco JL. Tracheotomy in the first year of life. *Ann Otol Rhinol Laryngol.* 1990;99:896–901.

258. Bove El, Fry WJ, Gross WS, et al. Hypotension and hypertension as consequences of baroreceptor dysfunction following carotid endarterectomy. *Surgery.* 1979;85:633–637.

259. Wenig BI, Heller KS. The syndrome of inappropriate secretion of antidiuretic hormone (SIADH) following neck dissection. *Laryngoscope.* 1987;97:467–470.

260. Streeten DHP, Moses AM, Miller M. *Harrison's Principles of Internal Medicine,* 9th ed. New York: McGraw-Hill; 1980; 1691–1694.

261. Sterns RH, Riggs JE, Schochet SS Jr. Osmotic demyelination syndrome following correction of hyponatremia. *N Engl J Med.* 1986;314:1535–1542.

262. Brown JS, Ward-Boothe RP. Arterio-venous malformation following a radical neck dissection. *Int J Oral Maxillofac Surg.* 1989;18:239–240.

263. Lorz M, et al. Clavicular fractures after radical neck dissection. *HNO.* 1991;39:147–150.

264. Fini-Storchi O, Lo Russo D, Agostini V. "Pseudotumors" of the clavicle subsequent to radical neck dissection. *J Laryngol Otol.* 1985;99:73–83.

265. Gorman JB, Stone RT, Keats TE. Changes in the sternoclavicular joint following radical neck dissection. *Am J Roent.* 1971;111:584–587.

266. Cantlon GE, Gluckman JL. Sternoclavicular joint hypertrophy following radical neck dissection. *Head Neck.* 1983;5:218–221.

267. Fleming TJ. Osteoradionecrosis associated with definitive radiation therapy for head and neck malignancies. *J Prosthet. Dent.* 1983;49:675–679.

268. Langlands AO, Souter WA, Samuel E, Redpath AT. Radiation osteitis following irradiation for breast cancer. *Clin Radiol.* 1977;28:93–96.

269. Stofman GM, Cohn JR, Lowry LD, Jabourian Z. Osteoradionecrosis of the head and neck: A case of a clavicular-tracheal fistula secondary to osteoradionecrogis of the sternoclavicular joint. *Ann Otol Rhinol Laryngol.* 1988;97:545–549.

270. John DG, Carlin WV. An unusual case of surgical emphysema. *J Laryngol Otol.* 1986;100:1209–1211.

12 Use of Prophylactic Antibiotics in Otolaryngology

Anna M. Pou, M.D., Jonas T. Johnson, M.D.

COST

Wound infections comprise the largest single group of postoperative infectious complications of surgery and are the second most frequent nosocomial infection. In the United States, at least 920,000 of the 23 million patients who undergo surgery each year develop a wound infection.[1]

Antibiotics are the second most commonly used class of drugs in the United States. In 1978, the sale of antibiotics was estimated to be $1 billion, excluding the costs of retail and distribution.[2] Approximately 30% of antibiotics prescribed in hospitals are used in surgical prophylaxis.[3] The misuse of antibiotics has contributed to the high cost. Shapiro et al[4] evaluated the use of antibiotics in 20 short-stay hospitals in Pennsylvania. He found that 1 of every 10 patients received antibiotic prophylaxis and that this prophylaxis was continued until the day of discharge in most patients. Almost all of these patients were on surgical services.

In the field of otolaryngology, the need for prophylactic antibiotics in major contaminated head and neck (H&N) surgery is accepted. In several prospective, randomized, clinical trials the postoperative wound infection rate with placebo approaches 100%.[5-7] It has been shown in the fields of gynecology and general surgery that the establishment of specific protocols involving prophylactic antibiotics decreased the overall use of antibiotics, the postoperative infection rate, and, therefore, the cost.[8,9]

There are few studies evaluating the cost-effectiveness of prophylactic antibiotic use in H&N surgery.[10,12] Mandell-Brown estimated the dollar cost of a wound infection following major contaminated H&N surgery. The average stay of each infected patient was increased from 17.9 to 32.6 days with additional costs of $10,255.16 per patient infection. In an attempt to update costs, Johnson et al[12] conducted a retrospective analysis of patients at The Eye and Ear Institute of Pittsburgh who developed wound infections following H&N surgery between August 1986 and December 1987. The dollar cost per infection per person was found to be $12,155.05. Johnson et al also compared the cost of 1 day versus 5 days of antibiotic prophylaxis because many physicians extend the use of antibiotics in the perioperative period. Using Cefoperazone as an example, 4 doses per 100 patients costs $9825.00 as compared to $47,990.00 for 20 doses per 100 patients.

In a more recent study by Blair et al,[11] similar cost-benefit analysis was performed on patients undergoing clean H&N procedures. A retrospective analysis of 192 patients undergoing uncontaminated neck dissections was performed. Although there was no statistically significant difference in infection rate in patients receiving perioperative antibiotics as compared to those who did not receive antimicrobials, an infection prolonged the hospital stay by an additional 15 days. Again, the dollar cost incurred by these infections is much greater than the cost of perioperative antibiotics. It is important to remember that cost alone is not an acceptable rationale for the use of perioperative antibiotics in clean surgery in view of possible repercussions, such as the emergence of resistant strains and pseudomembranous enterocolitis.

CLASSIFICATION OF WOUNDS

By classifying wounds according to the likelihood and degree of contamination, one can assess the potential for postoperative infections. Wounds are classified as clean, clean contaminated, contaminated, and dirty, according to the risk and degree of contamination at the time of operation. Clean wounds are usually elective. Contamination from the lumen of the respiratory, alimentary, and genitourinary (GU) tracts is not encountered. There is no inflammation encountered, and there is no break in aseptic technique. These wounds are closed primarily but may be drained with a closed system. Clean wounds have an infection rate of 1% to 5%. Clean-contaminated wounds are operations in which the oropharyngeal cavity, respiratory, alimentary, or GU tract is entered under controlled conditions. Most otolaryngologic procedures fall into this category. The infection rate documented in the literature for this category is 8% to 11%, although a 28% to 87% infection rate has been demonstrated in major head and neck cases (Table 12–1). Contaminated wounds include those in which gross spillage from the gastrointestinal tract occurs, acute nonpurulent inflammation is encountered, or there is a major break in sterile technique. Fresh traumatic wounds are included in this group, which carries an infection rate of 15% to 17%. Dirty wounds are those in which the organisms causing the postoperative infection are present in the wound prior to operation. These include old traumatic

159

Table 12-1. Infection Rate in Prospective Randomized Placebo-controlled Trials in Patients Undergoing Major Contaminated Head and Neck Surgery

STUDY	INFECTION RATE WITH PLACEBO
Piccart et al (1983)[89]	28%
Dor & Klastersky (1973)[5]	36%
Seagle et al (1978)[90]	48%
Eschelman et al (1971)[17]	50%
Sanginus et al (1988)[91]	55%
Raine et al (1984)[92]	75%
Johnson et al 1984)[7]	78%
Becker & Parell (1979)[6]	87%

Difference is accounted for by lack of consistency among trials in patient selection, technique and magnitude of surgical resection, and objective definition of infection.

wounds, an existing abscess, and a perforated viscus. This degree of contamination carries an infection rate of greater than 27%.[13] Host factors and local wound factors also play an important role in determining the risk of infection in addition to the degree of contamination.

Perioperative chemoprophylaxis is used when there is definite risk of infection (ie, when tissue planes are likely to be exposed to bacterial contamination during the procedure). The value of perioperative chemoprophylaxis in clean H&N surgery is not supported.[14,15] Antibiotic use in dirty or traumatic wounds is considered therapeutic rather than prophylactic.[16]

Most otolaryngologic procedures are performed in a clean-contaminated field. Although sinonasal and otologic procedures are occasionally performed in a contaminated field and stapedectomy and cochlear implantation may take place in a potentially contaminated field, routine antibiotic prophylaxis has not been proven to be efficacious in these cases.[17-20]

TIMING AND ROUTE

The effectiveness of prophylactic antibiotics depends on the time at which the drug is administered, the route of administration, and the use of an agent with activity against the most common offending pathogens. Miles[21] investigated the inflammatory response using an animal model. He found that injection with noradrenalin or liquoid or the presence of hypovolemic shock increased the degree of inflammation only if the noxious stimulus was administered within a few hours after inoculation with bacteria. An injection with penicillin or streptomycin inhibited the inflammatory response to the inoculum if administered during this same critical period. Thus, Miles suggested that the final outcome of an infected lesion is determined by events occurring in the early phase of the inflammatory response. Using an animal model, Burke[22] found that antibiotics were most efficacious when given before bacteria enter the bloodstream or tissue, and they have no effect if given 3 hours after inoculation has occurred. These findings have also been supported by clinical trials.[23-25]

Stone et al[23] demonstrated the rate of infection in intraabdominal operations to be equal to that of placebo if prophylaxis was administered 1 to 4 hours after the surgical incision. Classen et al[25] also corroborated these findings in a large prospective, randomized trial involving 2847 patients undergoing various clean and clean-contaminated surgical procedures. The lowest infection rate was seen when patients received antibiotics 0 to 2 hours prior to surgery (0.6%). The risk of infection increased with each hour that passed following surgical incision until the agent was administered. Surgical wound infections developed in 1.4% of those patients receiving antibiotics within 3 hours following surgical incision and in 3.3% of patients receiving antibiotics more than 3 hours postincision.

To achieve optimum efficacy, the antibiotic must be present in the tissue before it is exposed to bacterial contamination. The route of administration determines the rate at which the agent will reach therapeutic levels. Alexander and Alexander[26] demonstrated in an animal model that the intravenous (IV) push method achieved the earliest level in wound fluid, but the highest sustained antibiotic concentration was achieved with intramuscular (IM) injections. When contamination occurs prior to initiation of antimicrobial therapy (ie, trauma), simultaneous administration of antibiotics via IV push and IM injections are recommended followed by continuous IV infusion in patients with shock and intermittent IM injections in normotensive patients. Although the wound fluid analyzed was not in the H&N, it is reasonable to assume that adequate tissue levels would be achieved in this region due to its high vascularity. Parenteral administration of antibiotics in H&N prophylaxis is the traditional route of administration.

The efficacy of topical antibiotics used in contaminated H&N surgery is currently under investigation. The benefits of topical antimicrobial prophylaxis have been realized in colorectal surgery and penetrating abdominal wounds for a long time.[27,28] Previous animal studies have also demonstrated the efficacy of the combined use of systemic and topical antibiotics.[29,30] Robinson[31] investigated the use of topical antibiotics alone in 22 patients undergoing laryngectomies with or without radical neck dissections. The patients were divided into two groups; one half received antibiotics and the remaining half did not. The wound was sprinkled with 1 g of ampicillin and 1 g of carbenicillin before skin closure. The wound infection rate was reduced from 64% in the control group to 18% with the use of topical antibiotics.

The use of clindamycin mouthwash was evaluated in two studies using healthy volunteers.[32,33] Both trials demonstrated that a single dose of mouthwash can quantitatively reduce both aerobic and anaerobic bacterial counts in the oral cavity. These counts remained low for up to 4 hours after rinsing. By reducing the bacterial load with a topical antibiotic, systemic antibiotics may be more efficacious. In a placebo-controlled trial using an animal model, Bergamini et al[30] showed that combination of topical and systemic antibiotics resulted in the lowest infection rate when a high level of bacterial contamination was present. When bacterial contamination was low, there was no additional reduction in infection rate when compared with the use of systemic antibiotics alone. The use of topical clindamycin can be compared to prepping the skin and bowel prior to surgery. This practice seems reasonable considering that the bacterial content in the oral cavity is highest upon arising[34] and most H&N surgical procedures are done early in the morning.

To date there is only one study evaluating the use of topical antibiotics alone in contaminated H&N surgery.[35] Ten patients undergoing total laryngectomy plus neck dissection were administered mouthwash containing 1.5 g of clindamycin preoperatively and another dose 6 to 8 hours postoperatively. The neck was irrigated intraoperatively with a clindamycin-containing solution following neck dissection and pharyngeal contamination of the wound. Cultures were obtained from the oral cavity and neck viscera prior to and following antibiotic irrigation. No patients developed a postoperative wound infection. Preoperative antibiotic mouthwash reduced the aerobic and anaerobic bacterial counts in intraoperatively cultured neck sites by 99%. Intraoperative irrigation reduced the bacterial counts by an additional 90%. Gram-positive aerobes and anaerobes remained reduced in number up to 3 to 4 days following surgery, but the incidence of *Hemophilus species* was increased by 71% on oral cavity cultures postoperatively. The significance of this is unknown because no patient developed a wound infection.

Further studies are needed to evaluate the use of topical antibiotics alone in contaminated H&N surgery. The results of the previous study are encouraging, and the addition of topical to parenteral antibiotics may reduce the incidence of postoperative wound infections in high-risk groups. Furthermore, topical therapy is less toxic and less costly than parenteral agents.

RHINOLOGY

The need for routine antibiotic prophylaxis in nasal surgery has not been demonstrated. The reasons most frequently given to justify the use of antibiotic prophylaxis in this setting include the following: Mucosal incisions are made in a contaminated field; nasal packing is a foreign body predisposing the patient to infection of the surrounding soft tissues; the routine use of nasal packing increases the risk of sinusitis by causing mucosal edema and occlusion of ostia[18]; and the presence of infection when an allograft or cartilage graft is used can result in disfigurement.[36] Nevertheless, results of several studies have failed to demonstrate the need for antibiotic prophylaxis in a variety of rhinologic procedures.[17,18,37] There was no difference in the amount of nasal crusting, bleeding, edema, pain, ecchymosis, synechiae formation,[18] and postoperative sinusitis[17,18] in patients receiving antibiotics compared to those who received placebo or in those in whom antibiotics were withheld.

Two small clinical trials were designed to evaluate the efficacy of parenteral and local antibiotics in preventing septicemia and local infections when nasal packing is employed. Herzon,[38] in a prospective, randomized trial, used antibiotic-

impregnated gauze (oxytetracycline and polymyxin B) in half of the patients requiring a posterior nasal pack. Systemic antibiotics (penicillin) were administered to all patients while packing was in place. Cultures of the nasal packing were obtained in all patients. The patients treated with combined therapy showed light growth of a single organism, usually gram positive, as opposed to heavy colonization with gram-negative rods, as seen in the patients treated with systemic antibiotics alone. The odor was also decreased when packing was removed in those patients treated with combined therapy. The incidence of bacteremia was 12%. Two patients in each group had positive blood cultures. However, three of four patients displayed no clinical signs of sepsis. Only one person grew the infecting organism in both blood and nasal packing cultures. This patient developed sepsis secondary to a spontaneous esophageal perforation and mediastinal abscess felt to be unrelated to treatment. In addition, 73% of bacteria isolated in this study were resistant to the systemic antibiotic used, raising the possibility that use of an empiric agent led to the emergence of resistant strains of bacteria. In a prospective, randomized, placebo-controlled trial by Derkay et al,[39] 20 patients requiring posterior nasal packing received placebo versus cefazolin sodium. Antibiotic-impregnated gauze (bacitracin) was used in all patients. No patients developed infectious complications. As seen in the previous study, there was elimination of the offensive odor when cefazolin was used in addition to antibiotic-impregnated gauze, and the culture results were similar. In both studies, the incidence of infectious complications was low regardless of the use of parenteral antibiotics. It appears that the routine use of systemic antibiotic prophylaxis in patients with nasal packing does not reduce infectious complications but eliminates the odor. Derkay et al[39] speculate, however, that the high concentration of bacteria encountered in patients with nasal packing and no parenteral antibiotics may occasionally lead to clinically significant septicemia, and further study is warranted.

Bacteremia following septoplasty and rhinoplasty does not appear to occur commonly.[40,41] Although 46% of patients grew *Staphylococcus aureus* from preoperative nasal cultures in one study, no patients developed staphylococcal bacteremia.[40] Furthermore, the incidence of toxic shock syndrome following nasal surgery is very low and cannot be prevented by the administration of systemic antibiotics.[42]

There are no clinical trials to date evaluating the efficacy of perioperative antibiotics in septorhinoplasties employing allografts or cartilage grafts, although a survey of over 1718 plastic surgeons revealed that > 50% of these physicians used antibiotic prophylaxis in > 50% of cases.[36] Empiric antibiotic prophylaxis use in these cases is justified based on a risk-benefit analysis in which an infection resulting in the loss of the graft may result in disfigurement.

OTOLOGY

The routine use of prophylactic antibiotics is not necessary in otologic surgery. In a placebo-controlled, prospective study of 4000 patients undergoing a variety of otologic procedures, the use of antibiotic prophylaxis did not appear to be beneficial.[43] Cephalothin or cefazolin in comparison to placebo was used prophylactically in clean middle ear cases and surgeries for chronic otitis media, whereas oxacillin versus placebo was used in patients undergoing neurotologic procedures. There was no statistically significant difference in the postoperative infection rate or graft success rate in the antibiotic groups compared to those who received placebo. In addition, it was found that the infection rate was unaffected by duration of procedure, patient age, and preoperative condition of the ear. Although there was a higher incidence of infections and graft failure in those with contaminated or infected ears preoperatively, the use of antibiotics did not alter the outcome. This agrees with the findings of Eschelman et al,[17] who found that the use of penicillin or ampicillin versus placebo in 107 patients undergoing otologic surgery did not affect the infection rate. Strong[37] reviewed 287 general otolarygologic cases. Prophylactic antibiotics were not used in any of these cases. One hundred seventy-three cases were otologic in nature. Four of these patients developed postoperative infections, none of which developed permanent sequelae. In myringoplasty surgery, Donaldson and Snyder[44] found that the addition of systemic sulfamethoxazole to topical antibiotics did not alter the flora of the ear canal or influence the success of the procedure.

Although unproven, the empiric use of antibiotics is common in surgery involving placement of a prosthetic device. Wound infection following cochlear implantation may lead to wound breakdown and exposure of the device. In addition, infection in this area carries the risk of meningitis. A survey was conducted at 17 centers worldwide examining the use of antimicrobial prophylaxis in 1030 cochlear implantation procedures.[20] A variety of antibiotics were used (cephalosporin, amoxicillin, penicillin, cotrimoxazole, ciprofloxacin) for a mean duration of 7 days with a range of 2 to 15 days. Overall, 56.4% of physicians used antibiotics and 43.6% did not. The overall infection rate was 2.9%. Infection resulted in device removal in 4.5% in the antibiotic group compared with 0.9% infection rate in the untreated group. Most cases of infection were attributed to technical problems. There were no cases of meningitis. Infection resulting in removal of a cochlear implant does not appear to be dependent on antibiotic prophylaxis, and therefore the routine use of prophylaxis is not recommended.

Prophylactic antibiotic use does not appear to be efficacious in otologic surgery. Wound infection is prevented more effectively by starting with a dry ear and using good surgical technique.

NEUROTOLOGY

The neurotologist performs procedures that are long in duration, often exposing the dura and central nervous system (CNS). These operations are associated with the risks of cerebrospinal fluid (CSF) leak, meningitis, and wound infections.

Kartush et al[45] studied the effects of perioperative IV antibiotics and topical bacitracin irrigation on these postoperative complications in 236 patients who underwent either translabyrinthine resection of acoustic tumors (72%) or retrolabyrinthine vestibular nerve resection (28%). Topical bacitracin was chosen because of its lack of ototoxicity, lack of topical toxicity to brain tissue,[46] appropriate bactericidal effect, and low incidence of allergic reactions.[47] Patients were divided into four groups: perioperative IV antibiotics alone; topical bacitracin irrigation alone; combination IV and topical; and no antibiotics. It was found that bacitracin irrigation reduced the incidence of wound infection from 9% to 2%, the rate of CSF leak from 12% to 5%, and the combined complication rate from 22% to 9%. Furthermore, the irrigation-only group showed a significant reduction in wound infection (0%) compared to the IV-only group (9%). There was no significant reduction in the incidence of wound infection and CSF leak with the bacitracin-only group compared to the bacitracin-plus-IV-antibiotic group. There was no significant reduction in the rate of meningitis for any treatment group. It is suggested that bacitracin may allow the wound to better tolerate a transient CSF leak without dehiscence and infection, therefore allowing the CSF leak to close without surgical intervention. These results suggest that the use of a topical antimicrobial (such as bacitracin) alone is sufficient to prevent infectious complications in patients undergoing neurotologic procedures. Further studies are necessary to confirm these findings. The neurosurgical literature also supports the use of both IV and topical prophylactic antibiotics in major clean cases and those cases involving craniotomy.[48,49]

CRANIAL BASE

Patients undergoing cranial base procedures represent a high-risk group for postoperative infections. These operations frequently result in a large defect, with contamination of intracranial contents by flora of the upper aerodigestive tract and with resulting meningitis, brain abscess, or osteomyelites. To date there has been one study analyzing the role of perioperative antibiotic prophylaxis in these patients. Carrau et al[50] conducted a retrospective analysis of the role of antibiotic prophylaxis in 95 patients undergoing 100 clean-contaminated cranial base procedures over a 2-year period. All antibiotics were started prior to the skin incision. Intraoperative irrigation with bacitracin (50 mg/mL) or streptomycin (50 μg/mL) was employed in all patients. Seven patients (7%) developed an infection at the surgical site. Opening of the dura and sinuses occurred in all cases. An increase in infection was noted in patients receiving antibiotics for less than or equal to 24 hours as compared to those receiving antibiotics for longer than 24 hours. These authors suggest that a single broad-spectrum cephalosporin for 48 hours be used. Prolonged administration of antibiotics may be necessary due to continued contamination of the surgical site and CSF by bacteria following surgery. Additional clinical trials are necessary to determine the efficacy of antibiotic prophylaxis in cranial base surgeries.

TONSILLECTOMY

Recent clinical trials demonstrate that antibiotic prophylaxis is effective in reducing postoperative morbidity in both the pediatric and adult populations undergoing tonsillectomy. Telian et al[51] compared the effects of ampicillin/amoxicillin to placebo in children undergoing tonsillectomy. Ampicillin or placebo was administered intravenously at the time of operation and 12 and 24 hours postoperatively. These patients continued to receive oral amoxicillin or placebo for 7 days. The antibiotic group was found to have a lower incidence of fever, pain, mouth odor, lassitude, and poor oral intake following tonsillectomy. These children also returned to their usual daily activities earlier than did the placebo group. The morbidity associated with the use of antibiotics was extremely low; one definite drug rash and one clinical case of thrush developed in 45 patients receiving antibiotics. On the other hand, postoperative bleeding occurred in 3 of 40 patients receiving placebo requiring readmission. One patient in the antibiotic group with preexisting medical problems required readmission for intravenous antibiotics, hydration, and control of asthma. This patient refused his antibiotics prior to readmission. Six patients in the placebo group were withdrawn secondary to clinical signs of infection, including high fever, pain, lassitude, and mouth odor. These patients improved on amoxicillin, and readmission was not necessary.

Preoperative and postoperative cultures of the tonsils and tonsillar fossae were obtained. Overgrowth of resistant organisms was not a problem postoperatively. Three patient cultures grew *Hemophilus influenza* resistant to ampicillin/amoxicillin. Furthermore, only 10% of coagulase positive *Staphylococcus* isolated were sensitive to ampicillin/amoxicillin. It was not determined if these resistant organisms contributed to postoperative morbidity. Similar findings were also reported by DeDio et al,[52] who studied the flora of tonsils and adenoids in the pediatric group. *Hemophilus*, beta-hemolytic streptococcus, *Staphylococcus aureus*, and *Streptococcus pneumoniae* were identified as possible pathogens. *Hemophilus species*, other than influenza type B, were recovered in 54% and *Staphylococcus aureus* in 46% of cultures. It was previously seen in this patient population that only 8% of all *Staphylococcus aureus* isolated were sensitive to penicillin or amoxicillin. In addition, 17% to 20% of all *Hemophilus species*, not influenza type B, were beta-lactamase producers.

Although the efficacy of antibiotic prophylaxis in reducing postoperative morbidity following tonsillectomies in children has been demonstrated, the need for antibiotic coverage against these beta-lactamase-producing organisms is questioned. Jones et al[53] tested the hypothesis that cefaclor, with its broad-spectrum activity against beta-lactamase-producing strains of *Hemophilus* and coagulase positive *Staphylococcus*, would be more efficacious than amoxicillin in reducing postoperative morbidity in posttonsillectomy patients. No difference in severity and duration of postoperative symptoms or complications was found. Although *Staphylococcus aureus* was isolated more frequently from the amoxicillin-treated group (9%), there was no stastically significant difference

in postoperative morbidity. It was recommended that cefaclor be reserved for pediatric patients who demonstrate a prolonged recovery period despite treatment with amoxicillin.

Grandis et al[54] also demonstrated a decrease in postoperative morbidity in the adult posttonsillectomy population receiving antibiotics. One hundred and one patients completed a prospective, randomized, double-blind, placebo-controlled trial with either an antibiotic (ticarcillin disodium and clavulanate potassium) or placebo (saline) administered intravenously at the time of surgery and for 12 hours postoperatively. Patients subsequently received placebo or antibiotic (amoxicillin and clavulanate potassium) for an additional 7 days. These antibiotics were chosen because a higher incidence of *Bacteroides species* and beta-lactamase-producing bacteria were isolated from core tonsil cultures in adult patients.[55] Patients in the antibiotic group experienced decrease in mouth odor (2.5 days vs 4.2 days), tolerated a regular diet sooner (postoperative days 3 to 5), and resumed their normal daily activities earlier than the placebo group. There was no statistically significant difference in the severity or duration of fever or pain. Postoperative tonsillar fossae cultures showed quantitatively less growth in those patients receiving antibiotics than placebo. Moreover, *Candida albicans* was not recovered more frequently from the antibiotic group than the placebo group, indicating that superinfection was not a problem. Antibiotic prophylaxis in pediatric and adult patients undergoing tonsillectomy has been shown to reduce postoperative morbidity. The use of ampicillin/amoxicillin in the pediatric population and a beta-lactamase inhibitor (such as ticarcillin disodium and clavulanate potassium or amoxicilin and clavulanate potassium) in the adult population is recommended. The duration of antibiotic treatment is unknown, and currently a 7-day course is recommended.

TRAUMA

Because the term *prophylaxis* implies that the antibiotic be present in the tissue prior to bacterial contamination, use of antibiotics in trauma is actually therapeutic rather than prophylactic. As a rule, traumatic wounds are considered to be contaminated. However, it is the amount of bacteria present that determines the development of an infection. The critical number of bacteria necessary to infect tissue is estimated to be 100,000 organisms per gram of tissue.[56] Soft-tissue injuries of the head and neck involving crush injuries; wounds contaminated with body secretions, pus, and soil; wounds with devitalized tissue; and those patients receiving treatment 3 hours or more following injury have a high degree of contamination. These individuals should receive antibiotics at the time of initial evaluation and resuscitation.[56-59] Depressed immune function, hypermetabolic state, devitalized tissue, and shock predispose and potentiate infection in the trauma patient.[58]

Although traumatic wounds are heavily contaminated, infection is not inevitable. In addition to antibiotic therapy, other issues should be considered. These wounds should be examined aseptically by emergency room personnel wearing masks and gloves. Contamination by the examiner is a potential source of bacteria.[56] Antibiotic administration should not be substituted for proper wound care. Debridement is considered by many to be the single most important treatment of traumatic wounds.[59] Devitalized tissue hinders the wound's ability to fight infection by serving as a culture medium and by inhibiting leukocyte function and phagocytosis of bacteria.[59,60]

The administration of tetanus toxoid is imperative in the treatment of trauma victims and should be given in addition to antibiotics. In a review of 369 cases of clinical tetanus, 5.7% of wounds originated in the head and neck region with a 57.1% mortality rate.[61] One case report of tetanus following a nondisplaced noncomminuted zygomatic fracture developed as a result of a superficial laceration overlying the fracture in a patient who did not receive tetanus toxoid.[62]

FACIAL FRACTURES

The use of antibiotic prophylaxis has been shown to reduce significantly the infection rate in compound mandibular fractures.[63,64] In a prospective, randomized trial analyzing the efficacy of antibiotic prophylaxis in all facial fractures, perioperative use of cefazolin sodium reduced the incidence of postoperative infections; the infection rate was 42.2% in the placebo group compared to 8.9% in the antibiotic-treated group. There were no infections seen in the subgroups of zygomatic, maxillary, and subcondylar fractures. All infections were seen in patients who sustained mandibular fractures involving the angle of the mandible and parasymphyseal region, except for one case of meningitis.[63] Similar results regarding compound mandibular fractures were obtained by Zallen and Curry.[64] In a prospective, randomized, placebo-controlled trial, the infection rate was reduced from 50.0% to 6.0% in patients administered antibiotics.

LARYNGOTRACHEAL INJURIES

Penetrating and blunt injuries to the anterior neck may be associated with injury to the trachea, larynx, pharynx, esophagus, major vessels, and spinal cord. Infections following laryngotracheal injuries can result in compromise of the airway and voice. Le May[65] reviewed 25 cases of penetrating missile wounds to the trachea and larynx and found that 60% had perforation of the pharynx or esophagus. Cervical contamination by the pharyngeal contents or saliva must be assumed with these injuries.[66] Wound infections in 49 patients with laryngotracheal injuries developed in 20% of patients sustaining a crushing injury to the thyroid cartilage and in 15% whose treatment was delayed 24 to 72 hours postinjury.[67] No infections in other groups were seen. A 6% infection rate was reported by Trone et al[68] despite the routine use of antibiotics. Due to the morbidity and serious sequelae of infection in this area, including mediastinitis, a 10- to 14-day course of antibiotics is recommended.[65,66,68] Administration of antibiotics under these circumstances is therapeutic.

BASILAR SKULL FRACTURES

Basilar skull fractures often result in otorrhea or, more commonly, rhinorrhea.[69] Prospective and retrospective studies demonstrate antibiotics to be ineffective in preventing CNS infections. In several large, retrospective studies, the reported incidence of meningitis varied from 2% to 25% irrespective of the use of antibiotics.[70-72] In one retrospective analysis, patients receiving antibiotics actually developed a higher rate of meningitis (16%) than those who received no chemoprophylaxis (3.0%).[73]

Ignelzi et al[74] studied the efficacy of antibiotic prophylaxis in the treatment of basilar skull fractures in 129 patients over a 2-year period, 43 of whom had rhinorrhea or otorrhea at the time of presentation. In those patients receiving antibiotics, 2 of 54 patients developed a major CNS infection, one resulting in death and the other with serious neurological sequelae. The latter patient was infected with an organism that was resistant to the empiric antibiotic used. There were no infectious complications in the group of 50 patients that did not receive antibiotics. Furthermore, cultures of the nasopharynx revealed a significant change in the flora of patients receiving chemoprophylaxis, with an increase in gram-negative rods which were resistant to the agent given. These findings again support the suggestion that antibiotic prophylaxis may lead to the selection of resistant organisms or may allow the increase in number and virulence of organisms normally found in the nasopharynx by disturbing the degree of bacterial antagonism that exists.[75] Klastersky et al[76] also demonstrated that antibiotic prophylaxis administered to patients with otorrhea or rhinorrhea secondary to trauma to the head and face was not beneficial. In a double-blind study, penicillin versus placebo was administered to patients admitted for otorrhea/rhinorrhea. Only one patient in the placebo group developed meningitis. This patient was later found to have a retained intraventricular foreign body. Basilar skull fractures have a low incidence of meningitis which appears to be unaffected by chemoprophylaxis. Close clinical observation and initiation of treatment with the development of clinical signs of meningitis in this patient group are recommended.

BITES

Animal bites are a common problem in the United States. Dog bites account for approximately 80% of all animal bite injuries.[77] Canine flora is polymicrobial. A bacteriologic study of wound infections following dog bites revealed aerobic pathogens (74%), including *Streptococcus viridans*, *Staphylococcus aureus*, and *Pasteurella multocida*, and anaerobic bacteria (41%), including *Bacteroides species* and *Fusobacterium species*.[78] Sharp debridement and irrigation of animal bites is necessary following injury. Puncture wounds are never closed.[57]

The use of prophylactic antibiotics in retrospective studies has revealed conflicting results. Mathog et al[79] infrequently used antibiotics following animal bite injuries and saw only two infections; infection occurred in one patient treated with antibiotics and in another in which antibiotics were withheld. Chambers and Payne[80] also found prophylactic antibiotics to be of no benefit in this patient group. Schultz and McMaster[81] studied 116 patients sustaining dog bite injuries to the head and neck. All patients received antibiotic prophylaxis, and the infection rate was 6%. On the other hand, Thomson and Svitek[82] showed an infection rate of 29% despite the use of chemoprophylaxis. He felt that this high infection rate may be due to inadequate wound debridement and irrigation. This contention is supported by the observation that puncture wounds and lacerations had high infection rates, whereas avulsions and large soft-tissue defects did not. This is believed to be a consequence of more extensive wound care that is routinely administered to the latter type of injuries.

Two prospective, placebo-controlled studies were conducted which found antibiotic prophylaxis to be ineffective. No significant difference in infection rate existed between the treated and untreated groups. Elenbaas et al[83] conducted a prospective, double-blind, placebo-controlled trial using oxacillin. No infections occurred in the placebo-treated group, although two infections involving the hand occurred in the treatment group. This suggested that infection was due to the inability of the wounds to drain spontaneously and hence could not have been prevented by prophylactic antibiotics. In a placebo-controlled trial by Callahan,[84] prophylactic penicillin V potassium did not alter the infection rate compared to placebo in the low-risk wounds, such as deep lacerations and wounds of the scalp and face. The infection rate of debrided versus nondebrided wounds in this trial was 2% versus 62.5%, which again emphasizes the need for adequate debridement. Empiric antibiotic treatment is recommended only in animal bites in which debridement is insufficient and tissue damage is extensive (Table 12-2).

In contrast, human bites have a higher bacterial inoculum than animal flora. This was demonstrated by Brook,[85] who

Table 12-2. Recommended Empiric Antibiotic Therapy for Bite Wounds*

ROUTE	ANIMAL BITES	HUMAN BITES
Oral	Amoxicillin-clavulanate potassium or dicloxacillin	Amoxicillin-clavulanate potassium or amoxicillin plus dicloxacillin
Parenteral	Cefoxitin or penicillin G plus β-lactamases-resistent penicillin or ticarcillin-clavulanate potassium	Cefoxitin or first-generation cephalosporin plus β-lactamase-resistant penicillin or ticarcillin-clavulanate potassium

From Brook.[85]

*Empiric antibiotic therapy is recommended in animal bite wounds in which debridement is insufficient and tissue damage is extensive. Empiric antibiotic therapy is recommended in all human bites to the head and neck. The course of treatment is 10 days.

cultured the number of mean bacterial isolates per wound in human bites (5.4) compared to animal bites (2.8). Increased bacteria in wounds from human bites likely reflects the higher concentration of anaerobic bacteria in the oral cavity. The greatest concentration of bacteria is found in the gingival crevices and in plaque on teeth. This debris contains 10^{10} bacteria per gram wet weight.[56] Predominant organisms isolated from human bite wounds are anaerobes, particularly *Bacteroides species*, *Staphylococcus aureus*, alpha-hemolytic streptococcus, and *Eikenella corrodens*.[85,86] Beta-lactamase-producing bacteria have been isolated in as many as 41% of wounds, including *Bacteroides species* and *Staphylococcus aureus*.[85] *Group A streptococcus*, *Stalphylococcus aureus*, and *Eikenella corrodens* are usually associated with infectious complications.[86]

No prospective, randomized, placebo-controlled trials analyzing the effect of antibiotics in human bites to the head and neck have been documented in the literature. Zubowicz and Gravier[87] did find that mechanical wound care alone is not sufficient for the treatment of human bites to the hand. The infection rate in 15 patients receiving oral placebo was 46.7% (7/15) compared to 0% in those receiving Ceclor or intravenous Kefzol and penicillin. All patients underwent aggressive debridement and irrigation at the time of initial evaluation. Although anatomic differences exist, antibiotic treatment of human bites to the head and neck is likely beneficial. All human bites to the head and neck should receive an empiric course of antimicrobial therapy[56,88] (Table 12-2).

HEAD AND NECK SURGERY

It has been shown by many investigators that the use of perioperative prophylactic antibiotics is imperative during major H&N surgery in which the wound is contaminated by saliva. The postoperative infection rate following these procedures is reported to be 28% to 87% (Table 12-1). The wide range in incidence of postoperative wound infections is accounted for by the lack of consistency among trials regarding patient selection, technique, magnitude of surgical resection, objective definition of infection, and the inclusion of nosocomial infections such as pneumonia. Patients undergoing contaminated H&N procedures have fewer wound infections following the administration of perioperative antibiotics (Table 12-3). Although the role of perioperative antibiotics is controversial in uncontaminated H&N surgery, two studies have demonstrated the lack of efficacy of antibiotics administered in patients undergoing parotidectomy, thyroidectomy, submandibular gland excision,[14] and uncontaminated neck dissections.[15]

The duration of prophylaxis is also crucial in preventing postoperative wound infections. Although controversy does exist, most agree that a short course of prophylaxis (24 hours) is as effective as prolonged prophylaxis (2 to 7 days) (Table 12-4). In a study by Mombelli et al,[95] the prolonged use of carbenicillin resulted in increase isolation of *Klebsiella species* from postoperative wound cultures. This suggests that prolonged use can select for resistant strains of microorgan-

Table 12–3. Antibiotics with Proven Efficacy in Prevention of Wound Infection: 1-Day Administration Only

ANTIBIOTIC	DOSE	INFECTION RATE (%)
Cefazolin[93]	500 mg	7/20 (35)
Cefazolin[94]	2 g	5/59 (8.5)
Carbenicillin[95]	10 g	7/72 (9.7)
Moxalactam[94]	2 g	2/59 (3.4)
Moxalactam[96]	30 mb/kg	1/16 (6.2)
Clindamycin[97]	600 mg	2/52 (3.4)
Clindamycin[97] plus gentamicin	600 mg 1.7 mg/kg	2/52 (3.4)
Clindamycin[98] plus gentamicin	300 mg 1.7 mg/kg	2/29 (7)
Cefaperazone[7]	2 g	4/39 (10)
Cefotaxime[7]	2 g	3/32 (9)

isms. Findings in the general surgical literature also support the use of a short versus a long course of empiric antibiotics, even in the case of trauma.[23,25] However, in a study by Sawyer et al,[100] a statistically significant decrease in the incidence and severity of postoperative wound infections was demonstrated in patients receiving at least 7 days of metronidazole plus cefazolin following major contaminated H&N surgery. Due to the small number of cases (50) and the arbitrary endpoint of treatment days, further investigation is needed to determine the efficacy of prolonged metronidazole treatment.

The antibiotic of choice has not been identified. Regimens that have been found to be efficacious in controlled clinical trials include clindamycin plus gentamicin,[97,98] cefoperazone,[99] cefotaxime,[7] high-dose cefazolin,[94] and moxalactam.[96] Disagreement as to which antibiotic regimen should be used is influenced by the type of organisms one believes are pathogenic. Organisms cultured from wound infections represent those found in the oral cavity and oropharynx.[101,106] Infection can result from perioperative contamination via a mucosal incision but, most significantly, a persistent postoperative leakage of saliva.[107] The bacteriology of these infections has been analyzed both qualitatively and quantitatively to encourage the selection of an antimicrobial agent that will be most effective.[101-106]

The value of preoperative, intraoperative, and postoperative wound cultures in predicting the bacteriology of wound infections is unclear. Becker et al[103] attempted to identify patients at high risk for developing wound infections by obtaining cultures preoperatively (skin, oropharynx, and nares) and intraoperatively (surgical wound following closure of the pharyngeal defect and irrigation). They found that these cultures were not predictive of high-risk patients because only 35% of infected wounds had a potential pathogen isolated both preoperatively and intraoperatively. In addition, patients in whom *Staphylococcus aureus* was recovered from preoperative nasal and skin cultures did not demonstrate increased likelihood for developing postoperative staphylococcal infections. In a later study, Becker and Welch[104] analyzed the quantitative bacteriology results of closed-suction wound drainage in contaminated surgery. Again, there was poor correlation between the quantity of bacteria in the closed-suction drainage and the development of a wound infection. The species of bacteria cultured from the drainage did not necessarily reflect those subsequently found in wound infections. Rubin et al[101] conducted a retrospective analysis of the bacterial content of wound infections developing in 23 of 354 patients who participated in a series of antibiotic trials while undergoing contaminated H&N surgery. Polymicrobial infections occurred in 96% of cases. Aerobic bacteria accounted for 91% of organisms, anaerobes comprised 74%, and fungi comprised 48% of organisms isolated. Theoretically, the infecting organisms isolated should be inhibited by the antibiotics used in these trials, but this was not the case. The flora isolated in both early (days 1 to 5) and late postoperative infections (after day 5) were not significantly different. Anaerobic bacteria were recovered from patients who received antibiotics effective against anaerobes as well as from those who did not receive adequate anaerobic coverage. This finding supports the pathogenic role of anaerobes in causing postoperative wound infections. Earlier studies demonstrating the role of anaerobes in postoperative infections include the presence of anaerobic bacteremia in patients with concomitant anaerobic wound infections.[7,108] Nonpathogens may interfere with therapy directed at pathogenic bacteria, as evidenced by the failure of infecting organisms to respond to appropriate antimicrobial therapy.[109] The isolation of fungi from 48% of the wounds probably represented colonization because all infections resolved without antifungal therapy.

Table 12–4. Trials Comparing Brief versus Prolonged Antibiotic Administration

AUTHORS	DURATION (DAYS)	ANTIBIOTIC	NO. OF PATIENTS	INFECTION RATE (%)
Mombelli et al[95]	1		72	7/72 (9.7)
	4	Carbenicillin	68	4/68 (5.9)
Fee et al[96]	1		16	1/16 (6)
	2	Moxalactam	15	0/15 (0)
Johnson et al[98]	1	Clindamycin	29	2/29 (7)
	5	plus gentamicin	27	1/27 (4)
Johnson et al[99] (flap reconstruction)	1		53	10/53 (18)
	5	Cefoperazone	56	14/56 (25)
Sawyer et al[100]	2	Metronidazole	25	8/25 (32)
	7–10	plus cefazolin	25	5/25 (20)

Gram-negative aerobic organisms are frequently recovered from infections following major H&N surgery. Because saliva contains 10^8 bacteria/mL,[110] 90% of which are anaerobes, the presence of aerobic gram-negative organisms in these infections is not expected. The recovery of gram-negative aerobes from hospitalized patients has long been recognized,[111] but their role as a pathogen in H&N infections and the need for antibiotic coverage directed against these organisms is controversial.

Aerobic gram-negative bacilli (AGNB) have been cultured postoperatively in wound infections, although they were seldom isolated from preoperative skin and oropharyngeal cultures or intraoperative wound cultures.[5,102,103,112] These organisms have been shown to originate from the GI tract and may appear in the H&N via bacterial translocation.[113,114] Swift et al[102] demonstrated that although AGNB were ubiquitous to the oropharyngeal mucosa following H&N surgery, there was a low incidence of sepsis. This is probably due to the absence of these organisms from the oropharynx at the time of surgery when tissues are most susceptible to microbial invasion. Swift et al also speculated that infection may ensue when wounds are not closed adequately.

The role of AGNB in establishing infections caused by anaerobic bacteria has been investigated. *Escherichia coli*, a member of the Enterobacteriaceae family, produces Vitamin K, which is an essential growth factor for bacteroides.[115] In addition, Maddocks[109] postulated that nonpathogens inhabiting the normal body flora may develop mechanisms to protect pathogens from host defenses in mixed infections. Therefore, by using antibiotic prophylaxis with AGNB coverage, the rate of wound infections may decrease due to the loss of these protective factors.

Studies have been conducted to evaluate the need for AGNB coverage in these patients with conflicting results. Johnson et al[97,98] found that there was no statistically significant difference in the wound infection rate between patients receiving clindamycin alone versus clindamycin plus gentamicin, although the latter regimen is effective against AGNB. This agrees with the findings of others, who noted that the addition of an aminoglycoside (gentamicin, tobramycin, or netilmicin) did not alter the infection rate when compared to the use of a cephalosporin or clindamycin[89,116,117] alone. However, recent studies by Gerard et al[118] and Weber et al[106] support the need for AGNB coverage. In a prospective, randomized trial involving 113 patients undergoing major H&N surgery, clindamycin plus amikacin was compared to the use of ticarcillin plus clavulanic acid. There was a reduction in the infection rate from 36% to 10% with the addition of an aminoglycoside.[118] These results may be due in part to the prolonged postantibiotic effect (PAE) of aminoglycosides against AGNB and gram-positive organisms as compared to the lesser PAE of beta-lactam antibiotics.[119] The PAE refers to the recovery period or period of persistent suppression of bacterial growth following minimal antimicrobial exposure. In addition, it has been found that clindamycin causes decreased adherence of bacteria to mucosal membranes by inducing the formation of functionally aberrant bacterial adhe-

sions.[120] Weber et al[106] compared the effects of ampicillin/sulbactam to the effects of clindamycin alone on the number of postoperative wound infections in 212 patients undergoing H&N surgery. The infection rate was found to be significantly lower in the group receiving coverage against AGNB (ampicillin/sulbactam). Nineteen microorganisms were isolated from 14 patients treated with ampicillin/sulbactam, and six of these organisms were AGNB. Thirty-six organisms were isolated from 29 patients treated with clindamycin, 29 of which were AGNB. Weber suggests that the lower recovery rate of AGNB in those treated with ampicillin/sulbactam may be due to the bactericidal activity of beta-lactam antibiotics or to their superior penetration into the upper respiratory tract. It has been demonstrated that some enterobacteriaciae (AGNB) produce penicillinase, thereby destroying the bactericidal activity of certain antibiotics. By combining an antibacterial agent with an inhibitor of the enzyme that destroys it, such as ampicillin/sulbactam, this effect can be overcome in mixed infections. Therefore, the lower infection rate seen with the use of ampicillin/sulbactam may be attributed to the penicillinase effect of sulbactam.[109] Additional clinical trials are necessary to determine the clinical significance of AGNB. A metaanalysis of prophylactic antibiotics in H&N surgery suggest that a 1-day course of clindamycin may be most effective in this group of patients.[121]

Some patients are felt to be at high risk for developing postoperative wound infections following oncologic H&N surgery. Potential risk factors previously identified are related to tumor size and stage of disease, closure using flaps, nutritional status and alcohol consumption, duration of surgical procedure, intraoperative risk such as proper surgical technique, classification of procedure, and antibiotic used.[97,98,106,116,122-124] Univariate and logistic regression analysis of 63 wound infections identified the following factors to be most predictive of infection: the classification of surgery, the choice of antibiotic, the presence of concomitant disease, and the N stage.[122] Factors such as duration of surgery and complexity of surgery, including flap repair and tracheostomy, correlate with a higher infection rate because these factors are usually associated with clean-contaminated procedures in patients with advanced disease.[97,122] The effects of previous radiation therapy on the incidence of wound infection have been analyzed, and results are conflicting.[122,123,125,126] Overall, the incidence of postoperative infections is not statistically significant among patients receiving preoperative radiation therapy, although the infections that do develop can be more severe.[126] These patients are at risk for a prolonged hospital stay due to their overall health status and extent of surgical resection. Because it is known that patients with prolonged hospital stays become colonized or infected with AGNB, these patients may be among those that benefit from AGNB coverage.

It is critical that the antibiotic selected be administered in a dose such that the peak serum concentration exceeds the minimal inhibitory concentration (MIC) needed to eliminate the microorganisms likely to be encountered. The finding that high-dose cefazolin (2 g) is more effective than low-dose cefazolin (0.5 g) in reducing postoperative wound infections

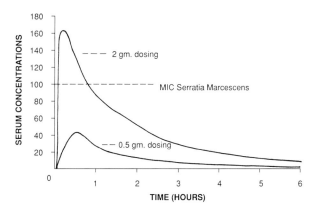

Figure 12–1. Relationship of cefazolin dosing to MIC of *Serratia marcescens* (from Johnson et al[94]).

in patients undergoing H&N surgery supports this theory.[94] In a sequential, prospective, randomized, double-blind trial, low-dose cefazolin was found to be relatively ineffective in reducing postoperative infectious complications when compared to clindamycin-gentamicin, cefaperazone, and cefotaxime.[97,127] Low-dose cefazolin (0.5 g) resulted in peak serum levels lower than the MIC of *Serratia marcescens*, whereas high-dose cefazolin (2.0 g) achieved peak serum levels above the MIC (Fig. 12–1).[128] This shows clearly that the efficacy of an antibiotic is dependent on appropriate antibiotic dosage.

PROSTHETICS

Antimicrobial prophylaxis is most useful as a means of reducing the risk of wound infection in clean-contaminated cases. Prophylaxis is generally not indicated for clean procedures unless infection is associated with life-threatening or severe consequences, as in the case of orthopedic and cardiovascular surgery when prosthetic (implant) devices are used.[129] The Centers for Disease Control (CDC) and the American Heart Association (AHA) have standard guidelines for antimicrobial prophylaxis for the prevention of bacterial endocarditis in high-risk patients undergoing dental, oral, and upper respiratory tract procedures, although no adequate controlled clinical trials exist. There are no standard guidelines for antimicrobial prophylaxis for patients with orthopedic implants undergoing similar procedures, although it is reasonable to assume that these devices may also become infected under the same conditions. Upper respiratory tract procedures that cause transient bacteremia include tonsillectomy and/or adenoidectomy, rigid bronchoscopy procedures or biopsies that involve respiratory mucosa, esophageal dilatation, and incision and drainage of infected tissue.[130,131]

Using an animal model, transient bacteremia produced by intravenous injection of both aerobic and anaerobic bacteria resulted in infected joint protheses. The authors concluded the following: Hematogenous spread of bacteria resulted in total joint prosthesis infection comparable to that caused by local inoculation; both aerobes and anaerobes have the same ability to cause hematogenous spread of infection to a total

joint replacement; an implant has a higher risk of infection in the early postoperative period (0 to 6 weeks) than in the late postoperative period (≥ 6 weeks).[132] The assumption that bacteremia during routine H&N and dental procedures can infect a prosthetic joint is supported by these findings.

Jaspers and Little[133] found that 93% of orthopedic surgeons recommend giving antibiotics to their patients with artificial joints undergoing dental procedures, although much controversy exists due to the lack of controlled clinical trials. Tsevat et al[134] performed a cost-benefit analysis evaluating antibiotic prophylaxis in patients with artificial joints undergoing dental procedures. The probability of developing an artificial joint infection from transient bacteremia during dental procedures was estimated to be 9.3/100,000. Although no controlled clinical trials exist, we recommend that empiric antimicrobial prophylaxis be used in patients with orthopedic devices in place undergoing any H&N procedure known to cause transient bacteremia.

CONCLUSION

The appropriate use of antimicrobial prophylaxis is critical in reducing the risk of postoperative wound complications, in addition to preventing antibiotic-related side-effects and increased cost. Antibiotic prophylaxis is most efficacious when the antibiotic is present in the tissue before bacterial contamination occurs. Parenteral administration of antibiotics in H&N surgery is the traditional route of administration, although the use of topical antibiotics alone may prove to be equally efficacious. The use of antibiotics (prophylactically, empirically, or as treatment) is routinely recommended in the following: major clean-contaminated H&N cases; any H&N procedure causing transient bacteremia in patients with risk factors for endocarditis or in patients with orthopedic implants; neurotologic procedures (topical); tonsillectomy; nasal surgery employing a graft; epistaxis requiring a posterior nasal pack; cranial base surgery; compound mandibular fractures; laryngotracheal injuries; animal bites that are extensive or poorly debrided; and all human bites. The antimicrobial agent used should be effective against normal oropharyngeal flora. The need for AGNB coverage in major clean-contaminated H&N surgery remains in question. A short course (24 hours) of antibiotic prophylaxis is efficacious in preventing postoperative infections in most H&N surgical procedures, although in some cases the use of antibiotics may extend for 2 to 10 days (cranial base surgery, epistaxis using posterior nasal packing, tonsillectomy, trauma, and animal and human bites).

REFERENCES

1. Haley RW, Culver DH, Morgan WM, White SW, Emori TG, Hooton TM. Identifying patients at high risk of surgical wound infection: A simple multivariate index of patient susceptibility and wound contamination. *Am J Epidemiol.* 1985;121: 206–215.

2. Kossmann CE. Antibiotic cost containment. *J Tenn Med Assoc.* 1980;72:723-728.

3. Shapiro M. Perioperative prophylactic use of antibiotics in surgery: Principles and practice. *Infect Control.* 1982;3:38-40.

4. Shapiro M, Townsend TR, Rosner B, Kass EH. Use of antimicrobial drugs in general hospitals. *N Engl J Med.* 1979; 301:351-355.

5. Dor P, Klastersky J. Prophylactic antibiotics in oral, pharyngeal and laryngeal surgery for cancer: A double blind study. *Laryngoscope.* 1973;83:1992-1998.

6. Becker GD, Parell GJ. Cefazolin prophylaxis in head and neck cancer surgery. *Ann Otol.* 1979;88:183-186.

7. Johnson JT, Yu VL, Myers EN, Muder RR, Thearle PB, Diven WF. Efficacy of two third-generation cephalosporins in prophylaxis for head and neck surgery. *Arch Otolaryngol.* 1984; 110:224-227.

8. Shapiro M, Schoenbaum SC, Tager IB, Muñoz A, Polk F. Benefit-cost analysis of antimicrobial prophylaxis in abdominal and vaginal hysterectomy. *JAMA.* 1983;249:1290-1328.

9. Olson M, O'Connor M, Schwartz ML. Surgical wound infections: A 5-year prospective study of 20,193 wounds at the Minneapolis VA Medical Center. *Ann Surg.* 1984;199:253-259.

10. Mandell-Brown M, Johnson JT, Wagner RL. Cost-effectiveness of prophylactic antibiotics in head and neck surgery. *Otolaryngol Head Neck Surg.* 1984;92:520-523.

11. Blair EA, Johnson JT, Wagner RL, Carrau RC, Byzakis J. Cost benefit analysis of antibiotic prophylaxis in clean head and neck surgery. *Arch Otolaryngol.* 1992.

12. Johnson JT, Wagner RL, Leonard MN. Economical considerations of antibiotic prophylaxis for head and neck surgery. In: Meyers AD, Eiseman B, eds. *Cost-Effective Otolaryngology.* St. Louis: BC Decker, Inc. 1990:223-230.

13. Howard JM, Barker WF, Culbertson WR, et al. Postoperative wound irradiation of the operating room and various other factors. *Ann Surg.* 1964;160:1-192.

14. Johnson JT, Wagner RL. Infection following uncontaminated head and neck surgery. *Arch Otolaryngol.* 1987;113:368-369.

15. Carrau RL, Byzakis J, Wagner RL, Johnson JT. Role of prophylactic antibiotics in uncontaminated neck dissections. *Arch Otolaryngol Head Neck Surg.* 1991;115:194-195.

16. Altemeier WA. Surgical infections: Incisional wounds. In: Bennett JV, Brackman PS, eds. *Incisional Wound, Hospital Infections.* Boston, Mass: Little, Brown and Company; 1979: 287-306.

17. Eschelman LT, Schleuning AJ, Brummett RE. Prophylactic antibiotics in otolaryngologic surgery: A double-blind study. *Trans Am Acad Opth Otol.* 1971;75:387-394.

18. Weimert TA, Yoder MG. Antibiotics and nasal surgery. *Laryngoscope.* 1980;90:667-672.

19. Leonard JR. Prophylactic antibiotics in human stapedectomy. *Laryngoscope.* 1967;77:663-680.

20. Robinson PJ, Chopra S. Antibiotic prophylaxis in cochlear implantation: Current practice. *J Laryngol Otol.* 1989;18:20-21.

21. Miles AA. Nonspecific defense reactions in bacterial infections. *Ann NY Acad Sci.*1956;66:356-369.

22. Burke JF. The effective period of preventive antibiotic action in experimental incisions and dermal lesions. *Surgery.* 1961; 50:161-168.

23. Stone HH, Hooper CA, Kolb LD, Geheber CE, Dawkins EJ. Antibiotic prophylaxis in gastric, biliary and colonic surgery. *Ann Surg.* 1976;184:443-452.

24. Galandiuk S, Polk HC, Jagelman DG, Fazio VW. Re-emphasis of priorities in surgical antibiotic prophylaxis. *Surg Gynecol Obstet.* 1986;169:219-222.

25. Classen DC, Evans S, Pestontnik SL, Horn SD, Menlove RL, Burke JP. The timing of prophylactic administration of antibiotics and the risk of surgical-wound infection. *N Engl J Med.* 1992;326;281-286.

26. Alexander JW, Alexander NS. The influence of route of administration on wound fluid concentration of prophylactic antibiotics. *J Trauma.* 1976;16:488-495.

27. Nichols RL, Broido P, Condon RE, et al. Effect of preoperative neomycin-erythromycin intestinal preparation on the incidence of infection complications following colon surgery. *Ann Surg.* 1973;178:453-462.

28. Fabian TC, Hoefling SJ, Strom PR, Stone HH. Use of antibiotic prophylaxis in penetrating abdmonial trauma. *Clin Ther.* 1982;5:38-47.

29. Gingrass RP, Close AS, Ellison EH. The effect of various topical and parenteral agents on the prevention of infection in experimental contaminate wounds. *J Trauma.* 1964;4: 763-783.

30. Bergamini TM, Lamont PM, Cheadle WG, Polk HC. Combined topical and systemic antibiotic prophylaxis in experimental wound infection. *Am J Surg.* 1984;147:753-756.

31. Robinson JMP. Wound infection following laryngectomy: The effect of topical ampicillin and carbenicillin. *J Laryngol Otol.* 1976;90:415-424.

32. Elledge ES, Whiddon RG, Fraker JY, Stambaugh KI. The effects of topical oral clindamycin antibiotic rinses on the bacterial content of saliva on healthy human subjects. *Otolaryngol Head Neck Surg.* 1991;105:836-839.

33. Kirchner JC, Edberg SC, Sasaki CT. The use of topical oral antibiotics in head and neck prophylaxis: Is it justified? *Laryngoscope.* 1988;98:26-29.

34. Nolte WA. Oral ecology. In: Nolte WA, ed. *Or Microbiology,* 2nd ed. St. Louis, MO: CV Mosby Co; 1973:3-44.

35. Grandis JR, Vickers RM, Rihs JD, et al. The efficacy of topical antibiotics prophylaxis for contaminated head and neck surgery. *Laryngoscope.* 1994;104:719-724.

36. Krizek TJ, Gottlieb LJ, Koss N, Robson MC. The use of prophylactic antibacterials in plastic surgery: A 1980's update. *Plast Reconstr Surg.* 1985;76:953-963.

37. Strong MS. Wound infection in otolaryngologic surgery and the inexpediency of antibiotic prophylaxis. *Laryngoscope.* 1963;173:165-183.

38. Herzon FS. Bacteremia and local infections with nasal packing. *Arch Otolaryngol.* 1971;94:317-320.

39. Derkay CS, Hirsch BE, Johnson JT, Wagner RL. Posterior nasal packing: Are intravenous antibiotics really necessary? *Arch Otolaryngol Head Neck Surg.* 1989;115:439-441.

40. Silk KL, Ali MB, Cohen BJ, Summersgill JT, Raff MJ. Absence of bacteremia during nasal septoplasty. *Arch Otolaryngol Head Neck Surg.* 1991;117:54-55.

41. Slavin SA, Rees TD, Guy CL, Goldwyn RM. An investigation of bacteremia during rhinoplasty. *Plast Reconstr Surg.* 1983;1:196-198.

42. Toback J, Fayerman JW. Toxic shock syndrome following septorhinoplasty. *Arch Otolaryngol.* 1983;109:627-629.

43. Jackson CG. Antimicrobial prophylaxis in ear surgery. *Laryngoscope.* 1988;98:1116-1123.

44. Donaldson JA, Snyder IS. Prophylactic chemotherapy in myringoplasty surgery. *Laryngoscope.* 1966;176:1201-1214.

45. Kartush JM, Cannon SC, Boirab Di, Graham MD, Schmaltz S, Kemink JL. Use of bacitracin for neurotologic surgery. *Laryngoscope.* 1988;98:1050-1054.

46. Teng P, Cohen I, Meleney FL. Bacitracin in neurosurgical infections. *Surg Gynecol Obstet.* 1951;92:53-63.

47. Zintel HA, Ma RA, Nichols AC, Ellis H. The absorption, distribution, excretion and toxicity of bacitracin in man. 1949; 218:439-445.

48. Malis Li. Prevention of neurosurgical infection by intraoperative antibiotics. *Neurosurgery.* 1979;5:339-343.

49. Blomstedt GC, Kyttä J. Results of a randomized trial of vancomycin prophylaxis in craniotomy. *J Neurosurg.* 1988;69: 216-220.

50. Carrau RL, Snyderman C, Janecka IP, Sekhar L, Sen C, D'Amico F. Antibiotic prophylaxis in cranial base surgery. *Head Neck.* 1991;3:311–317.
51. Telian SA, Handier SD, Fleisher GR, Baranak CC, Wetmore RF, Potsic WP. The effect of antibiotic therapy in recovery after tonsillectomy in children: A controlled study. *Arch Otolaryngol Head Neck Surg.* 1986;112:610–615.
52. DeDio RM, Tom LWC, McGowan KL, Wetmore RF, Handler SD, Potsic WP. Microbiology of the tonsils and adenoid in a pediatric population. *Arch Otolaryngol Head Neck Surg.* 1988;114:763–765.
53. Jones J, Handier SD, Guttenplan M, et al. The efficacy of cefaclor vs amoxicillin on recovery after tonsillectomy in children. *Arch Otolaryngol Head Neck Surg.* 1990;116:590–593.
54. Grandis JR, Johnson JT, Vickers RM, et al. The efficacy of perioperative antibiotic therapy on recovery following tonsillectomy in adults: Randomized double-blind placebo-controlled trial. *Otolaryngol Head Neck Surg.* 1992;106:137–142.
55. Brook I, Foote PA Jr. Comparison of the microbiology of recurrent tonsillitis between children and adults. *Laryngoscope.* 1986;96:1395–1388.
56. Edlich RF, Thacker JG, Buchanan L, Rodeheaver GT. Modern concepts in treatment of traumatic wounds. *Adv Surg.* 1979;13:169–197.
57. Lawson W. Management of soft tissue injuries of the face. *Otolaryngol Clin North Am.* 1982;15:35–48.
58. Yurt RW, Shires GT. Prophylaxis and treatment of infection in trauma. In: Mandell GL, Douglas RG, Bennet JE, eds. *Principles and Practice of Infectious Disease,* 3rd ed. New York: Churchill Livingstone; 1990:825–830.
59. Haury B, Rodeheaver G, Vensko J, Edgerton MT, Edlich RF. Debridement: An essential component of traumatic wound care. *Am J Surg.* 1978;135:238–242.
60. Mandell GL. Bactericidal activity of aerobic and anaerobic polmorphonuclear netrophils. *Infect Immunol.* 1974;9:337–341.
61. Communicable Disease Center; Public Health Service; U.S. Department of Health, Education, and Welfare. *Tetanus Surveillance.* Report No. 1, February 1, 1968.
62. Robson MC, Frank DH, Heggers JP. Tetanus resulting from osteomyelitis of the zygoma. *Plast Reconstr Surg.* 1980;65:679–682.
63. Chole RA, Yee J. Antibiotic prophylaxis for facial fractures. *Arch Otolaryngol Head Neck Surg.* 1987;113:1055–1057.
64. Zallen RD, Curry JT. A study of antibiotic usage in compound mandibular fractures. *J Oral Surg.* 1975;33:431–434.
65. LeMay SR Jr. Penetrating wounds of the larynx and cervical trachea. *Arch Otolaryngol.* 1971;94:557–566.
66. Shumrick DA. Trauma of the larynx. *Arch Otolaryngol.* 1967;86:109–114.
67. Harris HH, Tobin HA. Acute injuries of the larynx and trachea in 49 patients. *Laryngoscope.* 1970;80:1376–1384.
68. Trone TH, Schaefer SD, Carder HM. Blunt and penetrating laryngeal trauma: A 13-year review. *Otolaryngol Head Neck Surg.* 1980;88:257–261.
69. Schneider RC, Thompson JM. Rhinorrhea as a source of recurrent attacks of meningitis. *Ann Surg.* 1957;145:517–529.
70. Appelbaum E. Meningitis following trauma to the head and face. *JAMA.* 1960;173:1818–1822.
71. Leech PJ, Paterson A. Conservative and operative management for cerebrospinal-fluid leakage after closed head injury. *Lancet.* 1973;1:1013–1016.
72. Lewin W. Cerebrospinal fluid rhinorrhea in closed head injuries. *Br J Surg.* 1954;42:1–18.
73. MacGee EE, Cauthen JC, Brackett CE. Meningitis following acute traumatic cerebrospinal fluid fistula. *J Neurosurg.* 1970;33:312–316.
74. Ignelzi RJ, VanderArk GD. Analysis of the treatment of basilar skull fractures with and without antibiotics. *J Neurosurg.* 1975;43:721–726.
75. Weinstein L. The spontaneous occurence of new bacterial infections during the course of treatment with streptomycin or penicillin. *Am J Med Sci.* 1947;214:56–63.
76. Klastersky J, Sadeghi M, Brihaye J. Antimicrobial prophylaxis in patients with rhinorrhea or otorrhea: A double-blind study. *Surg Neurol.* 1976;6:111–114.
77. Maetz HM. Animal bites: A public health proble in Jefferson County, Alabama. *Public Health Rep.* 1979;94:528–534.
78. Goldstein EJC, Citron DM, Finegold SM. Dog bite wounds and infection: prospective clinical study. *Ann Emerg Med.* 1980;9:508–512.
79. Mathog RH, Wurman LH, Pollak D. Animal bites to the head and neck in plastic and reconstructive surgery of the face and neck. In: Sisson GA, Tardy ME, eds. *Plastic and Reconstructive Surgery of the Face and Neck,* vol. 2. New York: Grune & Stratton; 1977:105–113.
80. Chambers GH, Payne JF. Treatment of dog-bite wounds. *Minn Med.* 1969;52:427–430.
81. Schultz RC, McMaster WC. The treatment of dog bite injuries, especially those of the face. *Plast Reconstr Surg.* 1972;49:494–500.
82. Thomson HG, Svitek V: Small animal bites: The role of primary closure. *J Trauma.* 1973;13:20–23.
83. Elenbaas RM, McNabney WK, Robinson WA. Prophylactic oxacillin in dog bite wounds. *Ann Emerg Med.* 1982;11:248–251.
84. Callaham M. Prophylactic antibiotics in common dog bite wounds: A controlled study. *Ann Emerg Med.* 1980;9:410–414.
85. Brook I. Human and animal bite infections. *J Fam Pract.* 1989;28:713–718.
86. Goldstein EJC, Citron DM, Wield B, et al. Bacteriology of human and animal bite wounds. *J Clin Microbiol.* 1978;8:667–672.
87. Zubowicz VN, Gravier M. Management of early human bites of the hand: A prospective randomized study. *Plast Reconstr Surg.* 1991;88:111–114.
88. Stucker FJ, Shaw GY, Boyd S, Shockley WW. Management of animal and human bites in the head and neck. *Arch Otolaryngol Head Neck Surg.* 1990;116:789–793.
89. Piccart M, Klastersky J. Antimicrobial prophylaxis of infections in head and neck cancer surgery. *Scand J Infect Dis.* 1983;39:92–96.
90. Seagle MB, Duberstein LE, Gross CW, Fletcher JL, Mustafa AQ. Efficacy of cefazolin as a prophylactic antibiotic in head and neck surgery. *Otolaryngol.* 1978;86:568–572.
91. Saginus R, Odell PF, Poliquin JF. Antibiotic prophylaxis in head and neck cancer surgery. *J Otolaryngol.* 1988;17:78–80.
92. Raine CH, Bartzokas CA, Stell PM, Gallway A, Corkill JE. Chemoprophylaxis in major head and neck surgery. *J R Soc.* 1984;77:1006–1009.
93. Brand B, Johnson JT, Myers EN, Thearle PB, Sigler BA. Prophylactic perioperative antibiotics in contaminated head and neck surgery. *Otolaryngol Head Neck Surg.* 1982;90:315–318.
94. Johnson JT, Yu VL, Myers EN, Wagner RL, Sigler BA. Cefazolin vs moxalactam? *Arch Otolaryngol Head Neck Surg.* 1986;112:151–153.
95. Mombelli G, Coppens L, Dor P, Klastersky J. Antibiotic prophylaxis in surgery for head and neck cancer: Comparative study of short and prolonged administration of carbencillin. *J Antimicrob Chemother.* 1981;7:665–671.
96. Fee WE, Glenn M, Handen C, Hopp ML. One day vs two days of prophylactic antibiotics in patients undergoing major head and neck surgery. *Laryngoscope.* 1984;94:612–614.

97. Johnson JT, Yu VL, Myers EN, Wagner RL. As assessment of the need for gram-negative bacterial coverage in antibiotic prophylaxis for oncological head and neck surgery. *J Infect Dis.* 1987;155:331–333.

98. Johnson JT, Myers EN, Thearle PB, Sigler BA, Schramm VL Jr. Antimicrobial prophylaxis for contaminated head and neck surgery. *Laryngoscope.* 1984;94:46–51.

99. Johnson JT, Schuller DE, Silver F, et al. Antibiotic prophylaxis in high-risk head and neck surgery: One-day or five-day therapy. *Otolaryngol Head Neck Surg.* 1986;95:554–557.

100. Sawyer R, Cozzi L, Rosenthal Di, Maniglia AJ. Metronidazole in head and neck surgery—the effect of lengthened prophylaxis. *Otolaryngol Head Neck Surg.* 1990;103:1009–1011.

101. Rubin J, Johnson JT, Wagner RL, Yu VL. Bacteriologic analysis of wound infection following major head and neck surgery. *Arch Otolaryngol Head Neck Surg.* 1988;114:969–972.

102. Swift AC, Bartzokas CA, Corkill JE. The clinical significant of the gastro-oral pathway of intestinal bacteria after after head and neck cancer surgery. *Clin Otolaryngol.* 1987;12:455–249.

103. Becker GD, Parell CJ, Busch DF, Finegold SM, Acquarelli MJ, Citron DM. The non-value of preoperative and intraoperative cultures in predicting the bacteriology of subsequent wound infection in patients undergoing major head and neck cancer surgery. *Laryngoscope.* 1980;90:1933–1940.

104. Becker GD, Welch WD. Quantitative bacteriology of closed-suction wound drainage in contaminated surgery. *Laryngoscope.* 1990;100:403–406.

105. Johnson JT, Yu VL. Role of aerobic gram-negative rods, anaerobes, and fungi in wound infection after head and neck surgery: Implications for antibiotic prophylaxis. *Head Neck.* 1989;11:27–29.

106. Weber RS, Raad I, Frankenthaler R, et al. Ampicillin-sulbactam vs clindamycin in head and neck oncologic surgery: The need for gram-negative coverage. *Arch Otolaryngol Head Neck Surg.* 1992;118:1159–1163.

107. Newman RK, Weiland FL, Johnson JT, Rose PR, Gumerman LW. Salivary scan after major ablative head and neck surgery with prediction of postoperative fistulization. *Ann Otol Rhinol Laryngol.* 1983;92:366–368.

108. Sweeney G, Watson JD, McGrego IA, Sleigh JD. Successful prophylaxis with tinidazole of infectin after major head and neck surgery for malignant disease. *J Plast Surg.* 1984;37:35–42.

109. Maddocks JL. Indirect pathogenicity. *J Antimicrob Chemother.* 1980;6:307–309.

110. Bartlett JG, Gorback SL. Anaerobic infections of the head and neck. *Otolaryngol Clin North Am.* 1976;9:655–678.

111. Johanson WG, Pierce AK, Sanford JP. Changing pharyngeal bacterial flora of hospitalized patients. *N Engl J Med.* 1969;281:1137–1140.

112. Becker GD, Parell GJ, Busch DF, Finegold SM, Acquarelli MJ. Anaerobic and aerobic bacteriology in head and neck cancer surgery. *Arch Otolaryngol.* 1978;104:591–594.

113. Deitch EA, Bridger RM. Effects of stress and trauma on bacterial translocation from the gut. *J Surg Res.* 1987;42:536–542.

114. Swift AC, Bartzokas CA, Corkill JE. The gastro-oral pathway of intestinal bacteria after head and neck cancer surgery. *Clin Otolaryngol.* 1984;9:263–269.

115. Finegold SH. *Anaerobic Bacteria in Human Disease.* New York: Academic Press, Inc; 1977:34–40.

116. Goode RL, Abramson N, Fee WE, Levine P. Effect of prophylactic antibiotics in radical head and neck surgery. *Laryngoscope.* 1979;89:601–607.

117. van Laethem Y, Lagast H, Klastersky J. Anaerobic infections in cancer patients: Comparison between therapy oriented strictly against anaerobes or both anaerobes and aerobes. *J Antimicrob Chemother.* 1982;10:137.

118. Gerard M, Meunier F, Dor P, et al. Antimicrobial prophylaxis for major head and neck surgery in cancer patients. *Antimicrob Agent Chemother.* 1988;32:1557–1559.

119. Craig WA, Gudmundsson S. The postantibiotic effect. In: Lorain V. ed. *Antibiotics in Laboratory Medicine.* Baltimore, MD: Williams & Wilkins; 1986:515–536.

120. Beachey EH, Eisenstein Bi, Ofek I. Adherence of bacteria. In: Eickenberg O, Hahn H, Opferhuck W, eds. *Influence of Antibiotics on the Host-Parasite Relationship.* Berlin: Springer-Verlag; 1982:171–182.

121. Velanovich V. A meta-analysis of prophylactic antibiotics in head and neck surgery. *Plast Reconstr Surg.* 1991;87:429–433.

122. Robbins KT, Favrot S, Hanna D, Cole R. Risk of wound infection in patients with head and neck cancer. *Head Neck.* 1889;12:143–148.

123. Brown BM, Johnson JT, Wagner RL. Etiologic factors in head and neck wound infections. *Laryngoscope.* 1987;97:587–590.

124. Ketcham AS, Bloch JH, Crawford DT, Lieberman JE, Smith RR. The role of prophylactic antibiotic therapy in control of staphylococcal infections following cancer surgery. *Surg Gynecol Obstet.* 1962;114:345–352.

125. Yoder MG, Krause J, Kwyer TA. Infection and noninfection complications in head and neck surgery. *Otolaryngol Head Neck Surg.* 1979;87:797–806.

126. Johnson JT, Bloomer WD. Effect of prior radiotherapy on postsurgical wound infection. *Head Neck.* 1989;11:132–136.

127. Johnson JT, Yu VL. Antibiotic use during major head and neck surgery. *Ann Surg.* 1988;207:108–111.

128. Johnson JT. Antimicrobial prophylaxis for contaminated head and neck surgery. Presented at the Eastern Section of the Triologic Society; January 28, 1983; New York.

129. Garner JS, Jarvis WR, Emori TG, Horan TC, Hughes JM. CDC definitions for nosocomial infections, 1988. *Am J Infect Cont.* 1988;16:128–140.

130. Kay D. Prophylaxis for infective endocardiatis: An update. *Ann Intern Med.* 1986;104:419–423.

131. Dajani AS, Bisno AL, Chung KJ, et al. Prevention of bacterial endocarditis: Recommendations by the American Heart Association. *JAMA.* 1990;264:2919–2922.

132. Blomgren G. Hematogenous infection of total joint replacement. *Acta Orthopaedic Scand.* 1981;187:1–64.

133. Jaspers MT, Lehte JW. Prophylactic antibiotic coverage in patients with total arthroplasty: Current practice. *JADA.* 1985;111:943–948.

134. Tsevat J, Durand-Zaleski I, Pauker SG. Cost-effectiveness of antibiotic prophylaxis for dental procedures in patients with artificial joints. *Am J Publ Health.* 1989;79:739–743.

13 Complications of Salivary Gland Surgery

Michael J. Kaplan, M.D.

Preventing complications of salivary gland surgery begins with a thorough understanding of the complex regional anatomy of the parotid and submandibular areas and, in some instances, the adjacent infratemporal fossa, temporomandibular joint, and external ear canal. Next, familiarity with the wide spectrum of pathophysiology—malignant tumors, benign tumors, and infectious and inflammatory processes—will both guide appropriate selection of patients as well as preoperative evaluation and postoperative management.

This chapter will review complications in the diagnosis and evaluation of the patient with a possible parotid or submandibular gland problem, and it will discuss the prevention and management of surgical complications (Table 13–1). The complications of salivary gland tumors originating in the infratemporal fossa or in the oral cavity and oropharynx are discussed in other chapters. Although numerous complications and sequellae may occur, three in particular are more troubling to patient and surgeon: a consequential error in diagnosis (one resulting in an unindicated procedure or a different operation), facial paralysis, and recurrent tumor.

DIAGNOSIS AND EVALUATION COMPLICATIONS AND THE USE OF MAGNETIC RESONANCE IMAGING/ COMPUTED TOMOGRAPHY AND FINE-NEEDLE ASPIRATION

Differential Diagnosis

It is not uncommon for a patient to present to his or her physician with a newly noted, usually asymptomatic, firm periparotid mass. This mass is often 1 to 3 cm in size. Most of these will prove to be a parotid tumor, usually benign. The differential diagnosis, however, is long and includes a prominent anatomic structure (such as a transverse process of C-1, masseter hypertrophy, or elongated styloid process); systemic or inflammatory conditions (such as bacterial lymphadenitis, Sjogen's disease, benign lymphoepithelial lesions and cysts—sometimes associated with HIV and chronic sialadenitis from ductal obstruction); first bronchial cleft abnormalities; and metastases to intraglandular or extraglandular lymph nodes.

Table 13–1. Complications of Parotid and Submandibular Surgery

Diagnostic evaluation errors and complications
  Patient selection
  Options in diagnostic imaging
  Pitfalls in FNA
Surgical complications
  Nerve injury
    Parotid surgery: facial nerve injury
    Parotid surgery: greater auricular nerve sacrifice and neuroma
    Submandibular surgery: facial nerve, lingual nerve, hypoglossal nerve
  Hematoma
  Seroma
  Sialocele, saliva leak
  Infection
  Flap necrosis
Late complications and events
  Esthetic deformity
  Gustatory sweating (Frey's syndrome)
  Complications related to the external auditory canal
  Complications related to chewing
  Recurrent pleomorphic adenoma
  Recurrent malignant tumor

Facial or scalp skin tumors occasionally metastasize to these parotid nodes, as do pharyngeal squamous cell carcinomas (SCC). Prostate, renal cell, lung, and breast carcinomas and other tumors all rarely metastasize to the parotid area or ramus of the mandible. Oral cavity and pharyngeal SCC commonly metastasize to the submandibular triangle. If the entire parotid appears enlarged, and especially if the findings are bilateral, it should be recalled that some infiltrative processes may do this (alcoholism is the most common) and it is rarely a drug reaction.

A complete history may lead to obvious clues about the nature of the parotid or submandibular mass. A complete head and neck examination and pertinent general exam, as well as a chest x-ray, may similarly suggest a primary cancer elsewhere. Often, however, the only finding is an asymptomatic mass. The next step is likely to be a radiological imaging study, a fine-needle aspiration (FNA) biopsy, or a parotidectomy—but which one? In other words, when will either radiological imaging or an FNA assist the physician?

Imaging

When the parotid mass is small and the patient is otherwise healthy, it is usually unnecessary to obtain radiological information or an FNA prior to planned parotidectomy. For larger or recurrent tumors or for parapharyngeal space masses, magnetic resonance imaging (MRI) or, to a lesser extent, computed tomography (CT) offers accurate preoperative assessment of extraparotid involvement. This may suggest unresectability or may assist the planning of both the surgeon and radiation oncologist. MRI or CT may also demonstrate nodal involvement and the relationship of the tumor to the carotid sheath. The superior multiplanar imaging and contrast resolution of MRI compared to CT is most evident in the parapharyngeal space; for more superficial tumors, CT may be adequate.[1,2]

Although the appearance on MRI may suggest that a tumor is malignant or highly infiltrative and such information may be helpful in planning surgery and counseling the patient, histologic diagnosis is not the goal of radiological imaging. Benign and low-grade malignancies usually show low signal intensity on T1-weighted images and high signal intensity on T2-weighted images, reflecting their higher seromucinous secretions. High-grade tumors frequently reveal low signal intensity in both T1- and T2-weighted images and often have poorly defined margins. Fibrosis and sialolithiasis exhibit thickening of the deep cervical fascia and infiltration of subcutaneous fat; signal intensities are usually low on both T1- and T2-weighted images. Such information must be correlated with the clinical setting. If true pathologic preoperative information is needed, then clearly FNA is necessary.

Other radiological imaging techniques have been used such as ultrasonography, sialography, CT sialography, and radionuclide scans. An ultrasound, in the setting of parotitis, may demonstrate an abscess in need of drainage. Sialography may demonstrate a calculus in the parotid duct. A submenticovertical plain film may demonstrate a stone in a submandibular duct. Because Warthin's tumors (and oncocytomas) are detected with technitium-99 radionuclide imaging, this technique had been advocated as a diagnostic tool. Especially for patients in whom surgery would be high risk, the demonstration that a tumor is benign is particularly important. However, FNA is superior to radionuclide scanning for this purpose because a pathologic diagnosis is obtained, distinguishing the rare malignant oncocytoma from the common Warthin's tumor. Prior to the use of MRI, CT sialography was sometimes used in distinguishing primary parapharyngeal space (PPS) tumors from deep-lobe parotid tumors extending into the PPS. MRI, however, is superior in making this distinction.[5]

Fine-Needle Aspiration Biopsy

Fine-needle aspiration using a 23-gauge or 25-gauge needle has become a valuable diagnostic tool in many centers.[6–9] It is well tolerated, safe, and inexpensive. With experience, results correlate with final histology at least as well as frozen sections[10,11] and, with good communication between cytopathologist and surgeon, are rarely misleading. For this reason, the role of frozen section, always controversial, is probably fairly limited in salivary gland surgery: checking for margins in a known malignancy and checking for involvement of an enlarged node if this knowledge would lead the surgeon to proceed with a neck dissection.

Although certainly not always indicated, an FNA may assist the surgeon in several clinical situations. First, if a mass near the parotid is felt not to be of salivary origin, a surgical procedure other than parotidectomy may be planned, such as excision of a possible skin adnexal mass or a lymph node. An FNA that shows salivary pathology in this scenario demonstrates the need for parotidectomy, reducing the chance of an inappropriate parotid biopsy, tumor enucleation, or facial nerve injury that might have been the result of the lesser procedure. Second, the confirmation that a mass is a primary malignancy may assist the surgeon in counseling the patient, obtaining preoperative consultations from radiation oncology and other specialties, or obtaining an MRI. Certain histologies, such as squamous cell carcinoma and high-grade mucoepidermoid carcinoma, have a higher incidence of cervical nodal metastases. If the surgeon would do a prophylactic neck dissection in such a case, an FNA would be helpful. Some surgeons might obtain a CT to investigate nodal status in this situation, planning on a neck dissection only if there are enlarged nodes or planning to obtain either an FNA or a frozen section for such nodes. If a metastasis or lymphoma is demonstrated on FNA, whether suspected or not, the medical evaluation is likely to be expanded prior to or instead of parotidectomy. Third, the confirmation that a tumor is benign may alleviate concern in an anxious patient or offer a nonsurgical option in a surgically high-risk patient. If none of these reasons to obtain a FNA exist, as is frequently the case in a small parotid mass in an otherwise healthy patient, then its cost is usually unwarranted.

Although it is not infrequent that the cytopathologist is unable to make a complete and accurate diagnosis, a misleading diagnosis is unusual. In particular, a false-positive for malignancy is rare. An incomplete or unhelpful diagnosis may be a result of an unsatisfactorally prepared specimen or a geographic miss. In such cases, no clinical information is derived, and the FNA might be reattempted. A CT-guided FNA may be helpful in parapharyngeal tumors. More commonly, a descriptive but incomplete diagnosis is a result of difficulty caused by the underlying histology. The two most common situations that may pose difficulty are mucoepidermoid carcinomas and cellular mixed tumors with either nuclear atypia or with no stroma. Cystic lesions, lymphoid lesions, and rare tumors may also be difficult.

When nuclear atypia is evident along with biphasic mesenchymal (usually fernlike stroma) and epithelial elements typical of pleomoiphic adenoma, the relatively common pleomorphic adenom—not malignancy—is likely correct. Pleomorphic adenoma may also be difficult to diagnose when either the stroma or the epithelial cells are missing. The presence of intracellular mucin, squamous cells, or cystic changes may also pose diagnostic problems.

Cohen et al[12] reviewed the experience of the University of California, San Francisco, with 34 mucoepidermoid carcinoma (MEC) FNA specimens. Intermediate cells (in 79%) or both overlapping epithelial cells (91%) and squamous cells (77%) correlated best with the diagnosis of MEC, with a predictive value of over 98% using stepwise logistic recession analysis. High-grade MEC was best distinguished from low-grade lesions based on the presence of nuclear atypia (89% vs 19%), necrosis (28% vs 6%), and stringy extracellular mucin (44% vs 81%). Mucoepidermoid carcinomas with cystic changes may be difficult to distinguish from atypical benign cysts that contain mucin and necrotic debris.

Overall, among experienced cytopathologists, FNA is accurate. Qizilbash et al[13] reported 160 FNAs, of which 91% were satisfactory specimens. None of the 77 benign or nontumor cases were interpreted as being malignant, and 90% were complete and accurate. There were three false-negatives among the 14 malignant cases, with two lymphoma diagnoses attributed to early personal inexperience. Nettle and Orrel,[14] reviewing 25 malignant and 74 benign cases, reported a single false-positive and five false-negatives: an 80% specificity and 99% sensitivity for a malignant diagnosis. Overall, 68% were complete and accurate, with only 6/99 misleading. As with Cohen[12] and Jayaram,[15] mucoepidermoid carcinoma and unusual pleomorphic adenomas usually presented the most difficulty in interpretation.

When confronted with a diagnostic dilemma, the cytopathologist and the clinician should discuss the descriptive cytopathologic diagnosis and the clinical differential diagnosis. As in all tests, clinical judgment is necessary. FNA technique and interpretation requires considerable experience; success has clearly improved as experience has been gained. If the cytologic diagnosis does not concur with the clinical situation, further investigation may be needed before planning treatment.

Complications of FNA are rare. A small hematoma at the FNA site may occur and usually resolves in a few days. Facial paralysis has not been reported. Using 23- to 25-gauge needles, tumor seeding in the needle track has not been reported in the head and neck, and only two cases have been reported in any site.[16,17]

SURGICAL COMPLICATIONS

Nerve Injury

PAROTID SURGERY: FACIAL NERVE INJURY

Regardless of the indication for the surgery, the keys to the prevention of facial paralysis are identification and preservation of the branches of the facial nerve. This is easier when there is no inflammation and no prior surgery or prior irradiation, the process is limited to the superficial lobe, and the tumor is small. In such cases, careful surgical dissection is usually sufficient. Many surgeons find it helpful to have

available a disposable nerve stimulator to assist in identification of branches. When there has been prior surgery or irradiation, or in cases of chronic sialadenitis, intraoperative nerve monitoring via electromyography provides much improved—and often much needed and essential—assistance in nerve detection.[18]

The facial nerve exits the temporal bone through the styomastoid foramen. This foramen lies just posterior to the styoid process base and just anterior to the digastric ridge, the attachment of the posterior belly of digastric muscle (Fig. 13–1). The inferior end of the tympanomastoid suture is 6 to 8 mm lateral to the stylomastoid foramen. It is at this location, after first identifying the tragal pointer, that it is most common to identify the facial nerve.

If this posterior approach to the facial nerve is to be used, it is generally best to separate the tail of the parotid from the anterior border of the stemocleidomastoid muscle. This facilitates identifying the posterior belly of the digastric muscle and tracing it to the digastric ridge. The parotid is then dissected from the cartilage of the external auditory canal. The anteroinferior end of this cartilage is the tragal pointer. The facial nerve is located about 1 cm deep and slightly inferior. The tympanomastoid suture line is palpated, as is the styoid process. Careful dissection with a fine-point hemostat in the direction of the facial nerve, assisted if necessary by a nerve stimulator, will identify the nerve.

Alternative approaches to identification of the facial nerve must be considered when dissection near the stylomastoid foramen is expected to be difficult. One such situation is a large tumor in the tail of the parotid extending toward the pes. In addition, if a prior parotidectomy has been done, it is likely that there will be considerable scarring in this area.

Proximal to the most common point of identification, the descending portion of the facial nerve within the temporal bone may be located via a mastoidectomy. Sometimes removal of only the mastoid tip may afford the slight extra room for dissection to find the nerve, obviating the need for a formal mastoidectomy.

A third general approach is to locate a distal branch of the nerve and trace it retrograde back to the pes. Among the options, identification of the marginal mandibular nerve is the most common. It may be found by locating the posterior facial vein inferior to the parotid and tracing it superiorly. The marginal mandibular nerve crosses just superficial to the vein. Slightly more distal, the marginal mandibular nerve may be located crossing the anterior facial vein or overlying the fascia of the submandibular gland. The buccal branch is usually the next easiest peripheral branch to find because it lies just superior to the palpable parotid duct overlying the posterior part of the masseter muscle.

Once the facial nerve is identified, it is followed to the pes, where it branches. Because there is considerable variation in the branching patterns of the nerve, it is important to follow each branch as far as necessary toward the periphery to facilitate removal of the tumor with a cuff of normal gland around it. A curved mosquito hemostat is used to create tunnels over each branch, dividing the overlying parotid tissue

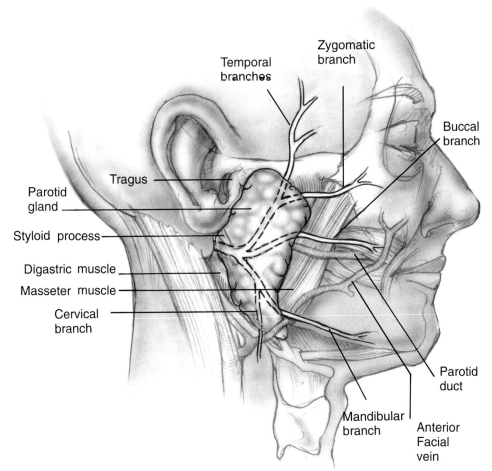

Figure 13-1. Branches of the facial nerve.

and connecting the tunnels. Tumors arising from or extending deep to the plane of the branches of the facial nerve are said to be "deep lobe." Retracting branches superiorly and inferiorly may be necessary to dissect such tumors. Division of the stylomastoid ligament affords additional exposure toward the parapharyngeal space.

If a major branch of the nerve is transected intraoperatively, it should be repaired at the end of the procedure. This may have been a result of a difficult dissection or may have been necessary to remove a malignant tumor. A simple microsurgical neurorrhaphy between the two ends should be done if it can be done without tension. A cable graft is the next best choice. The greater auricular nerve, if available, is often a wise choice for the donor nerve because the size match is likely to be good and one often has two or more distal branches available to anastamose to distal stumps of the facial nerve. The sural nerve, although larger in caliber, is another alternative if the greater auricular nerve is unavailable or inappropriate because of possible tumor involvement. If the facial nerve was involved by tumor, it is wise to check by frozen section the proximal and distal ends to enhance the chance of their being free of tumor before proceeding with the neurorrhaphy.

The management of facial paralysis depends in part on the branches involved, whether it is partial or complete, and for how long it is expected to persist. Paralysis of the marginal

mandibular branch and the branches to the orbicularis oculi is most likely to be symptomatic. Marginal mandibular nerve weakness results in incomplete lower lip depression, leading to possible lip biting and oral incompetence, with drooling. Paralytic ectropion, conjunctivitis, exposure keratitis, and epiphora are the result of obicularis oculi paralysis. Initial management is aimed at the prevention of corneal ulcers by keeping the conjunctiva moist. Artificial tears instilled frequently during the day and lubricating ointment at night are often effective. A self-humidifying transparent plastic bubble chamber over the eye is also used by many. Taping closed the upper lid at night may be tolerated by the patient instead. If recovery is expected to be delayed (or paralysis is permanent), an upper lid gold weight may be placed at or soon after surgery. Alternatively, a lateral tarsorrhaphy may be done. Signs and symptoms that should lead to ophthalmologic consultation include a scratchy foreign-body sensation, neovascularization of the cornea, conjunctivitis, or keratitis. If there is a weak corneal reflex suggestive of a fifth nerve deficit, the anesthetic cornea may not develop early symptoms. These patients should be followed closely by an ophthalmologist as well.

In addition to the aforementioned reparative and protective measures, numerous surgical procedures are available to attempt either to improve the esthetic asymmetry caused by unilateral permanent facial paralysis or reinnervate the

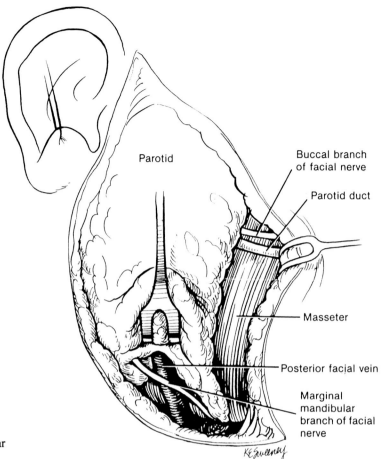

Figure 13–2. Marginal mandibular branch of the facial nerve.

affected muscles. The corner of the lip may be elevated with a static or dynamic temporalis muscle sling. A hypoglossal-facial nerve anastamosis may be used when there is no proximal facial nerve stump, but this is uncommon following parotid surgery. In other sources one may review the discussions regarding cross-face nerve transplantation and masseter muscle transfers. The indications for several relevant facial plastic procedures, including rhytidectomy, blepharoplasty, and brow lift as well as options to improve lower eyelid ectropion, are also discussed elsewhere.

PAROTID SURGERY: GREATER AURICULAR NERVE SACRIFICE
AND NEUROMA

During a parotidectomy, the greater auricular nerve is usually sacrificed. The numbness of the earlobe is permanent. This is an expected sequella of the operation. At times, the branch to the earlobe may be preserved because it courses superiorly on the stemocleidomastoid muscle. Patients should be specifically advised about this expectation preoperatively and reminded postoperatively to be cautious about possible sequellae of being unable to feel extremes of temperature (frostbite, hairdryers, etc).

Often months or even years following surgery, a small (< 0.5 to 1.5 cm) mass, often painful, may be palpated over the stemocleidomastoid muscle at the amputated greater auricular nerve. The initial presentation of this neuroma may be solely

radiating pain from a trigger point in the area. Because the differential diagnosis includes recurrent tumor, FNA may assist in making the diagnosis. Excision of a symptomatic neuroma should relieve the pain. If asymptomatic and the diagnosis is not uncertain, it may be followed clinically.[19]

SUBMANDIBULAR SURGERY: FACIAL NERVE, LINGUAL NERVE,
AND HYPOGLOSSAL NERVE

The facial nerve, lingual nerve, and hypoglossal nerves are preserved in submandibular surgery unless they are involved by tumor. The marginal mandibular branch of the facial nerve courses just superficial to the fascia overlying the gland and should be specifically sought and preserved by raising this fascia, with the nerve, toward the inferior border of the mandible. The anterior facial vein may be used to assist in this procedure. The nerve crosses superficial to the vein posteroinferior to the gland. Ligating the vein at this site and retracting the superior ligature will also retract the marginal mandibular nerve. Even when the nerve is preserved, the corner of the lip may not depress normally due either to inadequate function of the transected platysma muscle or temporary neuropraxia of the nerve from trauma or devascularization.

The hypoglossal nerve is found between the hyoglossus and mylohoid muscles. It is not essential to dissect this nerve to complete a submandibular gland excision, but it is nearby

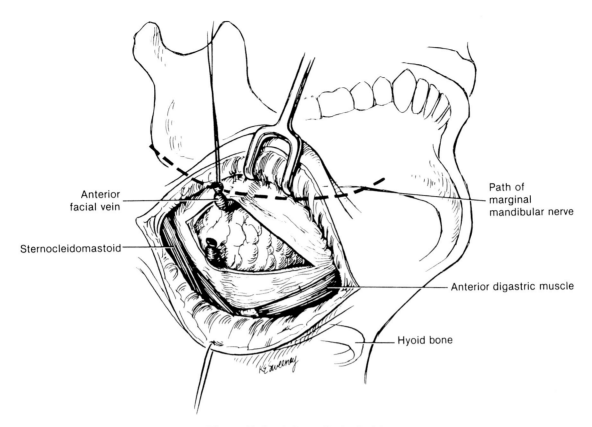

Figure 13–3. Submandibular incision.

as one ligates the external maxillary (facial) artery. Inferior retraction of the anterior belly of the digastric muscle and tendon should expose the nerve.

Ipsilateral loss of the hypoglossal nerve is usually well tolerated if there are no other neuromuscular deficits associated with speech or swallowing; the hypoglossal nerve is sacrificed, for instance, in a hypoglossal-facial anastamosis for facial reanimation following proximal facial nerve loss. The protruded tongue points to the affected side, and speech will transiently be affected. If, however, other aspects of swallowing are compromised, the additional loss of XII may be severe. If indicated, a deglutition study with a modified barium swallow and evaluation by a speech therapist may be helpful.

Anterior retraction of the mylohyoid muscle, while retracting the submandibular gland inferiorally, exposes the lingual nerve and submandibular ganglion as well as the submandibular (Wharton's) duct. When ligating the ganglion, care must be taken to avoid clamping the lingual nerve. Venous bleeding should be handled with ligatures or bipolar electrocautery to avoid heat injury to the nerve. Injury to the lingual nerve results in hypesthesia of the anterior two thirds of the tongue. The patient may occasionally repeatedly bite the tongue as a result.

Hematoma

Adequate intraoperative hemostasis using bipolar electrocautery and ligatures prevents most postoperative hematomas.

If the posterior facial vein had to be ligated to resect a deep-lobe tumor, there may be increased venous pressure, making complete hemostasis more difficult. Similarly, appropriate efforts should be made to correct any preoperative bleeding tendency, such as drug related ones. To coapt the skin flap, active closed-suction drainage (or, by some, passive drainage and a pressure dressing) is continued for 24 to 48 hours postoperatively.

A hematoma should be suspected if there is facial swelling over the surgical field, usually accompanied by pain. The suction tubes may fail to drain this adequately because blood may have clotted within them; maintaining constant or frequent suction on them during closure may reduce the incidence of this etiology of hematoma formation.

Often a hematoma will require reexploration and evacuation. The facial nerve is identified and preserved because any bleeding vessels are ligated or cauterized with bipolar electrocautery, and the wound is reclosed over active drains.

Seroma

Following removal of the drains, occasionally fluid will accumulate beneath the flap. Aspiration, using aseptic technique, is indicated. Determining the amylase content will likely distinguish a seroma from a sialocele (high amylase in a sialocele), but distinguishing between the two is not critical because the initial management is identical. A pressure dressing will help if effective pressure can be maintained. Repeat aspiration for reaccumulation is also likely to be helpful; occasionally several aspirations are needed. If no progressive reduction in the amount of fluid aspirated is seen, then slightly opening the incision in a dependent location, accompanied by a pressure dressing, is indicated.

Sialocele, Saliva Leak

A salivary leak may manifest as clear drainage (with a high amylase content) from the incision or drain site or as a sialocele beneath a healed flap. It is likely that this is more common if Stensen's duct has been ligated. Either a sialocele or a salivary leak is likely to respond within a week or two to treatment by a pressure dressing, although maintaining an effective pressure dressing may be difficult. Aspiration of a sialocele may be helpful or may have been the method of diagnosis, distinguishing it from a seroma. As in a seroma, repeat serial aspiration under sterile conditions, is also often helpful.

A salivary fistula that persists is problematic but may still respond to a prolonged pressure dressing.[20] Reducing salivary flow with anticholinergics, such as transdermal scopolamine, has been reported to be successful.[21] Tympanic neurectomy to reduce the parasympathetic innervation to the parotid has been used. Low-dose irradiation is successful but risks radiation-induced tumors years later. Unless irradiation is otherwise planned, there are likely to be safer alternatives. Completion parotidectomy is likely to be successful, but even with electromyographic nerve monitoring there is a significant chance of facial nerve injury.

Infection

Postoperative wound infections following parotid or submandibular gland surgery done for tumor are unusual. The use of perioperative antibiotics is controversial: Although most surgeons do not use them for this procedure (unless the indication for surgery is chronic sialadenitis or abscess), some do. Johnson and Wagner[22] failed to demonstrate a reduced infection rate by their use. Platt et al,[23] in a much larger series of herniorrhaphy and breast surgical procedures, showed a small reduction in the already low rate of wound infection.

As in almost all wound infections, cellulitis is treated with empiric antibiotics, and pus requires incision, drainage, culture, and tailoring of initial antibiotic selection based on Gram's stain and subsequent bacterial sensitivity. Initial empiric treatment should be based on coverage of oral flora (which may ascend via the parotid duct), possible skin contamination, and, if used, the perioperative antibiotic regimen. Pending culture and sensitivity results, any of the following antibiotic regimens may be a reasonable choice: ceftizoxime (cefuroxime or cefotetan); a first-generation cephalosporin plus metronidazole; or clindamycin. Because staphylococcus species are the most common when there is pus, nafcillin or another penicillinase-resistant synthetic penicillin is also likely to be a good initial choice in abscesses.

Flap Necrosis

Appropriate planning and handling of the parotidectomy skin flap usually avoids this rare complication. The flap should be extended inferior to the earlobe only as far posterior as needed to accomplish the surgical goal, before curving anteriorly toward the greater cornu of the hyoid—usually this is no farther posterior than the coronal plane of the anterior edge of the mastoid tip. Intraoperatively the flap should be kept moist and handled gently. Closure is often gentlest using a small double hook rather than forceps. Despite proper technique, flap necrosis occasionally occurs—usually just posteroinferior to the earlobe at the most posterior portion of the flap. As in other skin flaps, arterial supply may be compromised by advanced atherosclerosis, diabetes, tobacco use, and prior irradiation. Infection may also contribute to flap necrosis or be the result of it.

As in most local skin flaps, initial management is debridement, wet-to-dry dressings, and antibiotics (if there is evidence of cellulitis). Subsequently, if the wound is too large to close by secondary intent, a split-thickness skin graft usually suffices. In occasional cases, such as after a neck dissection and skin excision because of tumor involvement, wound breakdown requires more elaborate and more rapid closure because of its extent or because of carotid artery exposure.

Complications Related to the External Auditory Canal

The external auditory canal may become swollen postoperatively, especially if it has been entered dissecting the tragal cartilage. Blood may have entered the canal during the procedure as well. Any of these may lead to external otitis. Preventing blood from entering the canal by occluding it with sterile cotton or petrolatum gauze is often prudent. Cleaning the canal of blood at the end of a procedure may be necessary. If external otitis occurs, the canal must be cleaned of debris and antibiotic eardrops instilled; if the canal is so swollen to preclude a view of the tympanic membrane, a wick is used initially as well.

LATE COMPLICATIONS AND EVENTS
Esthetic Deformity

The major esthetic deformity noted postoperatively relates to facial nerve paralysis, discussed earlier. Rarely, other concerns may be the scar itself, the hollow cavity secondary to removal of the gland, or potential difficulty with heavy pierced earrings in an anesthetic earlobe. Careful realignment of the incision, especially placement of the earlobe, with good plastic surgical technique usually leads to a barely visible hairline scar. The rare keloid or hypertrophic scar may require further treatment, such as steroid injections or reexcision. If a highly noticeable hollow depression remains many months following surgery, a careful discussion of the risks of facial nerve injury, wound infection (especially if there was postoperative irradiation), masking recurrence, and likelihood of success should be included in the discussion of whether attempts should be made to improve this. This is unlikely to be an issue following superficial parotidectomy alone. Free abdominal dermis fat, rotated adjacent sternocleidomastoid muscle, and free muscle flaps have all been used to improve facial contour caused by a large soft-tissue defect in the parotid bed.[24]

Gustatory Sweating (Frey's Syndrome)

Frey's syndrome (gustatory sweating, or auriculotemporal syndrome) is postparotidectomy facial sweating and skin flushing while eating. It may also be seen in the distribution of the amputated greater auricular nerve or branches of the cervical nerves. Gustatory rhinorrhea has also been rarely reported. Symptoms usually occur months to a few years postoperatively, although a delay as long as 17 years has been reported.

Minor's starch/iodine test can be used to measure the extent of the gustatory sweating. The skin is painted with an iodine solution and allowed to dry, and starch powder is then dusted on. The patient then uses a sialagogue for a few minutes. Dark blue-black spots will appear where sweat has dissolved the starch powder, which reacts with the iodine.

The likely pathophysiology is aberrant regeneration of postganglionic secretomotor parasympathetic nerve fibers (originating in the otic ganglion) misdirected through severed axonal sheaths of postganglionic sympathetic fibers feeding the sweat glands. For Frey's syndrome, these sympathetic fibers are to the sweat glands of the skin in the dissected field, and for gustatory rhinorrhea, they are of the nasal mucous glands.

Such facial sweating can be documented in almost all patients using Minor's starch/iodine test and has been described in 30% to 65% of patients,[26,27] suggesting that the symptoms and signs are minor enough in many patients that they are either unaware of or not bothered by them. The majority of patients are clearly insufficiently symptomatic to choose medical intervention. When socially bothersome, however, an initial trial of applied antiperspirant once or a few times daily should be tried. Topical glycopyrrolate is another effective preparation, with a longer lasting effect from each application and few anticholinergic side-effects.[27]

Numerous surgical treatments have been proposed to improve the symptoms of Frey's syndrome, but reports generally are of few patients, and no procedure appears to have acquired wide acceptance. The basis for surgical treatment is either (1) to reduce parasympathetic innervation to the otic ganglion, from whence the postganglionic fibers misdirected to the sweat glands emerge; or (2) to place an autologous barrier between the skin sweat glands and deeper tissue. Tympanic neurectomy intends to interrupt the preganglionic parasympathetic fibers of the tympanic plexus, whose fibers then pass via the lesser petrosal nerve to the otic ganglion. Tympanic neurectomy has been reported to improve symptoms in about two thirds of patients. It is, however, difficult to section all such fibers via this approach because fibers in

the tympanic plexus may lie deeper within otic capsule bone or may run with the chorda tympani. Additional sectioning of the chorda would be expected to improve success at the price of loss of taste to the anterior two thirds of the tongue. The basis of subdermal placement of fascia lata, free or microvascular interposition of a dermal fat graft, and rotation of the sternocleidomastoid muscle is blocking access of regenerating fibers to the skin sweat glands. Few such procedures have been done, and reoperation risks injury to the facial nerve. Efforts to decrease the incidence of Frey's syndrome at the initial procedure are similarly based on presumably reducing access of regenerating fibers to the sweat glands. Maintaining a thick skin flap[28] and preserving the superficial musculoaponeurotic system[29-31] have both been suggested, with some documentation of success.

A preoperative discussion and supportive care are appropriate and usually sufficient to handle this sequela in most cases. If necessary, topical applications should be considered next, and only in severe cases should surgical options be considered. That few surgical corrective cases have been done, often with short follow-up reported, should be discussed, as should the potential complications of proposed surgical intervention.

Complications Related to Chewing

Slight difficulty chewing following parotidectomy is not uncommon and is the result of inflammation of the masseter muscle and subcondylar tissue near the temperomandibular joint. It is usually self-limited. Following radiation, however, trismus may become more severe. A simple mouth-opening stretching exercise that may prove helpful is pushing the thumb on the maxillary incisors and the middle finger on the mandibular incisors. Serial increase in the number of tongue depressors interposed between the upper and lower teeth similarly stretches the pterygoid muscles. Available, but expensive, are mechanical devices that accomplish the same with much greater leverage. In severe cases, consultation with an oral surgeon is advisable, and repeated lysis under anesthesia may be needed.

Recurrent Pleomorphic Adenoma

Prevention of recurrence of pleomorphic adenoma lies in complete removal of the tumor with a cuff of normal tissue at the time of the initial surgical procedure. When properly done without tumor spillage or capsular dissection, the incidence of recurrence appears to be less than 1% to 2%; with lesser procedures such as enucleation the incidence has been reported to be 30% and higher.[32-35] Recurrences usually occur years following initial surgery. Once recurrent, over 25% of pleomorphic adenomas will recur again, and usually at decreasing time intervals. Multicentricity is unusual initially but is common with recurrences.[36] For this reason a total parotidectomy should be the surgical procedure if surgery is elected. Fee et al[34] reported that 52% of such patients sustained temporary weakness and 8% permanent weakness of

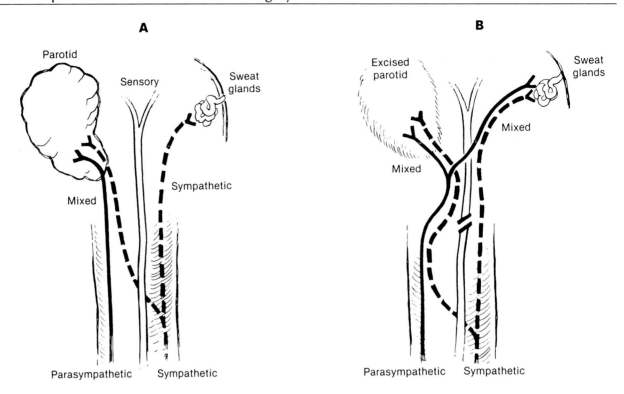

Figure 13-4.   Proposed mechanism of gustatory sweating. **(A)**. Normal. **(B)**. Frey's syndrome.

greater than 20% of the face. Conley and Clairmont[35] similarly reported 57% with some facial weakness when the facial nerve was dissected. Facial nerve monitoring is likely to reduce the increased incidence of transient or permanent facial paralysis. If surgery is elected, the facial nerve must be sacrificed as part of a radical parotidectomy in about 14% of cases to remove the tumor.[35]

Because of this risk to the facial nerve, especially if radical parotidectomy appears to be the indicated surgical procedure, a second option is irradiation. Dawson[37] has reported success in treating recurrent pleomorphic adenoma with radiation therapy. Others have added irradiation when there was tumor spillage or capsular disruption at the initial procedure.[38] The potential benefit of irradiation in avoiding iatrogenic facial nerve injury and reducing the incidence of subsequent tumor recurrence must be weighed against the known risk, albeit low, of subsequent radiation-induced tumors.

A third option to be considered is observation. An FNA is probably indicated if this option is considered, to be as sure as possible that the diagnosis is not carcinoma-ex-pleomorphic adenoma. Atypicality in the FNA requires careful comminication between cytopathologist and surgeon. MRI may be helpful to delineate the extent and multicentricity of the recurrence. MRI often helps the surgeon judge how high the potential surgical risk to the facial nerve is. If benign recurrent tumor is documented and the surgical risk to the facial nerve, as explained by the surgeon, is judged by the patient to be too high, he or she may opt (at least for the present) for a nonsurgical option. Subsequent events, such as the rate of growth of the recurrent tumor or local symptoms, may cause the physician and patient to reassess.

The management of recurrent pleomorphic adenoma requires judgment by and communication between doctor and patient. The age, health, occupation, and desires of the patient are important considerations. Tumor considerations, including multicentricity, extent of tumor, and its rate of growth, may affect the surgeon's assessment of the surgical risk to the facial nerve. Radiation may be considered to control tumor and prevent facial nerve injury. If only partially successful, at least it may have put off surgery, allowing the patient more time with normal facial movement. In the future, knowledge of the genetics of pleomorphic adenoma may affect the clinical decision of whether to add irradiation. Observation—aware of the risk of carcinoma-ex-pleomorphic adenoma and of eventual more extensive surgery—may often appear most appropriate. Clearly, this is a difficult decision which must be individualized for each patient and reassessed as the clinical situation changes.

Accumulating cytogenetic evidence suggests that there are three main cytogenetic subtypes of salivary gland pleomorphic adenomas that are distinguishable clinically and that may represent different etiologic entities.[38-44] These three groups show, respectively, no karyotypic abnormality, a break point at 8q12, and breakpoints at 12q13-15. The 8q12 group, for instance, was much younger than the normal karyotype group (39 vs 51 yo), and atypical histology was rarely seen in the normal group and not seen in the 12q13-15 group.[39] As the correlation between the cytogenetic differences and clinical course of pleomorphic adenoma strengthens, it may become appropriate to investigate whether a particular subgroup would benefit from radiation therapy initially or for recurrences.

Recurrent Malignant Tumor

Kaplan and Johns[45] updated Johns's earlier critical review of prognostic variables affecting management. Key factors affecting recurrence and survival included stage, histology, lymph node metastases and distant metastases, and local extension (including skin involvement and facial paralysis). Radiation therapy has been well documented to reduce recurrences and improve survival, and in selected cases high-LET (linear energy transfer) irradiation appears to have a role. Based on that review and using the 1988 American Joint Committee on Cancer staging system, we summarized principles of treatment for salivary gland malignancies as shown in Table 13–2.

Even when surgical resection has been adequate and appropriate postoperative irradiation is done, recurrences are common. Although properly not a postoperative complication, recurrent tumor is usually the single most serious adverse event following salivary gland surgery. Larger size, local extension (facial paralysis and skin or muscle extension), high-grade tumors, and positive nodes are tumor-related predisposing factors. Recurrence rates are less than 15% in small, low-grade mucoepidermoid carcinomas and acinic cell carcinoma; and they are between 40% and 70% for such high-grade tumors as adenoid cystic carcinoma, adenocarcinoma, undifferentiated carcinoma, and carcinoma-ex-pleomorphic adenoma (see ref 45 for a more thorough discussion). Long-term follow-up (10 to 20 years) is necessary because recurrences may appear many years following initial presentation.

Life expectancy is markedly reduced following recurrence of malignant tumor. Kagan,[46] reviewing 109 recurrences in 56 patients, found a 3.7-year median survival from the time of first recurrence. Five-year survival is reported between 15% and 50%.

An in-depth discussion of treatment of recurrent disease is beyond the scope of this chapter. Surgical re-resection (with likely facial nerve sacrifice) may at times be possible. Resection of a solitary pulmonary metastasis of adenoid cystic carcinoma should be considered if there appears to be local control in the parotid. Irradiation or reirradiation with high LET should be considered.[50] Among the roughly 320 patients with recurrent or inoperable salivary gland malignancies treated in this manner, including a prospective randomized trial,[51] the local control rate has been 67% versus 17% to 25% using conventional irradiation with photons and electrons.[52-56] The role of chemotherapy is uncertain,[57] although complete response rates of 10% have been reported for adenoid cystic carcinoma using adriamycin, 5-fluorouracil, and cisplatin.

SUMMARY

Prevention of complications from salivary gland surgery begins with a thorough understanding of the pathophysiology of inflammatory and infectious processes and the management principles for the benign and malignant tumors which affect these glands. Familiarity with the potential role of diagnostic and evaluation aids—notably FNA and MRI—is especially helpful when the diagnosis is uncertain or a likely malignant tumor is large. Superficial parotidectomy, total parotidectomy, and submandibular gland excision are surgical procedures that can be done with low morbidity when the surgeon is experienced in the various ways to prevent nerve injury. Wound infections are unusual. Most perioperative complications are appropriately and successfully managed conservatively. Eye protection is key in transient facial nerve paresis. When there is no preoperative paresis, permanent facial paralysis should be distinctly uncommon. However, it will sometimes occur, even with electromyographic nerve monitoring, when surgery is done for recurrent disease or

Table 13–2. Management Principles for Treatment of Salivary Gland Malignancies

STAGE/HISTOLOGY	I, LOW GRADE (0–4 cm, no local extension)	I, HIGH GRADE	II–IV w/N0M0 (local extension and/or >4 cm)	ANY T, N1–3 (positive nodes)
Surgical procedure (extent of parotidectomy)	Superficial (partial) or total as needed)	Superficial (partial) or total as needed	To fit disease: may require mastoid tip, mandible, muscles	To fit disease
(If submandibular tumor:)	Submandibular triangle resection	Wide excision submandibular triangle	Supraomohyoid neck dissection is likely; skin, muscles to fit disease	Radical or modified radical neck dissection; skin, muscles to fit disease
VII nerve Submandibular: V, XII	Preserve	Preserve	Preserve functioning branches if possible*	Preserve functioning branches if possible*
Neck dissection	No	No†	No†	Yes
Postoperative RT (4 Mev)	No, unless positive margins	Yes	Yes‡	Yes‡

From Kaplan and Johns.[45]

*Resected VII branches requiring reconstruction should be reconstructed immediately, usually with a cable graft.

†If positive nodes are found at surgery, neck dissection is indicated. In SCC, some would include a neck dissection; others would not because postoperative RT is included.

‡High-LET radiation should be considered when there are macroscopic positive margins, in unresectable tumors, and for previously irradiated tumors.

chronic inflammation; and it may be appropriate to sacrifice branches of the facial nerve (or V or XII) for some malignant tumors. Familiarity with the various options for more permanent eye protection and for facial reanimation is crucial to limit the potentially debilitating functional and esthetic consequences of these neurological deficits. Finally, the surgeon well versed in the evaluation, surgery, and care of patients with salivary gland disorders must be able to counsel and reassure effectively without minimizing or exaggerating the risks of various options.

REFERENCES

1. Cross RR, Shapiro MD, Som PM. MRI of the parapharyngeal space. *Radiol Clin North Am* 1989;27:353-378.
2. Som PM, Sacher M, Stollman AL, Biller HF, Lawson W. Common tumors of the parapharyngeal space: Refined imaging diagnosis. *Radiology.* 1988;169:81-85.
3. Swartz JD, Rothman MI, Marlowe FI, Berger AS. MR imaging of parotid lesions: Attempts at histopatholic differentiation. *J Comp Assist Tomogr.* 1989;13:789-796.
4. Som PM, Biller HF. High-grade malignancies of the parotid gland: Identification with MR imaging. *Radiology.* 1989;173:823-826.
5. Byrne MN, Spector JG, Garvin CF, Gado MH. Preoperative assessment of parotid masses: A comparative evaluation of radiologic techniques to histopathologic diagnosis. *Laryngoscope.* 1989;99:284-292.
6. Abele JS, Miller TR, Knoll R. Fine needle aspiration diagnosis of salivary glands. In Abele JS, Miller TR, eds. *Seventh Annual Symposium on Fine Needle Aspiration.* San Francisco: University of California; 1987.
7. Frable WJ. *Thin Needle Aspiration Biopsy.* Philadelphia: WB Saunders; 1983.
8. Frable MAS, Frable WJ. Fine-needle aspiration biopsy of salivary gland lesions. *Laryngoscope.* 1991;101:245-249.
9. Shaha AR, Weber C, DiMaio T, et al. Needle aspiration biopsy in salivary gland lesions. *Am J Surg.* 1990;160:373-376.
10. Cohen MB, Ljung BM, Boles R. Salivary gland tumors. Fine-needle aspiration vs frozen-section diagnosis. *Arch Otolaryngol Head Neck Surg.* 1986;112:867-869.
11. Layfield LJ, Tan P, Glasgow BJ. Fine needle aspiration salivary glands: Comparison with frozen sections and histologic findings. *Arch Pathol Lab Med.* 1987;111:346.
12. Cohen MB, Fisher PE, Holly EA, Ljung B-M, Lowhagen T, Bottles K. Fine needle aspiration biopsy diagnosis of mucoepidermoid carcinoma. Statistical analysis. *Acta Cytol.* 1990;34:43.
13. Qizilbash AH, Siamos J, Young JEM, Archibald SD. Fine needle aspiration biopsy cytology of major salivary glands. *Acta Cytol.* 1985;29:503.
14. Nettle WJ, Orrell SR. Fine needle aspiration in the diagnosis of salivary gland lesions. *Aust N Z J Surg.* 1989;59:47.
15. Jayaram N, Ashin D, Raajwanshi A, Radhika S, Banerjee CK. The value of fine-needle aspiration biopsy in the cytodiagnosis of salivary gland lesions. *Diag Cytopathol.* 1989;5:439.
16. Ferrucci JT Jr, Wittenberg J, Margolies MN. Malignant seeding of the tract after thin needle aspiration biopsy. *Radiology.* 1979;130:345.
17. Sinner WN, Zajicek, J. Implantation metastasis after percutaneous transthoracic needle aspiration biopsy. *Acta Radiol Diagn.* 1976;17:473.
18. Olsen KD, Daube JR. Intraoperative monitoring of the facial nerve: an aid in the management of parotid gland recurrent pleomorphic adenomas. *Laryngoscope.* 1994;104:229-232.
19. Hobsley M. Amputation neuroma of the greater auricular nerve after parotidectomy. *Br J Surg.* 1972;59:735-736.
20. Wax M, Tarshis L. Post-parotidectomy fistula. *J Otolaryngol.* 1991;20:10-13.
21. Talmi YP, Finkelstein Y, Zohar Y. Reduction of salivary flow with transdermal scopolamine: A four-year experience. *Otolaryngol Head Neck Surg.* 1990;103:615-618.
22. Johnson JT, Wagner RT. Infection following uncontaminated head and neck surgery. *Arch Otolaryngol Head Neck Surg.* 1987;113:368-369.
23. Platt R, Zalenik DF, Hopkins CC. Perioperative antibiotic prophylaxis for herniorrhaphy and breast surgery. *New Engl J Med.* 1990;332:153-160.
24. Nosan DK, Ochi JW, Davidson TM. Preservation of facial contour during parotidectomy. *Otolaryngol Head Neck Surg.* 1991;104:293-298.
25. Boddie AW, Guillamondegui OM, Byers RM. Gustatory rhinorrhea developing after radical parotidectomy—a new syndrome. *Arch Otolaryngol.* 1976;102:248-250.
26. Gordon AB, Fiddian RV. Frey's syndrome after parotid surgery. *Am J Surg.* 1976;132:54-58.
27. Hays LL, Novack AJ, Worsham JC. The Frey's syndrome: A simple, effective treatment. *Otolaryngol Head Neck Surg.* 1982;90:419-425.
28. Singleton CT, Cassisi NJ. Frey's syndrome: Incidence related to skin flap thickness in parotidectomy. *Laryngoscope.* 1980;90:1636-1639.
29. Casler JD, Conley J. Sternocleidomastoid muscle transfer and superficial musculoaponeurotic system application in the prevention of Frey's syndrome. *Laryngoscope.* 1991;101:95-100.
30. Yu LT, Hamilton R. Frey's syndrome: Prevention with conservative parotidectomy and superficial musculoaponeurotic system preservation. *Ann Plas Surg.* 1992;29:217-222.
31. Bonanno PC, Casson PR. Frey's syndrome: A preventable phenomenon. *Plas Reconstr Surg.* 1992;89:452-456.
32. Grage BG, Lober PH, Shahon DB. Benign tumors of the major salivary glands. *Surgery.* 1961;50:625.
33. Hanna DC, et al. Management of recurrent salivary gland tumors. *Am J Surg.* 1976;132:453-458.
34. Fee WE Jr, Goffinet DR, Calcaterra TC. Recurrent mixed tumors of the parotid gland—results of surgical therapy. *Laryngoscope.* 1978;88:265-273.
35. Conley J, Clairmont AA. Facial nerve in recurrent benign pleomorphic adenoma. *Arch Otolaryngol.* 1979;105:247-251.
36. Conley J. Problems with reoperation of the parotid gland and facial nerve. *Otolaryngol Head Neck Surg.* 99:480-488, 1988;99:480-488.
37. Dawson AK. Radiation therapy. *Int J Radiat Oncol Biol Phys.* 1989;16:819-821.
38. Samson MJ, Metson R, Wang CC, et al. Preservation of the facial nerve in the management of recurrent pleomorphic adenoma. *Laryngoscope.* 1991;101:1060-1062.
39. Bullerdiek J, Wobst G, Meyer-Bolte K, et al. Cytogenetic subtyping of 220 salivary gland pleomorphic adenomas: Correlation to occurrence, histological subtype, and in vitro cellular behavior. *Cancer Gen Cytogen.* 1993;65:27-31.
40. Kazmierczak B, Thode B, Bartnitzke S, Bullerdiek J, Schloot W. Pleomorphic adenoma cells vary in their susceptibility to SV40 transformation depending on the initial karyotype. *Genes, Chromosomes Cancer.* 1992;5:35-39.
41. Sahlin P, Mark J, Stenman G. INT1 and GLI genes are not rearranged or amplified in benign pleomorphic adenomas with chromosome abnormalities of 12q13-15. *Cancer Gen Cytogen.* 1992;58:85-88.
42. Sreekantaiah C, Sandberg AA. Clustering of aberrations to specific chromosome regions in benign neoplasms. *Int J Cancer.* 1991;48:194-198.

43. Rommel B, Bullerdiek J, Bartnitzke S, Schloot W. No rearrangement of c-mos in salivary gland pleomorphic adenomas with 8q12 aberrations. *Cancer Gen Cytogen.* 1990;49:165–169.
44. Sandros J, Stenman G, Mark J. Cytogenetic and molecular observations in human and experimental salivary gland tumors [see comments]. *Cancer Gen Cytogen.* 1990;44:153–167.
45. Kaplan MJ, Johns ME. Malignant neoplasms. In: Cummings et al, eds. *Otolaryngology—Head and Neck Surgery.* St. Louis, MO: Mosby, 1992;1043–1078.
46. Kagan AR, et al. Recurrences from malignant parotid salivary gland tumors. *Cancer.* 1976;37:2600–2604.
47. Rafla-Demetrious SR. *Mucous and Salivary Gland Tumors.* Springfield, IL: Charles C Thomas Publishers; 1970.
48. Hollander L, Cunningham MP. Management of cancer of the parotid gland. *Surg Clin North Am.* 1973;53:113.
49. Rodriquez-Bigas MA, et al. Recurrent malignant salivary gland neoplasms. *J Surg Oncol.* 1989;42:92–95.
50. Koh W, et al. Fast neutron radiation for inoperable and recurrent salivary gland cancers. *Am J Clin Oncol.* 1989;12:316–319.
51. Griffin TW, et al. Neutron vs photon irradiation of inoperable salivary gland tumors: Results of an RTOG-MRC cooperative randomized study. *In J Radiat Oncol Biol Phys.* 1988;15:1085–1090.
52. Batterman JJ, Mijnheer BJ. The Amsterdam fast neutron therapy project: A final report *Int J Radiat Oncol Biol Phys.* 1986;12:2093–2099.
53. Catterall M, Errington RD. The implications of improved treatment of malignant salivary gland tumors. *Int J Radiat Oncol Biol Phys.* 1987;13:1313–1318.
54. Saroja KR, et al. An update on malignant salivary gland tumors treated with neutrons at Fermilab. *Int J Radiat Oncol Biol Phys.* 1987;13:1319–1325.
55. Duncan W, Orr JA, Arnott SJ, Jack WJL. Neutron therapy for malignant tumors of the salivary glands—a report of the Edinburg experience. *Radiother Oncol.* 1987;8:97–104.
56. Griffin BR, et al. Fast neutron radiotherapy for advanced malignant salivary gland tumors. *Radiother Oncol.* 1988;12:105–111.
57. Kaplan MJ, Johns ME, Cantrell RW. Chemotherapy and radiation therapy for advanced salivary gland tumors. *Otolaryngol Head Neck Surg.* 1986;95:165–170.

14 Complications of Thyroid and Parathyroid Surgery

Jesus E. Medina, M.D., F.A.C.S., Edgar M. Boyd, Jr., M.D.

The risk of complications of surgery of the thyroid and parathyroid glands varies depending on the extent of the operation (ie, lobectomy vs subtotal or total thyroidectomy). In general, however, complications of this type of surgery are rare, but when they occur they may be life threatening or cause the patient severe functional impairment. The risk of complications is usually greater when a reoperation is required.

INTRAOPERATIVE BLEEDING

Hemorrhage is a concern during any surgical procedure; however, bleeding to any extent is not desirable during thyroid and especially during parathyroid surgery. Blood in the operative field increases the probability of injuring the recurrent laryngeal nerve; in addition, the resulting tissue staining makes it more difficult to identify the parathyroid glands.

It is therefore wise to avoid or to identify and ligate potential sources of bleeding that are obvious, such as the vein or veins in the suprasternal space of Lewis, the anterior jugular veins, the thyroid ima, and the middle thyroid veins. The next potentially troublesome spot in the course of a thyroidectomy is usually the area of the superior pole of the thyroid. Adequate exposure and careful ligation of individual vessels is paramount to avoid bleeding in this area; to improve exposure, it may be necessary to divide the sternothyroid muscle near its superior insertion. Next, bleeding can occur in the process of preserving the parathyroid glands. More often than not, small, thin-walled vessels need to be divided close to the parathyroid or as they enter the thyroid capsule. These vessels are easily torn when divided between clamps or during tying; thus, it may be preferable to isolate them gently, pass fine ligatures around them, tie the ligatures, and then divide the vessel between them. Finally, as the thyroid lobe is mobilized medially and before it can be removed, profuse bleeding can occur from small branches of the inferior thyroid artery, which course medial to the recurrent laryngeal nerve, in the area of the suspensory ligament of Berry. The proximity to the nerve usually precludes the use of electrocautery, and clamping may be cumbersome because of the proximity or adherence of the thyroid to the trachea. Clamping and ligation of these vessels can be facilitated by dividing the thyroid isthmus and dissecting the lobe off the trachea in a lateral direction. With the recurrent laryngeal nerve exposed and the lobe retracted anteriorly, clamps can be applied easily through the ligament of Berry's area.

POSTOPERATIVE BLEEDING AND SEROMA

Postoperative bleeding occurs after less than 2% of all thyroidectomies.[1,2] Small or moderate-size collections of blood in the wound are usually inconsequential; however, large hematomas can be life threatening due to airway compromise. A hematoma, contained under pressure by the strap muscles, can compress the trachea; furthermore, it has been postulated that the resulting increase in venous pressure produces laryngeal edema and airway obstruction.

Postoperative bleeding may result from faulty intraoperative hemostasis or from increased venous pressure caused by coughing or gagging prior to or after extubation.

Neither drains nor bulky dressings prevent hematomas. In fact, the latter may delay the diagnosis of a condition in which early recognition and immediate treatment is critical.[3]

Once the presence of a hematoma is recognized, the wound should be explored immediately in the operating room. If a delay is anticipated or there is any question about airway jeopardy, the skin incision and the closure of the strap muscles should be opened at the bedside, and the hematoma should be evacuated. The patient should then be returned to the operating room, as soon as possible, to control the bleeding.

Personal experience indicates that seromas occur more often when the thyroidectomy wound is not drained. As with hematomas, bulky dressing are of no benefit in the prevention of wound seromas. Seromas can usually be managed without surgical intervention. If the seroma is small, it may reabsorb over a period of several days. However, this may lead to the development of scar tissue and fibrosis. It is preferable to aspirate a seroma under sterile conditions. The seroma may recur, requiring repeated aspiration. If multiple aspirations are needed or if the seroma is large, it is necessary

184

to insert a drain and connect it to a closed-suction drainage system. This lessens the likelihood of bacterial contamination from the skin through repeated aspirations. If the seroma becomes infected, a passive drainage system, such as a Penrose or other nonsuction drain, may be indicated.

INJURY TO THE RECURRENT LARYNGEAL NERVE

Partial or complete transaction of the recurrent laryngeal nerve should be rare in the absence of pathology that distorts the anatomy of the region or actually involves the nerve. Even experienced surgeons, however, report inadvertent injury to the nerve and permanent vocal cord paralysis in about 1% of the cases.[1,2] Therefore, it is fitting to reflect about avoiding inadvertent injury to the nerve, what to do when such an injury occurs and vocal cord paralysis is detected in the postoperative period, and what to do when accidental transaction of the nerve is discovered by the surgeon in the operating room.

Avoiding Injury to the Recurrent Laryngeal Nerve

To assist surgeons in identifying and preserving the recurrent laryngeal nerve, several methods of intraoperative electrophysiological monitoring of the laryngeal musculature have been described. Stimulation of the nerve can be monitored using an electrode placed endoscopically into the thyroarytenoid muscle.[4] A simpler method uses a disposable nerve stimulator to stimulate the alleged recurrent laryngeal nerve while an assistant palpates the arytenoid cartilage and the posterior cricoarytenoid muscle, noting the presence or absence of motion during the stimulation.[5] A more recent technique utilizes an endotracheal tube that has a circumferential electrode attached to it. If there is electrical activity in the laryngeal musculature, this will be sensed and an electromyographic signal will be elicited; this signal can be coupled with a sound signal to alert the surgeon.[6]

These techniques may be useful when peforming a reoperation in the area of the thyroid. It is neither practical nor cost-effective to utilize them routinely in primary thyroid or parathyroid surgery.

It cannot be overemphasized that the two elements of greatest importance in avoiding injury to the recurrent laryngeal nerve are a thorough knowledge of the anatomy of the region and a meticulous surgical technique. Although a detailed description of anatomy and surgical technique is beyond the scope of this chapter, the reader will find the following pointers useful in avoiding this complication:

1. Awareness of the possibility of an aberrant recurrent laryngeal nerve. The nerve on the right side has a nonrecurrent course in 0.2% to 0.4% of individuals.[7] Even though the literature commonly cites that a nonrecurrent inferior laryngeal nerve is not possible on the left side, this anomaly has been described in association with malformations of the aortic arch.[8] To avoid injuring a nonrecurrent nerve, it is best to begin mobilization of the thyroid lobe by dissecting along the internal jugular vein and the common carotid artery and then dissecting the loose areolar tissue medial to the carotid. If this dissection is carried out in a layer-by-layer manner, up to the level of the prevertebral fascia and before proceeding medially, a nonrecurrent nerve can be uncovered with relative ease. It will course medially and inferiorly, from its origin high in the vagus nerve and behind the carotid, toward the larynx.

2. The position of the recurrent laryngeal nerve is somewhat different on the right than it is on the left side. The course of the nerve between the thoracic inlet and the larynx is oblique, from lateral to medial, on the right side and vertical on the left. The nerve is more consistently located in the tracheoesophageal groove on the left side (77%) than on the right (65%). It is located lateral to the trachea in 33% of individuals on the right side and in 22% on the left.[9]

3. It is preferable to identify and expose the recurrent laryngeal nerve during thyroid and parathyroid surgery. Farrar[7] reported that when this is done, the incidence of injury to the nerve was 2.1% to 3.9% in comparison to 6% when the nerve is not routinely exposed.[10]

4. The inferior thyroid artery is not a reliable landmark for identification of the recurrent laryngeal nerve because of the numerous variations in the relationship between these two structures.[11] A more constant relationship exists between the inferior cornu of the thyroid cartilage and the recurrent laryngeal nerve, as it has been described eloquently by Wang.[12]

5. The nerve is at greatest risk of injury in the vicinity of the suspensory ligament of Berry. The nerve runs posterior to the ligament and then enters the larynx.

6. It is important to be aware of the possibility of thermal injury to the nerve by using electrocautery, monopolar or bipolar, in the vicinity of an uncovered nerve. Particular attention should be paid when mobilizing the upper pole before exposing the recurrent nerve. The loose areolar tissue medial to the upper pole allows for easy dissection down to the area of Berry's ligament, where bleeding can occur. The inattentive surgeon may think that the nerve is not close and cauterize the area, causing a thermal injury to the nerve.

Postoperative Vocal Cord Paralysis

If a unilateral vocal cord paralysis is detected after a thyroid or parathyroid operation, management depends on the surgeon's recollection of the operation and the patient's symptoms. If the surgeon knows that the nerve is intact and feels that the problem is neuropraxia, treatment may not be necessary as long as the patient is not symptomatic. It is likely that nerve function will return up to a year after the operation. On the other hand, if the patient has incapacitating aspiration (as is often the case in elderly individuals with vocal cord paralysis), the surgeon may be forced to medialize the cord a few days after surgery. This can be accomplished in the following ways:

1. *Injecting teflon.* Although this is a time-honored method of medializing the surface of a paralyzed cord, it is not desirable in this situation. For all practical purposes, a well-done injection of teflon is not easily reversible in the event that motility of the cord returns.[13] In addition, the teflon paste may no longer be comercially available.
2. *Injecting Gelfoam or collagen.* These materials provide temporary medialization.
3. *Performing a type I thyroplasty.* This can be done using local anesthesia, and it permits a more precise medialization of the cord and can be reversed at any time if the motility of the vocal cord returns.[14]

The patient with a bilateral vocal cord paralysis will typically present with varying degrees of inspiratory stridor and a normal or near-normal voice. Management will depend on the degree of respiratory embarrassment. If the patient is not in distress, a watchful trial of racemic epinephrine, intravenous steroids, or both may be appropriate. Minimizing mucosal edema caused by the endotracheal intubation may preclude further manipulation of the airway. It is more likely, however, that the patient will be in respiratory distress. The surgeon will then face the dilemma of whether to perform a tracheostomy immediately or to intubate the patient for several days. A tracheostomy through a fresh thyroidectomy wound is frought with the prospect of infection of a relatively extensive wound. This is of particular concern when paratracheal or upper mediastinal dissections are performed in conjunction with the thyroidectomy. The alternative—keeping the patient intubated for 3 to 5 days—seeks to allow the skin flaps to stick down and initial wound healing to take place. A tracheostomy performed then may be less likely to cause a serious infection.

If the paralysis of both vocal cords persists for several weeks, an attempt could be made to reinnervate the posterior cricoarytenoid muscle using a nerve-muscle pedicled graft (ie, the ansa hypoglossi and a small piece of the omohyoid muscle).[15] Because this technique does not interfere with any future spontaneous recovery of vocal cord motility, it can be utilized at any time. Unfortunately, it has not been successful in everyone's hands.

Management of a bilateral vocal paralysis that persists for 10 to 12 months is aimed at reestablishing the airway. This can be accomplished by performing an arytenoidectomy, lateralizing the vocal cord, or both. Currently, one of the preferred techniques of arytenoidectomy is endoscopic, utilizing the CO_2 laser.[16] However, an arytenoid can be removed using conventional laryngoscopy instruments or, openly, through a laryngofissure or a pharyngotomy approach.[17] The vocal cord is lateralized by placing a suture around the vocal process of the arytenoid and pulling the vocal cord laterally.[18] The patient should know that the success of any of these techniques, in terms of restoring the airway, is inversely proportional to the quality of the resulting voice. The better the airway, the breathier the resulting voice.

Management of the Severed Recurrent Laryngeal Nerve

If the nerve is accidentally severed during the operation, the surgeon faces the controversial decision of whether to anastomose the nerve. The recurrent laryngeal nerve innervates adductor and abductor laryngeal muscles. These components cannot be identified and anatomosed separately. Consequently, misdirection in axon regrowth can result in synkinesis of the laryngeal musculature due to simultaneous activation of antagonistic muscles. It has been observed that this causes bulging of the vocal cord, which may compromise the airway, and spasms of the adductor muscles, which produce voice spaticity.[19] On the other hand, Green and Ward recently reported a well-documented case in which reanatomosis of a recurrent laryneal nerve, sectioned during thyroidectomy, resulted in adequate glottic closure and a normal voice.[20] This controversy will likely be resolved as patients who undergo reanastomosis of the nerve are studied with modern laryngological techniques. In the meantime, it would make theoretical sense to reanastomose the nerve and sever, if possible, the posterior branch of it to eliminate reinnervation of the abductor muscles. An additional option consists of anastomosing the ansa hypoglossi to the distal end of the severed recurrent laryngeal nerve. This technique has been reported to restore tone and bulk to the ipsilateral laryngeal musculature and a normal voice.[21]

SUPERIOR LARYNGEAL NERVE INJURY

The true incidence of this complication is unknown because there is no simple objective method to diagnose it. Furthermore, injury to this nerve produces only subtle changes in voice quality. These changes may not be apparent to the patient unless he or she is a singer or a frequent public speaker and notices inability to produce high pitched sounds or easy fatigability of the voice. Given the vulnerability of the nerve caused by its proximity to the superior thyroid vascular pedicle, it is likely that injury to it occurs frequently.

The superior laryngeal nerve is usually located medially to the superior thyroid artery. However, Mooseman and DeWeese[22] noted that in 15% of individuals the nerve was adherent to the superior thyroid artery or its branches, and in 6% it was entrapped while looping around or between the arterial branches above the superior pole of the thyroid gland. To avoid inadvertent damage to the nerve, it is essential to expose adequately the upper pole of the thyroid and the superior thyroid vessels. This is facilitated by retracting and, if necessary, dividing the stemothyroid muscle.[23] Gentle retraction of the vascular pedicle allows visualization of the external branch of the superior laryngeal nerve as it courses along the surface of the cricothyroid muscle and enters it. Cross-clamping the entire superior thyroid pedicle or indiscriminant use of electrocautery in this area should be avoided. It is preferable to ligate individual vessels close to the surgical capsule of the gland.

POSTOPERATIVE HYPOCALCEMIA

Hypocalcemia after thyroidectomy or parathyroidectomy may be caused by hypoparathyroidism or less frequently by the so-called bone hunger syndrome.

Hypoparathyroidism

Hypoparathyroidism is one of the most common and most dreaded complications of thyroid and parathyroid surgery. It can result from either inadvertent surgical removal of the parathyroid glands or from compromising their vascular supply. Fortunately, in most instances postoperative hypoparathyroidism is a temporary condition. When it is permanent, however, it cannot be cured at the present time; thus, the patient is committed to lifelong symptomatic treatment with calcium, vitamin D, or both. To avoid this complication, the surgeon must make every effort to preserve one or more viable parathyroid glands, particularly in the course of performing a total or a subtotal thyroidectomy.

Location of the Superior Parathyroids

Knowledge of the anatomy and embryology of the parathyroids is essential to identify them at the time of surgery. The superior parathyroids are derived from the fourth branchial arch. They are usually situated cephalad to the crossing point between the recurrent laryngeal nerve and the inferior thyroid artery. According to Wang,[24] who has performed one of the most extensive anatomic dissection studies of the parathyroids, the superior parathyroid glands are found most commonly (77%) at the level of the cricothyroid junction posteriorly, where they are in close proximity to and occasionally hidden by the recurrent laryngeal nerve and the adjacent vessels. Twenty-two percent of the superior parathyroid glands are located behind the superior pole of the thyroid gland and invariably beneath the thyroid capsule. The remaining 1% of the superior parathyroid glands are found encased in fatty tissue behind the pharynx or the cervical esophagus (Fig. 14–1A and 14–1B).

Location of the Inferior Parathyroids

The inferior parathyroid glands are derived from the third branchial arch and are, in general, situated more anteriorly than the upper parathyroids. They are usually found on the posterior lateral surface of the lower pole of the thyroid, anterior and medial to the recurrent laryngeal nerve (42%).[10] Thirty-nine percent of the inferior parathyroid glands are found in the lower neck or the thoracic inlet, within the thyrothymic ligament. Less common locations include the fibrofatty tissues lateral to the lower pole of the thyroid (15%)

and the mediastinal thymus (6%). Other possible locations are within the carotid sheath, the posterior mediastinum, or the thyroid gland.

Avoiding Injury to the Parathyroids

When performing a subtotal or a total thyroidectomy for a unilateral tumor, the surgeon's main concern during the removal of the opposite lobe should be to identify the parathyroids and preserve their vascular supply. To this end, meticulous bloodless technique is imperative and the use of magnifying glasses may be helpful.

After dividing the middle thyroid vein, which facilitates medial rotation of the thyroid lobe, an attempt should be made to identify the parathyroids. This is done before ligating the upper pole vessels or the inferior thyroid artery. Likewise, no initial attempt is made to identify the recurrent laryngeal nerve. This will ensure preservation of the blood supply of the parathyroids, which is derived most often from the inferior thyroid artery. Preservation of the blood supply can be accomplished by direct visualization and dissection of the supplying vessels or by ligating the branches of the inferior and superior thyroid arteries close to the thyroid capsule instead of ligating the main vessels proximally. As the vessels and the parathyroids are dissected away from the thyroid, the recurrent laryngeal nerve is identified.

If the vascular pedicle of a parathyroid is compromised and the color of the parathyroid turns gray or blue, it should be removed. A small portion of it is submitted for frozen section to confirm that it is a parathyroid. The remainder of the gland is minced into tiny pieces and autotransplanted into the sternocleidomastoid muscle or a muscle in the forearm.

Incidence of Hypoparathyroidism

The incidence of hypoparathyroidism varies depending on the experience of the surgeon, the extent of surgery, and whether transient and permanent disorders are separated in the report. The incidence of hypoparathyroidism reported by community hospitals in which surgery is performed by several surgeons with varying degrees of experience is higher than that of centers with specialized teams in thyroid and parathyroid surgery.[25] Permanent hypocalcemia following treatment of primary hyperparathyroidism is higher (37%) when a subtotal parathyroidectomy is performed than when only enlarged glands are removed (1.2%).[26] The reported incidence of hypoparathyroidism after total and subtotal thyroidectomy varies from 0.6% to 40%.[27,28] A reasonable estimate by Waldstein is that transient hypoparathyroidism occurs in 3% to 5% and permanent hypoparathyroidism in 1% to 2% of total thyroidectomies.

There is also a wide variance in the reported incidence of hypoparathyroidism depending on whether diagnosis is made on clinical grounds or based on determinations of total serum calcium levels, ionized calcium, or parathyroid hormone levels.

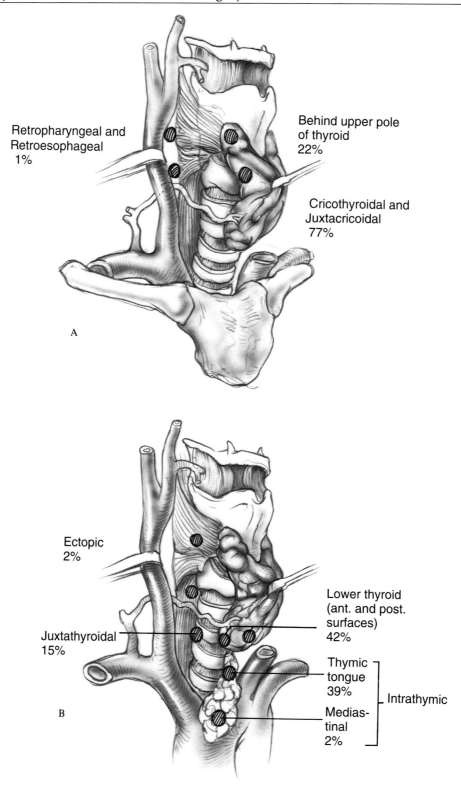

Figure 14–1. **(A).** The most common locations of the superior parathyroid glands. **(B).** The most common locations of the inferior parathyroid glands.

Management of Hypoparathyroidism/Hypocalemia

Awareness of the basic concepts of parathyroid physiology and calcium metabolism facilitates understanding of the principles of treatment of hypoparathyroidism. Calcium exists in three forms in the serum and other body fluids: (1) ionized or free calcium, (2) calcium complexed with organic acids, and (3) protein-bound calcium. The free and complexed calcium, also referred to as non-protein-bound or ultrafilterable calcium fraction, comprises 50% of the serum calcium.[29] The other 50% is protein bound. Ninety-five percent of the ultrafilterable fraction is in the form of free calcium, and the remaining 5% is in the form of complexed calcium. Only the free or ionized calcium is physiologically active. Determinations of total serum calcium often fail to reflect the level of ionized calcium levels, especially in patients with a changing serum albumin concentration, alkalosis, or acidosis. Consequently, determination of the serum level of ionized calcium is the most reliable way to monitor parathyroid function and to guide calcium replacement therapy following thyroidectomy or parathyroidectomy.

The parathyroid hormone (PTH) regulates the level of ionized calcium in the extracellular body fluids. When the level of ionized calcium decreases, secretion of PTH is stimulated. PTH, in turn, stimulates osteoclastic activity, which releases calcium and phosphorus into the extracellular fluids. PTH also increases the renal tubular reabsorption of calcium and magnesium. In addition, PTH increases the renal synthesis of calcitriol, the active form of vitamin D. As a result, the absorption of calcium in the intestine is indirectly stimulated by PTH.

Patients undergoing parathyroidectomy or total thyroidectomy should be closely observed for symptoms or signs of hypocalcemia. In addition, serum calcium levels should be checked every 12 to 24 hours. If hypocalcemia is detected, management will depend on whether the patient is symptomatic.

Symptomatic Hypocalcemia

Clinical manifestations of hypocalcemia may appear between 1 and 7 days after surgery. The symptoms and signs of hypocalcemia result from increased neuromuscular excitability caused by low levels of ionized calcium. The initial symptoms consist of perioral paresthesias, tingling of the extremities, and anxiety. At this stage, tetany can be induced by diagnostic maneuvers such as controlled hyperventilation, tapping the facial nerve over the stylomastoid area (Chvostek sign), or occluding the arterial blood supply to the arm for 3 minutes (Trousseau sign) (Fig. 14–2). If the hypocalcemia is not treated, the patient will develop potentially life-threatening manifestations, such as carpopedal spasm, tetany, seizures, and laryngeal spasm.

As soon as the patient becomes symptomatic, calcium should be given intravenously. Before doing this, it is advisable to obtain a blood sample for ionized calcium and phosphate levels. The calcium preparations available for

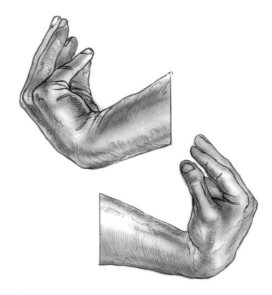

Figure 14–2. Trousseau's sign: Carpal spasm seen in patients with hypocalcemia after occlusion of the arterial supply to the arm as with a tourniquet or blood pressure cuff. It is typified by flexion of the hands at the wrists and of the fingers at the metacarpophalangeal joints and extension of the fingers at the phalangeal joints.

parenteral use and the appropriate dosages are outlined in Table 14–1. The advantages and disadvantages of these preparations are summarized in Table 14–2. Because most patients who become symptomatic will require calcium supplementation for a period of at least several weeks, oral calcium supplemments should be initiated as soon as it is feasible. The preparations commercially available, their elemental calcium content, and their dosage are shown in Tables 14–1 and 14–2.

If normal calcium levels cannot be maintained with the recommended doses of oral calcium, oral therapy with vitamin D is instituted. (See Table 14–1 for the appropriate preparations and doses.) The patient should be monitored closely for the possibility of vitamin D intoxication, and the dose of calcium and vitamin D should be adjusted on the basis of serum and urine calcium levels. In addition, it is desirable to decrease the serum levels of phosphorus because hyperphosphatemia depresses the serum calcium level. This can be accomplished by minimizing intake of foods high in phosphorus, such as dairy products and chocolate, and by administering aluminum hydroxide gel to bind dietary and intestinal phosphate and reduce its absorption.

Alternatively, Chlorthalidone, a thiazidelike diuretic, has been found effective in maintaining normal calcium levels without using vitamin D; it is used in combination with a low-sodium diet.[30]

Asymptomatic Hypocalcemias and Latent Hypoparathyroidism

It is common practice not to treat asymptomatic hypocalcemia in the early postoperative period. Although this may initially benefit the patient by stimulating recovery of parathyroid

Table 14–1. Calcium and Vitamin D Preparations for Parenteral and Oral Use

PREPARATION	ELEMENTAL CALCIUM	HOW SUPPLIED	DOSAGE
Parenteral Preparations			
10% calcium chloride	1.36 mEq per mL	10-mL vial 10-mL syringe	10 mL IV q 4–8 hours. Rate not more than 1 mL per minute.
Calcium lactate plus calcium glycerophosphate (Calphosan)	50 mg calcium lactate 50 mg calcium glycerophosphate	60-mL multidose vials	10 mL IM 1 to 4 timer per week
10% calcium gluconate	0.465 mEq per mL	10-mL vial 10-mL syringe	10 mL IV q 4–8 hours
Oral Preparations			
Oral calcium gluconate	2.3 mEq per 500 mg	500-mg tablets	1000–2000 mg per day
Oral calcium carbonate	40% elemental calcium	500-mg tablets	1000–2000 mg per day
Oral calcium lactate	13% elemental calcium	600-mg tablets	4 tablets prior to meals and at bedtime
Vitamin D_2 (Calciferol)		Drops 8000 U/mL. Injection 500,000 units/mL. Tablets 50,000 units per tablet.	25,000 to 50,000 units per day
Calcitriol (Rocaltrol)		0.25- and 0.5-μg tablets	0.5 to 1 μg per day
Calcifediol (Calderol)		20- and 50-μg tablets	50–100 μg per day

Table 14–2. Advantages and Disadvantages of Calcium and Vitamin D Preparations

PREPARATION	ADVANTAGES	DISADVANTAGES
Calcium chloride	Rapid correction of hypocalcemia	Irritating to tissues, cannot be injected IM, GI upset if given PO.
Calcium gluconate	Nonirritating to tissues, can be given IM, IV, or PO	IM form should not be used due to tissue necrosis.
Calcium glycerophosphate plus calcium lactate (Calphosan)	pH of 7. Injections are without pain, inflammatory response, or sloughing.	Cannot use if the patient is digitalized. Cannot use IM in infants and young children.
Oral calcium lactate	Contains twice as much calcium by weight compared to calcium carbonate	Less palatable than calcium carbonate. May not be commercially available.
Vitamin D_2 (Calciferol)	Inexpensive, effective for treating chronic hypocalcemia.	Slow onset of action. Prolonged half-life.
Calcitriol	Short onset of action	Expensive
Calcifediol	Short onset of action	Expensive

function, chronic hypocalcemia may eventually cause symptoms such as weakness, paresthesias, emotional instability, anxiety, or depression. Physical examination may reveal cataracts; trophic changes of the skin, nails, and hair; and sometimes Parkinsonism. This latent hypoparathyroid state may become more severe when calcium requirements are increased, such as during pregnancy. It can also be aggravated by anticonvulsant therapy (phenytoin and phenobarbital increase hepatic conversion of vitamin D into less active compounds), estrogen therapy (estrogens prevent bone resorption, and lower serum calcium), or steroids (decrease intestinal absorption, bone resorption and renal tubular absorption of calcium).

Treatment of latent hypoparathyroidism consists of administration of oral calcium supplements. If this does not correct the calcium and phosphorus levels, vitamin D, aluminum hydroxide, and possibly oral magnesium are begun. The preparations available are described in Tables 14–1 and 14–2.

In every case of hypoparathyroidism it is important to check thyroid function periodically. Hypothyroidism makes treatment of hypoparathyroidism less effective.

Bone Hunger Syndrome

This syndrome is characterized by postoperative hypocalcemia due to rapid absorption of calcium into demineralized bone in certain patients with hyperthyroidism and hyperparathyroidism. Patients with Grave's disease and hyperthyroidism have decreased gastrointestinal absorption of calcium. To maintain normal serum calcium levels, calcium is constantly resorbed from bone. After the thyroid is removed, hypo-calcemia will occur because calcium is rapidly taken up by the calcium-deficient/hungry bone. A similar phenomenon has been observed in patients with hyperparathyroidism who have preoperative radiological evidence of osteitis. Unlike patients in whom postoperative hypocalcemia is due to hypo-parathyroidism, patients with this syndrome will have low levels of serum phosphorus.

In addition to administering calcium intravenously and orally as needed to maintain normal serum levels, some of these patients also have deficits of magnesium, which will require replacement.

THYROTOXIC STORM

The syndrome of thyrotoxic storm or crisis is a rare, life-threatening complication of hyperthyroidism. It is a state of acute decompensation of the cardiovascular, gastrointestinal, hepatorenal, and central nervous systems in a thyrotoxic patient.[31] The incidence of thyrotoxic storm is reported to be only 1% to 2% of all hospitalizations for thyrotoxicosis; however, the reported rate of mortality ranges from 28% to 100%. The pathogenesis of thyrotoxic storm is not well understood. It appears to be caused by a combination of markedly elevated free thyroxine levels, decreased hepatic clearance of iodothyronines, and increased formation of iodothyronines triggered by a condition of medical, surgical, or dietary stress in a thyrotoxic patient. Thus, it is not unusual for the manifestations of a thyrotoxic storm to become apparent in the operating room or in the recovery room. The signs and symptoms of thyrotoxic storm are tachycardia, hyperthermia, diaphoresis, nausea, vomiting, tremor, extreme anxiety, altered mental status, and symptoms of congestive heart failure. If treatment is not instituted promptly and succesfully, the patient will progress to lethargy and coma. Fortunately, the majority of patients undergoing thyroid surgery today are euthyroid or are on thyroid suppressive medications.

Prevention of Thyrotoxic Storm

To prevent a perioperative thyroid storm, various combinations of medications may be utilized preoperatively to bring the patient as close to a euthyroid state as possible. Only in the event of a life-threatening emergency should a patient undergo surgery under general anesthesia without proper medical treatment of hyperthyroidism.[32] Preoperative treatment of hyperthyroid patients may include antithyroid drugs, organic iodine, beta-adrenergic blockers, and steroids.

The antithyroid drugs which may be utilized are propylthiouracil and methimazole. Propylthiouracil (PTU) is a member of the thioamide group of antithyroid drugs and may be considered as the prototype. The mechanism of action is the inhibition of the formation of thyroid hormone by interfering with the incorporation of iodine into tyrosyl residues of thyroglobulin. PTU also decreases the peripheral conversion of T_4 into the more metabolically active T_3 and inhibits the

coupling of the iodotyrosyl residues to form iodothyronines. Methimazole is a drug related to propylthiouracil which decreases the synthesis of thyroxine. The average onset of action for both of these drugs is 8 days. An average of 6 to 7 weeks of treatment is necessary to achieve a euthyroid state. The most common side-effect of these drugs is transient dermatitis, which is dose related. The most serious side-effect of this class of drug is agranulocytosis, which is not dose related.

Iodide administered orally (Lugol's solution) is effective in reducing the hyperplasia of the thyroid gland. In addition, it inhibits thyroid hormone synthesis and secretion. Iodine should be given for 7 to 10 days prior to surgery.

Beta-adrenergic receptor blockers are effective in controlling the peripheral manifestations of hyperthyroidism and thyrotoxic storm. The combination of propanolol 80 mg every 8 hours and potassium iodide 60 mg every 8 hours is effective in attenuating the cardiovascular manifestations of hyperthyroidism and in reducing the circulating plasma levels of T_3 and T_4.[33]

Corticosteroids given for 1 week before surgery have been shown to decrease secretion of thyroid-stimulating hormone (TSH), thus inhibiting thyroid function.[34]

Treatment of Thyrotoxic Storm

The treatment of thyrotoxic storm consists of various measures to return the body to a state of normal homeostasis. The specific therapy consists of sympatholytic drugs, corticosteroids, thionamides, and iodide. A patient in thyrotoxic storm has a markedly increased sympathetic tone. Propanolol has proven to be the drug of first choice in most instances of storm.[25] Propanolol may be given intravenously at a rate no faster than 1 mg per minute for a total dose of 2 to 10 mg.[25] The cardiac and psychomotor manifestations of storm are controlled within minutes when the drug is given intravenously, and the effects last several hours.

Hydrocortisone, administered intravenously in a dose of 100 to 300 mg, is highly effective in treating hyperpyrexia associated with thyroid storm.[25] Thyroid storm is not accompanied by an overt adrenal insufficiency, yet hydrocortisone results in prompt defervescence and reduction of toxicity, even when used alone.[25] Nevertheless, it is recommended that both hydrocortisone and propanolol be used concurrently in any patient when storm is overt.[25]

Sodium iodide in an intravenous dose of 1 to 2 g has a traditional and important role in thyroid storm. Although it is effective, it should not be relied on as the only form of therapy because of the greater potency of sympathetic blockade and steroid therapy.[25]

The administration of refrigerated intravenous fluids, placing the patient on a cooling blanket, or alcohol baths are beneficial in treating hyperthermia. With hyperthermia, the patient will have an increased oxygen demand, and appropriate measures should be taken to ensure that the patient remains well oxygenated.

Although the cardiac manifestations and other physiological abnormalities are best left to be treated by the anesthesiologist, the surgeon should be familiar with the signs, symptoms, and treatment of thyrotoxic storm.

Delayed Chronic Complications

The incidence of hypothyroidism is variable. Patients undergoing a total or subtotal thyroidectomy will become hypothyroid unless thyroid hormone is supplemented. Patients undergoing thyroid lobectomy become hypothyroid, particularly during periods of increased metabolism, such as pregnancy. This is also a common occurrence when hemithyroidectomy patients are treated with radiation therapy. Therefore, the surgeon should remain alert and inquire about symptoms suggestive of decreased thyroid function. Thyroid replacement is usually done with levothyroxine (Synthroid) at an initial dose of 0.1 mg per day. The final dose is adjusted on the basis of T_4, and TSH levels.

Although Synthroid is commonly thought of as a physiological form of thyroid hormone, it is actually a salt form of T_4, and prolonged use may have undesirable effects. Binodi et al, reported that long-term therapy with levothyroxine can affect cardiac function and is associated with an increased left ventricular hypertrophy rate, an increase in the average heart rate, and an increase in atrial premature contractions.[36] Furthermore, the left ventricular systolic function was enhanced with higher values of fractional shortening. In addition, it has been reported that long-term use of Synthroid in females under the age of 65, produces an increased risk of ischemic heart disease.[37] This is controversial, however. Petersen and Bengtsson have reported no side effects from long-term therapy in women.[38]

It is also thought that long-term Synthroid therapy may increase the risk of osteoporosis. However, two recent studies show that there is no change in the incidence of osteoporosis or its side-effects in women taking long-term Synthroid.[37,38] Cytomel has distinct advantages over Synthroid. Cytomel is the salt form of T_3 and has more metabolic activity than T_4. The onset of action with Cytomel can be detected in 4 to 6 hours, with a maximum response in 2 days or less.[39] The half-life of Cytomel is 2 days or less because it is less avidly bound to protein.[39] Synthroid is highly protein bound, with a half-life of 6 to 7 days.[39] Because of the shorter half-life, Cytomel has less potential for long-term side-effects than Synthroid. The shorter half-life may also be beneficial if the patient requires a thyroid scan, in that the clearance time for Cytomel is much less than for Synthroid. The recommended starting dose for Cytomel is 25 μg postoperatively per day. The daily dose may then be increased by 12.5 or 25 μg every 1 to 2 weeks. The usual maintenance dose is 25 to 75 μg daily. As with Synthroid, the final dose is suggested on the basis of T_4 and TSH levels.

Other Unusual Complications

Injury to the trachea or the esophagus during thryroidectomy is extremely rare.[35] If the trachea is entered in the course of a thyroidectomy, the tracheal defect is repaired primarily and the wound is drained adequately. This will prevent subcutaneous emphysema or pneumomediastinum in the event of an air leak. Likewise, if the esophagus is entered, a feeding tube is inserted, the esophageal wall is repaired properly, and the wound is drained. Pneumomediastinum and pneumothorax are also rare complications of thyroid or parathyroid surgery. They usually occur in the course of resecting extensive substernal goiters or during complicated parathyroid explorations. The key to a prompt institution of treatment is the surgeon's awareness of the possibility of these complications.

REFERENCES

1. Shemen L, Strong EW. Complications after total thyroidectomy. *Otolaryngol Head Neck Surg.* 1989;101:472–475.
2. Van Heerden JA, Groh MA, Grant CS. *Surgery.* 1987;101:224–227.
3. Wihlborg O, Bergljung L, Martenson H. To drain or not to drain in thyroid surgery. *Arch Surg.* 1988;13:40–41.
4. Lipton RJ, McCaffrey TV, Litchy WJ. Intraoperative electrophysiologic monitoring of laryngeal muscle during thyroid surgery. *Laryngoscope.* 1988;98:1292–1296.
5. Gavilan J, Gavilan C. Recurrent laryngeal nerve: Identification during thyroid and parathyroid surgery. *Arch Otolaryngol Head Neck Surg.* 1986;112:1286–1288.
6. Sercarz JA, Berke GS, Rothschiller J, Min Y. Fabrication of a custom electrode endotracheal tube. *Laryngoscope.* 1991;101:1024–1025.
7. Farrar WB. Complications of thyroidectomy. *Surg Clin North Am.* 1983;6:1353–1361.
8. Droulias V, Harlaftis S, Tzinas S, Gray SW, Akin JT. Recurrent laryngeal nerves. *Am Surg.* 1976;42:629–634.
9. Hunt PS. A reappraisal of the surgical anatomy of the thyroid and parathyroid glands. *Brit J Surg.* 1968;55:63–66.
10. Reeve, TS. The recurrent and external laryngeal nerves in thyroidectomy. *Med J Aust.* 1969;1:380–382.
11. Beahrs OH. Complications of surgery in the head and neck. *Surg Clin N Amer.* 1977;57:823–829.
12. Wang D. The use of the inferior comu of the thyroid cartilage in identifying the recurrent laryngeal nerve. *Surg Gynec Obst.* 1975;140:91–94.
13. Dedo H. Avoidance and treatment of complications of Teflon injection of the vocal cord. *J Voice.* 1988;2:90–92.
14. Isshiki N. Recent advances in phonosurgery. *Folia Phoniatr* 1980;32:119–130.
15. Tucker H. Laryngeal reinnervation for unilateral vocal cord paralysis. *Ann Otol Rhinol Laryngol.* 1981;90:457–459.
16. Eskew JR, Bailey BJ. Laser arytenoidectomy for bilateral vocal cord paralysis. *Head Neck Surg.* 1983;91:294–298.
17. Downey WL, Keenan WG. Laryngofissure approach for bilateral abductor paralysis. *Arch Otolaryngol.* 1968;88:513.
18. Kirchner F. Endoscopic lateralization of the vocal cord in abductor paralysis of the larynx. *Laryngoscope.* 1989;89:1179.
19. Crumley RL. Repair of the recurrent laryngeal nerve. *Otol Clin North Am.* 1990;23:553–563.
20. Green DC, Ward PH. The management of the divided recurrent laryngeal nerve. *Laryngoscope.* 1990;100:779–782.
21. Crumley RL. Voice quality following laryngeal reinnervation by ansa hypoglossi transfer. *Laryngoscope.* 1986;96:611–616.
22. Mooseman DA, DeWeese MS. The external laryngeal nerve as related to thyroidectomy. *Surg Gynec Obstec.* 1968;126:1011–1016.
23. Calderelli DD. Complications of thyroid surgery: Nonmetabolic complications. In: Falk SA, ed. *Thyroid Disease.* New York: Raven, 1990:599–607.

24. Wang C. The anatomic basis of thyroid surgery. *Ann Surg.* 1976;3:271–275.
25. Waldstein SS. Medical complications of thyroid surgery. *Otol Clin North Am.*
26. Bruining HA. *Surgical Treatment of Hyperparathyroidism: With an Analysis of 267 Cases.* Assen, The Netherlands: Royal Van Gorcum; 1971.
27. Clark OH. Total thyroidectomy. *Ann Surg.* 1982;196:361–367.
28. Herranz-Gonzales J, Gavilan J, Martinez J, Gavilan C. Complications following thyroid surgery. *Arch Otolaryngol Head Neck Surg.* 1991;117:516–518.
29. Falk, et al. Hypocalcemia. *Arch Otolaryngol Head Neck Surg.*
30. Porter RH. Treatment of hypoparathyroid patients with chlorthalidone. *N Eng J Med.* 1978;298:577–581.
31. Peele ME, Wartofsky L. Complications of thyroid surgery: Thyrotoxic storm. In: Falk SA, ed. *Thyroid Disease.* New York: Raven;1990;625–630.
32. Wu W, Choi JJ. General anesthesia in thyroid surgery. In: Falk SA, ed. *Thyroid Disease.* New York: Raven; 1990;571–584.
33. Feek CM, Sawyers SJ, Irvine WJ. Combination of potassium iodide and propanolol in preparation for thyroid surgery. *N Engl J Med.* 1980;302:883–885.
34. Wilbur JF, Tiger RD. The effect of glucocorticoids on thyrotropin secretion. *J Clin Invest.* 1969;48:2096–2103.
35. Guillamondegui OM. Surgery of the thyroid and parathyroid gland. In: Johns M, ed. *Complications in Otolaryngology—Head and Neck Surgery.* Philadelphia: BC Decker; 1986:180.
36. Binodi B, Fazio S, et al. Cardiac effects of longterm thyrotropin suppressive therapy with levothyroxine. *J Clin Endocrinol Metab.* 1993;77:334–338.
37. Leese GP, Jung RT, Guthrie C, et al. Morbidity in patients on L-thyroxine: A comparison of those with normal TSH to those with suppressed TSH. *Clin Endocrinol.* 1992;37:500–503.
38. Petersen K, Bengtsson C, Lapidus L, et al. Morbidity, mortality, and quality of life for patients treated with levothyroxine. *J Arch Int Med.* 1990;150:2077–2081.
39. Haynes RC. Meral. Thyroid and antithyroid drugs. In: Goodman, Gillman, eds. *The Pharmacological Basis of Therapeutics,* 7th ed. New York: Macmillan; 1985.
40. Rossi RL, Cady B. Surgical anatomy. In: Cady B, Rossi RL, eds. *Surgery of the Thyroid and Parathyroid Glands,* 3rd ed. Philadelphia: WB Saunders Co; 1991:26–27.

15 Complications of Radiotherapy for Head and Neck Neoplasms

James T. Parsons, M.D., William M. Mendenhall, M.D., Rodney R. Million, M.D.

The effects of irradiation on normal tissues usually are divided into (1) acute effects, which are present both during a course of irradiation and in the immediate postirradiation period, and (2) late effects, which become manifest months to years after treatment. Although patients are concerned mostly about acute side effects, clinicians mainly fear late sequelae because the latter may be chronic and progressive, as opposed to acute effects, which are self-limited.

The severity of acute effects generally does not predict the severity of late effects. A patient with moderate or severe acute side effects may not have late injury, whereas another with minimal acute reaction may develop severe late complications.

Radiotherapy regimens that employ a small number of large-dose fractions (eg, one or two fractions a week) are notable for producing mild acute reactions but severe late effects.

In general, tissues with rapidly dividing cell populations (eg, mucous membrane and skin epithelium) respond acutely, and those with slowly proliferating or nonproliferating cells (eg, connective tissue and spinal cord) are affected later.

Carcinomas tend to respond like rapidly proliferating normal tissues, so that radiotherapy regimens that produce few acute effects are usually less likely to cure the cancer.

There are two major schools of thought regarding the mechanism of late injury: One theory states that irradiation injury of the microvasculature is responsible; the other holds that late damage results from parenchymal or stromal cell death.[1]

ACUTE EFFECTS

Mucous Membranes

ORAL CAVITY, PHARYNX, AND LARYNX

With five 200-cGy fractions per week, mucosal erythema develops within 1 week. At about 2 weeks, the reddened mucous membrane develops small white patches, 2 to 3 mm in diameter, called mucositis or false membrane formation. Mucositis represents caking of dead surface epithelial cells, fibrin, and polymorphonuclear leukocytes on a moist background. Patients usually note a sore throat at 1½ to 2 weeks.

In many patients, the patches of mucositis become confluent by the third week.

Mucositis is sensitive to changes in daily dose of radiation. At 170 to 180 cGy five times weekly, the maximal reaction usually is only intense erythema, with an occasional patch of mucositis, even when large volumes are irradiated (eg, for cancer of the nasopharynx or advanced cancer of the oral cavity); in this situation, the cell killing and repopulation of mucous membrane stem cells are essentially in equilibrium. If the daily dose is more than 200 cGy and the treatment volume is large, cell killing exceeds the proliferative capacity of the mucous membrane stem cells; almost all patients develop confluent mucositis by the third week, which produces severe discomfort and often limits adequate nutrition. At the University of Florida, doses of 225 cGy per fraction are used only for very limited fields (eg, early vocal cord cancer).

The soft palate, tonsillar pillars, buccal mucosa, lateral border of the tongue, pharyngeal walls, and portions of the larynx readily develop mucositis. Other sites, such as the hard palate, gingival ridges, dorsum of the tongue, and true vocal cords, either develop no mucositis during treatment or develop it only after very high doses.[2] Coutard[3] noted that mucositis often first appears over the tumor itself, sometimes as early as 5 to 7 days into treatment (ie, a week before the appearance of mucositis over the normal mucous membranes). This early reaction is frequently dubbed tumoritis and is most often observed when treating carcinomas of the soft palate and anterior tonsillar pillar.

Sore throat is usually greatest 2½ to 3 weeks into therapy; thereafter, the pain may diminish, even though therapy is continued. While patients are under treatment, the mucous membranes should be examined at least weekly because the distribution of the mucosal reaction confirms adequate tumor coverage and acts as a biological dosimeter.

Patients with gold-crown dental restorations develop pronounced mucositis on the adjacent buccal mucosa and oral tongue, secondary to backscattered low-energy electrons. Because the range of these electrons is short, excessive mucositis can be prevented by placing a few millimeters of moistened gauze or paraffin between the mucosa and the teeth. During a course of radiation therapy that encompasses the oral cavity, the topical broad-spectrum antimicrobial chlorhexidine (15 mL, swish and gargle for 30 seconds, then expectorate, three to four times each day) is routinely prescribed and reduces the severity of oral mucositis.[4] The substance is bound to the mucosal surfaces and is slowly released. It is effective against anaerobic and aerobic bacteria as well as against *Candida*. Therapy is continued after irradiation until the soreness subsides. Chlorhexidine has little role in preventing mucositis in the larynx or hypopharynx because it must remain in contact with the mucosal surfaces to be effective.

The mucous membranes normally heal dramatically 2½ to 3 weeks after external-beam therapy, although occasionally patients require a longer time to heal. Until then, little change is obvious, either objectively or subjectively; the sore throat then suddenly subsides and improves rapidly over the next 2 to 3 days. After a month, the mucosa is healed in 90 to 95% of patients, and sore throat is absent or minimal.

The mucositis produced by a 7-day radium implant appears 7 to 10 days after removal, and is maximal about 2 weeks after removal. The reaction usually subsides by 6 weeks, unless the implanted volume was large, in which case complete healing sometimes requires several months.[5]

NASAL CAVITY

High-dose irradiation of the anterior nares produces a brisk mucosal reaction. The moist mucosal surfaces tend to adhere to each other during the healing phase; unless measures are taken to prevent formation of synechiae, stenosis of the anterior nares may occur within 1 or 2 months after treatment. Because of their rigid, bony framework, the surfaces of the posterior nares are not in apposition, and posterior stenosis does not occur. During the first month after treatment, patients are advised to pass a long, cotton-tipped applicator stick covered with petrolatum along the length of the nasal cavity and to douche the nasal cavity with a dilute saline solution (Fig. 15–1). Both procedures should be performed twice daily until healing is complete, after which the petrolatum may be discontinued if the patient desires. Regular douching is recommended indefinitely because this helps clear the crusts and debris that tend to collect on the dry membranes. If at the time of the first follow-up examination patients are already developing stenosis, the synechiae can usually be lysed with the use of topical anesthesia; patients then are asked to use the applicators more frequently and to return to the clinic on a weekly basis until the problem is resolved. If complete stenosis develops, surgical division is necessary.

Conjunctiva

During a course of ^{60}Co irradiation for cancer of the paranasal sinuses, patients typically develop mild or moderate symptoms of conjunctivitis (foreign-body sensation and occasionally photophobia) and lid irritation. Unless all of the lacrimal tissue have received a high dose, these symptoms resolve within 4 to 6 weeks after treatment.

Sense of Taste

Taste loss begins about 1 week into the course of irradiation and then progresses rapidly between 2000 and 4000 cGy. Salivary dysfunction precedes taste loss and, unlike taste loss, occurs without any apparent threshold.[7] Conger[8] suggests that taste loss is due to damage to the microvilli of the taste cells, and he has performed electron microscopic studies in mice that show loss of microvilli after irradiation. After therapy is finished, most patients report some improvement in taste acuity within 20 to 60 days.

Salivary Tissue

The major salivary glands account for 70% to 80% of the salivary flow; the remaining flow comes from minor salivary glands scattered throughout the mouth. Under resting conditions, the flow from the submandibular glands is at least as great as that from the parotid glands, or possibly greater;[9,10] the sublingual glands contribute only 2% to 5%.[11] Under conditions of stimulation (eg, eating or drinking), the parotid glands become the main contributors. In addition to decreased flow, irradiation produces an increase in salivary sodium concentration, a decrease in pH level, and an increase in oral yeast flora.[12,13] Clinical symptoms correlate with the amount of salivary tissue irradiated.

XEROSTOMIA

If only the submandibular and sublingual glands are treated, most patients note little subjective difference in their saliva; even in this setting, however, the salivary flow is altered so that dental caries becomes a problem and fluoride prophylaxis is necessary. If one or both parotid glands are irradiated along with the submandibular glands, the sensation of dryness is noted after only a few treatments. During a course of ^{60}Co irradiation, Mossman[7] noted 50% loss of flow in patients after 1000 cGy, followed by continual, but less rapid, loss as treatment progressed. If the parotid glands are irradiated and the submandibular glands are spared, moisture may be preserved.[10,11]

The saliva first becomes thick, sticky, and ropy. Continued use of tobacco and alcohol produces an additional drying effect. Patients are instructed to rinse and gargle with a salt-and-soda solution several times daily, both during the course of irradiation and until mucosal healing is complete. The solution consists of a teaspoon each of table salt and baking soda in a quart of water, and it serves to refresh the mouth, decrease the pain from mucositis, and loosen the thick, tenacious saliva. Commercial preparations of artificial saliva are available but few patients use them, often stating that the solutions have an unpleasant taste.

SIALADENITIS

Within 12 hours of the first treatment, about 5% of patients develop a transient, usually painless, enlargement of

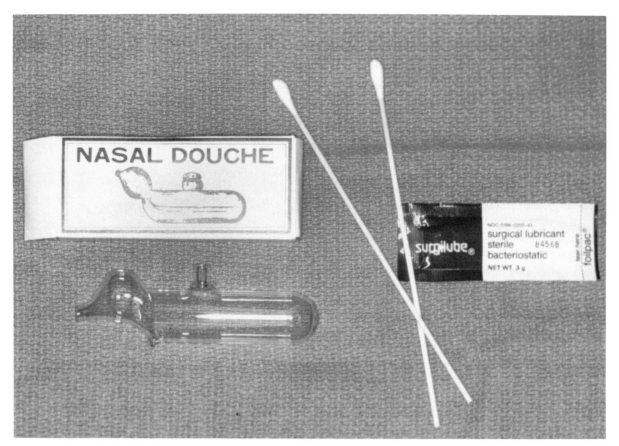

Figure 15–1. Nasal douche device and long cotton-tipped applicators used by patients after high-dose irradiation to the nose (from Parsons[6]).

one or more of the salivary glands within the treatment portal. Usually, symptoms are limited to a "tight" sensation. Systemic symptoms are minimal or nonexistent. Patients often are alarmed and call the physician just after eating, thinking that the cancer is growing rapidly in the neck. The swelling has been noted more frequently in the submandibular glands than in the parotid glands, but either may occur and one or both sides may be affected. The swelling usually disappears within 1 or 2 days despite continuation of treatment. Simultaneous with the swelling and its resolution is a rise and fall in the serum amylase level.[14] The physician should warn patients in advance. Patients are advised to drink plenty of water and to use sialagogues during the acute phase; antibiotics are not necessary.

Skin and Subcutaneous Tissues

In the orthovoltage era, treatment plans were dictated by the limits of skin tolerance. Today, the skin is rarely a major dose-limiting tissue. High-energy x-rays are skin-sparing; that is, the buildup characteristics of the absorbed dose are such that the skin receives a low dose relative to deeper structures. Skin-sparing is lost or reduced when tissue-equivalent material, called bolus, is placed on the skin; when the beam enters the body tangentially, rather than perpendicular to the skin surface; or when the lead blocks and blocking tray used to shape the x-ray fields are too close to patients. When tumor actually invades the skin and subcutaneous tissues, or when tumor cells have been seeded in surgical scars, skin-sparing is undesirable and steps are taken to ensure an adequate skin dose.

When parallel-opposed ^{60}Co fields are treated to tumor doses in the range of 7000 to 7500 cGy (five 180- to 200-cGy fractions per week), acute skin effects are limited to erythema, peeling, and tanning. Erythema often is noted first around hair follicles because the invaginations of epidermis receive a higher dose than cells on the skin surface; follicular erythema more often is seen in the lower neck fields than in the primary fields. Peeling (or dry desquamation) of the skin results from radiation killing of basal cells in the epidermis. Scales of skin (which are sometimes dark because radiation stimulates melanin production) result from caking of dead cells, a situation analogous to that seen on the mucous membranes (mucositis). As with a sunburn, patients note increased sensitivity to touch and complain of itching and drawing until healing is complete, 2 to 3 weeks after completion of therapy.

If the skin has been irradiated tangentially or with bolus, then the capacity of the basal cell layer to repopulate the epidermis may be exceeded and patients may develop areas of complete epidermal denudation, called moist desquamation, a medical euphemism for a radiation burn. The dermis is exposed and oozes serum. Although the appearance alarms physicians unfamiliar with the reaction, healing occurs spontaneously within 2 to 4 weeks, depending on the area involved and unless infection supervenes. Areas of moist desquamation should be kept clean; remove crusts by soaking with a dilute hydrogen peroxide solution. Gentian violet (1% aqueous solution) can be applied for its bactericidal and fungicidal properties as well as for the eschar that it forms. Reepithelialization occurs from the periphery of the field and, if the dose has not been too great, from single surviving cells in the middle of the field.[15] Such reactions are rarely encountered with the radiotherapy techniques used today. Epilation of the beard usually begins during the third week of treatment. Sweat and sebaceous glands cease to function.

LATE EFFECTS

Salivary Tissue

XEROSTOMIA

Xerostomia causes discomfort, alters taste acuity, contributes to deterioration of oral hygiene, and promotes dental decay. The remaining saliva has an altered electrolyte content and reduced pH level. Histologically, the heavily irradiated gland is obliterated and largely replaced by collagen.

Loss of salivary function is usually complete and permanent after doses higher than approximately 3500 cGy. In patients with extremely low flow rates before radiotherapy, lesser doses cause permanent dryness. Marks et al[16] found that only one fifth of patients whose parotid glands had received 4000 to 6000 cGy had any measurable parotid flow after salivary stimulation; above 6000 cGy, none of 24 parotid glands had measurable flow. Although occasional patients report improvement in the sensation of dryness several years after treatment, objective recovery of salivary flow has not been documented in such cases. If the salivary tissue received less than 3000 to 3500 cGy, often some function returns during the 6 months after therapy. Young patients are more likely than older patients to recover salivary flow. Minor changes in field size and shape may preserve some salivary flow.

The decrease in flow after irradiation follows an exponential decay curve. A certain dose reduces flow by about the same percentage, not by the same absolute amount, in two patients. A patient whose initial salivary flow rate is 0.2 mL/min would require a reduction of only 50% to reach a minimal flow rate (0.1 mL/min), whereas a patient whose flow rate is 1.0 mL/min would require a 90% reduction to reach the same level of flow. The latter patient would require about three times more irradiation than the former to reach 0.1 mL/min. Based on resting collections from all of the salivary glands, Mira et al[11] showed that during courses of irradiation that included almost all of the salivary tissue, 3500 to 4000 cGy was capable of inducing minimal flow (≤ 0.1 mL/min) in patients with high initial flow rates (0.9 to 1.5 mL/min); 500 to 1500 cGy resulted in minimal flow in patients with low (0.15 to 0.40 mL/min) initial flow rates.

Patients with significant xerostomia get some symptomatic relief by using one of the commercially available artificial saliva preparations. These solutions have a pH of about 7.0 and a consistency similar to saliva. Some patients carry a bottle of artificial saliva with them at all times, others use plain or flavored glycerin to lubricate their mouths, but most use water.

SIALADENITIS

Submandibular or parotid gland infection is sometimes seen after high-dose irradiation. Sometimes fever is present and patients may have marked pain and tenderness; in other patients the pain is intermittent. At the University of Florida, 6 of 419 patients who received high-dose, twice-a-day irradiation for cancers of the oral cavity, oropharynx, larynx, or hypopharynx developed sialadenitis at 1½, 2, 3, 4, 5, and 7 months postirradiation, respectively. Purulent debris could be easily expressed from Wharton's or Stensen's ducts in all patients. This complication probably is due to relative obstruction to flow in the heavily irradiated gland, inspissation of salivary secretions, and some degree of dehydration. Minimally syptomatic patients can be treated as outpatients with oral antibiotics, hydration, and sialagogues. Febrile or markedly symptomatic patients are treated with intravenous antibiotics. All six patients at the University of Florida responded to treatment, with resolution of symptoms over a period of several days to weeks.

Sense of Taste

Subjective recovery of preirradiation taste acuity is usually complete by 60 to 120 days after treatment.[8] Some patients state that their taste is never as sharp as before treatment, but it is usually adequate. Mossman et al[17] noted that many patients who have no subjective complaints of taste loss have measurable losses (most commonly for salt and bitter) when sophisticated testing is performed. On rare occasions, patients report little or no improvement for many months or years after treatment. At least part of this subjective loss is due to xerostomia, which itself affects taste acuity. Mossman and Henkin,[18] as well as Silverman and Thompson,[19] suggest that zinc therapy is useful in ameliorating symptoms in some patients whose sense of taste does not completely return to normal after therapy; the trials were not controlled and the tentative results require verification by other investigators.

Teeth

The pathologic changes that occur in the teeth secondary to irradiation are mainly due to diminished salivary flow, rather than being a direct effect on teeth or surrounding bone. The teeth are affected regardless of whether they are inside or outside of the radiation field. If the salivary glands are not irradiated, caries do not occur as a result of treatment.

During and immediately after treatment, patients have a sore throat and a dry, sticky mouth; they stop eating a rough diet and change to a soft, high-carbohydrate diet that has little detergent value and favors the growth of plaque. Patients have a tendency to stop routine dental care because the tissues are tender. In association with radiation-induced xerostomia, the normal oral microflora shifts markedly to a highly cariogenic microbial population.[20] Unless stringent measures are taken to protect the teeth, rampant dental caries begin to develop as early as 3 to 6 months after treatment and progress to complete destruction of all the teeth over a period of 3 to 5 years.

The histological character of radiation caries is similar to that of dental caries; the two lesions differ, however, in several important aspects. The lesions that develop after irradiation are more widespread; frequently a generalized attack on enamel occurs, beginning as fine, punctate defects that progress to larger lesions. Patients complain of hot-cold hypersensitivity and sensitivity to sweet foods.[21] Typical dental caries occur mainly on the proximal surfaces and fissures, sites not easily reached by saliva and therefore prone to food retention. The lesions induced by radiation, by contrast, occur mostly on the buccal, palatal, or lingual surfaces and on the incisal and occlusal edges of the teeth. Under normal circumstances, all of these surfaces are readily bathed by saliva[21] and are usually resistant to caries. The edges of the teeth may appear as though they have been finely sanded or filed; the concentric layers around the pulp sometimes are seen in cross section.[22]

As the late effects of radiation progress over several months, shrinkage of the periodontal tissues occurs, leading to exposure of cementum. Decay occurs at the exposed cervical portion of the tooth, usually beginning on the labial or buccal surfaces, then extending superficially around the neck of the tooth to produce an annular lesion that eventually results in complete amputation of the crown. The root remains in the alveolar cavity and is slowly eliminated.[22] Before irradiation, the dentulous patient should be evaluated by a dentist.

Masticatory Muscles and Temporomandibular Joint

High-dose irradiation to voluntary muscles may produce fibrosis, particularly when cancer has invaded and partially destroyed the muscles. Fibrosis of the muscles of mastication (temporalis, masseter, and pterygoid muscles) may cause trismus. Many patients with advanced cancer of the head and neck have trismus at the time of diagnosis, secondary to local tumor extension into the pterygoid musculature. This symptom may worsen in the postirradiation period if significant pterygoid muscle fibrosis develops. The temporomandibular joint itself is reasonably resistant to the ankylosis secondary to irradiation; the risk of injury increases if the joint has been invaded by tumor. The use of large daily fractions increases the risk of impairment of motion at the temporomandibular joint. Because no simple treatment of severe trismus exists, avoiding the problem is paramount. If severe trismus develops, dental extractions might be necessary to permit feeding.

Patients who have received both surgery and irradiation are at greater risk of developing trismus than patients treated by either modality alone. High-risk patients, and especially those in whom trismus is already beginning to develop, should perform exercises several times daily to increase the interarch distance; exercises should begin as soon as practical in the postoperative period and should continue both during and after irradiation. One technique is to have patients insert a number of stacked tongue blades between the teeth, then successively wedge additional blades into the stack until slight pain is encountered. Alternatively, a tapered cork can be inserted between the teeth to a point where minimal discomfort is reached; over a period of days to weeks, patients attempt to place the cork farther and farther into mouth. Another technique uses a clothespin onto which a rubber band is tightly wound to open the mouth forcibly (Fig. 15–2). The

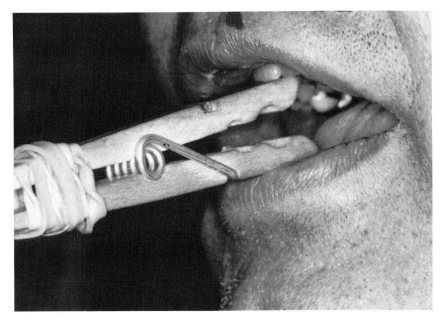

Figure 15–2. Trismus secondary to extensive squamous cell carcinoma of paranasal sinuses with invasion of pterygoid musculature. During the course of irradiation, the patient used a clothespin, onto which a rubber band had been tightly wound, to exercise and gradually increase the interincisor distance. Conscientious efforts should be made to reverse existing trismus or prevent its occurrence after irradiation because it is difficult to manage once established (from Parsons[6]).

exercises usually are done for about 30 seconds every 2 hours. The distance between the upper and lower incisors should be measured and patients should increase this distance by using the exercises to break down existing fibrosis. Most patients can function well with an interincisor distance of 35 mm for dentulous patients, or an interalveolar distance of 50 mm for edentulous patients. Early evaluation by a dentist is helpful in preventing or solving these problems.

Soft Tissue and Bone Necrosis

Radiation necrosis is a destruction of normal tissue. Necrosis is believed to be due to the avascular effect of radiation. After healing of the acute reaction of the mucous membrane, the epithelium is thinner than normal. The clinical appearance is that of a pale, hypotrophic epithelium through which telangiectatic vessels may be seen. Such mucosa is more susceptible than normal to mechanical injury and to the noxious effects of alcohol and tobacco. Necrosis usually begins with breakdown of this damaged mucosa, leaving a small ulcer.

If ulceration occurs on soft tissues that have no underlying bone, the result is a soft tissue necrosis. If it occurs on soft tissues of the gingiva and no obvious sequestration or bone necrosis exists, the ulcer is called bone exposure; if serious injury to the underlying bone occurs, bone necrosis, or osteoradionecrosis, is said to be present. Although the terms bone exposure and osteoradionecrosis frequently are used indiscriminately, few exposures progress to severe bone necroses.

BONE EXPOSURE AND OSTEORADIONECROSIS OF THE MANDIBLE AND MAXILLA

If the area of exposure is less than 1 cm, actual necrosis of the underlying bone and sequestration may not occur or may be minimal; roentgenograms appear normal. Small exposures heal spontaneously after a period of weeks to months. On the other hand, if the bone exposure enlarges and persists for a long period, bone necrosis followed by sequestration may occur, A segment of mandible or, rarely, maxilla is exposed, with apparently dead bone. Histologically, true osteoradionecrosis is characterized by damage to the cellular elements of bone, as well as vascular changes. The marrow space is infiltrated by inflammatory cells and loose connective tissue.[23] Roentgenograms show an irregular lytic defect that frequently extends beyond the clinically apparent area of destruction. Severe necroses may lead to orofacial fistulae and pathologic fractures.

To better define the pathogenesis of osteoradionecrosis, Marx[24] performed cultures and stains for microorganisms in the en bloc resection specimens of 12 osteoradionecrotic mandibles. In contrast with specimens obtained from infected jawbone grafts or patients with osteomyelitis (in which both the bony surface and medullary portions of the bone contained microorganisms), bones that were affected by osteoradionecrosis contained microorganisms only as surface contaminants (ie, no infectious process was demonstrated deep in the bone). Marx concluded that hypocellularity and hypovascularity, not infection, were the initiating agents after irradiation.

Although a direct effect of radiation on bone itself exists, most bone, including the mandible, tolerates high doses of radiation without serious problems, so long as the tissues overlying the bone remain intact and the bone is not subjected to excessive stress or trauma. Although occasional patients develop mandibular necroses beneath normal-appearing mucous membranes, 95% of necroses are associated with soft tissue necrosis and bone exposure. Patients occasionally develop a small sinus tract through which purulent debris spontaneously drains; such patients may have only mild or moderate pain despite radiographic evidence of lytic bone destruction. The jawbone may be tender to palpation and may give the examiner the impression that it is soft and expanded.

Compared with the maxilla, the gingiva of the mandible has a tenuous blood supply. The mucosal covering is thin and constantly traumatized (eg, by eating or by wearing dentures). Once mandibular necrosis occurs, it is difficult to obtain healing. Necroses of the maxilla occur less often and generally heal more rapidly.

Most spontaneously occurring bone problems first appear 3 to 12 months after irradiation; those that occur after trauma (usually dental extraction) are related in time to the traumatic event.

The mylohyoid ridge, which is normally prominent and covered by a thin gingival mucosa, and the anterior arch of the mandible are frequent sites of bone exposure. In some patients, bone exposure over the mylohyoid ridge is seen after dental extractions before irradiation owing to too-tight mucosal closure that stretches and thins the overlying mucosa. Most cases heal promptly, resulting in no significant delay of irradiation. If delayed healing occurs, irradiation must sometimes begin despite the exposure; usually healing continues during the irradiation. Exposure on the anterior arch of the mandible has become less common in recent years at our own institution as a result of greater emphasis on primary surgery, as opposed to irradiation, for most cases of oral cavity cancer. Posterior exposures, at the angle or ascending ramus of the mandible, sites that are well covered by muscle, are rare. If posterior necrosis does occur, it may result in severe infection and trismus.[22]

Although patients who have been edentulous for many years are still at risk of developing mandibular necrosis, overall risk is significantly less than in dentulous patients. A policy of selected tooth removal reduces the risk of necrosis, especially if patients have advanced periodontal disease in the mandibular molars or a history of poor dental compliance.[25] Indiscriminate extraction of all teeth within the treatment volume, however, is not indicated and probably increases the risk of necrosis, particularly in patients with healthy dentition and a history of good dental compliance. After irradiation, extraction of nonrestorable teeth within the high-dose irradiation volume is to be avoided unless all other measures are unsuccessful and patients have severe pain. Many times painful teeth can be successfully treated by root canal therapy.[26] The risk of postirradiation necrosis is much greater for mandibular than for maxillary extractions, although delayed healing is not unusual, even in the maxilla. Radiation caries in teeth that are outside the field of irradiation do not predispose patients to osteoradionecrosis because the bone at these sites has not received high-dose radiation; healing is usually normal after extraction.

Marx et al[27] randomly assigned patients, who required dental extractions from mandibles that had received high-dose irradiation (≥ 6000 cGy 6 months to 15 years before extraction), to receive either penicillin before and after extraction or hyperbaric oxygen (HBO) treatment before and after extraction. Hyperbaric oxygen treatment consisted of 20 dives at 2.4 atm with 100% humidified oxygen for 90 minutes each session, followed by extraction, then 10 more dives. Thirty-seven patients with 137 wound sockets were treated with penicillin. Thirty-seven patients with 156 wound sockets were treated with HBO. Thirty-one wound sockets (23%) in 11 patients (30%) developed osteoradionecrosis in the antibiotic group compared with four wound sockets (3%) in 2 patients (5%) in the HBO group. In addition, the necroses that occurred in the antibiotic group were clinically and radiographically more severe and more often resulted in surgical resection than those occurring in the HBO group.

Occasionally patients have unerupted molars. If well covered, these teeth usually do not cause a problem in the postirradiatior period. If a tooth is partially erupted, it should be extracted if high-dose irradiation is anticipated.[28] In actual practice, most partially erupted third molars occur in younger patients whose tumors, usually lymphomas, require lesser doses of irradiation so that postirradiation surgery can be accomplished at a later date with little risk. Impacted third molars are not extracted before irradiation because a prolonged period of healing is required when the bone defect is large.

Destruction of tissue by tumor increases the likelihood of necrosis; patients whose tumors involve the gingiva are at increased risk for bone exposure after irradiation. Patients who continue to smoke and drink after irradiation are also at increased risk. High doses, large treatment volumes, large dose fractions, and the addition of a radical neck dissection all place patients at greater risk. Patients whose treatment includes an interstitial implant also are more likely to develop necrosis. Of 315 patients who received irradiation for carcinomas of the oral cavity or oropharynx at the University of Florida between September 1964 and August 1976, about 5% of the 198 patients whose treatment was by external-beam irradiation alone developed bone necrosis of mild or moderate severity (ie, spontaneous healing in less than or more than 6 months, respectively); 1% developed severe osteoradionecrosis requiring mandibular resection. Of 117 patients whose treatment consisted of external-beam irradiation and a radium implant, the rate of development of mild or moderately severe necrosis was 18%. Severe necroses occurred in 3%.[29]

Management. In the 1960s, it was common practice to perform mandibulectomies on patients with bone exposure. From experience it is now known that 85% to 90% of bone exposures heal spontaneously after conservative treatment. Even large, moderately severe necrosis may eventually respond. Conservative measures often are more successful in cases of osteoradionecrosis induced by denture trauma or preirradiation dental extractions than those occurring after postirradiation extractions, or those that occur spontaneously in association with retained teeth.[26]

The key to treating minor bone exposures is patience. Several months are required for healing to occur; the area may enlarge before it starts to heal. If the bone is rough or protrudes above the level of the gingiva, the oral surgeon files it down to promote healing and to prevent irritation of the tongue. If patients wear dentures, the dentures either should be discontinued or at least should be relieved over the site of exposure to avoid causing further trauma. If the exposure is larger than 1 cm, it is preferable to discontinue the denture until healing is complete.

Surprisingly, most of these patients do not have major discomfort; pain usually is controlled with analgesics such as aspirin and local care. Continued alcohol ingestion retards healing. A 2- to 3-week course of antibiotics sometimes reduces discomfort. A local anesthetic, such as viscous lidocaine applied with a cotton-tipped applicator, helps to control the pain. Under conservative management, most small areas of exposure eventually heal with little or no loss of bone. Local debridement of moderate-sized necroses is done by the oral surgeon when necessary. Small sequestra can be removed in the office. It is not unusual for patients to report that a sequestrum was spontaneously extruded while at home, and when next examined, the area is completely healed.

The late 1970s saw a dramatic increase in the use of HBO for treating osteoradionecrosis and soft tissue necrosis.[30-32] Patients treated by HBO at the University of Florida have had close follow-up by an oral surgeon, sometimes on a daily or every-other-day basis, with meticulous local care and frequent debridement until improvement was noted. Hyperbaric oxygen treatment alone, without an aggressive surgical approach, has been shown to arrest, but often not completely resolve, the process. Since 1983, an HBO program similar to that developed by Marx[31] at Wilford Hall US Air Force Medical Center (San Antonio, Tex) has been in use at the University of Florida. The protocol does not apply to patients with minor bone exposures, which continue to be treated with less expensive and more conservative approaches, unless the lesion is clearly progressing or causing marked pain. The Wilford Hall protocol consists of three stages:

Stage I comprises 30 dives (2.4 atm of 100% oxygen, 90 minutes a day, once a day, 5 days a week), after which patients are reexamined. If the wound shows definite clinical improvement, such as a decrease in the amount of exposed bone, granulation tissue covering the exposed bone, resorption of nonviable bone, and absence of inflammation, patients complete a full course of 60 dives to achieve full mucosal cover. If no clinical improvement occurs by 30 dives, as evidenced by extended or continued exposure of bone, absence of mucosal proliferation, or presence of inflammation, patients are identified as not responding to stage I, and are advanced to stage II.

In stage II, a transoral alveolar sequestrectomy is accomplished with a primary mucosal closure. Hyperbaric oxygen dives continue after surgery. If healing progresses without complication, dives continue up to a total of 60. If dehiscence of the wound occurs, leaving exposed bone, patients are identified as not responding to stage II, and are advanced to stage III. In patients whose initial presentation includes either pathologic fracture, orocutaneous fistula, or radiographic evidence of resorption to the inferior border of the mandible, an initial course of 30 dives is given, and patients directly enter stage III of treatment.

In stage III, after a minimum of 30 dives, the patients undergo a resection (transoral approach preferred), the margins of which are determined at the time of surgery by the presence of bleeding bone or by tetracycline fluorescence under ultraviolet light (Wood's lamp). The segments of mandible are stabilized with either extraskeletal pin fixation or maxillomandibular fixation. If oral dehiscence or orocutaneous fistula occurs, deepithelialization and primary closure are done. Hyperbaric oxygen dives are continued until healthy mucosal closure is evident, or a total of 60 dives is reached. Reconstruction, if it is to be done, is dependent on many variables.

Marx[31] entered 58 patients with refractory (after surgery, HBO treatment, and/or nonsurgical approaches elsewhere) osteoradionecrosis onto his protocol. Eleven had orocutaneous fistulae, 11 had pathologic fractures, and 33 had pain. All 58 cases were successfully treated (resolution of pain, retention or reconstruction of mandibular continuity, restoration of function, with maintenance of an intact mucosa over all bone for 18 months minimum). Resolution was achieved in stage I in 9 patients (16%), stage II in 8 patients (14%), and in stage III in 41 patients (71%). All 41 of the latter patients had successful reconstructive therapy. Marx concluded that HBO treatment alone for refractory cases was rarely (16%) successful because HBO treatment cannot resurrect dead bone. Eighty-five percent required some surgical removal of bone. He concluded, furthermore, that HBO treatment should play an increased role in the management of osteoradionecrosis, with antibiotics, local wound care, and irrigation as adjuncts.

TEMPORAL BONE NECROSIS

Osteoradionecrosis of the temporal bone is an unusual complication that may occur after high-dose irradiation of carcinomas of the middle ear, auditory canal, or mastoid, or after incidental irradiation to the normal external auditory canal and temporal bone (eg, in treating the nasopharynx or parotid tumors).

Ramsden[33] collected 29 cases of osteoradionecrosis of the temporal bone from four large medical centers over a 30-year period. Two main patterns of necrosis, localized and diffuse, were observed. The localized form was more common (18 patients) and usually resulted from incidental irradiation that

was directed at primary lesions at some distance from the ear. The most common finding was an area of exposed or dead bone in the external auditory meatus, usually in the floor or anterior wall (Fig. 15–3). Most patients complained of mild otalgia and offensive otorrhea. Sequestration was sometimes present on tomography. Conservative treatment (regular washing, ear drops, and analgesics) usually resulted in gradual separation of the sequestration after 1 to 4 years, after which healing occurred.

Patients with diffuse osteoradionecrosis (11 patients) had extensive involvement of a large part or all of the temporal

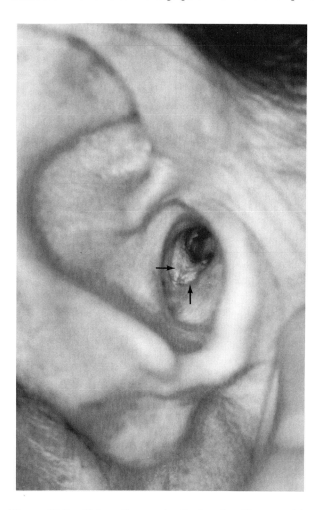

Figure 15–3. Osteoradionecrosis of external auditory canal in a 55-year-old woman 3½ years after superficial parotidectomy and postoperative irradiation of an adenoid cystic carcinoma of the parotid gland. Examination of the resected specimen revealed positive margins and extensive perineural spread. The dose to the temporal bone was 6850 cGy in 32 fractions by a continuous course. At 3½ years, the patient complained of pain and drainage from the right ear. There was exposed bone on the inferior and posterior walls of the external auditory canal (arrows). Infection and pain were controlled for several years with antibiotics, although the bone exposure persisted. At 8 years, the patient had increasingly severe pain. Computed tomography revealed an erosive process of the mastoid and adjacent squamous portion of the temporal bone. Computed tomographic-directed biopsy revealed no tumor. The patient was treated with antibiotics and a short course of HBO therapy. Acute symptoms resolved. The patient continued to have occasional discharge and intermittent pain (from Parsons[6]).

bone. In 10 of the 11 patients, the radiotherapy was directed primarily at the temporal bone, middle ear, or skin of the external meatus, pinna, or temporal region. Patients experienced severe, boring pain with profuse, pulsatile, and offensive otorrhea. Severe intracranial infection occurred in four patients (temporal lobe, cerebellar, or posterior fossa abscesses). Several patients developed other severe sequelae (trismus, cranial nerve palsies, dead ear, vertigo, or death). Treatment required an aggressive surgical approach.

Most reported cases of temporal bone osteoradionecrosis occur 5 years or more after irradiation.[33-37] In Ramsden's series,[33] 11 of 29 cases occurred 10 years or more after irradiation. Temporal bone necrosis often is related to technical factors (beam quality, total dose, and dose per fraction).[38]

Management.   In some cases, local treatment (local cleansing, antibiotics, and surgical débridement) is successful. However, in other patients a more aggressive approach, including extensive débridement, exploration of the mastoid, partial temporal bone resection, and abscess evacuation, is required. Moderately severe and severe problems also are treated with HBO.

SOFT TISSUE NECROSIS

Atrophy of the mucosa and its supporting stroma, reduced tissue vascularity, and tissue destruction by tumor all predispose patients to soft tissue necrosis. The risk of necrosis is increased by continued alcohol and tobacco consumption.

Most cases of pure soft tissue necrosis occur within 2 years. After interstitial therapy, most cases of necrosis appear within 5 to 8 months. Occurrence after 2 years generally is preceded by trauma to the mucosa.

Soft tissue necroses are most common after irradiation of lesions within the oral cavity or oropharynx; they are unusual after treatment of cancer of the nasopharynx and larynx but occasionally are seen after successful irradiation of cancer of the posterior pharyngeal wall. Necrosis is related to fraction size, total dose, volume, and use of interstitial treatment. Of 315 patients with squamous cell cancer of the oral cavity or oropharynx who received radical irradiation at the University of Florida between 1964 and 1976, mild (spontaneously healed within 6 months) or moderately severe (spontaneously healed but required longer than 6 months) soft tissue necroses were observed in about 10% of patients after external-beam irradiation alone, and in about 20% of those who received a combination of external-beam and interstitial irradiation. Severe soft tissue necroses (requiring an operation or prolonged hospitalization) were rare, occurring in 1 (0.5%) of 198 patients treated by external-beam therapy alone and 1 (1%) of 117 after external-beam plus interstitial irradiation.[29]

Management.   Necrosis must be distinguished from recurrent cancer. Although both conditions frequently ulcerate the mucosa, there are some clinical parameters that help to distinguish between the two. Recurrence of the primary cancer after irradiation almost always occurs at the center of the initial lesion. Ulceration outside the original cancer area usually is due to necrosis. Most cancer ulcers have a rolled margin, as opposed to the nearly flat, more sharply demarcated margins of necrosis. The induration around a tumor recurrence usually is a little more pronounced than around a necrosis. Both kinds of ulcer may enlarge but a cancer ulcer rarely decreases in size.

If physicians cannot decide whether the ulcer represents tumor recurrence or necrosis, patients are asked to return every 2 weeks for reexamination. If soft tissue necrosis is the most likely cause of the ulcer, biopsy is not performed because this may cause the necrosis to enlarge. If recurrent tumor is likely, biopsy is mandatory because the chance to perform surgical salvage is lost if one procrastinates too long. It is better to err on the side of biopsy when doubt exists. Our rate of success in the clinical diagnosis of necrosis versus recurrence is about 70%. In some areas, particularly the tongue, biopsy may have to be done under anesthesia because a deep biopsy is necessary to show recurrence. Negative biopsy results should be viewed with suspicion if there is a strong likelihood of recurrence and repeat biopsies are in order.

The management of soft tissue necrosis depends on the site involved and the severity of pain produced. In certain sites (eg, the lateral tongue or floor of the mouth) even a 1- to 2-mm superficial ulcer may be painful. Topical viscous lidocaine, 2%, may make patients comfortable enough to eat normally. Antibiotics such as tetracycline hydrochloride, 250 mg orally four times a day, may produce some relief of pain, particularly when the ulceration is deep and infected. It is essential that patients discontinue using alcohol and tobacco. If the area of necrosis is constantly traumatized by dentures, they should not be worn until healing has occurred. More than 95% of soft tissue necroses heal with conservative treatment, although several months are required. Cases that fail to respond to more conservative means may benefit from HBO treatment. Once healing has occurred, the scar appears pale and thin, and often is slightly depressed below the level of the surrounding mucosa; reappearance of necrosis at the same site is unusual.

Cartilage Necrosis

Numerous cartilaginous structures in the head and neck area, including the larynx, trachea, external ear, eustachian tube, and nose, are incidentally or intentionally irradiated to a high dose. The often-voiced fear of cartilage necrosis arose from the orthovoltage era, when vocal cord and skin cancers were treated with large daily fractions. Cartilage that is covered by a normal mucous membrane or skin usually tolerates conventionally fractionated high-dose irradiation. Although cartilage that has been compromised by tumor invasion, infection, or prior surgery is more vulnerable to radiation injury, these conditions themselves constitute no contraindication to irradiation because the risk of cartilage necrosis still is low.

Chondronecrosis generally occurs within the first posttreatment year but can be precipitated by trauma many years after treatment. Biopsies are sometimes the precipitating cause and should not be done after irradiation unless recurrence is suspected.[39,40] Cartilage necrosis often starts with necrosis of the soft tissues (skin or mucous membrane) overlying the cartilage.

LARYNGEAL CHONDRONECROSIS

Chondronecrosis of the larynx is rare, occurring in about 1% of patients who receive doses in the range of 6000 to 7000 cGy at 200 cGy per fraction. The risk increases with larger daily fractions (Table 15-1)[41-45] and larger treatment volumes; the risk is greater for supraglottic than for vocal cord carcinoma. For patients with cancer of the oral cavity, oropharynx, or nasopharynx, the larynx should not be included in the treatment portals.[46] Cartilage that has been compromised by partial laryngectomy would seem likely to develop necrosis after irradiation, but in practice it is rarely seen. Patients who continue to smoke or drink alcohol after treatment are at increased risk.

The symptoms and signs of cartilage necrosis (hoarseness, pain, edema, shortness of breath, tenderness over the cartilage, and foul breath) mimic those of recurrent cancer. Aspiration pneumonia, lung abscess, or laryngocutaneous fistula may result. Because most necroses and many recurrences occur within 1 year after treatment, time to onset is not helpful in distinguishing the two. Tumor recurrence is many times more common than cartilage necrosis; nevertheless, a strong suspicion of recurrence should exist before biopsy is undertaken. If patients have pain and marked edema, with or without obvious tumor regrowth, computed tomographic (CT) scan is performed for confirmation of the findings. If an obvious focal abnormality is noted on CT scan, then direct laryngoscopy and biopsy are indicated. If only edema but no focal abnormality is noted on CT scan, and no evidence of disease is noted at direct laryngoscopy, blind biopsies should not be performed as they may precipitate a chondronecrosis. In instances where patients have no pain, only moderate edema, an adequate airway, and CT scans showing no focal lesions, clinical follow-up alone is indicated. Even deep biopsy may fail to obtain representative tissue in

some recurrent cancers. Tracheotomy may be necessary for aspiration or edema. Antibiotic therapy is begun, and nasogastric or gastrostomy alimentation may be necessary. Hyperbaric oxygen therapy has been reported to be effective in the management of chondronecrosis. Ferguson et al[47] reported on eight patients who developed laryngeal chondronecrosis within 15 months of completing irradiation. One patient had a laryngocutaneous fistula, three patients had undergone tracheostomy, and the other four patients had severe pain, dysphagia, or tenderness over the cartilage. Patients received 40 dives (2 atm of 100% oxygen, 2 hours each, 6 days a week) plus antibiotics and humidity. Signs and symptoms of necrosis were dramatically relieved in seven patients; one patient required laryngectomy.

Antibiotics sometimes are successful in resolving the necrosis. If conservative measures are unsuccessful, laryngectomy is recommended because the problem is more apt to be tumor recurrence than necrosis.

CHONDRONECROSIS OF THE NOSE AND EAR

Even when nasal or ear cancers invade cartilage, necrosis is rare after conventionally fractionated therapy.[48,49] If necrosis does occur, it requires débridement and grafting.

Skin and Subcutaneous Tissues
SKIN

Because modern radiation therapy is conducted with supervoltage equipment, severe late skin changes are infrequent. Today, the only common indication for orthovoltage irradiation is skin cancer. After orthovoltage treatment, usually epidermal atrophy and sometimes telangiectasis occur. The skin is hairless and dry because the sweat and sebaceous glands cease to function. Some patients need to apply petrolatum regularly to keep the skin pliable and to prevent fissures from occurring. Acne does not occur in the irradiated field. Pigment changes also may occur; after very high doses, a thin, achromic, and telangiectatic scar may develop. Achromia results from melanocyte destruction; such areas readily sunburn. Occasionally, "tanning" or hyperpigmentation may persist

Table 15-1. Chondronecrosis after Irradiation of Laryngeal Cancer: Time-Dose Relations

STUDY	PRIMARY SITE	TUMOR DOSE (cGy)	FRACTION SIZE (cGy)	PATIENTS	PATIENTS WITH NECROSIS (%)
University of Florida[172]	Glottis (T1–T2)	5400 to 6525/ 4½ to 6 wk	225	174	1 (0.6)
Princess Margaret Hospital[43]	Glottis (T1)	5500/5 wk	210–230	283	0
M.D. Anderson Hospital[42]	Glottis and supraglottis	6000 to 7000/ 5½ to 7 wk	200–225	503	6 (1)
Rush Presbyterian-St Lukes[44]	Glottis (T1–T2)	6500/5 to 5½ wk	225–250	135	1 (0.7)
Liverpool[45]	Glottis and supraglottis	5500/3 wk	344	129	9 (7)
Penrose[41]	Glottis (T1–T2)	6100 to 6600/ 3½ to 4 wk	~300	16	1 (6)

for considerable periods. If the skin is severely damaged, it may ulcerate, especially after trauma; sometimes grafting is required.

Subcutaneous fibrosis usually appears within 6 to 12 months after treatment and is slowly progressive. Decreased pliability of the subcutaneous tissues exists. In severe cases, the tissues may have a woody texture and become fixed into a single hard mass in which the subcutaneous tissue is not separable from overlying skin or underlying muscle or bone. Patients with a great amount of adipose tissue in the subcutaneous layer tend to develop the most severe changes. Fibrosis is rarely painful.

Large areas of fibrosis may be accompanied by a tight, constrictive sensation. Obstructive lymphedema may be associated with fibrosis and may produce intermittent episodes of erysipelas.

High-dose irradiation of metastatic lymphadenopathy results in more subcutaneous fibrosis in the neck than does a comparable dose to a neck that has no palpable adenopathy; apparently, the fibrous stroma that replaces the tumor mass contributes to the reaction. Large daily fractions also increase the risk of subcutaneous fibrosis. Fat necrosis is rare.

Pharyngeal Stenosis

A rarely observed complication of high-dose irradiation consists of progressive fibrosis and eventual stenosis of the supraglottic larynx or pharynx, leading to severe dysphagia, aspiration, or airway problems.

Wound Healing

Wound healing is a complex, dynamic process involving an initial inflammatory-type response to tissue injury followed by proliferation of epithelial and endothelial cells, fibroblasts, and capillaries and later by synthesis, secretion, and eventually restructuring of collagen by fibroblasts.[50] Maximal mechanical wound strength is not attained for months, or even a year or more, after surgery. Irradiation can interrupt or delay the healing process at several points, especially at those points that depend on normal cell proliferation.[50]

A number of authors have performed animal experiments to study the effects of irradiation administered before wounding on (1) delay of gain in tensile strength[51-57]; (2) time to complete wound closure[58]; (3) histological progression of collagenesis[51,53,59,60]; and (4) incidence of postoperative wound infection.[61] The experiments studied the effects of various doses, usually administered as single fractions, given at various intervals before surgery. Although not all studies produced identical findings, most investigators agreed on the following:

1. Irradiation produces delays in complete healing and tensile strength. The greatest delays occur when irradiation immediately precedes wounding, or when it is administered less than 1 week before surgery. Delaying surgery beyond 3 weeks provides little additional advantage in terms of tensile strength.
2. The effect of irradiation on wound healing is dose related. Fractionated irradiation produces significant sparing in terms of wound strength, typical of late-responding tissue.[62]
3. The delay in tensile strength appears to be caused by delayed collagen synthesis, probably due to depletion of fibroblasts.
4. Preoperatively irradiated wounds are more susceptible to bacterial infection than nonirradiated wounds. The risk increases with dose and is particularly significant if the operative bed includes bacterial contaminants (as occurs when the aerodigestive tract is breached).
5. Once healing is complete, the scar is morphologically normal and final wound strength is the same as in unirradiated controls.

Although no evidence exists that delaying surgery beyond 3 weeks benefits tensile strength, frequently other practical considerations make longer delays (eg, 4 to 6 weeks) desirable, such as allowing time for mucositis to resolve, a positive nutritional state to be restored, and fixed nodal masses to shrink away from the carotid artery and base of skull.

In general, the incidence of complications is lower after postradiotherapy neck dissection than after resection of the primary lesion combined with a neck dissection. Additionally, neck dissection after twice-daily, compared with once-daily, irradiation is associated with a lower risk of wound complications after the same total dose.[63]

Chronic radiation effects result in tissues that are fibrotic, hypoxic, and susceptible to infection. Once these changes have occurred, they do not improve with time.[54] The doses that have been administered to the tissues before salvage surgery usually are 6000 to 7500 cGy. Both the high doses and existing fibrosis lead to a rate of complications that is higher than in planned preoperative irradiation cases.[58] Morbidity is increased by the same factors that increase late complications in general, namely, high total dose, large dose per fraction, large field size, and surgical procedures of great magnitude. Longer intervals to surgery and split-course irradiation techniques do not reduce the risk of complications.[64] Complications, when they occur, tend to be more severe in heavily irradiated patients than in unirradiated patients, leading to increased rates of fistulization, prolonged hospitalization, and carotid exposure.[65]

High doses administered immediately or within several days postoperatively significantly delay wound healing.[51,52]

If sufficient time (usually several weeks) has elapsed between surgery and irradiation, irradiation has no detectable effects on healing.[54] Occasionally, a patient in need of postoperative irradiation has an open, slow-healing wound and a decision must be made either to delay treatment and risk tumor recurrence or to proceed with irradiation and risk greater wound complications. In general, if the area of incomplete wound closure is not extensive and does not overlay a vital structure (eg, the carotid artery), irradiation is started at about 6 weeks. If the wound overlies the carotid artery, further delays are necessary, and the exact timing of irradiation must be individualized.[66]

Visual Apparatus

Although primary tumors of the eye (eg, melanoma, retinoblastoma) and optic nerve (eg, glioma) are rare, tumors that involve tissues adjacent to these structures are relatively common. Because many of these tumors are best treated with irradiation, the visual apparatus frequently receives incidental irradiation. When treating tumors of the paranasal sinuses with irradiation, varying portions of the eye are in the fields of treatment, depending on the degree to which the orbit is invaded.[67]

When orbital invasion is extensive, all of the orbital contents are irradiated, including the eyeball and all of the lacrimal tissue (Fig. 15–4A). If the administered dose is high, as when treating a carcinoma, a dry eye results and visual loss usually occurs within 6 to 10 months after treatment, owing to degeneration of the anterior segment of the eye, with resultant corneal ulceration and opacification. The direct effects of irradiation on the cornea also contribute to the problem. Lower doses, as used when treating lymphomas, result in only mild symptoms of a dry eye and cataract formation.

If orbital invasion is limited, so that most of the lacrimal tissue can be spared high-dose irradiation (Fig. 15–4B,C), severe dry eye problems do not occur, even when high doses are administered. If the dose to the eyeball itself has been high, however, visual loss due to posterior segment degeneration, radiation retinopathy, occurs, usually after a 2- to 3-year latency period. If low total doses are used, patients usually remain asymptomatic in the follow-up period with regard to dry eye complaints and retinal problems, but still are at risk for cataract formation.

Even when no orbital invasion is present, it is often necessary to include a portion of the contiguous orbit and the medial one fourth to one third of the eyeball in the irradiation field (Fig. 15–4D) because of the anatomic configuration of the sinuses and possible subclinical disease extensions through the thin bony walls that separate the sinuses from the orbit. Although visual loss secondary to eyeball injury is rare in this setting, a risk of blindness due to optic nerve injury still exists, usually after a 1- to 6-year latency period; the risk depends on the daily fraction size and total dose administered.

Patients should be evaluated before irradiation by an ophthalmologist knowledgeable in radiation complications.

Most potential complications can be anticipated, and patients should understand these risks. Lifelong ophthalmologic follow-up is advised. Before undertaking treatment, the ophthalmologist should discuss the treatment details with the radiation therapist because some pitfalls may be avoided by good communication. For example, if high-dose irradiation has been administered to the eyeball, cataract extraction should not be followed by prosthetic lens implantation. This is because the complication rate is increased and the expected benefits would be negligible as patients will almost certainly develop radiation retinopathy. Anterior-segment disease should be treated early and aggressively to avoid corneal complications. Even when vision is lost, vigorous attempts to save the eye are worthwhile for cosmetic reasons.

LACRIMAL APPARATUS

Although their mass is small in relation to the major lacrimal gland, the accessory lacrimal glands are believed to be responsible for the basal secretion of tears (Fig. 15–5).[68] Reflex secretion is from the main lacrimal gland.[69]

The tear film consists of a superficial lipid layer, derived from meibomian and Zeis gland secretions, which helps retard evaporation; a middle aqueous layer produced by the major and accessory lacrimal glands; and a deep mucinous layer that serves to wet the relatively hydrophobic corneal and conjunctival epithelium. The mucin layer is elaborated by conjunctival goblet cells. Deficiency of any of the three components leads to a loss of tear film stability (Fig. 15–6). A dry eye is the result, which leads to damage of the conjunctival and corneal epithelium (keratoconjunctivitis sicca). Because the corneal epithelium is endowed with numerous nerves, pain from a dry eye often is marked.

In a histopathologic study of eyes that were removed after irradiation, Karp et al[70] demonstrated atrophy of the meibomian and lacrimal glands. Because tumors most frequently invade the orbit through its floor (maxillary sinus) or medial wall (ethmoid sinus), the superolateral orbit (including the major lacrimal gland and much of the accessory lacrimal tissue in the upper lid) usually can be shielded, unless orbital invasion is extensive. During treatment, the eye is locally anesthetized and a lid retractor is inserted so that part of the upper lateral eyelid is displaced from the treatment field; maintaining the open-eye position during treatment also prevents bolus effect by the lids on the cornea and conjunctiva.

When the orbit is extensively invaded by carcinoma, high-dose irradiation of the entire orbit is necessary and generally results in severe dry eye syndrome. If the dose to the entire eye and lacrimal tissue exceeds 5000 cGy, prospects of maintaining vision are poor. Patients generally develop a red, painful, scratchy eye (foreign body sensation) and photophobia. Corneal ulceration, vascularization, and opacification may ensue (Figs. 15–7, 15–8).

In association with corneal ulceration, some patients develop acute anterior uveitis with severe pain, sometimes requiring hospitalization and intensive medical management with cycloplegics, mydriatics, narcotic analgesics, tranquilizers,

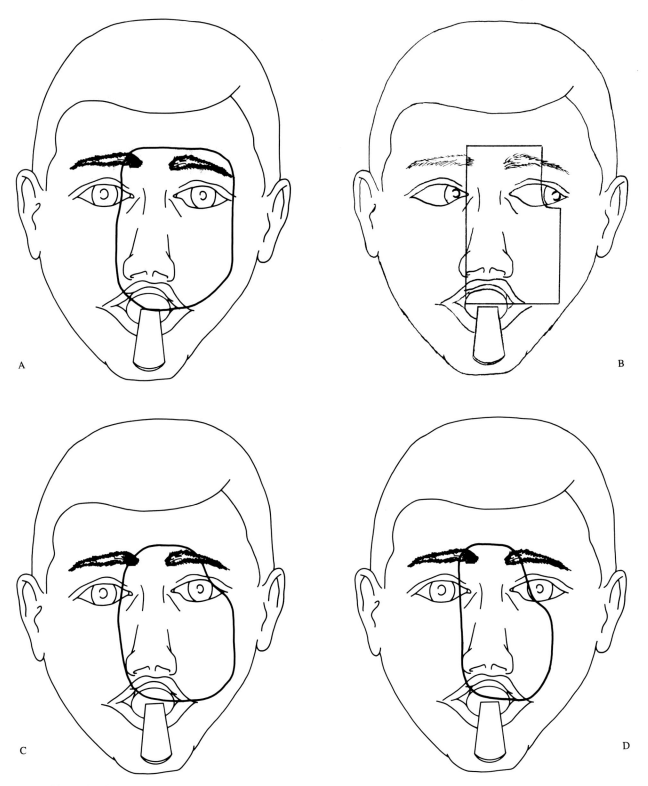

Figure 15–4. Anterior portals used to treat tumors of the nasal cavity and paranasal sinuses. **(A).** Extensive orbital invasion (eg, palpable orbital mass, proptosis, or blindness). No lacrimal shielding (from Parsons et al[67]). **(B).** Limited orbital invasion present. The major lacrimal gland is shielded. Patient is instructed to gaze laterally to displace lens from portal. This technique was discontinued at the University of Florida after 1970 (from Parsons et al[71]). **(C).** Limited orbital invasion present. The major lacrimal gland is shielded. This technique has been used at the University of Florida since 1971 (from Parsons et al[67]). **(D).** No orbital invasion (from Parsons et al[67]).

and antibiotic therapy as indicated.[71] Most patients tolerate doses in the range of 3000 to 4000 cGy (180 cGy per fraction) to the entire orbit with ^{60}Co without developing severe symptoms of a dry eye (Fig. 15-9).[71]

Treatment of a dry eye is symptomatic. For mild or moderate dry eye syndrome, artificial tears are used during the day and a sterile ophthalmic lubricating ointment is applied at night. Hydrophilic soft contact lenses sometimes are used as a protective bandage for corneal epithelial defects and may serve as a tear reservoir, but are not always well tolerated by patients who have severe dry eyes. Treatment of a painful, nonseeing eye is by evisceration or enucleation.

The Nasolacrimal Drainage System. The nasolacrimal duct usually is not affected by high-dose irradiation unless it has been disrupted by tumor or prior surgery. Stenosis of the lacrimal puncta or canaliculi after high-dose irradiation is more common.

EYELIDS

Ectropion or entropion is seldom seen. Loss of the eyelashes usually is not a significant cosmetic problem. on occasion, however, some of the eyelashes that regrow turn inward (trichiasis) and must be surgically removed.

CONJUNCTIVA

Conjunctival telangiectasia is common after high-dose irradiation. It produces no symptoms. Symblepharon is a rare,

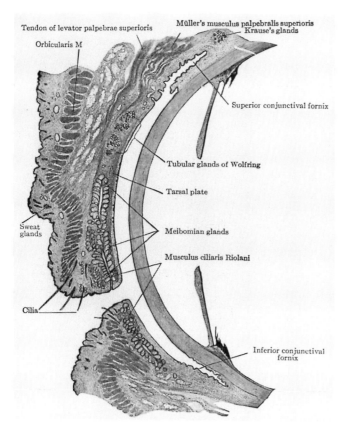

Figure 15-5. Sagittal section through the eyelids and eyeball. Note the location of the accessory lacrimal glands of Krause in the superior conjunctival fornix and the accessory lacrimal glands of Wolfring at the superior margin of the tarsal plate (from Scheie and Albert[68]).

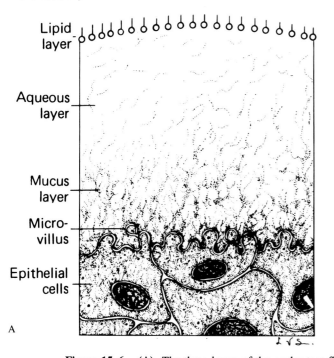

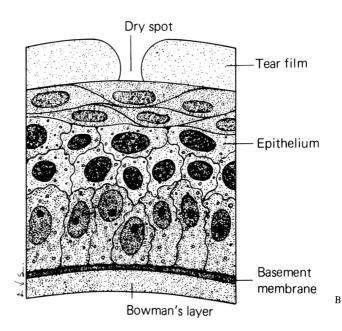

Figure 15-6. **(A).** The three layers of the ocular tear film covering the superficial corneal epithelium. **(B).** Loss of normal constituents of the tear film leads to rapid tear film breakup, with resultant dry spots that expose the corneal epithelium and lead to damage of its cells (from Tabbara KF. Tears. In: Vaughn D, Asbury T, Tabbara KF, eds. *General Ophthalmology.* 12th ed. East Norwalk, Conn: Appleton & Lange; 1989:68, 70).

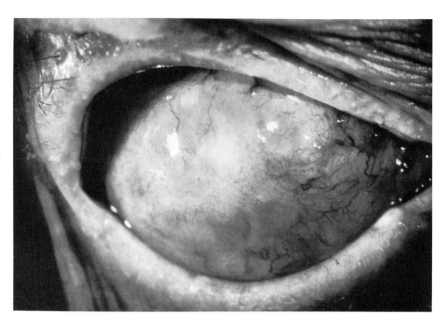

Figure 15-7. Eye of a 57-year-old man 3 years 10 months after treatment of an advanced adenoid cystic carcinoma of the ethmoid sinus, which extensively invaded the orbit and base of the skull. The entire eye and orbital contents received 6800 cGy in 38 fractions over 66 days by split-course irradiation. At the end of treatment, the patient had a severe dry eye syndrome with keratitis and conjunctivitis. By 9 months, the cornea was scarred and there was pannus formation. The patient developed rubeosis iridis and neovascular glaucoma (intraocular pressure, 60 mm Hg). Attempts to control pain by cyclocryotherapy were unsuccessful and enucleation was recommended (from Parsons et al[71]).

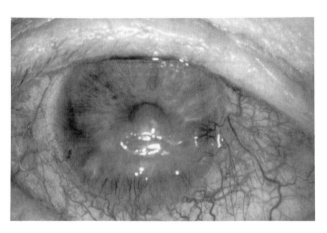

Figure 15-8. Right eye 1 year after treatment with split-course irradiation, 7250 cGy in 39 fractions over 9½ weeks, for adenocarcinoma arising in the orbit. None of the lacrimal tissue was shielded. Note vascularization and ulceration of the inferior and medial cornea. Cultures revealed *Staphylococcus aureus*. One month later, the intraocular pressure was 42 mm Hg. Cyclocryotherapy and retrobulbar alcohol injections failed to relieve severe pain; enucleation was required (from Parsons JT, Bova FJ, Fitzgerald CR, Hood I, Mendenhall WM, Million RR. Tolerance of the visual apparatus to conventional therapeutic irradiation. In: Gutin PH, Leibel SA, Sheline GE, eds. *Radiation Injury to the Nervous System.* New York, NY: Raven Press; 1991:283–302).

severe radiation injury in which the palpebral and bulbar conjunctiva are denuded of their epithelium and become adherent to one another.[72]

SCLERA

Perforation of the sclera is rare, even with extremely high local doses used in treating malignant melanomas of the choroid and ciliary body.[72]

RETINA

When the lacrimal apparatus is shielded from high-dose irradiation, permanent visual loss secondary to degeneration of the anterior segment of the eye usually is preventable; a risk of radiation injury to the retina still exists, however. The retina is supplied by an end-arterial system; that is, the arteries have practically no anastomoses with each other except at the capillary level. After arteriolar occlusion, the amount of collateral flow that can occur through capillary anastomoses is insufficient to prevent retinal damage.[73]

Manifestations of Radiation Retinopathy. Radiation retinopathy presents a clinical picture similar to that seen in diabetic retinopathy. Retinal injury after high-dose irradiation usually is not expressed clinically for 1½ to 3 years after irradiation, during which time visual acuity often remains normal. Subsequent deterioration is thought to occur because of progressive obliteration of small retinal vessels, resulting in retinal ischemia, edema, microaneurysm formation, capillary dilatation, hemorrhage, and retinal or nerve head neovascularization (Fig. 15-10).

It is theorized that the hypoxic retina elaborates a vasoproliferative factor similar to that thought responsible for new vessel formation in diabetic retinopathy. New vessels are situated on the retina, the optic disc, or both. As neovascularization progresses, the vessels invade the plane between the vitreous and retina, and eventually the vitreous itself. Patients with proliferative retinopathy tend to develop contracture of the vitreous gel; as the vitreous shrinks, neovascular fronds that have become attached to its posterior surface are pulled forward, producing preretinal or intravitreal hemorrhage,[74] or retinal detachment.

Macular edema occurs owing to incompetent perifoveal capillaries[74] and results in reduced central vision. Fluorescein angiography demonstrates leakage of dye. It often delineates focal retinal capillary nonperfusion or occluded branch arterioles; central retinal artery occlusion has also been described.[75-77] It seems that the capillaries are most susceptible to obliteration, followed by the smaller branch arterioles.

Some patients with radiation retinopathy develop a neovascular proliferation on the anterior surface of the iris, called rubeosis iridis. The cause may be the same as for posterior-segment neovascularization (ie, a vasoproliferative factor produced by the hypoxic retina). New blood vessels usually appear first at the pupillary margin, then progress to the angles, resulting in peripheral anterior synechiae and neovascular glaucoma, which is secondary to angle closure (Fig. 15–11). The vessels are also very prone to hemorrhage, leading to hyphema.

"Cotton-wool" exudates are a frequent result of retinal ischemia. Such lesions are not true exudates but instead are microinfarcts in the nerve fiber layer. True retinal exudates (also called hard or waxy exudates) also may be seen, and are presumably due to extravasation of fluid from abnormally permeable vessels. They are most common near microaneurysms and have a particular predilection for the region of the macula. Most commonly, there is a 2- to 3-year period during which the visual acuity remains normal or near normal; then, over several months, the vision progressively deteriorates.[78]

Visual loss usually is painless unless neovascular glaucoma develops. Pain from the latter condition usually is not well controlled by medical means, by retrobulbar injections of alcohol, or by cyclocryotherapy. Enucleation or evisceration of the painful eye is often necessary. The best estimate from available data is that a significant risk of severe retinal injury is present when retinal doses exceed 5000 cGy (at 180 to 200 cGy per fraction).

Management of Radiation Retinopathy. Even in the presence of severe retinopathy that results in blindness, maintenance of the eyeball is preferable to enucleation or evisceration unless the eye is painful. Efforts should be made to prevent neovascular (closed angle) glaucoma. In diabetic patients with proliferative retinopathy, panretinal laser photocoagulation eliminates the stimulus to new vessel formation in the anterior and posterior segments, reducing the risk of developing glaucoma.[79] Laser photocoagulation at the University of Florida on a small number of patients suggests that this therapy may be beneficial (Fig. 15–12).

Prevention of Radiation Retinopathy. All fields should be treated daily. Contours and isodose plans through the level of the eyes should be obtained. The dose per fraction should not exceed 180 to 190 cGy per day to the retina. If feasible, fields should be reduced to limit the retinal dose to 5000 cGy or less. In the last several years, physicians at the University of Florida have used hyperfractionation to reduce the risk of complications.

When only a portion of the eye is irradiated, its position during treatment is important. Until 1970, patients at the

University of Florida with ethmoid sinus carcinomas were instructed to gaze laterally to displace the lens from the treatment field (see Fig. 15–4B); the field edge was at or near the medial limbus. This position rotated the posterior pole, and thus most of the sensory retina, into the treatment field. Currently, patients are instructed to gaze straight ahead with the lids open to prevent bolus effect.

OPTIC NERVE

Optic Atrophy. Diagnosis of optic atrophy is based on the ophthalmoscopic appearance of a pale optic disc (due to reduced vascularity of the nerve head) and defective visual function (loss of visual acuity, visual field defects, or both). Fluorescein angiography reveals a loss of vessels in both the superficial and deep vascular networks.

Optic Neuropathy. Two types of neuropathy (anterior ischemic optic neuropathy and retrobulbar ischemic optic neuropathy) may be seen after irradiation. Both types are believed to be caused by vascular occlusive disease, with an interruption of blood supply to either the nerve head or the retrobulbar portion of the nerve, respectively. Patients with preexisting small vessel occlusive disease are at increased risk.

Ophthalmoscopic findings in anterior ischemic optic neuropathy are those of disc pallor and edema with splinter hemorrhages on or adjacent to the disc; the clinical picture is similar to that seen in patients with papilledema. In the University of Florida series, there was a 2- to 4-year latency period after irradiation in five affected eyes. Orally administered corticosteroids failed to halt progressive loss of vision over a period of several months. Disc pallor eventually resulted and was permanent. Brown et al[80] reported on six patients who developed a clinical picture of ischemic optic neuropathy at an average of 19 months after treatment with 3600 to 7000 cGy of external-beam irradiation to the area of the anterior optic nerve. In their series, the acute picture of nerve head swelling and peripapillary hemorrhages and exudates usually persisted for several months, followed in most instances by optic atrophy. However, in two patients, visual acuity improved from 20/200 at the onset of acute disc swelling to 20/30 and 20/40 over 10 weeks to 6 months, respectively; one of the patients received oral glucocorticosteroids and the other HBO therapy, but the authors were unconvinced that these therapies were responsible for the observed recovery.

Seven eyes in five patients at the University of Florida developed visual loss secondary to retrobulbar ischemic optic neuropathy, that is, proximal injury to the nerve without evidence of disc edema or hemorrhage. Time to onset was generally shorter than reported by Shukovsky and Fletcher,[77] who noted a 4- to 5-year latency interval. Visual difficulties were first noted at 11, 12, 14, 28, 42, 72, and 100 months and were thought by the patients to have occurred suddenly.

Three eyes initially lost vision in all fields at the onset of injury. In the other four eyes, the initial visual symptom was

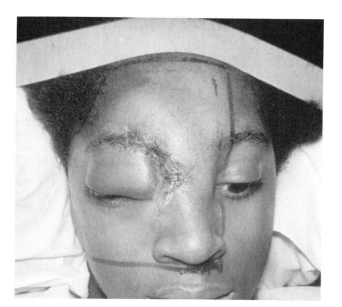

A

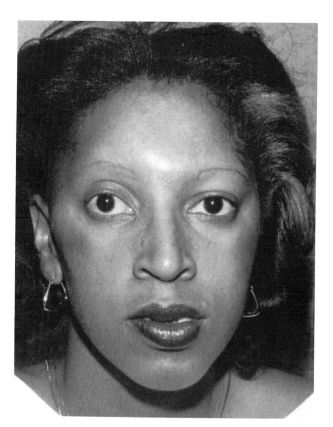

B

Figure 15–9. **(A).** Fifteen-year-old girl with an extensive orbital lymphoma. There were enlarged right preauricular and right jugulodigastric nodes. The right eye and entire lacrimal apparatus received 4000 cGy in 24 fractions over 34 days with ⁶⁰Co. **(B).** There was no evidence of disease at 12 years. A cataract was extracted at 4 years. The patient tolerates a hard contact lens over the right eye (visual acuity 20/30) and has spectacle correction over the left eye (visual acuity 20/20).

a field defect. In our series and other reported cases,[81-83] the defects noted most frequently have been altitudinal, similar to the defects most commonly observed in patients with vascular occlusive disease affecting the optic nerves. Within 2 weeks to 2 months after losing a portion of the visual field, the remaining field of vision also abruptly became affected

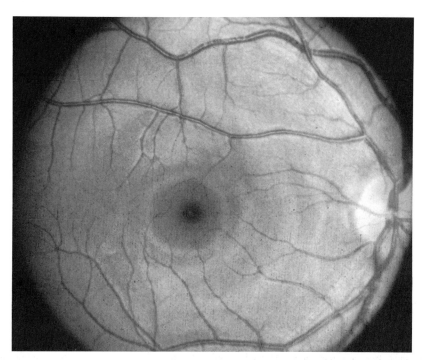

C

Figure 15–9 (continued). (C). The right fundus appears normal. Photograph was made at 8 years (from Parsons et al[71]).

in three of the four eyes; the fourth patient died 10 months after developing an altitudinal defect and had no progression of the deficit during the final 10 months of follow-up. Ophthalmoscopic examination shortly after the onset of symptoms usually revealed a normal-appearing disc or a disc with pallor of only one sector. There was eventual progression to a chalk-white disc (Fig. 15–13). Visual acuity became "count fingers at 1 or 2 feet" in two eyes, "light perception" in the third, and "no light perception" in the other 4 eyes.

The risk of injury correlates with daily fraction size as well as total dose. At approximately 165 to 190 cGy per fraction, a dose of 6000 to 7300 cGy produced injuries in 8% (2 of 24 patients) of long-term survivors. After daily doses of 195 cGy or greater, the risk within the same dose range was 41% (7 of 17 patients).[71]

Management of Optic Nerve Injury. Although a preliminary report on the use of HBO therapy for radiation-induced optic neuropathy was encouraging,[84] HBO had no demonstrable efficacy in a larger series. Roden et al[85] treated 13 patients who had delayed radiation injury to the optic nerves and/or chiasm after 4500 to 7200 cGy. Patients received HBO therapy consisting of repeated treatments with 100% oxygen at 2 atm for 2 hours; 11 patients received corticosteroids simultaneously. Treatment was undertaken as soon after diagnosis as possible; in 6 of 13 patients, therapy was begun within 1 month of recognized visual loss. No patient's vision improved during treatment or follow-up and many had continued deterioration of vision after HBO therapy. Patients whose treatment was initiated early had no better outcome than those treated later. No effective therapy currently exists. Efforts should be directed at prevention by portal reductions, where possible, hyperfractionation, and lower-dose irradiation combined with surgery rather than high-dose irradiation alone.

LENS

Radiation Cataracts. Depending on the dose and its fractionation, a radiation cataract may remain stationary at any stage of development and produce little or no visual impairment; conversely, it may progress to produce blindness. The time to onset of clinically detectable lenticular opacities is inversely related to dose. Fractionation lengthens the latency period. After low-dose irradiation, the latent period may be many years, whereas very intense exposures result in a progressive cataract within 6 months. Several patients at the University of Florida did not develop cataracts until 3 to 3½ years after 4000 to 7000 cGy to the lens with external-beam irradiation.

Bessel et al[86] reported life-table estimates of the probability of developing a cataract after fractionated irradiation of orbital lymphomas. For patients who received 1500 cGy to the germinative zone of the lens, 5- and 8-year probabilities of cataract formation were 12% and 28%, respectively. The 5-year probability for patients who received 3000 cGy was 64%; the authors concluded that it is likely that all of the latter patients eventually will develop cataracts.

Ear

SEROUS OTITIS MEDIA

Serous otitis media is a frequent complication of irradiation of cancer of the paranasal sinuses and nasopharynx, occurring in at least 15% to 20% of patients. Patients whose tumors involve the eustachian tube are at greater risk of developing posttreatment otitis than patients with normal ears, which suggests that fibrosis of previously damaged tissue may be contributory.

Usually otitis is transient and results from desquamated cells and debris, and edema of the mucous membrane lining

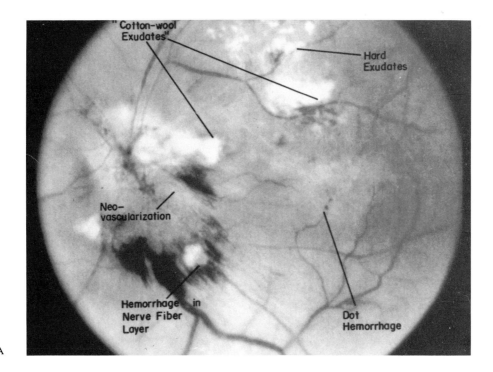

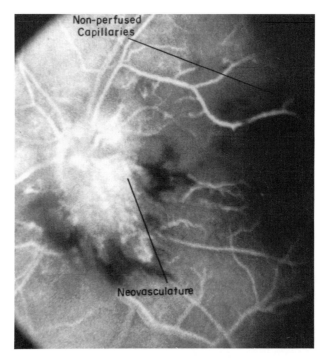

Figure 15–10.   (A). Appearance of left eye on ophthalmoscopic examination 2 years 8 months after irradiation of a low-grade fibrosarcoma of the left nasal cavity, paranasal sinuses, and orbit in a 42-year-old woman. The dose to the left retina was 6000 cGy in 32 fractions over 61 days by split-course technique; the lacrimal gland was shielded. Visual acuity remained 20/20 in the left eye for 2 years after irradiation, but by 2 years 7 months she had developed an edematous, congested optic disc; her visual acuity was 20/300. One month later, at the time of this photograph, there was a Marcus-Gunn pupil, and vision was "counts fingers"; the disc margins were hazy and there were cotton-wool spots, hard exudates, intraretinal and preretinal hemorrhages, and irregular, tortuous branch retinal arterioles (from Parsons et al[71]). **(B).** Fluorescein angiography showed irregular fluorescence of the large vessel walls superiorly, compatible with damage to these structures. There was an extensive fluorescein leak from neovascular tissue over the disc and an area of retinal capillary nonperfusion superior to the fovea. Several months later, the patient presented to her local ophthalmologist with severe pain secondary to neovascular glaucoma (40 mm Hg). Enucleation was performed. In addition to rubeosis iridis, the surgical specimen showed neovascular tissue arising from the surface of the nerve head and extending into the vitreous (from Parsons et al[71]).

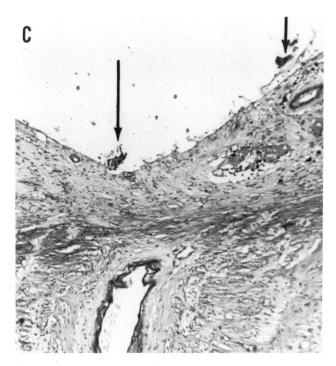

Figure 15–10 (continued). (C). Photomicrograph of the eye after enucleation showing cluster of small, thin-walled neovasculature protruding from the surface of the nerve head into the vitreous (arrows). The neovasculature corresponds to the area of leakage noted on fluorescein angiography (from Parsons JT, Bova FJ, Fitzgerald CR, Hood I, Mendenhall WM, Million RR. Tolerance of the visual apparatus to conventional therapeutic irradiation. In: Gutin PH, Leibel SA, Sheline GE, eds. *Radiation Injury to the Nervous System.* New York, NY: Raven Press; 1991:283–302).

the eustachian tube. Patients complain of a stuffy feeling in the ear and conductive hearing loss. Some cases resolve when oral decongestants are administered but others require myringotomy, usually within the first year after treatment. It is rarely necessary to perform myringotomy during a course of irradiation. Bacterial infection rarely supervenes.

SENSORINEURAL HEARING LOSS

Sensorineural hearing loss is a rarely reported complication of ear irradiation; its incidence is unknown but it may be more common than generally thought. Of 137 patients who underwent nasopharyngeal irradiation at the Massachusetts General Hospital between 1961 and 1969, 7 (54%) of 13 patients who had pretreatment and posttreatment audiometric evaluation were noted to have developed sensorineural hearing loss.[87] Because a selection factor existed (ie, patients who were evaluated were those who were having problems), the incidence of injury could not be established. Hearing losses ranged from 10 dB to almost total deafness; the most profound losses occurred after extremely high-dose treatment (more than 20,000 cGy). Small sensorineural hearing losses were noted during the first few years but the onset of severe losses was gradual and occurred 3 to 6 years after treatment. Small losses had flat audiometric patterns, whereas the more profound losses were most severe in the high-frequency range. The risk is greater in older patients.[87,88]

Few reports exist of histological studies of irradiated temporal bone. In an autopsy done at 1 year posttreatment, Leach[88] noted absence of the organ of Corti and atrophy of the spiral ganglion and cochlear nerve. Schuknecht and Karmody[35] described a patient who had temporal bone radionecrosis 8 years after irradiation; autopsy at 12 years showed atrophy of the organ of Corti, loss of some hair cells, atrophy of the basilar membrane, and loss of some of the cells of the spiral ganglion.

VESTIBULAR DISORDERS

Little is known about the effects of conventional fractionated radiation on vestibular function. Leach[88] described several patients who complained of vertigo in the postirradiation period, some of whom had abnormal results of ice-water caloric tests. In one patient, 1 year after treatment, absence of the macula (of the utricle) and cristae (of the semicircular canals), the structures in which hair cells transmit sensory information by way of the vestibular nerve to the central nervous system (CNS), was noted at autopsy.

Spinal Cord and Brain Stem
LHERMITTE'S SIGN

A transient radiation myelopathy, manifested by Lhermitte's sign, or the "barber chair" sign, occurs frequently in patients whose spinal cords are incidentally irradiated. The sign was first described during World War I in French military hospitals by Marie and Chatelin,[89,90] who noted it in soldiers who had experienced injuries to the head and neck area. Similar cases were described by Babinski and Dubois[91] and by Lhermitte[92] himself in 1918. The sign was first described in association with radiotherapy in 1948 by Boden.[93] It consists of a momentary, but very disturbing, electric-like shock that is triggered by flexion of the cervical spine. The sensation may be limited to the spine, but more commonly it radiates into the extremities, particularly the backs of the thighs. The distribution of the sensation does not correspond with the finite territory of any dermatome. The distribution usually is symmetrical and equal on both sides of the body. Symptoms usually appear 1 to 3 months after completion of irradiation and last from 1 month to as long as 8 or 9 months, with an average duration of 3 to 4 months. The symptoms usually subside gradually. The condition produces no muscle weakness, sphincter disturbance, or accompanying neurological signs. The character, latency period, and duration of symptoms are identical to those described after traumatic injury to the neck.

Lhermitte's sign is an early-appearing, benign form of myelopathy and should be distinguished from later-occurring, progressive radiation myelopathy. Lhermitte's sign rarely leads to progressive cord degeneration and transverse myelopathy. When the condition arises soon after completion of irradiation, healing almost always occurs without permanent damage. When the syndrome appears late (9 to 12 months), however, radiation myelitis may follow.[94]

Damage to the posterior columns is thought to be a prerequisite for Lhermitte's sign.[95] Jones[94] attributes the transient

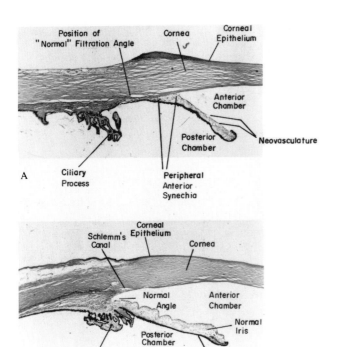

myelopathy to temporary demyelination. The minimum dose of radiation that produces Lhermitte's sign has not been clearly identified. A spinal cord dose as low as 3000 cGy in 25 fractions over 7 weeks by split-course irradiation to the Hodgkin's mantle field, with both fields treated daily, may produce mild symptoms.

The condition is self-limited, reversible, and requires no specific therapy. In two patients who were extremely symptomatic, a cervical collar was used for several months until symptoms resolved. Patients should be warned about the possible occurence of Liermitte's sign so they are not alarmed should symptoms occur.

TRANSVERSE MYELITIS

Radiation-induced transverse myelitis is a rare complication of brain stem and spinal cord irradiation. The process almost always is irreversible, and no effective therapy is known. Symptoms and signs of partial or complete transection of the cord appear 6 months to 2 years after irradiation (the earliest reported case occurred 4 months after treatment). The latent intervals tend to be shortest in patients whose spinal cords were retreated, patients whose cords received the highest doses, and possibly, pediatric patients.[96,97]

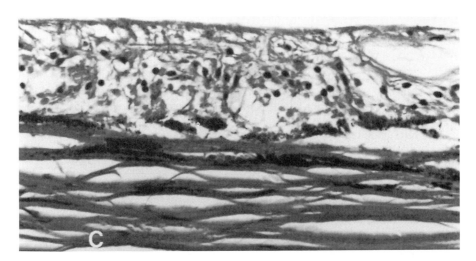

Figure 15–11. A 47-year-old man received 6500 cGy in 32 fractions over 44 days to the nasal half of his right eye for a poorly differentiated cancer involving the ethmoid sinus and orbit. The position of the eye during treatment was "lateral gaze." Until 14 months after treatment, he noted only epiphora, which had been present before treatment, and occasional flashes of light in the right eye; visual acuity remained 20/40. Three months later, there was severe sheathing of retinal arterioles and declining visual acuity. At 22 months, vision was "counts fingers" and the patient complained of ocular pain. Ocular tension was 44 mm Hg. Pain was progressive and unrelieved by narcotic analgesics and carbonic anhydrase inhibitors. Blood in the anterior chamber (hyphema) was noted. Enucleation was required. **(A).** The surgical specimen showed rubeosis iridis (note numerous dilated vessels on the anterior surface of the iris), ectropion uveae, and a broad, peripheral anterior synechia, which obliterated the filtration angle. **(B).** Normal iris and normal filtration angle for comparison with **A. (C).** The retina was in place. Retinal changes were most severe in those portions of the retina that received the highest dose. Microscopic section shows severe atrophy and disorganization of the nasal (irradiated) retina.

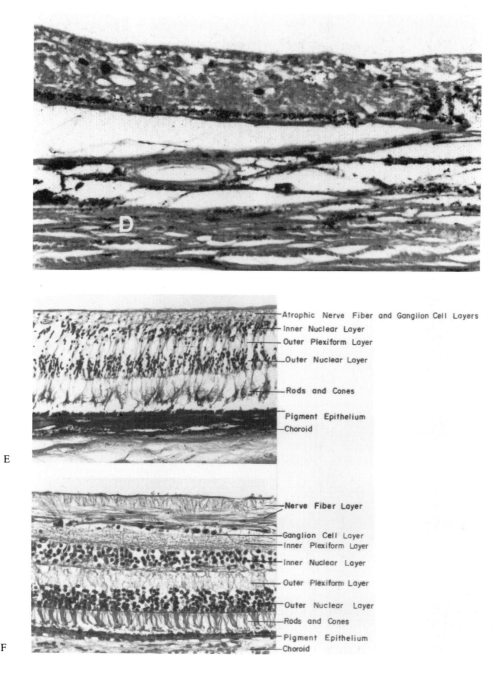

Figure 15–11. continued. **(D).** Microscopic section from another area of the nasal retina showed full-thickness retinal necrosis. **(E).** The temporal retina, which received a low dose of irradiation, showed only the effects of elevated intraocular pressure, rather than effects due to a direct action of irradiation. The nerve fiber layer was atrophic and the ganglion cells absent. Nuclei of the inner nuclear layer were decreased in number whereas those of the outer layer were preserved. **(F).** Appearance of normal retina for comparison with **C** through **E**. It should be noted that the histological changes secondary to irradiation are nonspecific (from Parsons et al[71]).

Typically, patients first develop paresthesia followed by steadily progressive sensorimotor disturbances, bowel and bladder dysfunction, and paraplegia or quadriplegia. The sensory symptoms usually begin in the lower extremities, then, over weeks to months, ascend to involve the trunk and upper limbs. The initial findings may, therefore, lead one to suspect a lesion lower in the cord.[98] Pain in the neck and arms is sometimes prominent, and the signs are usually asymmetrical at first. Horner's syndrome has been reported in a few patients.[99] Symptoms progress at a variable rate. Although the signs and symptoms may not progress beyond a certain stage, once present, they rarely disappear. The syndrome results in death in about two thirds of patients within 4 years[100] and the rest usually are severely incapacitated. Involvement of the sphincters implies a poor prognosis.[101] Complete transverse myelitis at the level of the upper cervical cord or brain stem results in death, usually secondary to bronchopneumonia. A number of patients with myelopathy developed the

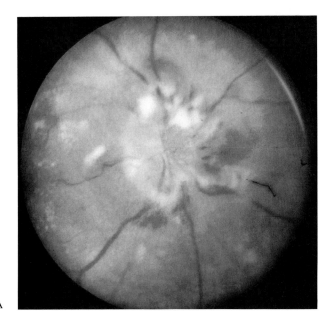
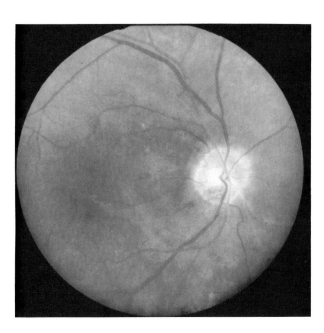

A   B

Figure 15–12. **(A).** Right eye of 66-year-old man 16 months after 4000 cGy to the posterior half of the right retina. Because of inhomogeneity in the dose distribution, the posterior pole of the eye received 5000 cGy to 5500 cGy in the area of the nerve head. Visual acuity was 20/100. There is extensive disc edema with surrounding hemorrhages and exudates. On fluorescein angiography, there were tremendously dilated capillaries on the optic disc with an extensive late leak with some areas of retinal nonperfusion. The patient underwent panretinal laser photocoagulation. By 4 months, the capillary dilation at the nerve head had diminished markedly. In the ensuing months, the hemorrhages and exudates gradually resolved. **(B).** At the time of this photograph (1 year after laser photocoagulation), the disc edema had dissipated. Visual acuity was 20/25 (from Parsons JT, Bova FJ, Fitzgerald CR, Hood I, Mendenhall WM, Million RR. Tolerance of the visual apparatus to conventional therapeutic irradiation. In: Gutin PH, Leibel SA, Sheline GE, eds. *Radiation Injury to the Nervous System.* New York, NY: Raven Press; 1991:283–302).

Brown-Séquard syndrome, with loss of voluntary movements and Babinski's sign on one side and loss of pain and temperature sensations on the opposite side; in some patients the syndrome remained stable, whereas in others it progressed.

Diagnostic workup should include lumbar puncture (including cytological study) and myelogram. The cerebrospinal fluid contains no excess of cells. The myelogram and the total protein values in the cerebrospinal fluid usually are normal in patients with radiation myelitis, but cord swelling, with complete blockage of contrast material, and marked elevations of protein have been reported.[102–105] Cord narrowing on myelography, presumably due to cord necrosis and atrophy, also has been reported.[98,106] Myelography aids in the diagnosis of extradural metastatic compressive lesions; CT scans and magnetic resonance imaging (MRI) help to exclude intradural or intramedullary tumor.[107] Cervical spine roentgenograms help rule out cord injury secondary to bony problems. The differential diagnosis also includes necrotizing myelopathy,[108] vascular lesions, and syphilis.

Boden[109] reported seven cases of brain stem myelitis after irradiation of tumors of the middle ear, nasopharynx, or parotid. The usual time to onset was about 1 year after treatment, and death followed in all patients within 1 to 6 months. The onset is sometimes preceded by acute stomach ulceration. Common signs and symptoms included nystagmus, cranial nerve palsies, ataxia, paralysis, and anesthesia. A common occurrence was unilateral seventh-nerve palsy and contralateral hemiplegia.

The white matter is more susceptible to radiation injury than the gray matter. A notable manifestation of myelopathy is demyelination, which may be due to injury to the oligodendrogliocyte (the myelin-forming cell of the CNS), and obliterative changes in small blood vessels or both.

TIME-DOSE-VOLUME CONSIDERATIONS FOR SPINAL CORD INJURY

Marcus and Million[110] evaluated the incidence of cervical spinal cord injury in 2901 patients with malignancies of the upper respiratory tract who received radiation therapy at the University of Florida between 1964 and 1987. A total of 1112 patients received a minimum incidental dose of 3000 cGy to at least a 2-cm length of the cervical cord with megavoltage irradiation, and had at least 1 year of follow-up (unless a neurological complication occurred before 1 year). One year was chosen as the period of minimum follow-up because about 70% of myelopathies occur between 6 and 12 months. Of the 1112 patients, 788 were observed for at least 2 years and 308 for at least 5 years. Continuous-course, once-a-day treatment was given to 709 patients, 170 received split-course irradiation, and 233 received twice-a-day irradiation (120 cGy twice a day with a minimum 4-hour interval between fractions). Most of the once-a-day patients received treatment at

180 to 200 cGy/d. Two patients (0.18%) developed radiation myelitis. One had received 4660 cGy at 173 cGy/d (continuous course) and the other had received 4907 cGy at 169 cGy/d (split course).

The incidence of myelitis for patients receiving 4000 to 4499 cGy was 0 of 442; for patients receiving 4500 to 4999 cGy, it was 2 of 471 (difference not significant); and for patients receiving 5000 cGy or more, the incidence was 0 of 75. The occurrence of myelitis did not correlate well with either total dose or fraction size; the results for 879 patients who received once-a-day irradiation by either continuous- or split-course techniques are shown in Table 15-2. None of 233 patients who received twice-a-day irradiation developed myelitis, including 18 who received doses of 5000 to 5400 cGy.

The incidence of myelitis, according to total dose versus length of spinal cord irradiated, is shown in Table 15-3. No obvious pattern of occurrence is seen. Seventy-eight patients received doses of 4500 cGy or greater to 9-cm or longer portions of the spinal cord without experiencing myelitis.

Several reports of high-dose (5700 to 6800 cGy) irradiation of the cervical spinal cord exist. McCunniff and Liang[111] reported on 144 patients with cancer of the head and neck treated at the Bowman Gray School of Medicine between 1971 and 1980 who, in the course of treatment, received doses ranging from 5600 to 6500 cGy to varying lengths of their cervical spinal cords. Treatment was by split course; a compensating filter was used in most patients to ensure dose homogeneity throughout the treatment volume. Portals included 3.5- to 15.0-cm lengths of the spinal cord. Treatments were administered 5 days each week. The fraction size (to the spinal cord) was usually less than 180 cGy/d. Eighty-two of the 144 patients had follow-up for more than 1 year, and 53 were observed for more than 2 years. Only one patient developed myelitis (6000 cGy at 200 cGy per fraction).

Baekmark[112] reported on 21 patients who had follow-up for more than 1 year after receiving 5700 cGy over 6 weeks by continuous-course irradiation (five fractions per week); none developed progressive myelopathy. Jeremic et al[113] reported on 72 patients who were observed for 2 years or more after cervical spinal cord doses of 5500 to 6800 cGy. Four patients (5.6%) developed permanent radiation myelitis.

Table 15-4 summarizes the data for 146 patients who received doses of 5500 cGy or more, in various fractionation schemes, to the cervical spinal cord.[111-113] Four (7%) of 60 patients treated with fractions of 190 to 200 cGy developed radiation myelitis. One (1%) of 86 patients treated with lower doses per fraction developed late radiation myelitis. Although lower doses per fraction seem to decrease the risk of radiation myelitis, extension of overall treatment time (eg, by split-course techniques) affords little or no additional protection.

Extension of the lateral portals to cover the entire neck results in irradiation of long lengths of cord and likely increases the risk of damage.[114] Guidelines at the University of Florida call for portal reductions off the spinal cord after doses of 4500 to 4680 cGy in 25 to 26 fractions (180 cGy per fraction); 4600 cGy in 23 fractions (200 cGy per fraction); or 4560 cGy in 38 fractions (120 cGy per fraction twice a day). If necessary, the dose to lymph nodes behind the plane of the spinal cord is then boosted with electrons or an anterior and posterior wedge pair, or the nodes are removed by neck dissection.

Higher doses are required, however, in certain circumstances (eg, advanced cancer of the nasopharynx or unresectable sarcomas encircling the spinal canal). In these circumstances, the risk of injury must be weighed against the consequences of uncontrolled tumor growth, and a 5%, or even 10%, probability of spinal cord injury becomes an acceptable risk.

Brain

Adverse effects of irradiation on the brain may be divided into three groups, depending on the time of appearance. Acute reactions occur during and immediately after a course of irradiation and generally consist of edema. In the absence of tumor in the brain, the syndrome is rare, and it will not be discussed. The early delayed syndrome usually is transient and appears weeks to months after irradiation. The syndrome was first described in 1929 by Druckmann,[115] and many names have been applied to it, including early delayed CNS syndrome, transitory CNS syndrome, acute transient leuko-encephalopathy, and somnolence syndrome. All apparently describe the same phenomenon. The late delayed reaction occurs months to years after irradiation.[116]

TRANSITORY CNS SYNDROME (EARLY DELAYED REACTION)

After irradiation of advanced tumors of the ethmoid or sphenoid sinuses or nasopharynx, about 10% of patients develop a clinically recognizable syndrome characterized by lethargy, nausea, occasional vomiting, headache, and dizziness; rarely, transient cranial nerve palsies or ataxia develop. The syndrome typically appears 2 to 3 months after treatment, lasts 2 to 6 weeks, then disappears spontaneously. Patients should be forewarned of this alarming problem because it appears about the time that they are beginning to recover from the acute effects of radiation. The syndrome is believed to result from transient demyelination, secondary to incidental brain irradiation. The latent period corresponds to the turnover time for myelin; the syndrome may be similar in etiology to Lhermitte's sign of the spinal cord.[117,118]

The differential diagnosis usually is recurrent tumor versus delayed transient CNS syndrome, the symptoms and signs of which may be similar. The time frame of CNS syndrome is characteristic and assists in making the correct diagnosis. Usually no CT scan abnormalities are present, although in one patient, Graeb et al[119] observed low-density changes that subsequently resolved and may have represented the early delayed reaction. Although no specific therapy is required, corticosteroids have been reported to relieve signs and symptoms in severe cases.[118,120]

Because of the transient nature of the early delayed reaction, little information exists on the histological features. Lampert et al[121,122] described two patients in whom the early delayed reaction was unusually severe, resulting in the death of both patients. Clinically, each case was characterized by the sudden

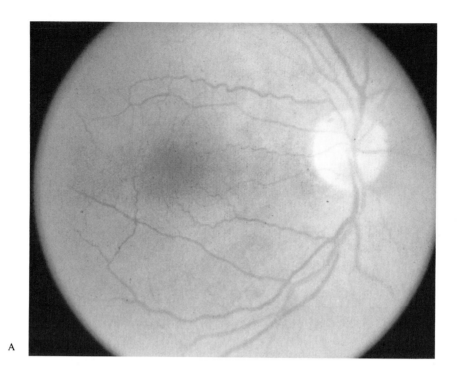

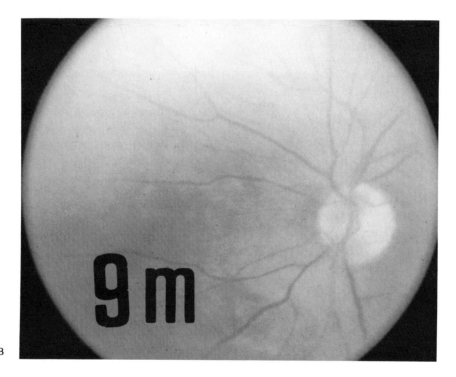

Figure 15–13.   Right **(A)** and left **(B)** fundi 9 months after treatment of squamous cell carcinoma of the nasal cavity and ethmoid sinuses in a 70-year-old man who received 6000 cGy in 30 fractions over 43 days followed by a radium needle implant for 2000 cGy. The left optic nerve received approximately 6200 cGy and the right optic nerve approximately 5900 cGy. Both fundi appeared normal.

onset of symptoms about 3 months after termination of irradiation. Autopsies showed plaques of demyelination within the field of irradiation that resembled the lesions of acute multiple sclerosis. Also present were perivascular lymphocytic and plasma cell infiltrates. Degenerative vascular changes (which are prominent in the late delayed reaction)

were not present.

LATE DELAYED REACTION

The late delayed reaction usually is irreversible, progressive, and sometimes fatal. Signs and symptoms depend on the area and volume of brain irradiated and resemble those of an

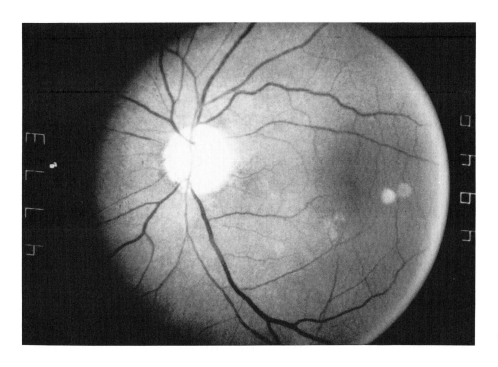

C

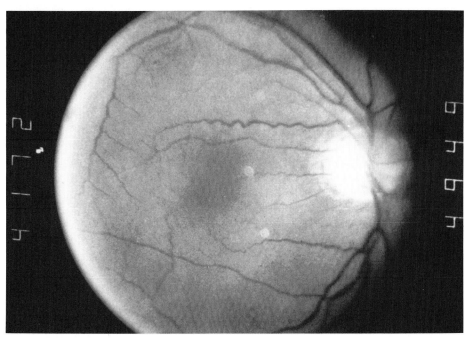

D

Figure 15–13 (continued). (C). At 11 months after treatment, there was optic atrophy of the left eye (visual acuity "hand motion"). Fluorescein angiography revealed a paucity of disc capillaries in both eyes. **(D).** At 14 months, the patient noted a visual field defect in the right eye. At this time there was an area of pallor on the temporal side of the disc. Visual acuity remained 20/20 in the right eye, but over the next 2 weeks, it became "no light perception" in both eyes (from Parsons JT, Bova FJ, Fitzgerald CR, Hood I, Mendenhall WM, Million RR. Tolerance of the visual apparatus to conventional therapeutic irradiation. In: Glutin PH, Leibel SA, Sheline GE, eds. *Radiation Injury to the Nervous System.* New York, NY: Raven Press; 1991:283–302).

intracranial mass.[116] The essential lesion is demyelination with loss of oligodendrogliocytes and focal or diffuse areas of white matter necrosis. Both small vessel and glial cell damage are responsible. Computed tomographic scan demonstrates hypodense areas that are most frequently observed in the periventricular areas; ventricular asymmetry or dilation and widening of the subarachnoid spaces (a reflection of cerebral cortical atrophy); and sometimes intracerebral calcification, which represents mineralizing microangiopathy. Magnetic resonance imaging is better at visualizing the abnormalities than CT scan; white matter damage is seen as an area of relatively high-signal intensity on T2-weighted

Table 15–2. Risk of Myelitis According to Total Dose and Dose Per Fraction in Patients Treated with Once-a-Day Irradiation (No. with Myelitis/No. at Risk) (University of Florida)

DOSE (cGy)	< 160 cGy/d	160–179 cGy/d	180–189 cGy/d	≥ 200 cGy/d
<4000	0/57	0/22	0/21	0/6
4000–4499	0/44	0/191	0/91	0/9
4500–4999	1/23	1/119	0/211	0/28
5000–5499	0/1	0/14	0/22	0/12
≥5500	0/2	n.d.	0/3	0/3

Abbreviation: n.d = no data.

Note: Seven hundred nine patients were treated by continuous-course irradiation; 170 patients were treated by split-course irradiation.

Data from Marcus and Million.[110]

Table 15–3. Risk of Myelitis According to Total Dose and Length of Cervical Spinal Cord Treated (No. with Myelitis/No. at Risk) (1112 Patients) (University of Florida)

LENGTH OF CORD (cm)*	DOSE (cGy)			
	< 4000	4000–4499	4500–4999	≥ 5000
2–4	0/41	0/77	0/85	0/14
5–6	0/51	0/202	1/212	0/31
7–8	0/13	0/94	1/109	0/17
9–10	0/13	0/44	0/54	0/10
>10	0/6	0/25	0/11	0/3

Note: Patients include continuous-course, split-course, once-day-, and twice-a-day irradiation techniques.

*Lengths were rounded to the nearest centimeter.

From Marcus and Million.[110]

images. Extensive brain damage is seen as areas of cystic degeneration, representing coagulative necrosis. Most patients whose brains are incidentally irradiated develop no MRI or CT scan abnormalities.[123] Most patients who have mild abnormalities remain asymptomatic, and some with extensive MRI changes also remain asymptomatic. The time interval to the development of frank CNS necrosis is generally 6 months to 2 years, although occasionally injury is seen later than 2 years.[124] Sequelae consist of impaired mental function in adults, learning disabilities in children, seizures, dementia, and death.

Frank necrosis is rare. In most reported cases, patients have received treatment with large (more than 200 cGy) daily fractions or multiple courses of therapy for cancer of the skin, middle ear, nasopharynx, paranasal sinuses, or brain. The incidence of the complication is difficult to determine because literature reports are anecdotal. Most radiation oncologists regard the maximum safe dose for large-volume brain irradiation in adults to be 5500 cGy in 30 fractions, 5 days per week, over 6 weeks; few data substantiate such a threshold, but the dose is a useful guideline.[125,126] Small volumes of brain tolerate 6000 to 6500 cGy.

Lee et al[127] reported on 9606 patients who received irradiation for nasopharyngeal carcinoma at the Queen Elizabeth Hospital, Hong Kong, 1964 through 1984. One hundred two patients (1%) developed temporal lobe necrosis. The patients received large-dose fractions (420 cGy twice weekly to 5040 cGy, with or without a boost, or 6000 cGy in 24 fractions of 250 cGy each). Eighty percent of the patients received a single course of treatment and the rest received a second course of treatment after recurrence. Symptoms included classic temporal lobe epilepsy (déjà vu, hallucinations, or

Table 15–4. Radiation Myelitis According to Total Dose to the Cervical Spinal Cord and Number of Fractions with >1 Year Follow-Up

SPINAL CORD DOSE (cGy)	FRACTIONS	AVERAGE FRACTION SIZE	PATIENTS	CASES OF MYELITIS (%)
5500–5700	28–30	190–196	24	1 (4)
5700	34	167	1	1
6000	30	200	36	3 (8)
6000	32	188	12	0
6000	35–37	163–171	9	0
6000	40	150	12	0
6120	34	180	1	0
6300	40	157	6	0
6331	43	147	1	0
6500	40	163	43	0
6800	40	170	1	0

Data from McCunniff and Liang,[111] Baekmark,[112] and Jeremic et al.[113]

"absence" attacks) in 32 patients; and dizziness, impaired memory, headache, confusion, generalized convulsions, or personality changes in 54 patients. There were no symptoms or signs in 16 patients, although 4 subsequently became symptomatic. The median latency interval for patients who had a single course of irradiation was 4 years, and for patients who had two radical courses of treatment, 18 months. Computed tomographic scan showed either fingerlike hypodense shadows (85 patients) or cysts in the temporal lobes (16 patients). Cerebral angiograms in three patients showed avascular space-occupying lesions with displacement of adjacent blood vessels. Twelve patients had histological confirmation. Findings consisted of coagulative necrosis, demyelination, fibrinoid changes of blood vessels, hemorrhage, and edema in the white matter. Surgical intervention did not benefit five patients in whom it was undertaken. Seventy-two patients were treated with corticosteroids, and improvement was noted in some patients with early lesions but not in patients with cystic necrosis.

No specific therapy for radiation-induced brain necrosis exists. Some necrotic foci act like mass lesions; resection of necrotic tissue may be lifesaving in this circumstance. Corticosteroid treatment may relieve surrounding cerebral edema.[120] The differential diagnosis includes recurrent cancer and other CNS disease that produces a similar clinical picture.

Cranial and Peripheral Nerves

The cranial and peripheral nerves are seldom regarded as major dose-limiting tissues in treatment planning. Injury is uncommon, even after high-dose therapy. In contrast, the brain stem and spinal cord frequently are the major dose-limiting tissues within a treatment volume.

The most frequent cranial nerve deficit after high-dose irradiation of pharyngeal cancer is hypoglossal nerve palsy.[128,129] Palsy is most likely in patients who develop extensive fibrosis in the neck after high-dose irradiation. The most common scenario is a patient who has a large subdigastric lymph node metastasis that has been successfully treated by irradiation alone, who then develops extensive fibrosis, presumably resulting in nerve entrapment and palsy 3 or more years after irradiation. Patients who undergo neck dissection after irradiation are, paradoxically, at less risk of the complication, presumably because the node and its mass of keratin, which eventually is replaced by a fibrous mass,[39] have been removed. Patients who have no lymph node metastasis are at lesser risk of hypoglossal nerve palsy but occasionally develop the problem if they develop severe fibrosis. Often patients are unaware of the deficit until tongue atrophy, fasciculation, and deviation are noted during a follow-up visit. Speech is not greatly impaired unless both nerves are affected, in which case difficulty in swallowing and aspiration also occur. Soft tissue necrosis in the glossotonsillar sulcus may lead to an early appearing hypoglossal nerve deficit.

The brachial plexus is included within the treatment volume when the lower neck is irradiated. Elective lymph node irradiation to the lower neck (5000 cGy at D_{max}) with an anterior cobalt 60 portal would produce a dose of 4000 to 4500 cGy to the brachial plexus (at 3 to 5 cm depth, depending on the patient's physical structure). Brachial plexus neuropathy is exceedingly rare after standard fractionated therapy and has been observed at the University of Florida in only one patient with cancer of the head and neck, who underwent a second course of irradiation for a late supraclavicular nodal failure, which brought the total dose to more than 13,000 cGy.

Pituitary Gland
ANTERIOR LOBE

The pituitary gland and hypothalamus are incidentally irradiated during treatment of tumors of the paranasal sinuses and nasopharynx. Sophisticated tests (eg, radioimmunoassay and stimulation tests employing synthetic hypothalamic hormones) that were unavailable to early investigators have shown that pituitary dysfunction is more common than previously thought. The exact incidence is still unknown because many of the patients have been selected for evaluation because of some clinical abnormality.

The pituitary of the child is thought to be more sensitive than that of the adult.[130,131] It has also been suggested that female patients are more susceptible than male patients to irradiation-induced hypopituitarism.[132]

Samaan et al[133] studied 110 patients with tumors of the nasopharynx or paranasal sinuses 1 to 26 years after irradiation to portals that included both the hypothalamus and pituitary gland. Patients were studied clinically and by biochemical endocrine testing, including tests before and after stimulation with insulin, luteinizing hormone–releasing hormone (LH-RH), and thyrotropin releasing hormone (TRH). Seventy-six patients (69%) showed one or more features suggestive of hypothalamic injury and 43 (39%) had evidence of primary pituitary deficiency. The percentage of patients with clinical and biochemical abnormalities increased as a function of time up to 10 years after treatment. Impairment can be demonstrated as early as 1 year after irradiation.[134] Other authors have similarly concluded that the hypothalamus more often is the site of injury than the pituitary gland.[131,134,135]

Growth hormone is the hormone most frequently affected by hypothalamic-pituitary irradiation.[130,136] The incidence of clinical growth hormone deficiency is less than the incidence of reduced growth hormone response to pharmacological stimuli.[135] Children who undergo radiotherapy should have their growth rate measured at regular intervals. Tests for growth hormone secretion are done only if the growth rate declines significantly.[137] Hormonal deficiencies must be detected before epiphyseal fusion occurs. The diagnosis of growth hormone deficiency in an adult is of academic interest only. The hormone need not be replaced.

The serum morning cortisol is used to screen patients for corticotropin deficiency. If the results are abnormal, more sophisticated testing is done.

Follicle-stimulating hormone (FSH) and LH regulate the development, reproductive functions, and hormonal secretions of the testicle and ovary. The screening test for gonadotropin insufficiency in male patients is serum testosterone. In female patients, basal and stimulated (LH-RH) FSH and LH values are obtained. Samaan et al[133] noted subnormal LH and FSH levels before and after administration of LH-RH in 33 patients, indicating a primary pituitary deficiency. Signs and symptoms included amenorrhea, impotence, absence of pubic and axillary hair, testicular atrophy, and decreased libido. Estrogen or testosterone therapy is done under the direction of an endocrinologist.

Hypothyroidism may result from irradiation of the thyroid (primary hypothyroidism) or pituitary (secondary hypothyroidism) gland. Twenty-one patients from the M.D. Anderson Hospital had diminished thyroid function as well as thyrotropin levels that were not elevated and failed to rise after administration of TRH, indicating pituitary deficiency.[133] Nine others with diminished thyroid function had low thyrotropin levels that showed a delayed rise after TRH administration, suggesting a hypothalamic problem.

Prolactin secretion is under the inhibitory control of the hypothalamus. In the presence of a hypothalamic lesion, the basal serum prolactin level is elevated. Forty-three of 110 patients from the M.D. Anderson Hospital showed hyperprolactinemia, presumably from hypothalamic injury.[133] Amenorrhea and galactorrhea result.[131,132]

Follow-up Policy. Adult patients are asked about impotence, libido, amenorrhea, oligomenorrhea, and galactorrhea. Children are observed by a pediatrician, who looks for evidence of decline in growth rate. Annual evaluations of thyroxine (T_4) , thyroid-stimulating hormone (TSH), and serum morning cortisol are performed in all patients. Testosterone levels are checked annually in male patients. Follicle-stimulating hormone and LH are checked in postmenopausal women. If any test results or symptoms suggest deficiency, patients are referred to an endocrinologist for detailed evaluation.

POSTERIOR LOBE

Diabetes insipidus has been reported after deliberate pituitary ablation by transsphenoidally implanted ^{90}Y pellets, which deliver tens of thousands of centigrays to the pituitary gland. The complication is not reported after standardly fractionated radiotherapy.

Thyroid and Parathyroid Glands
THYROID GLAND

Clinical hypothyroidism develops after lower neck irradiation in about 5% of adults and a somewhat higher proportion of children. The problem is more common in women than men.[138,139] Signs and symptoms may be classic but often are nonspecific and attributable to other causes. The chemical detection of hypothyroidism can be made some weeks before clinical symptoms or signs develop. Onset of hypothyroidism may occur within weeks of the completion of treatment but more often occurs months or years later. Frequency of development apparently is related to dose as well as to volume[140,141]; the isthmus of the gland should be shielded during lower neck irradiation, if practical to do so. The addition of a hemithyroidectomy after irradiation increases the risk of subsequent hypothyroidism.[139,142] The screening test is the serum T_4 level. A high serum TSH level confirms the diagnosis of primary hypothyroidism.

The prevalence of chemical hypothyroidism, as manifested by elevated TSH levels with normal T_4 levels, has been estimated to be as high as 20% to 25% after radiation therapy for cancer of the head and neck.[138] The addition of hemithyroidectomy increased the prevalence to 66% in the series by Vrabec and Heffron.[139] The condition may represent mild or developing hypothyroidism that has been compensated by increased TSH secretion. In some patients, TSH levels are only transiently elevated and return to normal[140,141,143]; other patients remain euthyroid for long periods while the serum TSH level is persistently high; and still others develop frank hypothyroidism.

Management of hypothyroidism consists of thyroid hormone replacement. Patients with compensated hypothyroidism (elevated TSH, normal T_4 levels) present a treatment question because the long-term effects of this condition are unknown. As a minimum, such patients should have their TSH and T_4 levels checked at regular intervals; some authors advocate replacement therapy. The possibility exists that thyroid neoplasia may be induced in these patients secondary to prolonged TSH stimulation, as has been observed in some animals.[130]

PARATHYROID GLANDS AND PARAFOLLICULAR CELLS

Serum calcium concentration is maintained in part by the interaction of parathormone (which is secreted by the parathyroid glands) and calcitonin (which is secreted by the parafollicular cells of the thyroid gland). Several retrospective studies have shown that decades after low doses of external irradiation to the neck, the prevalence of hyperparathyroidism is increased.[144] There are few data on the effect of higher radiation doses. Disorders of calcium and phosphorus homeostasis secondary to irradiation of these structures have not been noted in the University of Florida radiotherapy series. Holten and Peterson[145] studied serum levels of calcium, phosphate, and parathyroid hormone before, during, and every 3 to 6 months after treatment for 3 years in 29 patients whose parathyroid glands received 3700 to 6700 cGy; serum levels of parathyroid hormone showed a slightly increasing trend during the follow-up period. No patient developed hyperparathyroidism and there was no essential change in serum calcium concentration. A few reports have been made of parathyroid insufficiency after treatment with iodine-131 (^{131}I) for hyperthyroidism, suggesting that very high doses are required to impair function of the glands.[146]

Lung

After low neck irradiation, fibrosis of the apical segments of the lungs frequently is seen on routine follow-up chest roentgenograms, beginning 6 to 12 months after treatment. Fibrosis of the apices is of little functional consequence. The apical changes occasionally are misinterpreted on lung radiographs as mass lesions.

Chronic Lymphatic Obstruction, Lymphedema, and Erysipelas

Irradiation or neck dissection may produce chronic obstructive lymphedema that predisposes patients to erysipelas. At least one episode of erysipelas follows large-field irradiation of nasopharynx cancer in 5% to 10% of long-term survivors; it is seen less often after irradiation of other primary sites. The addition of a neck dissection increases the risk. Only 1 of the first 356 patients with 2 years of minimum follow-up who received twice-a-day irradiation for tumors of the larynx, oropharynx, or hypopharynx at the University of Florida developed erysipelas. The condition usually develops months or years after treatment. Rarely has it been seen during a course of treatment. The infections are similar to those occurring in edematous extremities after axillary or inguinal lymphadenectomy and irradiation. Some patients have repeated exacerbations. Group A β-hemolytic *Streptococcus* usually is the responsible organism.

Onset of the skin infection is abrupt; sometimes a history of an earlier upper respiratory tract infection exists. Although the infection initially is limited to the irradiated fields, it may later extend to unirradiated skin. The skin is hot, bright red, tense, and slightly raised. Fever, chills, and rarely, severe toxemia may occur. The infection typically spreads rapidly behind a well-demarcated border. Appropriate antibiotics are started without delay and usually without obtaining a culture. The disease process generally is rapidly reversed. Older or debilitated patients may become severely, systemically ill and require hospitalization and intravenous antibiotics.

Paranasal Sinuses

After high-dose irradiation of cancer of the nasal cavity and ethmoid and sphenoid sinuses, 5 (10%) of 48 patients at the University of Florida had one or more episodes of purulent sinusitis, unassociated with tumor recurrence.[147] One patient required nasal antrostomy at 16 months, after antibiotics failed to control infection. Another, who had intermittent episodes of purulent sinusitis, developed meningitis 4½ years after treatment. A third developed a 3-mm, asymptomatic fistula between the ethmoid sinus and anterior facial skin 7 years after treatment. A fourth underwent a negative Caldwell-Luc procedure to rule out recurrence 2 years after treatment, whereas the fifth was successfully treated with antibiotics alone.

Patients typically exhibit a purulent nasal discharge, headache, tenderness and pain over the sinus area, facial edema, conjunctival edema, and low-grade fever. The sinus does not transilluminate. Computed tomographic scan shows opacity. The differential diagnosis is recurrent cancer. Exploration is required for diagnosis and drainage if response to antibiotics is incomplete. When the sinuses are uninvolved by neoplasm, it is distinctly unusual for patients to develop radiation-induced sinusitis.

Large Arteries

Radiation-induced carotid artery disease is regarded as rare. Its exact incidence is unknown for the following reasons: (1) Few case reports have clinicopathologic correlation. (2) Irradiation is delivered at an age when atherosclerotic disease of carotid arteries is common. (3) Most reported cases of radiation-induced injury have occurred after a latent interval of 5 to 10 years or more, making an extended follow-up period mandatory to assess the risk. (4) Carotid narrowing may be clinically silent in the presence of good collateral flow.

Elerding et al[148] found a nonsignificant (P = .39) trend toward an increased risk of stroke in 910 patients who had received irradiation to at least one entire side of the neck, and who survived a minimum of 5 years after treatment of lymphoma or cancer primary to the head and neck. No apparent correlation between dose and incidence of injury existed.

Piedbois et al[149] reported on five patients who developed carotid artery narrowing or occlusion 3 to 11 years (mean, 6 years) after irradiation for head and neck cancer. All five patients had other atherosclerotic risk factors (smoking in five, hyperlipidemia in two, diabetes and high blood pressure in one); two of the patients had no significant arterial disease outside of the irradiated area. Stenoses were treated by bypass (four patients) or endarterectomy (one patient). One patient had to have reoperation 5 years later because of stenosis of the bypass. Functional results in the other four patients remained satisfactory at 3 to 7 years. Anastomotic leakage and cutaneous nonhealing were not encountered.

Histological changes include intimal thickening with or without superimposed thrombus, fragmentation of the internal elastic membrane, atheroma formation, fibrosis of the media, and adventitial fibrosis. Atheromatous narrowing may involve portions of the great vessels not usually involved with atherosclerosis.[150]

Vascular reconstruction may be indicated. After moderate doses (4500 to 5500 cGy) at Stanford University (Stanford, Calif), carotid endarterectomy was technically more difficult than in unirradiated patients but was accomplished without increased morbidity or mortality.[150] Although one might suspect that higher doses would significantly increase the operative risk, several patients from the University of Florida have undergone endarterectomy in heavily irradiated necks without serious complications.

In one heavily irradiated patient (dose unknown), Levinson et al[151] at the University of California, San Francisco, performed bilateral carotid endarterectomies and successfully bypassed both common carotid arteries from the level of the clavicle to the bulb by means of saphenous vein grafts. The only bypass reported by the Stanford group (after 12,000-cGy skin dose) was unsuccessful because of clot formation.

Percutaneous transluminal angioplasty has been used to recanalize heavily irradiated brachial and iliac vessels in a limited number of patients.[152,153] The technique avoids a surgical procedure in heavily irradiated tissue. Although we are not aware of patients who have undergone transluminal angioplasty for postirradiation carotid injuries, it could be considered.

Arterial rupture after irradiation fortunately is rare; rupture usually is precipitated by wound complications (necrosis, infection, dehiscence, or fistulae) after operation. Ruptured vessels show transmural necrosis of the vessel wall. The complication is dramatic and often fatal.[154]

Call et al[155] described carotid artery thromboses in three young patients (26 to 42 years of age) after 3800 to 7000 cGy. In each instance the occlusion occurred within 3 years after irradiation in the absence of atherosclerotic stenosis. The authors speculated that this earlier-appearing type of injury resulted from intimal damage, and suggested that patients who develop neurological symptoms or signs after neck irradiation should be evaluated for carotid or vertebral artery disease regardless of age, radiation dose, or interval from irradiation. If the ischemic nature of the symptoms appears definite, antiplatelet agents are recommended even if vascular studies are negative. If symptoms persist, the authors recommend consideration of antithrombotic therapy with warfarin.

Radiation-Induced Neoplasia after Therapeutic Irradiation

Despite extensive use of therapeutic irradiation for cancer of the head and neck, induction of malignancy fortunately is rare. Most reported cases have been sarcomas, usually osteogenic sarcomas or fibrosarcomas of bone, and less often soft tissue sarcomas.

The latent interval between irradiation and the development of cancer varies from several to many years. To qualify as a radiation-induced cancer, histological proof must exist of a new cancer and the lesion must be within the prior field of irradiation. Three aspects of the problem of radiation-induced neoplasia are explored: mucosal lesions, primarily squamous cell carcinomas; sarcomas; and thyroid neoplasia.

MUCOSAL CANCER

In 1975, Lawson and Som[156] analyzed 535 patients who had follow-up for 5 to 25 years after treatment of T1 vocal cord cancer by cordectomy or hemilaryngectomy (310 patients) or by irradiation (225 patients). Twelve (4%) of the surgery group and 18 (8%) of the radiotherapy group developed second primary laryngeal carcinomas (P = .017). Since their study, a large body of data from a number of institutions has failed to confirm the authors' conclusions that irradiation is likely to result in a higher incidence of subsequent cancer.

In a 1982 review of more than 200 cases of laryngeal cancer with more than 5 years of follow-up after irradiation, Harwood and Yaffe[157] found no such excess risk. At the M.D. Anderson Hospital, Kögelnik et al[158] reviewed the late clinical courses of patients who had received curative therapy for head and neck squamous cell carcinoma and lived for a minimum of 5 years without recurrence of cancer within that 5-year period. The clinical occurrences subsequent to 5 years were recorded in 1163 patients after surgery, irradiation, or combined treatment. Follow-up intervals ranged from 7½ to 25 years. The incidence of new cancer developing in the original disease site, the immediate vicinity of the original lesion, or sites remote from the primary lesion but still within the oral cavity and pharynx, was not higher in the patients who received irradiation alone or irradiation plus surgery when compared with patients who received operation alone. It was concluded that irradiation did not produce an excess of new squamous cell carcinomas compared with surgery. Data from the Fox Chase Cancer Center (Philadelphia, Pa) on almost 2000 patients who underwent surgery or irradiation for cancer of the oral cavity or oropharynx showed a slightly higher incidence of new upper aerodigestive cancer in the surgery group.[159]

Parker and Enstrom[160] evaluated 2151 patients for second primary malignancies of the head and neck after treatment of their first cancer of the head and neck at University of California, Los Angeles, between 1955 and 1979. Follow-up ranged from 5 to 30 years. No significant difference in the risk of developing a second cancer was noted in the group treated by irradiation compared with those treated by surgery.

Friedman et al[161] reported on 1856 patients with head and neck squamous cell carcinomas other than skin cancer who received treatment at the University of Illinois (Urbana, Ill) between 1960 and 1980. Four hundred twenty-two patients had follow-up for over 5 years. The incidence of second primary malignancies of the head and neck mucosa did not differ significantly between the groups treated by surgery, irradiation, or surgery plus irradiation.

It has been suggested that irradiation is contraindicated in cancer of the head and neck in patients younger than 40 years of age because of the risk of radiation-induced malignancy. Harwood and Yaffe[157] reported on 272 patients with cancer of the head and neck who were less than 30 years old when irradiated at the Princess Margaret Hospital; 58 had more than 10 years (up to 24 years) of follow-up. No second malignancy attributable to irradiation was observed.

SARCOMA

The rarity of radiation-induced sarcomas, the long latent period (mean, 10 to 12 years) to their development, and the difficulty in obtaining reliable long-term follow-up data make the task of estimating the true risk of cancer induction difficult.[162] Most series report one or two cases of radiation-induced bone sarcoma per 1000 5-year survivors.[159,163-165] Assuming a malignant induction in 1 patient of every 500 long-term survivors, then with an estimated 5-year survival rate of 40% for all irradiated patients with cancer of the head and neck, one case would be induced per 1250 patients treated. The younger the patient, the greater would be the risk of developing a new cancer because the at-risk period would be longer; whether children are more susceptible than adults to neoplastic induction, as is suspected by many authors, remains unproved but seems likely.

Other factors that increase the risk include orthovoltage irradiation, high doses, and multiple courses of treatment spread over many months or years.[157] Most authors concur that previously abnormal bone, such as that affected by fibrous dysplasia, is more prone to sarcomatous change than normal bone.[166-168] Whether the addition of chemotherapy to irradiation increases the risk is unknown. Most radiation-induced sarcomas are diagnosed at an advanced stage, have high-grade histological features, are located where radical surgery cannot be performed, respond poorly to chemotherapy, and as a consequence, have a dismal prognosis.[169,170]

THYROID CANCER

An association between radiation and thyroid neoplasia has long been recognized.[171] The latent period is usually 10 to 30 years. The mortality rate from these forms of thyroid cancer is very low, and the patients essentially have a normal life span. Almost all the reported cases have followed doses (6 to 1500 cGy) of radiation that are well below the levels delivered for squamous cell carcinomas (5000 to 7000 cGy). Doses above 2000 cGy are associated with a very low risk of induction of thyroid neoplasia compared with lower doses of radiation. This is probably because higher doses either completely destroy the follicular cells or, at least, render the surviving cells incapable of division. Such a situation is seen after ^{131}I therapy for hyperthyroidism; many patients become hypothyroid but few develop thyroid cancer.

REFERENCES

1. Kögelnik HD, Kärcher KH. Radiobiological considerations of late effects arising from radiotherapy. *Radiobiological Research and Radiotherapy: Proceedings of an International Symposium on the Radiobiological Research Needed for the Improvement of Radiotherapy*; November 22-26, 1976. Vienna: International Atomic Energy Agency; 1977;1:275-286.
2. Coutard H. Principles of x-ray therapy of malignant diseases. *Lancet.* 1934;227:1-8.
3. Coutard H. X-ray treatment of inoperable carcinoma of the larynx. *Surg Gynecol Obstet.* 1939;68:467-471.
4. Ferretti GA, Hansen IA, Whittenburg K, Brown AT, Lillich TT, Ash RC. Therapeutic use of chlorhexidine in bone marrow transplant patients: case studies. *Oral Surg Oral Med Oral Pathol.* 1987;63:683-687.
5. Martin CL, Martin JA. *Low Intensity Radium Therapy.* Boston, Mass: Little Brown & Co; 1959.
6. Parsons JT. The effect of radiation on normal tissues of the head and neck. In: Million RR, Cassisi NJ, eds. *Management of Head and Neck Cancer: A Disciplinary Approach.* 2nd ed. Philadelphia, Pa: JB Lippincott; 1994.
7. Mossman KL. Quantitative radiation dose-response relationships for normal tissues in man. II. Response of the salivary glands during radiotherapy. *Radiat Res.* 1983;95:392-398.
8. Conger AD. Loss and recovery of taste acuity in patients irradiated to the oral cavity. *Radiat Res.* 1973;53:338-347.
9. Enfors B. The parotid and submandibular secretion in man: quantitative recordings of the normal and pathological activity. *Acta Otolaryngol.* 1962;172(suppl):1-67.
10. Shannon IL, Trodahl JN, Starcke EN. Radiosensitivity of the human parotid gland. *Proc Soc Exp Biol Med.* 1978;157:50-53.
11. Mira JG, Wescott WB, Starcke EN, Shannon IL. Some factors influencing salivary function when treating with radiotherapy. *Int J Radiat Oncol Biol Phys.* 1981;7:535-541.
12. Dreizen S, Brown LR, Handler S, Levy BM. Radiation-induced xerostomia in cancer patients: effect on salivary and serum electrolytes. *Cancer.* 1976;38:273-278.
13. Kuten A, Ben-Aryeh H, Berdicevsky I, et al. Oral side effects of head and neck irradiation: correlation between clinical manifestations and laboratory data. *Int J Radiat Oncol Biol Phys.* 1986;12:401-405.
14. Kashima HK, Kirkham WR, Andrews JR. Postirradiation sialadenitis: a study of the clinical features, histopathologic changes and serum enzyme variations following irradiation of human salivary glands. *Am J Roentgenol Radium Ther Nucl Med.* 1965;94:271-291.
15. Coutard H. Roentgen therapy of epitheliomas of the tonsillar region, hypopharynx and larynx from 1920 to 1926. *Am J Roentgenol Radium Ther* 1932;28:313-331.
16. Marks JE, Davis CC, Gottsman VL, Purdy JE, Lee F. The effects of radiation on parotid salivary function. *Int J Radiat Oncol Biol Phys.* 1981;7:1013-1019.
17. Mossman KL, Shatzman A, Chencharick J. Long-term effects of radiotherapy on taste and salivary function in man. *Int J Radiat Oncol Biol Phys.* 1982;8:991-997.
18. Mossman KL, Henkin RI. Radiation-induced changes in taste acuity in cancer patients. *Int J Radiat Oncol Biol Phys.* 1978;4:663-670.
19. Silverman S Jr, Thompson JS. Serum zinc and copper in oral/oropharyngeal carcinoma: a study of seventy-five patients. *Oral Surg Oral Med Oral Pathol.* 1984;57:34-36.
20. Brown LR, Dreizen S, Handler S, Johnston DA. Effect of radiation-induced xerostomia on human oral microflora. *J Dent Res.* 1975;54:740-750.
21. Frank RM, Herdly J, Philippe E. Acquired dental defects and salivary gland lesions after irradiation for carcinoma. *J Am Dent Assoc.* 1965;70:868-883.
22. Del Regato JA. Dental lesions observed after roentgen therapy in cancer of the buccal cavity, pharynx and larynx. *Am J Roentgenol Radium Ther.* 1939;42:404-410.
23. Murray CG, Herson J, Daly TE, Zimmerman S. Radiation necrosis of the mandible: a 10 year study: Part I. Factors influencing the onset of necrosis. *Int J Radiat Oncol Biol Phys.* 1980;6:543-548.
24. Marx RE. Osteoradionecrosis: a new concept of its pathophysiology. *J Oral Maxillofac Surg.* 1983;41:283-288.
25. Beumer J, Harrison R, Sanders B, Kurrasch M. Preradiation dental extractions and the incidence of bone necrosis. *Head Neck.* 1983;5:514-521.
26. Beumer J, Harrison R, Sanders B, Kurrasch M. Osteoradionecrosis: predisposing factors and outcomes of therapy. *Head Neck.* 1984;6:819-827.
27. Marx RE, Johnson RP, Kline SN. Prevention of osteoradionecrosis: a randomized prospective clinical trial of hyperbaric oxygen versus penicillin. *J Am Dent Assoc.* 1985;111:49-54.

28. Murray CG, Herson J, Daly TE, Zimmerman S. Radiation necrosis of the mandible: a 10 year study. Part II. Dental factors; onset, duration, and management of necrosis. *Int J Radiat Oncol Biol Phys.* 1980;6:549–553.

29. Parsons JT, Bova FJ, Million RR. A re-evaluation of split-course technique for squamous cell carcinoma of the head and neck. *Int J Radiat Oncol Biol Phys.* 1980;6:1645–1652.

30. Davis JC, Dunn JM, Gates GA, Heimbach RD. Hyperbaric oxygen: a new adjunct in the management of radiation necrosis. *Arch Otolaryngol.* 1979;105:58–61.

31. Marx RE. A new concept in the treatment of osteoradionecrosis. *J Oral Maxillofac Surg.* 1983;41:351–357.

32. Myers RAM, Baker T, Cowley RA. Hyperbaric medicine: state of the art, 1979. *Am Surg.* 1982;48:487–494.

33. Ramsden RT. Osteoradionecrosis of the temporal bone. *J Laryngol Otol.* 1975;89:941–955.

34. Ma KH, Fagan PA. Osteoradionecrosis of the temporal bone: a surgical technique of treatment. *Laryngoscope.* 1988;98:554–555.

35. Schuknecht HF, Karmody CS. Radionecrosis of the temporal bone. *Laryngoscope.* 1966;76:1416–1428.

36. Thornley GD, Gullane PJ, Ruby RRF, Heeneman H. Osteoradionecrosis of the temporal bone. *J Otolaryngol.* 1979;8:396–400.

37. Wurster CF, Krespi YP, Curtis AW. Osteoradionecrosis of the temporal bone. *Otolaryngol Head Neck Surg.* 1982;90:126–129.

38. Wang CC, Doppke K. Osteoradionecrosis of the temporal bone: consideration of nominal standard dose. *Int J Radiat Oncol Biol Phys.* 1976;1:881–883.

39. Ackerman LV. The pathology of radiation effect of normal and neoplastic tissue. *Am J Roentgenol Radium Ther Nucl Med.* 1972;114:447–459.

40. Parsons JT, Mendenhall WM, Mancuso AA, Cassisi NJ, Stringer SP, Million RR. Twice-a-day radiotherapy for T3 squamous cell carcinoma of the glottic larynx. *Head Neck.* 1989;11:123–128.

41. Chahbazian CM, del Regato JA. Cobalt 60 teletherapy of early carcinoma of the vocal cords. *Am J Roentgenol Radium Ther Nucl Med.* 1967;99:333–335.

42. Fletcher GH, Barkley HT Jr, Shukovsky LJ. Present status of the time factor in clinical radiotherapy: Part II. The nominal standard dose formula. *J Radiol Electrol.* 1974;55:745–751.

43. Harwood AR, Hawkins NV, Rider WD, Bryce DP. Radiotherapy of early glottic cancer: I. *Int J Radiat Oncol Biol Phys.* 1979;5:473–476.

44. Kim JC, Elkin D, Hendrickson FR. Carcinoma of the vocal cord: results of treatment and time-dose relationships. *Cancer* 1978;42:1114–1119.

45. Stell PM, Morrison MD. Radiation necrosis of the larynx: etiology and management. *Arch Otolaryngol.* 1973;98:111–113.

46. Mendenhall WM, Parsons JT, Million RR. Unnecessary irradiation of the normal larynx. *Int J Radiat Oncol Biol Phys.* 1990;18:1531–1533.

47. Ferguson BJ, Hudson WR, Farmer JC Jr. Hyperbaric oxygen therapy for laryngeal radionecrosis. *Ann Otol Rhinol Laryngol.* 1987;96:1–6.

48. Del Regato JA, Vuksanovic M. Radiotherapy of carcinomas of the skin overlying the cartilages of the nose and ear. *Radiology.* 1962;79:203–208.

49. Parker RG, Wildermuth O. Radiation therapy of lesions overlying cartilage—I. Carcinoma of the pinna. *Cancer.* 1962;15:57–65.

50. Moss WT. Principles of combining radiation therapy and surgery. In: Moss WT, Cox JD, eds. *Radiation Oncology: Rationale, Technique, Results.* St Louis, MO: CV Mosby; 1989:58–67.

51. Dobbs WGH. A statistical study of the effect of roentgen rays on wound healing. *Am J Roentgenol Radium Ther.* 1939;41:625–632.

52. Gorodetsky R, McBride WH, Withers HR. Assay of radiation effects in mouse skin as expressed in wound healing. *Radiat Res.* 1988;116:135–144.

53. Lawrence W Jr, Nickson JJ, Warshaw IM. Roentgen rays and wound healing: an experimental study. *Surgery.* 1953;33:376–384.

54. Moore MJ. The effect of radiation on connective tissue. *Otolaryngol Clin North Am.* 1984;17:389–399.

55. Nickson JJ, Lawrence W Jr, Rachwalsky I, Tyree E. Roentgen rays and wound healing: II. Fractionated irradiation: an experimental study. *Surgery.* 1953;34:859–862.

56. Stajić J, Milovanović A. Radiation and wound healing: evolution of tensile strength in excised skin-wound of irradiated rats. *Strahlentherapie.* 1970;139:87–90.

57. Zelman D, Song IC, Porteous DD, Bromberg BE. The effect of total body irradiation on wound healing and the hematopoietic system in mice. *Bull NY Acad Med.* 1969;45:293–300.

58. Powers WE, Ogura JH, Palmer LA. Radiation therapy and wound healing delay: animals and man. *Radiology.* 1967;89:112–115.

59. Archer RR, Greenwell EJ, Ware T, Weeks PM. Irradiation effect on wound healing in rats. *Radiat Res.* 1970;41:104–112.

60. Stajić J, Jovanovic M. Radiation and wound healing: a study of the gain of collagen content in the damaged skin of irradiated rats. *Strahlentherapie.* 1969;138:361–364.

61. Ariyan S, Marfuggi RA, Harder G, Goodie MM. An experimental model to determine the effects of adjuvant therapy on the incidence of postoperative wound infection: I. Evaluating preoperative radiation therapy. *Plast Reconstr Surg.* 1980;65:328–337.

62. Gorodetskv R, Mou X, Fisher DR, Taylor JMG, Withers HR. Radiation effect in mouse skin: dose fractionation and wound healing. *Int J Radiat Oncol Biol Phys.* 1990;18:1077–1081.

63. Taylor JMG, Mendenhall WM, Parsons JT, Lavey RS. The influence of dose and time on wound complications following post radiation neck dissection. *Int J Radiat Oncol Biol Phys.* 1992;23:41–46.

64. Johansen LV, Overgaard J, Elbrønd O. Pharyngo-cutaneous fistulae after laryngectomy: influence of previous radiotherapy and prophylactic metronidazole. *Cancer.* 1988;61:673–678.

65. Johnson JT, Bloomer WD. Effect of prior radiotherapy on postsurgical wound infection. *Head Neck.* 1989;111:132–136.

66. Isaacs JH Jr, Thompson WB, Cassisi NJ, Million RR. Postoperative radiation of open head and neck wounds. *Laryngoscope.* 1987;97:267–270.

67. Parsons JT, Mendenhall WM, Bova FJ, Million RR. Irradiation techniques for head and neck cancer. In: Levitt SH, Khan FM, Potish RA, eds. *Levitt and Tapley's Technological Basis of Radiation Therapy: Practical Clinical Applications.* 2nd ed. Philadelphia, Pa: Lea & Febiger; 1992:203–231.

68. Scheie HG; Albert DM, eds. *Textbook of Ophthalmology.* 9th ed. Philadelphia, Pa: WB Saunders; 1977.

69. Jones LT. The lacrimal secretory system and its treatment. *Am J Ophthalmol.* 1966;62:47–60.

70. Karp LA, Streeten BW, Cogan DG. Radiation-induced atrophy of the meibomian glands. *Arch Ophthalmol.* 1979;97:303–305.

71. Parsons JT, Fitzgerald CR, Hood CI, Ellingwood KE, Bova FJ, Million RR. The effects of irradiation on the eye and optic nerve. *Int J Radiat Oncol Biol Phys.* 1983;9:609–622.

72. Brady LW, Shields J, Augusburger J, Markoe A, Karlsson UL. Complications from radiation therapy to the eye. *Front Radiat Ther Oncol.* 1989;23:238–250.

73. Anders B. Ocular circulation. In: Moses RA, ed. *Adler's Physiology of the Eye: Clinical Applications.* 7th ed. St Louis, Mo: CV Mosby; 1981:184–203.

74. Brown GC, Shields JA, Sanborn G, Augsburger JJ, Savino PJ, Schatz NJ. Radiation retinopathy. *Ophthalmology.* 1982; 89:1494–1501.

75. Bedford MA, Bedotto C, MacFaul PA. Radiation retinopathy after the application of a cobalt plaque: report of three cases. *Br J Ophthalmol.* 1970;54:505–509.

76. Hayreh SS. Post-radiation retinopathy: a fluorescence fundus angiographic study. *Br J Ophthalmol.* 1970;54:705–714.

77. Shukovsky LJ, Fletcher GH. Retinal and optic nerve complications in a high dose irradiation technique of ethmoid sinus and nasal cavity. *Radiology.* 1972;104:629–634.

78. Bagan SM, Hollenhorst RW. Radiation retinopathy after irradiation of intracranial lesions. *Am J Ophthalmol.* 1979;88: 694–697.

79. Wand M, Dueker DK, Aiello LM, Grant WM. Effects of panretinal photocoagulation on rubeosis iridis, angle neovascularization, and neovascular glaucoma. *Am J Ophthalmol.* 1978;86:332–339.

80. Brown GC, Shields JA, Sanborn G, Augsburger JJ, Savino PJ, Schatz NJ. Radiation optic neuropathy. *Ophthalmology.* 1982;89:1489–1493.

81. Boghen DR, Glaser JS. Ischaemic optic neuropathy: the clinical profile and natural history. *Brain.* 1975;98:689–708.

82. Crompton MR, Layton DD. Delayed radionecrosis of the brain following therapeutic X-irradiation of the pituitary. *Brain.* 1961;84:85–101.

83. Schatz NJ, Lichtenstein S, Corbett JJ. Delayed radiation necrosis of the optic nerves and chiasm. In: Glaser JS, Smith JL, eds. *Neuroophthalmology Symposium of the Bascom Palmer Eye Institute and University of Miami.* vol 8. St Louis, Mo: CV Mosby; 1978:131–139.

84. Guy J, Schatz NJ. Hyperbaric oxygen in the treatment of radiation-induced optic neuropathy. *Ophthalmology.* 1986;93:1083–1088.

85. Roden D, Bosley TM, Fowble B, et al. Delayed radiation injury to the retrobulbar optic nerves and chiasm. Clinical syndrome and treatment with hyperbaric oxygen and corticosteroids. *Ophthalmology.* 1990;97:346–351.

86. Bessell EM, Henck JM, Whitelocke RAF, Wright JE. Ocular morbidity after radiotherapy of orbital and conjunctival lymphoma. *Eye.* 1987;1:90–96.

87. Moretti JA. Sensori-neural hearing loss following radiotherapy to the nasopharynx. *Laryngoscope.* 1976;86:598–602.

88. Leach W. Irradiation of the ear. *J Laryngol Otol.* 1965;79: 870–880.

89. Marie P, Chatelin C. Note sur certains symptômes vraisemblablement d'origine radiculaire chez les blessés du crâne. *Rev Neurol.* 1917;24:143–144.

90. Marie P, Chatelin C. Sur certains symptômes vraisemblablement d'origine radiculaire chez les blessés du crâne. *Rev Neurol.* 1917;24:336.

91. Babinski J, Dubois R. Douleurs à forme de décharge électrique consécutives aux traumatismes de la nuque. *Presse Med.* 1918;26:64.

92. Lhermitte J. Hypertophie des muscles de la jambe consécutive à une lésion du nerf sciatizue par balle. *Presse Med.* 1918;26:64.

93. Boden G. Radiation myelitis of the cervical spinal cord. *Br J Radiol.* 1948;21:464–469.

94. Jones A. Transient radiation myelopathy (with reference to Lhermitte's sign of electrical parasthesia). *Br J Radiol.* 1964;37:727–744.

95. Butler WM, Taylor HG, Diehl LF. Lhermitte's sign in cobalamin (vitamin B12) deficiency. *JAMA.* 1981;245:1059.

96. Abbatucci JS, Delozier T, Quint R, Roussel A, Brune D. Radiation myelopathy of the cervical spinal cord: time, dose and volume factors. *Int J Radiat Oncol Biol Phys.* 1978;4:239–248.

97. Schultheiss TE, Higgins EM, El-Mahdi AM. The latent period in clinical radiation myelopathy. *Int J Radiat Oncol Biol Phys.* 1984;10:1109–1115.

98. Reagan TJ, Thomas JE, Colby MY Jr. Chronic progressive radiation myelopathy. *JAMA.* 1968;203:106–110.

99. Burns RJ, Jones AN, Robertson JS. Pathology of radiation myelopathy. *J Neurol Nerosurg Psychiatry.* 1972;35:888–898.

100. Schultheiss TE, Stephens LC, Peters LJ. Survival in radiation myelopathy. *Int J Radiat Oncol Biol Phys.* 1986;12:1765–1769.

101. Pallis CA, Louis S, Morgan RL. Radiation myelopathy. *Brain.* 1984;84:460–479.

102. Fogelholm R, Haltia M, Andersson LC. Radiation myelopathy of cervical spinal cord simulating intramedullary neoplasm. *J Neurol Neurosurg Psychiatry.* 1974;37:1177–1180.

103. Marty R, Minckler DS. Radiation myelitis simulating tumor. *Arch Neurol.* 1973;29:352–354.

104. Palmer JJ. Radiation myelopathy. *Brain.* 1972;95:109–122.

105. Worthington BS. Diffuse cord enlargement in radiation myelopathy. *Clin Radiol.* 1979;30:117–119.

106. Atkins HL, Tretter P. Time-dose considerations in radiation myelopathy. *Acta Radiol Ther Phys Biol.* 1966;5:79–94.

107. Margolis L, Smith ME, Fortuin FD, Chin FK, Liebel SA, Hill DR. Intramedullary tumor metastasis simulating radiation myelitis: report of a case. *Cancer.* 1981;48:1680–1683.

108. Ojeda VJ. Necrotizing myelopathy associated with malignancy: a clinicopathologic study of two cases and literature review. *Cancer.* 1984;53:1115–1123.

109. Boden G. Radiation myelitis of the brain-stem. *J Fac Radiol.* 1950;2:79–94.

110. Marcus RB Jr, Million RR. The incidence of myelitis after irradiation of the cervical spinal cord. *Int J Radiat Oncol Biol Phys.* 1990;19:3–8.

111. McCunniff AJ, Liang MJ. Radiation tolerance of the cervical spinal cord. *Int J Radiat Oncol Biol Phys.* 1989;16:675–678.

112. Baekmark UB. Neurologic complications after irradiation of the cervical spinal cord for malignant tumor of the head and neck. *Acta Radiol Ther Phys Biol.* 1975;14:33–41.

113. Jeremic B, Ljubodrag D, Ljiljana M. Incidence of radiation myelitis of the cervical spinal cord at doses of 5500 cGy or greater. *Cancer.* 1991;68:2138–2141.

114. Gillette EL, Gillette SM, Childs G, Ritt M, Powers B. Volume effects on canine spinal cord function (abstract). *Int J Radiat Oncol Biol Phys.* 1990;19(suppl):156.

115. Druckman A. Schlafsucht als folge der röntgenbestrahlung. Beitrag zur strahlenempfindlichkeit des gehirns. *Strahlentherapie.* 1929;33:382–384.

116. Sheline GE. Irradiation injury of the human brain: a review of clinical experience. In: Gilbert HA, Kagan AR, eds. *Radiation Damage to the Nervous System: A Delayed Therapeutic Hazard.* New York, NY: Raven Press; 1980:39–58.

117. Kramer S, Southard ME, Mansfield CM. Radiation effect and tolerance of the central nervous system. *Front Radiat Ther Oncol.* 1972;6:332–345.

118. Sheline GE, Wara WM, Smith V. Therapeutic irradiation and brain injury. *Int J Radiat Oncol Biol Phys.* 1980;6:1215–1228.

119. Graeb DA, Steinbok P, Robertson WD. Transient early computed tomographic changes mimicking tumor progression after brain tumor irradiation. *Radiology.* 1982;144:813–817.

120. Edwards MS, Wilson CB. Treatment of radiation necrosis. In: Gilbert HA, Kagan AR, eds. *Radiation Damage to the Nervous System: A Delayed Therapeutic Hazard.* New York, NY: Raven Press, 1980:129–143.

121. Lampert PW, Davis RL. Delayed effects of radiation on the human central nervous system. "Early" and "late" delayed reactions. *Neurology.* 1964;14:912–917.

122. Lampert PW, Tom MI, Rider WD. Disseminated demyelination of the brain following Co[60] (gamma) radiation. *Arch Pathol Lab Med.* 1959;68:322–330.

123. Dooms GC, Hecht S, Brant-Zawadzki M, Berthiaume Y, Norman D, Newton TH. Brain radiation lesions: MR imaging. *Radiology.* 1986;158:149–155.

124. Constine LS, Konski A, Ekholm S, McDonald S, Rubin P. Adverse effects of brain irradiation correlated with MR and CT imaging. *Int J Radiat Oncol Biol Phys.* 1988;15:319–330.

125. Bloom HJG. Intracranial tumors: response and resistance to therapeutic endeavors, 1970–1980. *Int J Radiat Oncol Biol Phys.* 1982;8:1083–1113.

126. Marks JE, Wong J. The risk of cerebral radionecrosis in relation to dose, time and fractionation: a follow-up study. *Prog Exp Tumor Res.* 1985;29:210–218.

127. Lee AWN, Ng SH, Ho JHC, et al. Clinical diagnosis of late temporal lobe necrosis following radiation therapy for nasopharyngeal carcinoma. *Cancer.* 1988;61:1535–1542.

128. Berger PS, Bataini JP. Radiation-induced cranial nerve palsy. *Cancer.* 1977;40:152–1542.

129. Cheng VST, Schulz MD. Unilateral hypoglossal nerve atrophy as a late complication of radiation therapy of head and neck carcinoma: a report of four cases and a review of the literature on peripheral and cranial nerve damages after radiation therapy. *Cancer.* 1975;35:1537–1544.

130. Fuks Z, Glatstein E, Marsa GW, Bagshaw MA, Kaplan HS. Long-term effects of external radiation on the pituitary and thyroid glands. *Cancer.* 1976;37:1152–1161.

131. Huang K. Assessment of hypothalamic-pituitary function in women after external head irradiation. *J Clin Endocrinol Metab.* 1979;49:623–627.

132. Lam KSL, Ho JHC, Lee AWM, et al. Symptomatic hypothalamic-pituitary dysfunction in nasopharyngeal carcinoma patients following radiation therapy: a retrospective study. *Int J Radiat Oncol Biol Phys.* 1987;13:1343–1350.

133. Samaan NA, Vieto R, Schultz PN, et al. Hypothalamic, pituitary and thyroid dysfunction after radiotherapy to the head and neck. *Int J Radiat Oncol Biol Phys.* 1982;8:1857–1867.

134. Lam KSL, Tse VKC, Wang C, Yeung RTT, Ma JTC, Ho JHC. Early effects of cranial irradiation on hypothalamic-pituitary function. *J Clin Endocrinol Metab.* 1987;64:418–424.

135. Shalet SM, Price DA, Beardwell CG, Jones PHM, Pearson D. Normal growth despite abnormalities of growth hormone in children treated for acute leukemia. *J Pediatr.* 1979;94:719–722.

136. Wara WM, Richards GE, Grumbach MM, Kaplan SL, Sheline GE, Conte F. Hypopituitarism after irradiation in children. *Int J Radiat Oncol Biol Phys.* 1977;2:549–552.

137. Duffner PK, Cohen ME, Voorhess ML, et al. Long-term effects of cranial irradiation on endocrine function in children with brain tumors: a prospective study. *Cancer.* 1985;56:2189–2193.

138. Posner MR, Ervin TJ, Miller D, et al. Incidence of hypothyroidism following multimodality treatment for advanced squamous cell cancer of the head and neck. *Laryngoscope.* 1984;94:451–454.

139. Vrabec DP, Heffron TJ. Hypothyroidism following treatment for head and neck cancer. *Ann Otol.* 1981;90:449–453.

140. Constine LS, Donaldson SS, McDougall IR, Cox RS, Link MP, Kaplan HS. Thyroid dysfunction after radiotherapy in children with Hodgkin's disease. *Cancer.* 1984;53:878–883.

141. Glatstein E, McHardy-Young S, Brast N, Eltringham JR, Kriss JP. Alterations in serum thyrotropin (TSH) and thyroid function following radiotherapy in patients with malignant lymphoma. *J Clin Endocrinol Metabl.* 1971;32:833–841.

142. Palmer BV, Gaggar N, Shaw HJ. Thyroid function after radiotherapy and laryngectomy for carcinoma of the larynx. *Head Neck.* 1981;4:13–15.

143. Shafer RB, Nuttall FQ, Pollak K, Kuisk H. Thyroid function after radiation and surgery for head and neck cancer. *Arch Intern Med.* 1975;135:843–846.

144. Tisell LE, Carlsson S, Fjälling M, et al. Hyperparathyroidism subsequent to neck irradiation. Risk factors. *Cancer.* 1985;56:1529–1533.

145. Holten I, Peterson LJ. Early changes in parathyroid function after high-dose irradiation of the neck. *Cancer.* 1988;62:1476–1478.

146. Holten I, Christiansen C. Unchanged parathyroid function following irradiation for malignancies of the head and neck. *Cancer.* 1984;53:874–877.

147. Parsons JT, Mendenhall WM, Mancuso AA, Cassisi NJ, Million RR. Malignant tumors of the nasal cavity and ethmoid and sphenoid sinuses. *Int J Radiat Oncol Biol Phys.* 1988;14:11–22.

148. Elerding SC, Fernandez RN, Grotta JC, Lindberg RD, Causay LC, McMurtrey MJ. Carotid artery disease following external cervical irradiation. *Ann Surg.* 1981;194:609–615.

149. Piedbois P, Becquemin JP, Blanc I, et al. Arterial occlusive disease after radiotherapy: a report of 14 cases. *Radiother Oncol.* 1990;17:133–140.

150. Silverberg GD, Britt RH, Goffinet DR. Radiation-induced carotid artery disease. *Cancer.* 1978;41:130–137.

151. Levinson SA, Close MB, Ehrenfeld WK, Stoney RJ. Carotid artery occlusive disease following external cervical irradiation. *Arch Surg.* 1973;107:395–397.

152. Guthaner DF, Schmitz L. Percutaneous transluminal angioplasty of radiation-induced arterial stenoses. *Radiology.* 1982;144:77, 78.

153. Saddekni S, Sniderman KW, Hilton S, Sos TA. Percutaneous transluminal angioplasty of nonatherosclerotic lesions. *Am J Roentgenol.* 1980;135:975–982.

154. Fajardo LF, Berthrong M. Vascular lesions following radiation. *Pathol Annu.* 1988;23:297–330.

155. Call GK, Bray PF, Smoker WRK, Buys SS, Hayes JK. Carotid thrombosis following neck irradiation. *Int J Radiat Oncol Biol Phys.* 1990;18:635–640.

156. Lawson W, Som M. Second primary cancer after irradiation of laryngeal cancer. *Ann Otol Rhinol Laryngol.* 1975;84:771–775.

157. Harwood AR, Yaffe M. Cancer in man after diagnostic or therapeutic irradiation. *Cancer Surg.* 1982;1:703–731.

158. Kögelnik HD, Fletcher GH, Jesse RH. Clinical course of patients with squamous cell carcinoma of the upper respiratory and digestive tracts with no evidence of disease 5 years after initial treatment. *Radiology.* 1975;115:423–427.

159. Seydel HG. The risk of tumor induction in man following medical irradiation for malignant neoplasm. *Cancer.* 1975;35:1641–1645.

160. Parker RG, Enstrom JE. Second primary cancers of the head and neck following treatment of initial primary head and neck cancers. *Int J Radiat Oncol Biol Phys.* 1988;14:561–564.

161. Friedman M, Toriumi DM, Strorigl T, Grybauskas VT, Skolnik E. Effects of therapeutic radiation on the development of multiple primary tumors of the head and neck. *Head Neck.* 1988;10(suppl):48–51.

162. Coleman CN. Adverse effects of cancer therapy. *Am J Pediatr.* 1982;4:103–111.

163. Hatfield PM, Schulz MD. Postirradiation sarcoma: including 5 cases after x-ray therapy of breast carcinoma. *Radiology.* 1970;96:593–602.

164. Phillips TL, Sheline GE. Bone sarcomas following radiation therapy. *Radiology.* 1963;81:992–996.

165. Steeves RA, Bataini JP. Neoplasms induced by megavoltage radiation in the head and neck region. *Cancer.* 1981;47:1770–1774.

166. Coia LR, Fazekas JT, Kramer S. Postirradiation sarcoma of the head and neck: a report of three late sarcomas following therapeutic irradiation for primary malignancies of the paranasal sinus, nasal cavity, and larynx. *Cancer.* 1980;46:1982–1985.

167. De Lathouwer C, Brocheriou C. Sarcoma arising in irradiated jawbones: possible relationship with previous non-malignant bone lesions: report of 6 cases and review of the literature. *J Maxillofac Surg.* 1976;4:8–20.
168. Tountas AA, Fornasier VL, Harwood AR, Leung PMK. Postirradiation sarcoma of bone: a perspective. *Cancer.* 1979;43:182–187.
169. Robinson E, Neugut AI, Wylie P. Review: clinical aspects of postirradiation sarcomas. *J Natl Cancer Inst.* 1988;80:233–240.
170. Smith LM, Mendenhall NP, Cicale MJ, Block ER, Carter RL, Million RR. Results of a prospective study evaluating the effects of mantle irradiation on pulmonary function. *Int J Radiat Oncol Biol Phys.* 1989;16:79–84.
171. Duffy BJ, Fitzgerald PJ. Thyroid cancer in childhood and adolescence: a report on 28 cases. *Cancer.* 1950;3:1018–1032.
172. Mendenhall WM, Parsons JT, Million RR, Fletcher GH. T1-T2 squamous cell carcinoma of the glottic larynx treated with radiation therapy: relationship of dose-fractionation factors to local control and complications. *Int J Radiat Oncol Biol Phys.* 1988;15:1267–1273.

16 Complications of Chemotherapy in the Treatment of Head and Neck Cancer

Stephen A. Bernard, M.D.

The use of chemotherapy in the management of head and neck cancer has continued to increase in the decade since the previous edition of this book was published.[1] At that time, chemotherapy for patients with head and neck cancer consisted of either single agents or combinations that were relatively modest in dose and schedule by current standards. The indications for drug therapy were either local disease where other treatment modalities had been exhausted or distant spread of disease. Patients were often already quite debilitated by their disease. Expected benefits were modest and were usually of brief duration.[2]

Locally advanced head and neck cancer is seen in 60% of the patients at time of diagnosis. The disease, at this stage, is cured only 20% of the time.[3] The need to define newer treatments that will improve the cure rate is still a challenge. Recent efforts with chemotherapy for these diseases have led to the utilization of more aggressive combination chemotherapy regimens, with or without irradiation (Table 16–1).

Regimens employing multiple drugs are now being evaluated in head and neck cancer as induction therapy to decrease tumor bulk prior to surgery or irradiation; and following surgery as an adjuvant to prevent distant and local reoccurrence.[3] Where the disease is unresectable at diagnosis or where risk factors for local recurrence are seen at time of surgery, there are now ongoing studies to evaluate the value of chemotherapy in combination with irradiation.

The application of these therapies as well as the continued search for newer agents in these diseases requires a focus not only on efficacy but also on the toxicity of these agents. The increased use of combinations of chemotherapy and

Table 16–1. Use of Chemotherapy and Other Systemic Therapies in Head and Neck Cancer

1. Induction or neoadjuvant therapy
2. Adjuvant therapy
3. Combined modality therapy with irradiation for locally advanced disease or residual disease after surgery
4. Palliation of locally recurrent disease or distant disease
5. Prevention of head and neck cancer

irradiation requires that the complications of combined chemoradiotherapy also be addressed. The failure of patients to continue on a therapy may not allow an accurate assessment of the potential additional benefit of these therapies.[4,5] Patients may also refuse definitive surgery following chemotherapy.[6] The need to reduce the amount of drug given because of toxicity may also lessen the effectiveness of the chemotherapy regimen.[4] Although a recent meta-analysis has not shown a major impact of these more aggressive regimens on survival, toxicity has often not been discussed in detail in the individual trials.[7] The death rate from these more aggressive treatments is infrequently described.[7] Quality of life analysis is increasingly used to assess the benefits of therapy for a disease, balanced against the impact on normal activities of the disease and its treatment. This type of analysis is also being done with treatment for head and neck cancer.[8–10]

Although the responses to treatment in various regions of the head and neck may vary, depending on the anatomy and biology of cancer in that region, differences in chemotherapy-related toxicity by region have not been emphasized. Obviously the consequences of sloughing of the mucosa vary by the site where this condition occurs. For example, there can be ulceration of the nose produced by 5-fluorouracil (5-FU), producing nose bleeds; in the oral cavity, the same ulceration produces pain with chewing and swallowing. 5-Fluorouracil typically affects the anterior oral cavity more than the oropharynx (Capizzi, personal communication, 1982).

Grading of chemotherapy-related toxicity has become more uniform. Currently all of the multi-institutional cooperative groups performing clinical trials in cancer have adopted and modified the World Health Organization (WHO) criteria.[11] These detailed systems classify toxicity on the basis of anatomic site and the functional impact and score toxicity for severity based on the impairment in function for that specific site.[12] For most organ sites, grades 3 or 4 are severe or life threatening. In the case of mucositis, grade 3 implies decreased oral intake and grade 4 is associated with no oral intake (Table 16–2). Milder toxicity is usually grade 1 or 2

Table 16–2. Grading of Mucositis and Neutropenia

Mucositis	
Grade 1:	Soreness, red
Grade 2:	Ulcers, able to eat solids
Grade 3:	Ulcers, liquid diet
Grade 4:	Not able to eat
Neutropenia ($\times$ 1000/mm³)	
Grade 1:	1.5–1.9
Grade 2:	1.0–1.4
Grade 3:	0.5–0.9
Grade 4:	<0.5

Data from Miller et al.[11]

and implies no major disturbance in organ function. Grade 5 indicates death due to toxicity at that organ site. Most of the older literature does not grade toxicity except in a subjective fashion. Comparison of treatment regimens, especially the more aggressive ones in use today, requires quantification of toxicities to allow more reliable comparisons that are reproducible between studies.

Any discussion of toxicity in head and cancer chemotherapy must also compare toxicity seen with drugs alone to those that are being seen with drug and irradiation combinations. Scheduling of the two modalities must also be considered because sequential administration of chemotherapy and radiotherapy may increase the side effects seen with concomitant administration of the two modalities.

Issues of both acute and chronic toxicity need to be considered. Although patients may not be cured of their disease, they may live longer before recurrence is seen. During this prolonged disease-free interval, there is increased potential for the development of toxicities that are seen with the additional period of survival.

The toxicities of chemotherapy when given by a different route of administration or schedule will also be addressed in this review. Intra-arterial chemotherapy has been utilized for head and neck cancer. Toxicity considerations have been important in the failure of this route to gain acceptance for the treatment of head and neck cancer.

Immunotherapy has now begun to be evaluated in head and neck cancer. Toxicities from these biological agents differ from those seen with chemotherapy and will be discussed.

The use of drugs or vitamins to prevent cancer has proven successful in head and neck cancer. Chemoprevention, using β-carotene or vitamin A, has been successful in ameliorating leukoplakia and preventing second malignancies.[13,14] In the initial trial of high-dose cis-retinoic acid for prevention of second malignances, however, 18% of the participants dropped out because of toxicity. An understanding of these problems and efforts to decrease the complications may allow for further benefits to be derived with this approach. A more recent study using lower doses of isotretinoin or β-carotene was much better tolerated.[15] The lower dose used as maintenance has shown an improvement in duration of control. Addressing toxicity by modifying the therapy has increased the adherence to the treatment.

TOXICITIES OF SPECIFIC AGENTS

Single agents that have shown activity in head and neck cancer are shown in Table 16–3. The individual agents are discussed below. A brief summary of toxicities is found in Table 16–4. Pharmacological considerations are reviewed as well as a brief discussion of drug-radiation interactions where appropriate.

Methotrexate: Pharmacology and Mechanism of Action

Methotrexate has been utilized most frequently as a single agent for advanced head and neck cancer. More recently it has been used in combination with other drugs and with radiation therapy.[16] The drug belongs to the class of chemotherapy compounds known as antimetabolites. It acts by binding to dihydrofolate reductase leading to a reduction in folate pools intracellularly.[17] This depletion causes a cessation of thymidylate synthesis and purine biosynthesis. Additionally, methotrexate is metabolized to polyglutamate derivatives that inhibit both dihydrofolate reductase and thymidylate synthase.[17] The drug acts on cells in S-phase when DNA synthesis is occurring. The drug has been given either before or after irradiation. There is little in vitro data to show benefit of this drug in combination with irradiation, further there is increased toxicity (vide infra).[18,19]

The drug is cleared by the kidney with 50 to 80% of the drug being excreted within the first 12 hours after administration.[20] Toxicity of methotrexate is related to the concentration of the drug and the duration of exposure.[1,17] The threshold level of methotrexate injury varies for individual tissues. The duration of exposure of tissues to the threshold level plays a critical role in producing cellular injury. High-dose methotrexate (1 or more g/m²) may increase the response rate in head and neck cancer.[21] The potential for injury is greater with these doses, which are usually several grams rather than milligrams. The injury is to a large extent prevented by the use of leucovorin. Renal excretion is variable and the level of methotrexate must also be monitored when high doses are used.

Table 16–3. Chemotherapy Agents Active in Head and Neck Cancer

AGENT	ACTIVITY (%)	REFERENCE
Methotrexate	20–50	1,20,31,132
Cisplatin	40–70	132
Bleomycin	20, 6–45	2,132
5-FU	15	2
Hydroxyurea	39	2
Vinblastine	29	2
Doxorubicin	24	2
Cyclophosphamide	36	2
Taxol	45	73

*Activity is defined by the proportion of complete and partial responses seen in the treated group.

Table 16–4. Side Effects Seen with Single Agents in the Treatment of Head and Neck Cancer

TOXICITY	AGENT
Acute	
Fever, nausea, and vomiting	Bleomycin, cisplatin, vinblastine, doxorubicin, taxol
Hypersensitivity	Cisplatin, can be suppressed; taxol (vehicle), can be pretreated; bleomycin, can be pretreated; methotrexate, pulmonary component; mitomycin, rare, acute dyspnea
Immediate	
Myelosuppression	Methotrexate, cisplatin, mild; carboplatin, moderate to severe
	5-FU, schedule dependent—most severe with bolus injection
	Taxol
	Mitomycin, prolonged
	Vinblastine
	Cyclophosphamide
	Doxorubicin
Mucositis	Methotrexate, dose dependent, preventable with leucovorin
	5-FU, schedule dependent, worst with bolus injection, may worsen with addition of leucovorin
	Bleomycin, dose dependent
	Doxorubicin
	Vinblastine
Extravasation	Vinblastine
	Doxorubicin
Delayed	
Renal	Methotrexate, prevented with leucovorin, fluids, alkalinization
	Cisplatin, prevented with fluids, ?diuretics
	Mitomycin, accompanied often by hemolytic anemia
	Ifosfamide, prevented with mesna
	Cyclophosphamide, prevented with hydration
Cardiac	Doxorubicin, cumulative dose dependent
	5-FU, with all schedules, rare
Pulmonary	Bleomycin, fibrosis at cumulative dose of 200 mg/m²
	Mitomycin, basilar fibrosis
	Cyclophosphamide, fibrosis
	Methotrexate, chronic changes
Neurological, special senses	Cisplatin, peripheral neuropathy, cumulative dose effect; rarely visual symptoms, loss of high-frequency hearing with cumulative doses
	5-FU, rarely cerebellar injury
	Taxol, peripheral injury
	Vinblastine, peripheral
Alopecia	Doxorubicin
	Vinblastine
	Taxol
	Ifosfamide
	Bleomycin
Dermatologic	5-FU, hyperpigmentation, phlebitis
	Doxorubicin, hyperpigmentation
	Bleomycin, rash, skin thickening, Raynaud's phenomenon
	Cisplatin, Raynaud's phenomenon
Late	
Radionecrosis	Methotrexate, rarely
	5-FU, rarely

Acute, within the first 24 to 48 h after administration; intermediate, within the first 1 to 2 weeks; delayed, over first several months of treatment; late, more than 6 months.

Methotrexate diffuses across the blood-brain barrier and into peritoneal or pleural fluid accumulations. In general, toxicity is increased where large fluid collections are present at the time of methotrexate administration. Third spacing of the drug occurs, which leads to prolonged exposure. Pleural and peritoneal effusions should be removed prior to drug administration.

Toxicities that are seen with methotrexate include bone marrow suppression. This usually occurs between 7 to 14 days after drug administration. There is a dose–response relationship such that higher doses are more likely to produce significant injury.[21] The usual low dose of methotrexate is 30 to 40 mg/m^2; intermediate doses are in the range of 250 to 500 mg/m^2.

Mucositis as well as other gastrointestinal toxicities such as nausea vomiting, and diarrhea are also seen. In a study by Ensley et al,[22] in which cisplatin and 5-FU were alternated with moderate-dose methotrexate as induction therapy for T$_4$ lesions of the head and neck, methotrexate produced much less gastrointestinal symptoms than the other regimen. Moderate mucositis was seen only 2% of the time. In another trial, using low-dose methotrexate, 40 mg/m^2, and randomizing patients to cisplatin or methotrexate, mucositis was seen 38% of the time. These patients had recurrent disease; side effects are more common in these patients than in those without prior therapy.[23] High-dose methotrexate can produce an acute chemical hepatitis that is usually reversible. Chronic administration of low doses of the drug is associated with hepatic fibrosis.

An acute type of lung injury can be seen with methotrexate. Clinically there is fever, dyspnea, eosinophilia, and pulmonary infiltrates. The exact mechanism is not known but is thought to be allergic. Patients respond to steroids and can be retreated without an exacerbations.[17]

Toxicities with radiotherapy, primarily mucositis, and the lack of benefit have limited the use of concomitant chemoradiotherapy.[18,19] In an older nonrandomized series, oral methotrexate with irradiation produced a higher incidence of radionecrosis compared with irradiation alone or methotrexate given intravenously; however, the radiation dose was also higher in the group receiving oral methotrexate.[16] Using moderate doses of irradiation with moderate doses (100 mg/m^2) of methotrexate, Gupta et al[24] have shown a nonsignificant increase in mucositis and no increase in late side effects—fibrosis—in a trial comparing patients randomized to receive radiotherapy with or without methotrexate. Renstschler et al[25] demonstrated that patients receiving methotrexate after irradiation develop intolerable mucositis at a lower concentration of the drug. The white blood cell (WBC) nadir may also be lower in the postirradiation group.

Cisplatin: Pharmacology and Mechanism of Action

Cisplatin is a platinum coordination compound that was initially described as an antibiotic in 1965. Subsequently it has demonstrated to be extremely active against a range of tumors, including head and neck cancer.[26] The drug is aquated, losing chloride ions, and rapidly binds to DNA. The drug acts as an alkylating agent and forms intrastrand and interstrand cross-links with DNA and nucleoproteins. Cisplatin is rapidly bound to protein and only a small amount (10%) remains as free drug. The drug is excreted via the kidney.[27] Cisplatin is usually administered with fluids, and frequently diuretics, to prevent renal injury, although the additional benefit of diuretics is not as certain. Mannitol, an osmotic diuretic, does increase the level of free platinum but does not increase excretion.[27,28] Toxicity of the drug, especially nephrotoxicity, may be in part dose related; types of toxicity and their severity are also schedule dependent.[29,30] Forastieree et al[30] demonstrated accumulation of filterable platinum with a continuous infusion technique. This increase in platinum concentration over time was believed to account for the increased myelosuppression and hypomagnesemia in this group of patients in contrast to the bolus group where the peak level of the drug was higher.

Cisplatin is highly effective as a radioenhancer, both in vitro and in clinical trials.[31,32] The exact mechanism is not clear but may be due to production of free radicals or inhibition of cellular repair mechanisms. Because cisplatin does not produce severe mucositis when used alone, this potential overlapping toxicity with combined chemoradiotherapy is less of a problem than when radiotherapy is combined with either 5-FU or methotrexate. On the other hand, both radiotherapy and cisplatin can cause injury to the gastrointestinal crypts, making the potential for nausea and vomiting and diarrhea worse. However, in an Eastern Cooperative Oncology Group (ECOG) trial of weekly low-dose cisplatin, with irradiation, hematologic toxicity was worse, but no increase in vomiting or mucositis was seen.[33]

Toxicity with cisplatin can be seen immediately after the drug is given, or over the next 1 to 2 weeks. Toxicities can also appear after several courses of the drug. Toxicities that are seen within 24 hours after drug administration include nausea and vomiting. Cisplatin is a strong emetogen and is the agent that is usually used to evaluate new antiemetics for their effectiveness in preventing this complication. Ensley et al[22] reported one patient who sustained a Mallory-Weiss tear from cisplatin-related nausea and vomiting; this complication has been previously seen in other patients. The drug acts on both serotonin receptors in the gut and also at the chemoreceptor trigger zone in the medulla.[34] Individuals who use alcohol frequently (more than five drinks per day) may have less nausea and vomiting with this drug than other patients. This phenomenon may occur because of damage to the chemoreceptor trigger zone from alcohol.[35] In addition to acute nausea and vomiting, cisplatin can produce both anticipatory nusea and vomiting prior to treatment and delayed nausea and vomiting (occurring after treatment) that can last for up to 72 to 96 hours. Aggressive use of antiemetics prophylactically may forestall the development of these problems.

Hypersensitivity reactions to cisplatin have also been reported. These include anaphylactoid reactions with respiratory symptoms, skin reactions including urticaria, and facial edema.[36,37] These reactions are partly histamine related; skin testing can be done. Pretreatment with antistamines can prevent the reaction.

Toxicities seen at 1 to 2 weeks include myelosuppression. This side effect is usually milder compared with other chemotherapeutic agents. There can, however, be increased myelosuppression at higher doses (100 to 120 mg/m^2) than in lower-dose range (20 to 75 mg/m^2). There can be mild to moderate anemia, unlike many of the other antineoplastics that generally produce depression of the WBC count and platelets more commonly.[26] Generally, the nadir from cisplatin is seen at 10 to 14 days with recovery within 1 week. Renal toxicity is also seen at 1 to 2 weeks; the injury is seen in both the proximal and distal tubule in animal models but is more often distal in humans.[38,39] The use of aminoglycosides and other nephrotoxins may augment this toxicity. The level of total platinum has been shown to correlate with the renal injury.[29] This level may vary, even in patients receiving the same dose. Subclinical renal injury may then result.

The duration of drug administration and the schedule of administration may play a role in the frequency and severity of the nausea and vomiting and renal injury seen with cisplatin. Administration of the drug over longer periods of time (3, 6, or 24 hours) may make the severity of nausea and vomiting milder than when the drug is given over 15 minutes or 1 hour. Belt et al[28] have also shown an increased rate of platinum excretion with a 6-hour cisplatin infusion, which could potentially decrease the renal injury. The renal injury to the tubule frequently produces leakage of magnesium and rarely sodium wasting.[40] This injury may be permanent and require careful attention to magnesium and potassium replacement during and after treatment.

Cisplatin is an alkylator and can produce injury to the seminiferous tubule. A decrease in sperm production was temporary in 40% of men treated for testicular cancer with cisplatin in one series.[39] The dose of cisplatin used for this disease is the same as with head and neck cancer; however, the drug dose is broken up into smaller doses over several days and the drug is repeated for three to four courses. The use one or two doses of cisplatin at the much higher single dose, as is often used in the treatment of head and neck cancer, has not been reported to cause azoospermia.

Late toxicities seen with cisplatin include neurotoxicity, both peripheral and central, and Raynaud's phenomenon. Peripheral nerve injury in one study was not related to prior history of alcohol exposure, diabetes, or prior neuropathy.[41] The neuropathy is initially sensory but there can be a significant loss of fine motor function, and in some individuals, severe gross motor function loss occurs. This latter finding is more common in high-dose regimens using 200 mg/m^2 over 5 days.[41] The first sign may be a loss of vibratory sensation at a cumulative dose of 300 ro 400 mg/m^2. The symptoms may be reversible if the drug is stopped. However, weakness may be permanent.

Loss of vision has also been reported. This can vary from blurring of vision to blindness. These symptoms are seen at various dose levels and often the cisplatin is given with other drugs. Generally the symptoms are reversible.[42]

Ototoxicity is of particular concern in the head and neck cancer patient. This side effect is seen with cisplatin in 30 to 50% of patients treated with the drug.[39,43] Infusion of the drug over several days may further increase the incidence.[30] High-frequency hearing loss is most common and is more frequently seen in children or older individuals who develop renal toxicity.[39]

Several chemotherapy agents have been reported to cause acute leukemia. These have primarily been alkylator agents that are radiomimetic. The cumulative dose of these drugs may play a role in the production of leukemia. There are several reports in the literature of cisplatin producing acute leukemia. A recent careful review by Greene[44] suggests that most of these reports included combinations of chemotherapy that contained drugs such as etoposide, a known carcinogen. Continued monitoring of patients receiving cisplatin will be needed to resolve this concern.[44]

Intra-arterial infusions of cisplatin have been used for several types of tumors including head and neck cancer. Neurological damage of adjacent nerves in the brachial or sacral plexus has been reported.[45] In a study by Forastiere et al,[46] the main toxicity was mucositis probably related to the floxuridine (FUdR) given with the cisplatin.

Carboplatin

Carboplatin is a coordination level II analog of cisplatin. The carboxylato-ligand is more slowly dissociated from the molecule and thus aquation is slower. Binding to plasma proteins is much slower than with cisplatin. Carboplatin is excreted more quickly with 68% excreted by 24 hours in contrast to cisplatin where only 25% of the drug is excreted in the same time period; nephrotoxicity is much less frequent.[47,48] The drug has a similar spectrum of antineoplastic activity against solid tumors as the parent compound, cisplatin. Carboplatin may achieve a higher tissue level of platinum; it has shown supra-additivity with irradiation in vitro.[32] Several trials have been reported with carboplatin in combination with other chemotherapy agents as well as with irradiation.[49-51] These are reviewed in the section on combined therapy. As a single agent, carboplatin has considerably more myelosuppression than cisplatin. In the initial phase I studies, the dose-limiting toxicities of the drug were thrombocytopenia (less than 100,000/μL) and leukopenia, which were seen in 84% of the patients at doses of 440 mg/m^2.[52] The recommended dose was 400 mg/m^2. No nephrotoxicity was seen, although this side effect can be seen with continued dosing. Hypomagnesemia was seen in 5 of 47 courses. No auditory toxicity was seen and only one patient developed neurotoxicity.[52]

Bleomycin: Pharmacology

Bleomycin, derived from fungal sources, belongs to the antibiotic class of antineoplastics. The drug has been used extensively in several tumors and has activity in head and neck cancer. It binds to DNA and produces single-strand breaks. Excretion of the drug is primarily renal. In patients with a creatinine clearance of less than 30 mL/min, excretion is reduced.[53]

TOXICITIES

Toxicities seen with bleomycin differ from other drugs in that myelosuppression is infrequently seen.[38] Acutely the drug produces fever in 20 to 40% of patients treated,[54] which may be accompanied by dyspnea and hypotension. These symptoms occur within 24 hours of administration and may respond to steroids.

The most serious long-term side effect of bleomycin is pulmonary fibrosis, which increases in incidence at a cumulative dose of 200 mg/m^2, although the problem can be seen at lower doses. This side effect occurs in 10% of the patients treated.[54] The use of diffusion capacity allows a quantitative measure of the decrease in lung capacity but is not predictive of the development of this problem. Clinically, patients develop dyspnea, cough, and fever; the earliest physical findings may be fine rales at the lung bases before the patient is symptomatic.[54] Age, underlying pulmonary disease, irradiation to the chest, and exposure to high concentrations of oxygen during general anesthesia may predispose to difficulties with this complication of bleomycin.[55] Other long-term side effects seen with this drug include skin thickening, especially over the joints of the hands, skin darkening, and Raynaud's syndrome.[38]

Several trials using bleomycin with irradiation in the treatment of head and neck cancer have used the drug in combination and are discussed below. A trial by Shanta and Krishnamurthi[56] randomized 157 patients to receive irradiation with or without bleomycin as the sole chemotherapy agent. The drug was given both intra-arterially and intravenously at doses of 10 to 15 mg three times a week up to a total dose of 150 to 250 mg. The drug was alternated with irradiation. Dosing continued until side effects were limiting. Severe mucositis was seen, which was diminished by dose reductions. Two patients developed skin ulcers, presumably in the area of irradiation. Fatal pneumonitis occurred in four patients.[56] The fatal pulmonary complications make this drug less attractive as a radioenhancer. A recent review of chemoradiotherapy by Jassem et al[57] notes that severe mucositis is a feature of many of the trials comparing bleomycin alone with the drug used with irradiation.

5-FU Pharmacology

5-Fluorouracil, an antimetabolite, is a substituted pyrimidine that was initially developed in 1957. The drug acts to both inhibit RNA and DNA synthesis directly by incorporation of metabolites into the respective molecules. The more important site of action is inhibition of thymidylate synthase with decreased production of thymidylate for DNA synthesis. This inhibition requires reduced folate as a cofactor.[58] The drug is metabolized in the liver to β-alanine, ammonia, and carbon dioxide. This reaction occurs quickly and the drug has a half life of 10 to 15 minutes.

Recently leucovorin has been given prior to 5-FU; this combination further inhibits thymidylate synthase and increases the cytotoxicity of 5-FU which is primarily used in the treatment of head and neck cancer in combination with other drugs or, most often, for radioenhancement. An extensive literature documents the increased cell kill with this agent when added to cell lines exposed to irradiation.[19] These studies have shown that the drug is most effective if given for prolonged periods of time during and after irradiation.[59] Clinical trials using the drug in combination with irradiation have also shown benefit at other sites for the combination of drug and radiation therapy.[19,60]

TOXICITIES

These side effects seen are highly schedule dependent. Because of rapid clearance, constant infusions over several days generally produce less myelosuppression than when the drug is given as a bolus on a daily schedule. Mucositis is the main toxicity seen with constant infusion at the usual dose range (1000 mg/m^2/d) employed in many current trials with head and neck cancer.[61] Byfield et al [60] have demonstrated that a level of 1000 ng/mL (which can be achieved by a 72-hour infusion of the drug at a dose of 45 to 50 mg/kg) produces grade 3 mucositis in head and neck cancer patients who were also receiving irradiation. A similar dose of drug with irradiation to other sites did not produce this degree of mucositis. Patients receiving the drug without irradiation could tolerate a level of 1600 ng/mL before grade 3 mucositis was seen.[60] A separate trial by Byfield et al[62] used 5-FU given at doses of 20 to 30 mg/kg over 5 days with irradiations. Each patient underwent dose escalation as tolerated during ongoing irradiation to 5000 cGy. There were rest periods after each 4 to 5 days of therapy of up to 9 days. Grade 2 mucositis was seen at the lowest dose of 20 mg/kg in five of six patients. At the next dose level four of nine patients developed grade 3 mucositis requiring a dose reduction and five of nine developed grades 1 and 2 (mild) mucositis.[62] All patients treated at 30 mg/kg (the highest dose level) developed grade 3 mucositis. With an increasing dose of chemotherapy given with irradiation, there is an increasing frequency of mucositis. Other side effects seen were mild phlebitis and hyperpigmentation over the infusion sites. In addition, there was mild nausea and occasional skin injury. The distribution of the mucositis was in the oropharynx rather than in the oral cavity as has been reported with 5-FU alone. This distribution corresponded to the radiation portals. Two patients developed fistulae after surgery for residual disease, both of whom had resolution of the fistulae.[62]

Myelosuppression is more frequent but usually mild at the typical doses (25 to 30 mg/kg or 400 to 500 mg/m^2) used for treatment at other sites when the drug is given alone as a bolus. However, if the drug is given with irradiation to areas of marrow production such as with pelvic irradiation, this side effect is more frequent and more severe.[63] Late side effects of the drug in combination with irradiation for head and neck cancer were reported by Lo et al.[64] They noted 5 of 68 patients who developed major complications that consisted of bone or soft tissue necrosis or fistula formation. One patient died of these complications. No major complications were seen in the patients receiving irradiation only. Minor complications such as ulcerations were similar in both groups.

Although most trials of 5-FU in head and neck cancer have used the higher dose continuous infusion regimens in combination with irradiation, a recent trial used a low-dose (200 to 300 mg/m^2) protracted infusion technique with irradiation.[65] The protracted infusion technique produces different side effects than either bolus or high-dose short-term continuous infusion. The predominant side effect seen is pain and redness of the palms and soles—ethrodysthesia. Lokich et al[66] initially used this technique and noted that 300 mg/m^2 was the optimum dose. In the study of Weppelman et al,[5] patients with head and neck cancer received irradiation also; the predominant side effect was mucositis and skin injury at a dose similar to that reported by Lokich et al [66] who used the drug alone. No hand/foot syndrome was seen. The maximum tolerated dose was 250 mg/m^2 for 12 weeks.

Other side effects seen with 5-FU include diarrhea and skin darkening. Ataxia due to cerebellar injury is occasionally seen. This side effect may be dose related. Recently, there have been a few patients who have developed angina, or myocardial infarction, or life-threatening arrhythmias either during or after administration of this drug. This side effect is rare, and has been reported in patients receiving both bolus and constant infusion 5-FU.[67]

5-FU and Leucovorin

Leucovorin has been given with 5-FU in a variety of schedules, including daily for 5 days or once weekly. The side effects are quantitatively different. Specific side effects that are seen with 5-FU and leucovorin are diarrhea, myelosuppression, and mucositis.[68] Daily administration for 5 days is associated with an increase in mucositis. The severity of the toxicity is also dependent on the dose of the two drugs.

Hydroxyurea: Pharmacology and Toxicity

Hydroxyurea is rarely given today as a single agent to patients with head and neck cancer. It has been employed as a radioenhancer[69] and the toxicity seen is discussed in the section on combinations of chemotherapy and radiotherapy below. The drug blocks ribonucleotide reductase and thus inhibits DNA synthesis. Approximately one half of the dose is metabolized in the liver. The primary toxicity of the drug is myelosuppression, which is dose related.[39]

Vinblastine: Pharmacology

Vinblastine (and other vinca alkaloids such as vincristine) is derived from the periwinkle plant. These drugs act by inhibiting the mitotic spindle. Although they are similar in origin and structure, there are differences in activity and toxicity. Vinblastine is usually given in combination with other chemotherapy agents (vide infra). It is excreted through the bile and doses must be modified for biliary obstruction.

TOXICITY

Vinblastine, unlike vincristine, causes significant myelosuppression. Nadirs are seen at 4 to 10 days with recovery by 7 to 21 days.[70] The drug causes mucositis and stomatitis. Diarrhea and nausea and vomiting are infrequent. Autonomic neuropathy is seen; there can be a paralytic ileus or abdominal cramps.. Peripheral neuropathy is less common than with vincristine; more common with this vinca is jaw pain or other neuromyopathic pains. Raynaud's phenomenon and hypertension have been reported. There can be aiopecia, which is usually mild; the drug can also produce a syndrome of inappropriate antidiuretic hormone release as with other vincas.

Extravasation of any vinca can cause considerable skin damage and ulceration. Prompt measures are required to minimize the injury. These usually consist of stopping the infusion, withdrawing any drug through the tubing, and removing the needle. Unlike other chemotherapy extravasations, where cold is now used, extravasation of vinblastine or other vincas is treated with warm compresses. Hyaluronidase is recommended by the manufacturer for this type of extravasation.

Doxorubicin (Adriamycino): Clinical Pharmacology and Toxicity

Doxorubicin is a fungally derived compound that intercalates into DNA. The drug, which is used infrequently in the current treatment of head and neck cancer, is metabolized in the liver and excreted into the bile. Biliary obstruction requires a dose reduction.

Side effects seen with this drug include nausea and vomiting and mucositis. Myelosuppression is seen as with other antibiotics at 7 to 10 days.[71] Alopecia occurs several weeks after the drug is used. Acutely, if the drug is extravasated, there can be the development of painful ulcers requiring skin grafting. Long-term administration causes cumulative damage to the myocardium and is usually dose limiting at 550 mg/m^2. Other risk factors for the development of cardiomyopathy, such as alcohol, may lower this threshold.[71] Scheduling of administration may be changed to delay the development of this toxicity.

Doxorubicin can interact with previously irradiated patients to produce a "recall" phenomenon with an exacerbation of the previous radiation injury.[71] This reaction can cause an acute inflammatory reaction or increased fibrosis.

Cyclophosphamide

Cyclophosphamide is a prodrug and is converted by the liver to the active metabolite. The drug is an alkylator. Typical side effects are moderate nausea and vomiting. There is usually mild to moderate myelosuppression. Excretion of another metabolite of cyclophosphamide causes hemorrhagic cystitis if hydration is not given. The drug can cause sterility and pulmonary fibrosis. Secondary malignancies have occurred.[72]

Taxol

Taxol is a new agent with a unique structure derived from the bark of the western yew.[73] The drug has shown activity in head and neck cancer.[74] It acts by increasing microtubule assembly, causing these structures to accumulate in the cell and inhibiting mitosis and other cell functions.[73] The drug is both metabolized in the liver and also excreted in the bile. There is extensive protein binding.[73]

Side effects are related to the drug and the Cremophor (polyoxyethylated castor oil) vehicle, which are needed to solubilize the drug. Anaphylaxis has been seen. This reaction is specifically related to the vehicle and premedication with antihistamines, steroids, and cimetidine are used to prevent the side effect. Myelosuppression is seen at a dose of 200 to 250 mg/m^2 when the drug is given over 24 hours. Shorter infusion times are being evaluated and may avoid some of the problems with myelosuppression. The drug causes peripheral neuropathy that is mainly sensory and increases in frequency with continued dosing. An initial dose of 250 mg/m^2 is associated with early onset of neuropathy.

In the initial trials with this agent, bradycardia was reported in 19%.[73] When patients are monitored while receiving this drug, more significant conduction disturbances have been seen. It is not clear whether these are drug related. Patients with underlying heart disease may not be candidates for taxol.

In a preliminary report by Forastier[74] taxol at a dose of 250 mg/m^2 in a group of patients with advanced head and neck cancer, the main toxicity was hematologic with grade 3 to 4 neutropenia in 89% of the 22 patients treated and grade 2 to 3 anemia in 56% of the patients. Eight patients were hospitalized for fever. There was one death due to neutropenia and one due to cardiac toxicity. A grade 1 sensory neuropathy was seen in two patients and a grade 2 neuropathy in three patients. The neuropathy was seen after two to four courses. Other side effects were alopecia and myalgias.[74]

Miscellaneous Agents

MITOMYCIN: PHARMACOLOGY

Mitomycin is an antibiotic derived from a fungal source. It possesses a quinone ring structure, like doxorubicin, and functions as an alkylator once activated by reduction of the quinone ring. The active compound forms DNA and DNA-protein cross links. If oxygen is present,the compound is reoxygenated to a less toxic form.[75] This feature makes the drug attractive for radioenhancement. Increased activity might be expected in less well-oxygenated tumor tissue; this has not always been described.[19] In vitro studies have shown additivity or surpa-additivity with radiation therapy. In solid tumor

models, there may be heterogeneity of drug distribution and of oxygen tension, making the overall reduction of tumor mass less than might be expected from in vitro studies.[75,76]

The drug is metabolized by the liver and cleared by the biliary system and also in part by the kidney. Patients with either biliary obstruction or renal insufficiency require dose modifications of mitomycin. Where the bilirubin level is greater than 3 or the creatinine is moderately elevated, the drug may be held. Clearance may be dose dependent.[71,77] The drug has been used as a single agent in the treatment of head and neck cancer; more recently it has been used for its radioenhancing effects in combined chemoradiotherapy.

Toxicities. Myelosuppression can be delayed with mitomycin and the nadir can be seen up to 8 weeks after the drug is administered. Scheduling of administration of the drug should take this delayed nadir into account. Myelosuppression is cumulative and may cause prolonged thrombocytopenia. The drug produces mild to moderate nausea and vomiting; anorexia can be seen. The drug can also produce fever occasionally. Early reports of toxicity indicated that mitomycin could also cause glomerulonephritis. This complication was described as mild.[43] More recently, the drug has been reported to produce renal failure and hemolytic anemia in a few patients. This microangiopathic hemolytic anemia–renal failure syndrome may be irreversible.[71,78]

Of concern in the head and neck patient population is the development of a pulmonary reaction. This acute syndrome can occur within 4 to 12 hours after the drug is administered and is manifested as bronchospasm. Chronic pulmonary toxicity can also be seen with the development of pulmonary fibrosis and a restrictive pattern on pulmonary function studies.[78] The threshold dose for this long-term complication is 50 to 60 mg/m^2 which represents two to three doses.[71] Combinations of mitomycin with bleomycin or vinca alkaloids have also produced this complication. This toxicity may be related to the production of superoxide radicals. Other toxicities seen with mitomycin include extravasation, including at a site distant from the infusion. We have seen this occur in patients with a poor nutritional status at a venipuncture site that was several weeks old.

A recent study by Weissberg et al[76] in patients with head and neck cancer compared radiotherapy to radiotherapy with mitomycin at a dose of 15 mg/m^2. Patients included both those with advanced local disease early disease for which therapy was given preoperatively. Side effects were characterized descriptively. Acute reactions were similar in both groups. A comparable incidence of fibrosis was also seen. An excess of pulmonary deaths was seen in the combined therapy group; the authors attribute this excess in part to chronic lung disease in this population.[76]

IFOSPHAMIDE

Ifosphamide is structurally similar to cyclophosphamide. The drug has shown activity in head and neck cancer. Side effects are similar to those with cyclophosphamide, but hemorrhagic cystitis is much more common. Vigorous hydration and treatment with mesna, a uroprotective, are needed to avoid this complication.

EDATREXATE

Edatrexate is another antifol that is being evaluated in head and neck cancer.[79] The drug is related to methotrexate. Increased entry of this compound into the cell, as well as increased polyglutamation, occurs when compared with methotrexate.[79] The principal side effect is mucositis.

COMBINATION CHEMOTHERAPY

Several recent reviews of combination chemotherapy for head and neck cancer have reviewed the efficacy of this technique.[61,80,81] Approaches used include combination chemotherapy alone prior to surgery or radiotherapy (induction therapy); after surgery and radiotherapy (adjuvant therapy); or concomitant with radiotherapy. In addition, combination chemotherapy is used for palliation of recurrent disease. Often these trials are single arm, phase II studies and are thus focused on efficacy issues; however, more recently, phase III randomized trials are increasingly being reported. Frequently, toxicity is now being evaluated in a quantitative manner rather than descriptively. Many of these patients have marginal nutritional status and poor overall medical status; often the patient population being reported has far advanced local disease or represent retreated patients. The types and severity of toxicity may differ in these subgroups.

Induction therapy may be better tolerated than adjuvant therapy given after definitive local therapy.[25,61,82,83] In the report by the Head and Neck Contracts Program,[82] only 13% were able to complete the planned postoperative course of cisplatin chemotherapy. Thirty-seven percent of the patients refused any further chemotherapy after their surgical procedure. Ervin et al[83] noted that only 10 of 26 patients received adjuvant therapy in contrast to the patients in the study receiving induction in a trial using both preoperative and postoperative chemotherapy. Toxicity was also different in the two groups with increased mucositis in the postoperative group. Both groups received the same chemotherapy. Other studies have not shown differences related to the timing of chemotherapy. Al-Sarraf et al[84] reported two separate nonrandomized phase II trials by the Radiation Therapy Oncology Group (RTOG) that looked at pre versus postoperative chemotherapy. Radiation was sequenced after chemotherapy in both groups. Toxicities with chemotherapy were similar in both studies.

Although drug combinations are usually selected to avoid common toxicities, the addition of more drugs may produce additional toxicities such that the combination as a whole is not tolerated as well, although the individual drugs alone are well tolerated at the doses used. In the four trials reported by Wittes et al,[85] in which additional drugs were added to a cisplatin and bleomycin regimen, overall toxicity was severe; the only significant overlapping toxicity was mucositis.

The impact of chemotherapy on surgical complications is infrequently commented upon. The Head and Neck Contract Program[82] found no increase of wound infection, fistula, or healing in the group receiving chemotherapy. No increase in postoperative complications was seen in the recent Veterans Affairs Laryngeal Cancer trial either.[86] Nonetheless, this remains an area of concern.[61]

In the next several sections, we have organized a discussion of combination therapy by whether the therapy is used for induction, adjuvant, or advanced disease because of the potential differences in patient tolerance. The sections are then subdivided by a predominant drug in the combination regimen. These trials may be briefly reviewed again under the discussion of one of the other drugs in the combination but we have tried to avoid redundancy as much as possible. Combined modality therapy is discussed after this section.

Induction Therapy, Overview of Toxicities

Induction therapy has frequently employed a platinum-based chemotherapy regimen, either in combination with 5-FU, bleomycin, methotrexate, or vinblastine.[82,83,85,87–90] In general, toxicities seen with the combinations reflect the dominant toxicities of the individual drugs. The frequency of the toxicities may vary because of deliberate scheduling of the drugs to avoid overlapping toxicities.[83] Ervin et al sequenced a combination of cisplatin and methotrexate, both nephrotoxins, so that the drugs were separated in time. Although nephrotoxicity was seen, the frequency was low and generally mild to moderate; 7% of the patients did experience severe renal toxicity. Twelve patients required dose attenuation because of renal toxicity.

Induction Therapy with Bleomycin and Drugs Other than Cisplatin

A trial with bleomycin, vincristine, 5-FU, and methotrexate has been reported by Price and Hill.[91] This study used bleomycin at a dose of 60 mg given as an infusion over 3 days. Patients with pulmonary disease, either by diffusion capacity or on x-ray, were excluded. Side effects included myelosuppression, mucositis, and peripheral neuropathy. All of these side effects were seen less than 10% of the time. The degree of myelosuppression was mild, with only one patient experiencing a WBC nadir of less than 2000/mm³. Other side effects seen in 5% or less of the patients included nausea and vomiting, alopecia, and anorexia. One death occurred in a patient who had renal disease and failed to receive leucovorin.[91]

Induction Therapy with Bleomycin and Cisplatin

A trial employing cisplatin at a dose of 187.5 mg/m² (approximately twice the usual dose of cisplatin) and bleomycin given as a 5-day infusion at a total dose of 60 U/m² has been reported by Haines et al.[89] Alopecia was seen in all patients. Nausea and vomiting were seen in 94%. In 20%, this side effect was severe enough (grade 3 or 4) that they required intravenous hydration. Sixteen percent of the patients had grade 3 or 4 thrombocytopenia; one patient developed epistaxis. Twenty percent of the patients had grade 3 or 4 neutropenia; one half of these patients required admission for neutropenic fever. All of these side effects are related to the cisplatin dose except alopecia. Overlapping toxicity with bleomycin should not be significant. Bleomycin was responsible for a decrease in diffusion capacity or other pulmonary function parameter in 24% (49) of the patients. One patient died of pulmonary toxicity. Because the patients also received surgery or radiation therapy, the contribution of either general anesthesia or irradiation is not clear. In the one bleomycin-related death, the patient received local irradiation.[89]

Seven patients were not able to continue chemotherapy owing to toxicity. These toxicities included a transient increase in serum creatinine, pulmonary toxicity, arterial embolism, ototoxicity, and atrial tachycardias. Long-term side effects included ototoxicity in 12 of 49 patients (25%) and neurotoxicity in 19 of 49 patients (39%). Again, these side effects are most likely related to the cisplatin.

Three trials have used bleomycin, methotrexate, and cisplatin.[83,92,93] These trials all employed differing doses of drugs with the bleomycin either given as an infusion in two studies and coming between the two nephrotoxins or as a series of bolus injections between the methotrexate and cisplatin. Side effects were in general much milder than in the high-dose cisplatin/bleomycin study by Haines et al.[89] Myelosuppression was seen less often and was less severe; however, six patients in the study by Ervin had dose attenuations due to myelosuppression. Severe thrombocytopenia in the trial by Ervin et al[83] occurred in 14% of the patients. Mucositis was seen 14% of the time in the trial by Ervin et al[83] but 20% of the time in the study by Zidan et al.[93] The patients in that trial may have had more advanced disease and received their radiotherapy immediately after the chemotherapy.

Severe pulmonary toxicity was seen only in the study by Ervin et al,[83] where one death occurred that was clearly related to bleomycin or methotrexate. In none of the studies did the dose of bleomycin reach the cumulative range of 200 mg/m². Most of the patients underwent surgery or radiotherapy or both. Presumably efforts were made to avoid additional toxicity by the use of lower oxygen concentrations with general anesthesia.[83] In the other trial using infusional bleomycin, two patients developed pleuritic chest pain and another had acute dyspnea.[92] Skin rashes were seen in a few patients. In the study by Wittes et al,[85] one patient developed exfoliation.

Nephrotoxicity was avoided in these studies by the use of leucovorin rescue. Neurotoxicity was seen only rarely; the dose of cisplatin was in the range of 60 to 100 mg/m².

Induction Therapy Using Methotrexate and Other Drugs

Ensley et al[22] have reported on a feasibility trial in which methotrexate administered at a moderate dosage was followed by 5-FU and then leucovorin rescue. These courses were alternated with cisplatin (100 mg/m²) and 5-FU (1000 mg/m² daily, infused for 4 days) given at a common dose and schedule. Six of the 46 patients dropped out owing to toxicity issues. Of the six, four had exacerbation of concurrent diseases. Three patients required a treatment delay because of myelosuppression and three were removed owing to grade 4 neutropenia with fever and hospitalization.[22] Toxicities seen were mucositis in 23% and diarrhea in 3%. One patient had severe diarrhea due to alcohol-related liver disease and difficulties with drug metabolism. One patient continued drinking and had severe myelosuppression. These problems reflect the difficulties in treating with intensive chemotherapy in a patient population with several intercurrent diseases and problems with alcohol abuse. Renal toxicity was seen in less than 10% of patients and was reversible except for a patient with occult lead nephropathy due to use of "moonshine" abuse.[22] Cumulative myelosuppression was seen so that by course 5 of this alternating regimen, 30% of patients had mild myelosuppression. Fifteen percent had moderate myelosuppression after the second course of methotrexate. Little nausea and vomiting were seen after each methotrexate course.

No severe neurotoxicity was seen; a desquamating skin rash occurred with the cisplatin and 5-FU in one patient but was not seen in the courses with methotrexate. In another trial of sequential methotrexate and 5-FU that was given without other drugs, and at similar doses to that of the trial by Ensley et al,[22] mild gastrointestinal toxicity was seen with treatment given every other week. When drugs were administered weekly, 5 of 36 patients experienced severe stomatitis.[94] Severe myelosuppression was only seen in one patient on one occasion. Leucovorin rescue was given with all courses.

Several trials with methotrexate, bleomycin, and cisplatin have been previously reviewed in the section on combination treatment with bleomycin. To summarize these combinations, nephrotoxicity was usually minimal, even with two nephrotoxins in the regimen. In the study of Ervin et al,[83] 7% of patients had severe renal toxicity; one patient in the study by Price and Hill[91] died when leucovorin was not given. This side effect was minimized by scheduling the drugs several days apart in all of these studies. In another study reported by Vokes et al,[4] methotrexate was given at a moderate dose followed 24 hours later by cisplatin and then 5-FU. Leucovorin was also given. Eight of the 38 patients developed a transient rise of the creatinine; only one of these patients had a creatinine of more than 4 mg/mL. In the trial by Ervin et al,[83] methotrexate accounted for only one fourth of the patients developing nephrotoxicity, with cisplatin responsible for the remaining cases of nephrotoxicity. Mucositis remains a problem in all of the trials with methotrexate. The addition of bleomycin did not increase the incidence greatly. Use of 5-FU accounted for severe mucositis in 30 to 35% of the patients in the study of Vokes et al.[4]

Lockhart and Clark[95] focused on the toxicities of the regimen reported by Ervin et al.[83] They noted that mucositis was seen in 30% of patients receiving the platinum, bleomycin, and methotrexate combination. Frank ulceration was seen in approximately three fourths of the group with mucositis. In addition 23% of the patients developed xerostomia and 37% taste alteration. Other intraoral complications included bleeding in 4 of 141 cycles, and infection with fungal, bacterial, or viral agents in 6 of 141 cycles.[95]

Induction Therapy with Cisplatin

Several of these trials have been reviewed in the sections on bleomycin and methotrexate. Only areas of toxicity pertinent to cisplatin will be discussed here. In the high-dose trial by Haine et al,[89] vigorous hydration and hypertonic saline were used to prevent nephrotoxicity; this side effect was only seen in one patient. More commonly, there was myelosuppression. Five of the patients required admission for fever. Long-term side effects included ototoxicity in 25% and neuropathy in 39% (19 of 49). Severe hearing loss was seen in 2 of the 12 patients affected. Mild muscle weakness was seen in 8 of the 19 and more severe weakness in 2 of the 19 patients reporting neurotoxicity.[89]

In contrast to the trial by Haines et al,[89] the trials by Tannock et al[92] and Zidan et al[93] used approximately one-third the dose of cisplatin. Only one patient developed neurotoxicity and one patient developed nephrotoxicity. Myelosuppression was mild except for three patients in the trial by Tannock et al[92] who had granulocytes below 1000/mm³.

Several studies with cisplatin and 5-FU as induction therapy have been reported.[6,70,86,88] In two of the trials, cisplatin at a dose of 100 mg/m² was given with 4 days of 5-FU by constant infusion at 1000 mg/m². In the study by the VA Laryngeal Cancer Study Group[86] patients who were randomized to chemotherapy received two courses of chemotherapy and then were reassessed. Fourteen of the patients who might have received an additional third course of treatmen did not because of either toxicity or refusal. Of the 166 patients treated with chemotherapy, 1 died of septicemia. Other toxicities were similar in the two groups—those receiving chemotherapy and then radiotherapy and those having surgery followed by radiotherapy.[86] Grade 2 mucositis was slightly more frequent in the chemotherapy group. The authors do not comment on whether the mucositis was scored before or during the radiotherapy that this group received. There was no increase in surgical complications in the chemotherapy group.[86]

In a trial by the RTOG, nausea and vomiting were severe in 10% of the patients and moderate in 50% of the patients.[6] Leukopenia was seen in one half of the patients but only 1 of 42 patients had severe leukopenia and none required

hospitalization. Other side effects that were frequently seen were anemia and stomatitis. This latter side effect was moderate in 5 of the 42 patients.[6] Compliance with chemotherapy was very good with only two of the patients refusing further treatment.

In three recent trials, leucovorin was added to the two-drug combination.[88,90,96] Cisplatin was given at a dose of 100 mg/m², either as a single dose or fractionated into 5 days. The doses of leucovorin and 5-FU all were at the higher end of the dose range for the combination of leucovorin and 5-FU. In the trial by Vokes et al,[88] grade 3 mucositis was seen in one half of the patients and one half of the patients required a dose reduction of 5-FU in the second course. Myelosuppression was generally mild as was nephrotoxicity. Other side effects seen were hand–foot syndrome, and two deaths due to toxicity including one that may have been related to 5-FU.

In the trial by Caty et al,[96] one third of the 30 patients had grade 3 mucositis and one patient had grade 4 toxicity. Six of the patients had grade 3 neutropenia. In the study of Clark et al,[90] 80 to 90% of the patients had grade 3 or higher mucositis; 20 to 25% had grade 3 diarrhea; and 50% had grade 3 nausea and vomiting. In this study the leucovorin was given at a higher dose than in the two previous trials, and continuously with the 5-FU infusion.

Induction Therapy with 5-FU

Most of these studies have been reviewed in the section on cisplatin. Although there may be additional benefit for the combination of cisplatin and 5-FU the frequency of mucositis is increased. Further escalation of the effects of 5-FU occurs with the addition of leucovorin. In the high-dose trial of cisplatin, even with the addition of bleomycin, mucositis was infrequent.[89] In the trials with infusional 5-FU added to cisplatin, mucositis occurred 30 to 80% of the time.[88,90,96]

A dose escalation trial with 5-FU and cisplatin given at a constant dose showed that the prevalence of mucositis was 38%.[97] This is within the range reported above. Allopurinol was also given and was believed by the authors to be partly protective.

Adjuvant Therapy

Adjuvant trials have employed similar regimens to those in the induction setting. Many of these studies combine both induction and adjuvant treatment in the same patient population. Often the same regimen is given in both settings.

The Head and Neck Contracts Program evaluated both a treatment arm with induction therapy consisting of cisplatin and bleomycin and a second arm with both induction therapy and maintenance (adjuvant) therapy with cisplatin alone for six monthly cycles. Only 9% of the patients completed the maintenance therapy, 45% received no adjuvant therapy. Many of these individuals refused further chemotherapy. In the patients who did receive adjuvant therapy, toxicities were similar to those of induction therapy—nausea and vomiting and myelosuppression. Mucositis was infrequent in either group.[82]

In contrast, in two trials employing higherdoses of cisplatin, either in combination with bleomycin and methotrexate or 5-FU, mucositis was more common in the adjuvant setting than during treatment with the same regimen during the induction period.[4,83] In the trial of Vokes et al only 61% of the dose of infusional 5-FU could be given in the adjuvant phase of the study whereas 86% of the calculated dose was given in the induction phase. Quantitatively, the severity of all toxicities was similar in the two phases. In the study by Ervin et al,[83] mucositis was twice as frequent in the adjuvant phase. Other toxicities were less severe in the adjuvant phases.

Rentschler et al[25] also demonstrated a reduction in tolerance for chemotherapy after radiation therapy and surgery. In this trial, employing escalating methotrexate doses given both before and after definitive local therapy, the mean dose of methotrexate that the patients received was 76 mg/m^2 prior to local therapy and 58 mg/m^2 after local therapy. Toxicities were not compared between the two phases but were relatively mild even without leucovorin rescue.

In a nonrandomized trial using only adjuvant chemotherapy, only 78% of the patients completed all chemotherapy consisting of cisplatin and 5-FU. In this RTOG study, toxicities were mild to moderate except for nausea and vomiting that were severe in 26% of the patients and stomatitis that was severe in 4% of the patients.[5]

In summary, adjuvant therapy using more aggressive regimens is often not given because of patient refusal after initial preoperative chemotherapy. Tolerance is often poorer, perhaps related to predisposition of the treated area to develop mucositis.

Combination Chemotherapy for Advanced Head and Neck Cancer

Initially, chemotherapy has been given to this group of patients who have otherwise failed other treatment modalities or where the tumor is not resectable. The toxicities of single agents in this group of patients have been reviewed already (vide supra). These patients, as a group, are often more debilitated by their disease. Toxicities that are seen are in general similar to those of other groups of patients receiving combination chemotherapy.

Patients receiving cisplatin-based regimens have generally had infrequent nephrotoxicity; mucositis has not been a factor unless 5-FU is given.[30,98,99] Differences in types of toxicities seen are related to the schedule of the drug with increased toxicity with constant infusions of 5 days duration.[30] Shorter infusion schedules may decrease the frequency of nausea and vomiting.[99]

Carboplatin has been used in this setting. In an initial trial at the University of Michigan, carboplatin was escalated to 420 mg/m^2 and given with 5-FU.[50] Dose-limiting grade 3 to 4 myelosuppression was seen at 360 mg/m^2. One half of

the patients at this dose had grade 2 myelosuppression. Prolonged myelosuppression was seen with treatments in 18% of the patients. Sixty-one percent of the patients had mucositis.[50] Other toxicities included nausea and vomiting and diarrhea. Chemical phlebitis was also frequently seen. In a trial by the Southwestern Oncology Group (SWOG), carboplatin given with 5-FU was compared with cisplatin and 5-FU and to weekly methotrexate.[49] The incidence of myelosuppression and the severity were worse in the cisplatin arm, in contrast to the single agent studies and the previous phase I trial where myelosuppression was seen more frequently with carboplatin. The frequency of stomatitis was similar in all three arms. Ototoxicity was more common in the cisplatin arm also.

Several trials using methotrexate combinations have been reported. Mild to moderate mucositis is seen. The frequency is not greater than in the induction trials.[100,101] The incidence and severity of side effects in this population do not seem to be increased despite the poorer overall status compared with other populations with head and neck cancer. There may be a predisposition to mucositis in those patients already treated with irradiation as judged by the adjuvant trials; this does not seem to be the case in the published reports in the advanced patients. Dose attenuation may be occurring as well as patient selection.

COMBINED CHEMORADIOTHERAPY

Combined modality therapy has been used to improve local control. Trials in which the drug is given prior to radiotherapy have been reviewed in the section on induction therapy. Chemotherapy given concomitantly with irradiation has been increasingly used to improve local control in head and neck cancer. Because these modalities can produce mucositis and other oral injuries, these side effects have been the most difficult to treat.

Several strategies have been used to avoid this toxicity. In general the drugs selected have both intrinsic activity against squamous cell carcinoma and produce radioenhancement. This latter property also increases the frequency of normal tissue injury.[102] Dose escalation trials have shown a clear relationship with the dose of the drug given and the incidence of toxicity.[56,62] Trials with single agent chemotherapy given with irradiation have been recently reviewed.[57,80,81]

Several randomized trials with methotrexate or bleomycin added to radiotherapy have been done.[16,24,103,104] Mucositis was excessive for either drug in combination with raiotherapy except for the trial by Pennachio et al[103] where 41% of the patients developed mild mucositis. The dose of bleomycin was lower in this study. A nonrandomized trial by Fu et al[102] using vincristine, bleomycin, and cyclophosphamide during radiotherapy and bleomycin, methotrexate, and cyclophosphamide after radiotherapy had a 20% (3 of 15) death rate due to treatment complications. Mucositis was severe and seen at doses of radiotherapy of 3000 to 4000 cGy. Treatment interruptions were necessary.

5-Fluorouracil has also been evaluated as a single agent with radiotherapy in head and neck cancer.[62,64,65] A randomized trial reported by Lo et al[64] used relatively low-dose bolus administration. There was no difference in mucositis or skin reaction in the two groups. Long-term complications such as fistula were increased in the combined group. Escalation of the drug dose by Byfield et al[62] has shown severe mucositis with high-dose infusions over 5 days. Weppelmann et al[65] used a protracted infusion technique in a nonrandomized trial; they showed that mucositis occurs with even a low dose of 5-FU if given for protracted periods of time. A dose could be found however, where the incidence and severity were acceptable.

Cisplatin has been given in a variety of schedules with radiotherapy.[57] Nausea and vomiting, fatigue, and long-term drug–radiation interactions limit the attractiveness of the use of weekly cisplatin or daily low-dose cisplatin.[33,105] Although low-dose infusions of cisplatin over 5 days have produced a small number of severe episodes of myelosuppression but no increase in mucositis, high-dose therapy over 5 days produces unacceptable neurotoxicity.[33,89]

Carboplatin has been given with radiotherapy in a nonrandomized trial.[51] Severe myelosuppression was seen at a dose level that was similar to that used in trials with the drug alone.[52] Eighty-one percent developed mucositis; there was no renal toxicity or ototoxicity. The effects of carboplatin and irradiation on skin flap survival have been evaluated in an experimental model. Kleiman et al[106] showed no decrease in skin flap survival after rats were given drug, irradiation, or the combination.

Mitomycin as a radioenhancer has been evaluated in one randomized trial in head and neck cancer.[76] Mucositis and skin reactions were not increased in frequency or severity in the combined group. Myelosuppression was seen more often in the combined group, 12% had severe leukopenia or thrombocytopenia. Long term, there were more pulmonary deaths in the combined group; Weissberg et al[76] ascribe these results to the number of individuals with underlying lung disease. However, both treatment modalities can produce injury to the lung.

Combined chemoradiotherapy using combination chemotherapy has employed combinations of bleomycin, methotrexate, and cyclophosphamide and combinations of mitomycin and 5-FU.[57,102] These trials have produced frequent and severe side effects in the oral cavity and an excess mortality.

Cisplatin and 5-FU both of which have radioenhancing properties as well as antineoplastic effects, have been used most frequently in the more recent literature.[57,107–109] In the trial by Adelstein et al,[108] grade 4 life-threatening myelosuppression occurred in 42% and hospitalization was required in 18% due to fever. Mucositis was almost universal; patients had an average weight loss of 11.7% of initial body weight. Twenty-one percent required hospitalization for nutrition and hydration due to the mucositis.[108] Vomiting, although nearly universal, responded to medical management in almost all patients. One patient developed cardiac ischemia during treatment. In the trial by Taylor et al,[107] which involved combined modality therapy for 1 week alternating with a 1-week rest period, an average weight loss of 10% was seen and forced feeding was required in 9%. Mucositis was dependent on the dose of 5-FU. Severe leukopenia was seen in 27% and transfusions were often required, although the exact incidence of anemia is not given. Symptomatic neurotoxicity was seen after 1 year of follow-up and limited further use of this regimen.[107] In the trial of Taylor et al[107] several patients had complications that reflected debilitation from the treatment or their underlying disease. One patient aspirated and died. Two patients died suddenly. One sustained a fall and vertebral collapse and the other had a cerebrovascular accident.

A trial using cisplatin, 5-FU, leucovorin, and hydroxyurea and radiotherapy has been reported by Vokes et al.[110] The trial was designed to escalate the dose of cisplatin. Myelosuppression was severe and required two changes in the treatment regimen and an inability to significantly escalate cisplatin. Eighty-eight percent had grade 3 or 4 myelosuppression with continued therapy, indicating that this effect was cumulative. An increase in mucositis was seen when the patients received 5-FU and leucovorin as opposed to the hydroxyurea-containing arm. Patients who had head and neck cancer had twice the frequency of severe mucositis as did those who had other types of cancer.

Efforts to avoid the significant increase in mucositis have utilized separation of the two treatment modalities. Sequencing of the chemotherapy and radiotherapy was reported by Price and Hill[91] and Siodlak et al[111] to produce much less toxicity, both acute and chronic. The regimen used methotrexate, cyclophosphamide, and bleomycin but at lower doses compared with the trial by Fu et al[102] using concomitant chemoradiotherapy in which a 20% mortality rate was reported.

Recently, Merlano et al[109] described a sequential approach with cisplatin and 5-FU alternating with three 2-week courses of radiotherapy. They compared this group to another group of patients receiving irradiation only. Severe mucositis was seen in only 19% of the combined group in comparison to 18% in the group that was randomized to receive radiotherapy only.[109] The dose of of 5-FU was 200 mg/m^2 given daily by infusion, a relatively low dose.

Simultaneous chemoradiotherapy using a cisplatin and 5-FU regimen has been compared with sequential therapy in a trial by Adelstein et al.[112] The simultaneous arm had a mean weight loss of 19% as compared with 10% in the sequential arm. The increased weight loss was believed to be due to more severe mucositis in the simultaneous arm.[112]

Two trials have used accelerated hyperfractionated radiotherapy together with cisplatin and 5-FU in an effort to decrease the contribution of radiotherapy to the mucositis.[113,114] In the trial reported by Wendt et al,[114] leucovorin was also given with moderate doses of the two drugs. The study by Weissler et al[113] employed a conventional cisplatin dose (100 mg/m^2) with a 4-day 5-FU (1000 mg/m^2) infusion. Grade 3 mucositis was seen in 34% of the patients treated by Wendt et al.[114] The mean weight loss was

6%. The reaction was worse during the treatment break, which occurred every 2 weeks but quickly resolved; only three patients required a treatment delay for mucositis.

In the trial by Weissler et al,[113] grade 3 or 4 mucositis was seen in 40% of the patients treated with irradiation only but 53% of the patients in the combined group. This group also received a larger dose of irradiation.[113] Of interest, grade 3 anemia was seen in 11% of the group receiving radiotherapy only in comparison to 7% of the combined arm.

Combined chemoradiotherapy continues to be evaluated; additional issues related to toxicity that require further exploration include the need for hospitalization for the chemotherapy, the impact on lifestyle, and late sequelae.

INTRA-ARTERIAL CHEMOTHERAPY

Intra-arterial chemotherapy has been used for head and neck cancer.[46,115] Drugs used with this technique have included most of the drugs that have been employed systemically. Complications include mucositis and leukopenia in these studies. Toxicities that are unique to this route of administration include cranial nerve injuries including transient blindness, scalp sloughing, and unilateral alopecia.[115] These toxicities coupled with modest efficacy have limited the application of this technique for head and neck cancer.[46]

BIOLOGICALS

Interferon and other biologically active peptides are being evaluated in the treatment of head and neck cancer.[116-119] These agents produce side effects that are related to their protein structure. These include fever, chills, arthralgias, headache, and fatigue. Other side effects that have been reported include myelosuppression and cardiovascular complications. Many of these side effects are dose related. Interleukin can also cause a capillary leak in the pulmonary circulation producing noncardiogenic pulmonary edema.[118] When interferon is added to chemotherapy, there can be an increase in the toxicities normally seen with the chemotherapy.[116]

CHEMOPREVENTION

Chemoprevention of second malignancies has been reported for patients with a previous head and neck cancer.[13] Regression of oral leukoplakia has also been reported.[15,120] In the prevention trial by Hong et al,[13] cis-retinoic acid at a high dose was used. Toxicities seen included dry skin, cheilitis, hypertriglyceridemia, and conjunctivitis. These side effects were severe in 2 to 12% of the patients. One third of the patients in the treatment group stopped therapy either because of noncompliance (14%) or toxicity (18%).[13] In the trial by Lippman et al,[15] high-dose tretinoin was given initially but

patients were maintained on either low-dose tretinoin or β-carotene. Similar side effects, as before, were seen in the high-dose phase of the study. Toxicities seen during the maintenance phase were generally milder and did not necessarily carry over from the induction phase. There were no differences in the frequency of severe, although uncommon, side effects in the maintenance between the two arms. Milder side effects were less common in the β-carotene group than in those receiving low-dose tretinoin.[15] Compliance was much better than on the previous trial with high-dose tretinoin given throughout the study. Benner et al[120] have reported a trial that used vitamin E as the chemopreventative agent. Toxicities were mild and included headache, fatigue, nausea, and diarrhea.

MANAGEMENT OF SELECTED CHEMOTHERAPY TOXICITIES
Mucositis and Other Oral Complications

Mucositis is the most common and the most troublesome side effect in the treatment of patients with head and neck cancer. Current combined modality therapy produces this complication in almost all patients. There may be an earlier onset and severity of this complication with combined modality therapy. Use of forced feeding has been required in some of the more recent trials. In addition to mucositis, there can be xerostomia, taste alteration, and decreased salivary flow.[95] Lockhart and Clark carefully evaluated patients receiving aggressive chemotherapy and demonstrated that these side effects can be seen without the addition of irradiation.

The frequency of mucositis varies with the intensity of the treatment and was seen as often as 70% of the time, even without irradiation in one series.[121] Others have reported an even higher incidence.[90] In patients without head and neck cancer, mucositis occurs less frequently and is generally milder; however, patients receiving more aggressive chemotherapy regimens for hematologic malignancies can have a comparable frequency and severity of this complication.[122]

Histologically, chemotherapy produces atrophy of the mucosa, which resolves over 1 to 2 weeks; degeneration of collagen and salivary glands; and decreased neutrophils.[123] Histological changes were most noticeable on the buccal and labial surfaces. There may also be reduced salivary flow and an increase in candida and *Staphylococcus aureus*.[124] Other frequent acute complications seen in the oral cavity include hemorrhage and infection.[122]

Management of Oral Complications

Management of these problems has generally focused on two area. First, efforts to ameliorate these side effects by the selection of chemotherapeutic agents and alterations in dose have been done. Scheduling of combined modality therapies to avoid overlapping toxicities is an active area of investigation. Second, there have been a variety of agents used in the mouth to decrease injury. Numerous nonrandomized studies claiming benefit for a variety of agents have been reported. Randomized trials have evaluated ice to decrease drug delivery to the area,[125] allopurinol to antagonize the effects of 5-FU,[126] and a suspension of sucralfate, diphenhydramine, and kaolin-pectin for radiotherapy-related mucositis.[127] In the study by Mahood et al,[125] both patients and physicians believed that the mucositis was less severe with the use of ice. Allopurinol was without benefit.

Several trials have used chlorhexidine prophylactically to reduce streptococcal species and candida that have been implicated in causing mucositis.[128,129] Although there is a reduction in the number of these organisms, the trial by Ferretti et al[129] showed reduction in mucositis in the group receiving chemotherapy but not in the group receiving radiotherapy to the head and neck region.

Infectious Complications

Infections can be seen in the head and neck cancer patients in the mouth and systemically following chemotherapy. Specific rates of infection in the mouth are less frequent than in patients with hematologic malignancies undergoing aggressive chemotherapy.[130] Severe neutropenia is not seen as often, nor does it last as long in the chemotherapy regimens used for head and neck cancer. With the use of more aggressive combination chemotherapy, there may be an increased frequency of oral infection, although this complication was not increased in frequency in the article by Lockhart and Clark[95] who reported an aggressive regimen employing cisplatin, bleomycin, and methotrexate.

Organisms that have been seen include bacteria, especially streptococcus and staphylococcus, herpes, and candida. Gram negative organisms are common in patients treated for acute leukemia.[122] Of concern is an increase of gram negative species in a trial with chlorhexidine.[129]

Systemic infection has been seen more often with the aggressive combination chemotherapy regimens employed recently.[107] Treatment of these infections requires broad spectrum antibiotics and is beyond the scope of this chapter.

Late Sequelae of Chemotherapy

Late complications of chemotherapy related to the patient with head and neck cancer include caries, osteoradionecrosis, permanent loss of taste, and skin and subcutaneous tissue changes. Most of these effects are seen with radiation therapy alone. The addition of chemotherapy has not shown an increase in the frequency of these complications in the series where this issue has been addressed.

REFERENCES

1. Capizzi R. Complications of chemotherapy for head and neck neoplasms. In: *Complications of Head and Neck Surgery.* New York, NY: Thieme Medical Publishers Inc; 1979:317–327.
2. Hong W, Bromer, R. Chemotherapy in head and neck cancer. *N Engl J Med.* 1983;308:75–79.
3. Vokes E, Weischselbaum R, Lippman S, et al. Head and neck cancer. *New Eng J Med.* 1993;328:184–193.
4. Vokes E, Moran WJ, Mick R, et al. Neoadjuvant and adjuvant methotrexate, cisplatin, and fluorouracil in multimodal therapy of head an neck cancer. *J Clin Oncol.* 1989;7:838–845.
5. Jacobs J, Pajak TF, Al-Sarraf M, et al. Chemotherapy following surgery for head and neck cancer. *Am J Clin Oncol.* 1989;12:185–189.
6. Jacobs J, Pajak TF, Kinzie J, et al. Induction chemotherapy in advanced head and neck cancer. *Arch Otolaryngol Head Neck Surg.* 1987;113:193–197.
7. Stell P, and Rawson NSB. Adjuvant chemotherapy in head and neck cancer. *Br J Cancer.* 1990;61:779–787.
8. Harwood A, Rawlinson E. The quality of life of patients following treatment for laryngeal cancer. *Int J Radiat Oncol Biol Phys.* 1983;9:335–338.
9. Pruyn J, DeJong PC, Bosman LJ, et al. Psychosocial aspects of head and neck cancer—a review of the literature. *Clin Otolaryngol.* 1986;11:469.
10. McNeil B, Weichelsbaum R, Pauker P. Speech and survival: tradeoffs between quality and quantity of life in laryngeal cancer. *N Engl J Med.* 1981;305:982–987.
11. Miller A, Hoogstraten B, Staquet M, et al. Reporting results of cancer treatment. *Cancer.* 1981;47:207–214.
12. Perry MC. *The Chemotherapy Source Book.* Baltimore, Md: Williams & Wilkins; 1990.
13. Hong W, Endicott J, Itri LM, et al. 13-cis-Retinoic acid in the treatment of oral leukoplakia. *N Engl J Med.* 1986; 315:1501–1505.
14. Hong W, Lippman SM, Itri LM, et al. Prevention of second primary tumors with isotretinoin in squamous-cell carcinoma of the head and neck. *N Engl J Med.* 1990;323:795–801.
15. Lippman S, Batsakis, JG, Toth B B, et al. Comparison of low-dose isotretinoin with beta carotene to prevent oral carcinogenesis. *N Engl J Med.* 1993;328:15–20.
16. Lustig RA, DeMare PA, Kramer S. Adjuvant methotrexate in the radiotherapeutic management of advanced tumors of the head and neck. *Cancer.* 1976;37:2703–2708.
17. Schilsky R. Antimetabolites. In: Perry M, ed. *The Chemotherapy Source Book.* Baltimore, Md: Williams & Wilkins; 1992:301–317.
18. Hill B. Overview of experimental laboratory investigations of antitumor drug-radiation interactions. In: Hill BT, Bellamy AS, eds. *Antitumor Drug-Radiation Interactions.* Boca Raton, Fla: CRC Press Inc; 1990:225–246.
19. Vokes E, Weischelbaum RR. Concomitant chemoradiotherapy: rationale and clinical experience in patient with solid tumors. *J Clin Oncol.* 1990;8:911–934.
20. Schilsky R. Clinical pharmacology of methotrexate. In: Ames M, Powis G, Kovach JS, eds. *Pharmacokinetics of Anticancer Agents in Humans.* Amsterdam: Elsevier Science Publishers BV; 1983:187–205.
21. Woods R, Fox RM, Tattersall MHN. Methotrexate treatment of advanced head and neck cancers: a dose response evaluation. *Cancer Treat Rep.* 1981;65(suppl 1):155–159.
22. Ensley J, Kish J, Tapazoglou E, et al. An intensive, five course, alternating combination chemotherapy induction regimen used in patients with advanced, unresectable head and neck cancer. *J Clin Oncol.* 1988;6:1147–1153.
23. Hong WK, Schaefer S, Issell B, et al. A prospective randomized trial of methotrexate versus cisplatin in the treatment of recurrent squamous cell carcinoma of the head and neck. *Cancer.* 1983;52:206–210.
24. Gupta NK, Pointon RCS, Wilkinson PM. A randomized clinical trial to contrast radiotherapy with radiotherapy and methotrexate given synchronously in head and neck cancer. *Clin Radiol.* 1987;38:575–581.

25. Rentschler R, Wilbur DW, Petti GH, et al. Adjuvant methotrexate escalated to toxicity for resectable stage III and IV squamous head and neck carcinomas—a prospective randomized study. *Clin Oncol.* 1987;5:278–285.

26. Prestayko AW, D'Aoust JC, Issell BF, et al. Cisplatin (cis-diamminedichloroplatinum II). *Cancer Treat Rev.* 1979; 6:17–39.

27. Patton TF, Repta AJ, Sternson LA. Clinical pharmacology of cisplatin. In: Ames MM Powis G, Kovachi JS, eds. *Pharmacokinetics of Anticancer Agents in Humans.* Amsterdam: Elsevier Science Publishers BV; 1983:155–186.

28. Belt RJ, Himmelstein KJ, Patton TF, et al. Pharmacokinetics of non-protein bound platinum species following administration of cis-dichlorodiammineplatinum. *Cancer Treat Rep.* 1979;63:1515–1521.

29. Campbell AB, Kalman SM, Jacobs C. Plasma platinum levels: relationship to cisplatin dose and nephrotoxicity. *Cancer Treat Rep.* 1983;67:169–172.

30. Forastiere AA, Belliveau JF, Goren MP, et al. Pharmacokinetic and toxicity evaluation of five-day continuous infusion versus intermittent bolus cis-diamminedichloroplatinum (II) in head and neck cancer patients. *Cancer Res.* 1988;48:3869–3874.

31. Coughlin CT, Richmond RC. Biologic and clinical developments of cisplatin combined with radiation: concepts, utility, projections for new trials, and the emergence of carboplatin. *Semin Oncol.* 1989;16(Suppl 6):31–43.

32. Double EB. Interactions between platinum coordination complexes and radiation. In: Hill BT, Bellamy AS, eds. *Antitumor Drug-Radiation Interactions.* Boca Raton, Fla: CRC Press Inc; 1990:171–190.

33. Haselow R, Warshaw MG, Oken MM, et al. Radiation alone versus radiation with weekly low dose cis-platinum in unresectable cancer of the head and neck. In: Fee W, Goepfert H, Johns ME, et al, eds. *Proceedings of the International Conference on Head and Neck Cancer.* Boston, Mass: BC Decker; 1988: 279–281.

34. Tyers MB, Bunce KT, Humphrey PPA. Pharmacological and anti-emetic properties of ondansetron. *Eur J Cancer Clin Oncol.* 1989;25(suppl 1):516–519.

35. D'Acquisto RW, Tyson LB, Gralla RJ, et al. The influence of a chronic high alcohol intake on chemotherapy-induced nausea and vomiting. *Proc Am Soc Clin Oncol.* 1986;5:257.

36. Khan A, Hill JM, Grater W, et al. Atopic hypersensitivity to cis-dichlorodiammineplatinum(II) and other platinum complexes. *Cancer Res.* 1975;35:2766–2770.

37. Wiesenfeld M, Reinders E, Corder M, et al. Successful retreatment with cis-dichlorodiamminieplatinum after apparent allergic reactions. *Cancer Treat Rep.* 1979:63:219–221.

38. Chabner BA, Myers CE. Clinical pharmacology of cancer chemotherapy. In: DeVita VT Jr, Hellman S, Rosenberg SA, eds. *Cancer: Principles and Practice of Oncology.* Philadelphia, Pa: JB Lippincott Co; 189:349–395.

39. Lyss AP. Enzymes and random synthesis. In: Perry MC, ed. *The Chemotherapy Source Book.* Baltimore, Md: Williams & Wilkins; 1992:398–412.

40. Hutchinson FN, Perez EA, Gandara DR, et al. Renal salt wasting in patients with cisplatin. *Ann Intern Med.* 1988; 108:21–25.

41. Moliman JE, Glover DJ, Hogan WM, et al. Cisplatin neuropathy. *Cancer.* 1988;61:2192–2195.

42. Cohen RJ, Cunco RA, Cruciger MP, et al. Transient left homonymous hemianopsia and encephalopathy following treatment of testicular carcinoma with cisplatin, vinblastine, and bleomycin. *J Clin Oncol.* 1983;1:392–393.

43. Dorr R, Fritz WL. *Cancer Chemotherapy Handbook.* New York, NY: Elsevier Science Publishers BV; 1980.

44. Greene MH. Is cisplatin a human carcinogen? *J Natl Cancer Inst.* 1992;84:306–312.

45. Kahn C, Messersmith RN, Samuels BL. Technical note: brachial plexopathy as a complication of intraarterial cisplatin chemotherapy. *Cardiovasc Intervent Radiol.* 1989;12:47–49.

46. Forastiere AA, Baker SR, Wheeler R, et al. Intra-arterial cisplatin and FUDR in advanced malignancies confined to the head and neck. *J Clin Oncol.* 1987;5:1601–1606.

47. Van Echo DA, Egorin MJ, Aisner J. The pharmacology of carboplatin. *Semin Oncol.* 1989;16(suppl 5):1–6.

48. Elfernik F, van der Vijgh WJF, Klein I, et al. Pharmacokinetics of carboplatin after IV administration. *Cancer Treat Rep.* 1987;71:1231–1237.

49. Forastiere AA, Metch B, Schuller KE, et al. Randomized comparison of cisplatin plus fluorouracil and carboplatin plus fluorouracil versus methotrexate in advanced squamous cell carcinoma of the head and neck: a Southwest Oncology Group Study. *J Clin Oncol.* 1992;10:1245–1251.

50. Forastiere AA, Natale RB, Takasugi B, et al. A phase I-II trial of carboplatin and 5-fluorouracil combination chemotherapy in advanced carcinoma of the head and neck. *J Clin Oncol.* 1987;5:190–196.

51. Jacobs MC, Eisenberger M, Oh MC, et al. Carboplatin (CBDCA) and radiotherapy for stage IV carcinoma of the head and neck: a phase I-II study. *Int J Radiat Oncol Biol Phys.* 1989;17:361–363.

52. Koeller JM, Trump DL, Tutsch KD, et al. Phase I clinical trial and pharmacokinetics of carboplatin (NSC 241240) by single monthly 30-minute infusion. *Cancer.* 1986;57:222–225.

53. Powis G. Effects of disease states on pharmacokinetics of anticancer drugs. In: Ames MM, Powis G, Kovach JS, eds. *Pharmacokinetics of Anticancer Agents in Humans.* Amsterdam: Elsevier Science Publishers BV, 1983:363–397.

54. Crooke ST. Bleomycin: a brief review. In: Carter SK, Crooke ST, eds. *Bleomycin: Current Status and New Developments.* New York, NY: Academic Press; 1978:1–8.

55. Bauer KA, Skarin AT, Balikian JP, et al. Pulmonary complications associated with combination chemotherapy programs containing bleomycin. *Am J Med.* 1983;74:557–563.

56. Shanta V, Krishnamurthi S. Combined bleomycin and radiotherapy in oral cancer. *Clin Radiol.* 1980;31:617–620.

57. Jassem J, Dewit L, Keus R, Bartelink H. Concomitant chemotherapy and radiotherapy. In: Snow GB, Clark JR, eds. *Multimodality Therapy for Head and Neck Cancer.* Stuttgart, Germany: Georg Thieme Verlag; 1992:126–146.

58. Ardalan B, Glazer R. An update on the biochemistry of 5-fluororuacil. *Cancer Treat Rev.* 1981;8:157–167.

59. Byfield JE. Useful interactions between 5-fluorouracil in man: 5-fluorouracil as a radiosensitizer. In: Hill BT, Belamy AS, eds. *Antitumor Drug-Radiation Interactions.* Boca Raton, Fla: CRC Press Inc; 1989:87–106.

60. Byfield J, Frankel SS, Sharp TR, et al. Phase I and pharmacologic study of 72-hour infused 5-fluororuracil and hyperfractionated cyclical radiation. *Int J Radiat Oncol Biol Phys.* 1984;11:791–800.

61. Morrison BW, Clark JR. Induction chemotherapy. In: Snow GB, Clark JR, eds. *Multimodality Therapy for Head and Neck Cancer.* New York, NY: Thieme Medical Publishers Inc; 1992:95–111.

62. Byfield JE, Sharp TR, Frankel SS, et al. Phase I and II trial of five-day infused 5-fluorouracil and radiation in advanced cancer of the head and neck. *J Clin Oncol.* 1984,2:406–413.

63. Thomas PRM, Lindblad AS, Stablein DM, et al. Toxicity associated with adjuvant postoperative therapy for adenocarcinoma of the rectum. *Cancer.* 1986;57:1130–1134.

64. Lo TC, Wiley AL, Ansfield FJ, et al. Combined radiation therapy and 5-fluorouracil for advanced squamous cell carcinoma of the oral cavity and oropharynx: a randomized study. *Am J Roentgenol.* 1976;126:229–235.

65. Weppelmann B, Wheeler RH, Peters GE, et al. A phase I study of prolonged infusion 5-fluorouracil and concomitant radiation therapy in patients with squamous cell cancer of the head and neck. *Int J Radiat Oncol Biol Phys.* 1991;20:357–360.

66. Lokich J, Bothe A, Fine N, et al. Phase I study of protracted venous infusion of 5-fluorouracil. *Cancer.* 1981;48:2565–2568.

67. Freeman NJ, Costanza ME. 5-Fluorouracil-associated cardiotoxicity. *Cancer.* 1986;61:36–45.

68. Poon MA, O'Connell MJ, Wieand HS, et al. Biochemical modulation of fluororuracil with leucovorin: confirmatory evidence of improved therapeutic efficacy in advanced colorectal cancer. *J Clin Oncol.* 1991;9:1967–1972.

69. Richards GJ, Chambers RG. Hydroxyurea in the treatment of neoplasms of the head and neck. *Am J Surg.* 1973;126:513–518.

70. Rowinsky EK, Donehower RC. Vinca alkaloids and epipodophyllotoxins. In: Perry MC, ed. *The Chemotherapy Source Book.* Baltimore, Md: Williams & Wilkins, 1992:359–383.

71. Riggs CJ. Antitumor antibiotics and related compounds. In: Perry M, ed. *The Chemotherapy Source Book.* Baltimore, Md: Williams & Wilkins; 1991:318–358.

72. Clamon GH. Alkylating agents. In: Perry MC, ed. *The Chemotherapy Source Book.* Baltimore, Md: Williams & Wilkins, 1992:286–300.

73. Rowinsky EK, Onetto N, Canetta R, et al. Taxol: the first of the taxanes, an important new class of antitumor agents. *Semin Oncol.* 1992;19:646–662.

74. Forastiere A. Taxol in head and neck cancer. *Cancer Invest.* 1993;11(suppl 1):9, 10.

75. Rockwell S, Sartorelli AC. Interactions between mitomycin C and radiation. In: Hill B, Bellamy AS, eds. *Antitumor Drug-Radiation Interactions.* Boca Raton, Fla: CRC Press Inc; 1989:125–139.

76. Weissberg J, Son YH, Papac RJ, et al. Randomized clinical trial of mitomycin C as an adjunct to radiotherapy in head and neck cancer. *Int J Radiat Oncol Biol Phys.* 1989;17:3–9.

77. Powis G, Ames MM, Kovach JS. Dose-dependent pharmacokinetics of anticancer drugs. In: Ames M, Powis G, Kovach JS, eds. *Pharmacokinetics of Anticancer Agents in Humans.* Amsterdam: Elsevier Science Publishers BV; 1983:49–69.

78. Doll D, Weiss RB, Issell BF. Mitomycin: ten years after approval for marketing. *J Clin Oncol.* 1985;3:276–286.

79. Grant S, Kris MG, Young CW, et al. Edatrexate, an antifolate with antitumor activity; a review. *Cancer Invest.* 1993;11:36–45.

80. Clark JR, Frei E. Chemotherapy for head and neck cancer: progress and controversy in the management of patients with MO disease. *Semin Oncol.* 1989;16(suppl 6):44–57.

81. Dimery IW, Hong WK, Overview of combined modality therapies for head and neck cancer. *J Natl Cancer Inst.* 1993;85:95–111.

82. Strong E. Adjuvant chemotherapy for advanced head and neck squamous carcinoma. *Cancer.* 1987;60:301–311.

83. Ervin TJ, Clark J, Weischelbaum RR, et al. An analysis of induction and adjuvant chemotherapy in the multidisciplinary treatment of squamous-cell carcinoma of the head and neck. *J Clin Oncol.* 1987;5:10–20.

84. Al-Sarraf M, Pajak T, Larramore G. Timing of chemotherapy as part of definitive treatment for patients with advanced head and neck cancer. An RTOG study. *Proc Am Soc Clin Oncol.* 1985;4:141.

85. Wittes R, Heller K, Randolph V, et al. Cis-dichlorodiammineplatinum(II)-based chemotherapy as initial treatment of advanced head and neck cancer. *Cancer Treat Rep.* 1979;63:1533–1538.

86. Department of Veterans Affairs Laryngeal Cancer Study Group. Induction chemotherapy plus radiation compared with surgery plus radiation in patients with advanced laryngeal cancer. *N Engl J Med.* 1991;324:1685–1690.

87. Schuller D, Laramore G, Al-Sarraf M, et al. Combined therapy for resectable head and neck cancer. *Arch Otolaryngol Head Neck Surg.* 1989;115:364–368.

88. Vokes EE, Schilsky RL, Weischelbaum RR, et al. Induction chemotherapy with cisplatin, fluorouracil, and high-dose leucovorin for locally advanced head and neck cancer: a clinical and pharmacologic analysis. *J Clin Oncol.* 1990;8:241–247.

89. Haines I, Bosl G, Pfister D, et al. Very high dose cisplatin with bleomycin infusion as initial treatment of advanced head and neck cancer. *J Clin Oncol.* 1987;5:1594–1600.

90. Clark JDA, Busse P, et al. Continuous infusion cisplatin, 5-FU and high dose leucovorin: an induction therapy for SCCHN with high rates of complete response and radiotherapy alone as primary site management. In: Salmon SE, ed. *Adjuvant Therapy of Cancer.* Philadelphia, Pa: WB Saunders Company; 1990;6:71–81.

91. Price LA, Hill BT. Safe and effective induction chemotherapy without cisplatin for squamous cell carcinoma of the head and neck. *Med Pediat Oncol.* 1982;10:535–548.

92. Tannock I, Payne D, Cummings B, et al. Sequential chemotherapy and radiation for nasopharyngeal cancer: absence of long-term benefit despite a high rate of tumor response to chemotherapy. *J Clin Oncol.* 1987;5:629–634.

93. Zidan J, Kuten A, Cohen Y, et al. Mutlidrug chemotherapy using bleomycin, methotrexate, and cisplating combined with radical radiotherapy in advanced head and neck cancer. *Cancer.* 1987;59:24–26.

94. Ringborg E, Ewert G, Kinnman J, et al. Sequential methotrexate-5-fluorouracil treatment of squamous cell carcinoma of the head and neck. *Cancer.* 1983;52:971–973.

95. Lockhart PB, Clark JR. Oral complications following neoadjuvant chemotherapy in patients with head and neck cancer. *Natl Cancer Inst Monogr.* 1990;9:99–100.

96. Caty A, Lefebvre JL, Mirabel X, et al. Induction chemotherapy by a combination of 5 FU-cisplatin-folinic acid in advanced head and neck squamous cell carcinoma. *Proc Am Soc Clin Oncol.* 1992;11:246.

97. Greenberg B, Ahmann F, Garewal H, et al. Neoadjuvant therapy for advanced head and neck cancer with allopurinol-modulated high dose 5-fluorouracil and cisplatin. *Cancer.* 1987;59:1860–1865.

98. Kish J, Weaver A, Jacobs J, et al. Cisplatin and 5-fluorouracil infusion in patients with recurrent and disseminated epidermoid cancer of the head and neck. *Cancer.* 1984;53:1819–1824.

99. Jacobs C, Bertino JR, Goffinet DR, et al. 24-hour infusion of cis-platinum in head and neck cancers. *Cancer.* 1978;142:2135–2140.

100. Vogl SE, and Kaplan BH. Chemotherapy of advanced head and neck cancer with methotrexate, bleomycin, and cis-diamminedichloroplatinum II in an effective outpatient schedule. *Cancer.* 1979;44:26–31.

101. Panasci L, Gravenor D, Black M, et al. Alternating combination chemotherapy using cisplatin-bleomycin with sequential methotrexate-5 FU plus leucovorin rescue in patients with head and neck cancer. *Cancer Treat Rep.* 1985;69(9):1015–1017.

102. Fu KK, Silverberg IJ, Phillips TL, et al. Combined radiotherapy and multidrug chemotherapy for advanced head and neck cancer: results of a radiation therapy oncology group pilot study. *Cancer Treat Rep.* 1979;63(3):351–357.

103. Pennachio J, Hong WK, Shapshay S, et al. Combination of cis-platinum and bleomycin prior to surgery and/or radiotherapy compared with radiotherapy alone for the treatment of advanced squamous cell carcinoma of the head and neck. *Cancer.* 1982;50:2795–2801.

104. Petrovich A, Block J, Kuisk H, et al. A randomized comparison of radiotherapy with a radiotherapy-chemotherapy combination in stage IV carcinoma of the head and neck. *Cancer.* 1981;47:2259–2264.

105. Shaake-Koning C, Van Den Bogaert, W, Dalesio O, et al. Effects of concomitant cisplatin and radiotherapy on inoperable non-small cell lung cancer. *N Engl J Med.* 1992;326:524–530.

106. Kleiman LA, Hasslinger B, Eddy H, et al. The effects of carbocisplatin and radiation on skin flap survival. *Arch Otolaryngol Head Neck Surg.* 1992;118:68–73.

107. Taylor SG IV, Murthy AK, Caldarelli DD, et al. Combined simultaneous cisplatin/fluorouracil chemotherapy and split course radiation in head and neck cancer. *J Clin Oncol.* 1989;7:846–856.

108. Adelstein, DJ, Sharan, VM, Earle AS, et al. Chemoradiation as initial management in patients with squamous cell carcinoma of the head and neck. *Cancer Treat Rep.* 1986;70:761–768.

109. Merlano M, Vitale V, Rosso R. Treatment of advanced squamous-cell carcinoma of the head and neck with alternating chemotherapy and radiotherapy. *N Engl J Med.* 1992;327:1115–1121.

110. Vokes EE, Moormeier JA, Ratain MJ, et al. 5-Fluorouracil, leucovorin, hydroxyurea, and escalating doses of continuous-infusion cisplatin with concomitant radiotherapy: a clinical and pharmacologic study. *Cancer Chemother Pharmacol.* 1992;29:178–184.

111. Siodiak M, Dalby JE, Bradley PJ et al. Induction VBM plus radiotherapy, versus radiotherapy alone for advanced head and neck cancer: long-term results. *Clin Otolaryngol.* 1989;14:17–22.

112. Adelstein DJ, Sharan VM, Earle AS, et al. Simultaneous versus sequential combined technique therapy for squamous cell head and neck cancer. *Cancer.* 1990;65:1685–1691.

113. Weissler MC, Melin S, Sailer S, et al. Simultaneous chemoradiation in the treatment of advanced head and neck cancer. *Arch Otolaryngol Head Neck Surg.* 1992;118:806–810.

114. Wendt TG, Hartenstein RC, Wustrow TPU, et al. Cisplatin, fluorouracil with leucovorin calcium enhancement, and synchronous accelerated radiotherapy in the management of locally advanced head and neck cancer: a phase II study. *J Clin Oncol.* 1989;7:471–476.

115. Cruz AB, McInnis WD, Aust JB. Triple drug intra-arterial infusion combined with X-ray therapy and surgery for head and neck cancer. *Am J Surg.* 1974;128:573–579.

116. Vokes EE, Ratain MJ, Mick R, et al. Cisplatin, fluorouracil, and leucovorin augmented by interferon alfa-2b in head and neck cancer: a clinical and pharmacologic analysis. *J Clin Oncol.* 1993;11:360–368.

117. Clayman GL, Young G, Taylor DL, et al. Detection of regulatory factors of lymphokine-activated killer cell activity in head and neck cancer patientstreated with interieukin-2 and interferon alpha. *Ann Otol Rhinol Laryngol.* 1992;101:909–915.

118. Schantz SP, Dimery I, Lippman SM, Clayman GL, et al. A phase II study of interleukin-2 and interferon alpha in head and neck cancer. *Invest New Drugs.* 1992;10(3):217–223.

119. Richtsmeier WJ, Koch WM, McGuire W P, et al. Phase I-II study of advanced head and neck squamous cell carcinoma patients treated with recombinant human interferon gamma. *Arch Otolaryngol Head Neck Surg.* 1990;116:1271–1277.

120. Benner SE, Winn RJ, Lippman SM. et al. Regression of oral leukoplakia with alpha-tocopherol: a community clinical oncology program chemoprevention study. *J Natl Cancer Inst.* 1993;85:44–47.

121. Archibald D, Lockhart PB, Sonis ST, et al. Oral complications of multimodality therapy for advanced squamous cell carcinoma of head and neck. *Oral Surg Oral Med Oral Pathol.* 1986;61:139–141.

122. Dreizen S. Description and incidence of oral complications. *Natl Cancer Inst Monogr.* 1990;9:11–15.

123. Lockhart PB, and Sonis ST. Alterations in the oral mucosa caused by chemotherapeutic agents. *J Dermatol Surg Oncol.* 1981;7:1019–1025.

124. Main BE, Calman KC, Ferguson MM, et al. The effect of cytotoxic therapy on saliva and oral flora. *Oral Surg.* 1984;58:545–548.

125. Mahood DJ, Dose AM, Loprinzi CL, et al. Inhibition of fluorouracil-induced stomatitis by oral cryotherapy. *J Clin Oncol.* 1991;9:449–452.

126. Loprinzi CL, Cianflone SG, Dose A, et al. A controlled evaluation of an allopurinol mouthwash as prophylaxis against 5-fluorouracil-induced stomatitis. *Cancer.* 1990;65:1879–1882.

127. Barker G, Loftus L, Cuddy P, et al. The effects of sucralfate suspension and diphenhydramine syrup plus kaolin-pectin on radiotherapy-induced mucositis. *Oral Surg Oral Med Oral Pathol.* 1991;71:288–293.

128. Epstein JB, McBride BC, Stevenson-Moore P, et al. The efficacy of chlorhexidine gel in reduction of Streptococcus mutans and Lactobacillus species in patients treated with radiation therapy. *Oral Surg Oral Med Oral Pathol.* 1991;71:172–178.

129. Ferretti GA, Raybould TP, Brown AT et al. Chlorhexidine prophylaxis for chemotherapy- and radiotherapy-induced stomatitis: a randomized double blind trial. *Oral Surg Oral Med Oral Pathol.* 1990;69:331–338.

130. Shira RB. Chemotherapy-associated oral infections in adults with solid tumors. *Oral Surg Oral Med Oral Pathol.* 1983;55(2):113–120.

131. Bertinoi J, Boston B, and Capizzi RL. The role of chemotherapy in the management of cancer of the head and neck: a review. *Cancer.* 1975;36:752–758.

132. Eisenberger M, Posada J, Soper W, et al. The current status of chemotherapy. In: Wittes R, ed. *Head and Neck Cancer.* Chichester: John Wiley & Sons Inc; 1985:181–220. Cancer Investigation and Management; vol 2.

17 Complications of Aesthetic Facial Surgery

Fred J. Stucker, M.D., F.A.C.S., Robert F. Aarstad, M.D., Denis K. Hoasjoe, M.D., F.R.C.S.(C)

Fundamental to the oath we have all taken is "Do no harm." This credo is maximally challenged in the field of aesthetic surgery. Most patients seeking aesthetic facial surgery are in good health and lack a major physical defect or deformity. Our task is to improve on this natural state and most certainly leave them in no worse condition physically or psychologically; "do no harm."

The first and perhaps the most important step in ensuring this goal, takes place during the initial consultation. Here, the patient's motives and expectations must be elicited. Simultaneously, an educational process ensues so that the patient is fully informed as to the reasonableness of the surgery as well as the possible complications. If this evaluation is satisfactorily carried out, then the chances of the surgery reaching a similar conclusion without complications are manifestly improved.

GENERAL CONSIDERATION

Why does the patient desire to have aesthetic facial surgery? There is a vast gulf between television personalities who wish to improve their on-camera appearance and partners in failing marriages who feel a facial rejuvenation will do the same for their marriage. The grossly psychologically unbalanced person must be ferreted out during the initial interview; however, some subtle but likely troublesome candidates can hopefully be identified through experience and intuition. Certain behavioral characteristics should alert the surgeon. Beware of the patient who:

- Is rude and/or demanding to your office staff prior to being seen.
- Misses appointments or reschedules a number of times or is late in arriving.
- Brings pictures of themselves or others of a much younger age as a point of reference for surgery.
- Has a long list of written questions.
- Effusely offers praise to you and/or denigrates past physicians.
- Has had a number of cosmetic procedures in the past.

- Has litigation pending bearing a real or imagined relation to the surgery requested.
- Is vague or declines to discuss past medical problems.
- Is taking tranquilizers or antidepressants.
- Is under psychotherapy.
- Focuses on a relatively minimal problem or overlooks a more blatant defect.
- Is undergoing a life change (ie, divorce, job loss, drug rehabilitation, etc).
- Is indecisive.

Also, if you personally do not like some patients, they more than likely feel the same toward you and it is best to avoid those situations.

What does the patient desire to have done? Once you have decided that the patient's motivations are legitimate and, contrary to the above, the majority are, their expectations must be evaluated. By selecting those patients with proper motivations for surgery, the majority of patients with unreasonable expectations will be eliminated. Hopefully, the remainder can be educated to expect reasonable results and also be prepared for surgery and the ensuing postoperative course. The educational process occurs by means of discussions, video presentations, and written handouts that should be documented in the medical chart. Well-motivated patients whose expectations are unrealistic must undergo an educational modification prior to proceeding with surgery. The educational process may involve a discussion of what is actually obtainable or evolve into other procedures that can be done to obtain a satisfying result. A discussion should also take place regarding the actual mechanics of the operative procedure, postoperative course, time for return to normal activities, and possible complications. The more the patient knows and thus better informed, the greater the chance the patient's expectations will be satisfactorily achieved.

GENERAL COMPLICATIONS

There are three areas of complications common to most surgical procedures; anesthesia, infection, and bleeding.

Volumes have been written and although there are a few specific problem areas in each procedure, some general considerations should be discussed.

Anesthesia

The majority of procedures in the head and neck area can be safely performed under local and/or regional anesthesia. For a number of reasons, but predominantly owing to patient and/or surgeon's preference, general anesthesia is increasingly utilized. It is generally believed that local anesthesia is faster, safer, helps decrease bleeding, and facilitates postoperative recovery. Also, the patient being conscious may be forewarned of impending complications. A predominant reason for utilizing local anesthesia is that it is the cost-effective alternative. This must be measured against contemporary techniques of general anesthesia that actually can speed up the procedure and improve the postoperative course. Excessive bleeding and other complications in an anesthetized unconscious patient are proving to be more myth than truth and probably depend more on technique than anesthetic agent.[1]

The cost saving of local anesthesia does remain a valid point. However, in many sections of the country and with increasing third party intervention as well as the threat of malpractice litigation for any untoward real or imagined mishaps, the use of an anesthesiologist for monitoring becomes more of a practical necessity than a medical one. Thus, any cost savings that could be passed on to the patient is sacrificed in the interest of contemporary expediency. Even in areas where this has not become a problem, it is incumbent on surgeons and their staff to have current advanced cardiac life support (ACLS) training and possess the necessary monitoring and resuscitative equipment and medication at hand.

The possible complications encountered in general and local and/or regional anesthesia can be found elsewhere, but a few general considerations should be kept in mind. The patient should be placed in a chaise lounge position with the head elevated to decrease/minimize bleeding and edema. Adequate use of a more dilute anesthetic agent rather than suboptimal quantity of a concentrated anesthetic agent not only decreases bleeding, but aids the surgery with hydrostatic dissection. The surgeon must be familiar with the anesthetic or sedative agents being utilized along with maximum dosages, side and adverse effects, and means to reverse them.

Infection

There is a low incidence of infection in uncomplicated surgery of the head and neck, especially aesthetic facial surgery owing to its excellent vascularity. Generally, the population is in good health; however, one must be wary of those patients with anemia, diabetes, immunologic problems, poor hygiene, and especially smokers that may predispose to infection. The general surgery literature has shown that shaving increases the risk of infection, especially if done several hours prior to surgery.[2,3] Therefore, if anything more than a little hair clipping is absolutely necessary, it is best done when prepping for surgery.

Surgical technique is one of the major determining factors for susceptibility to infection:

- Implants, be they allogaft, homogaft, or autograft, should be handled carefully and kept from contamination.
- Surgery should be carried out as expeditiously, atraumatically, and easily as possible in keeping with good technique.
- Clinical infection is the inoculum concentration or a product of infectious load × period of exposure.
- Dead space should be closed and any accumulation of fluid evacuated to avoid a breeding ground for infection.

Prophylactic antibiotics are controversial and the subject for heated discussion, but should be given according to the surgeon's best judgment and not dogmatically. If prophylactic antibiotics are to be given, they should be administered prior to the contamination (surgery) to be effective; if given more than 3 hours postcontamination they are ineffective.[4] Optimal use of antibiotics would be for 24 hours postoperatively and prolonged use of antibiotics has little efficacy unless there are implants or other mitigating circumstances.[5,6]

Bleeding

Prevention of bleeding commences with the initial interview, taking a history of past bleeding problems, and any medications that may aggravate bleeding as well as warnings to refrain from their use prior to surgery. It is not uncommon for someone with a postoperative hematoma, who has previously denied the use of medications, blatantly to admit to taking ASA daily as a routine. Nutrition-oriented patients on mega doses of vitamins may be taking large amounts of vitamin E that interfere with platelet adhesiveness.[7] The correct use of anesthetic agents and positioning can aid in preventing bleeding problems as do proper postoperative dressing, drains if required, and proper instructions to the patient to be compliant. Good surgical technique is the mainstay of hemostasis.

RHINOPLASTY

A patient requesting nasal surgery is seeking correction of either nasal function or appearance or both. It is incumbent on the surgeon to be aware of the problem and its solution as the patient perceives it. To do otherwise can result in a dissatisfied patient with a beautiful nose and poor function or improved airway and an unattended deformity. The nose may be pleasing to the operating surgeon but a source of consternation to the patient or his/her ethnic group. Therefore, know what needs to be done before setting a course of action.

Complications
HEMORRHAGE

Because the majority of these procedures are done on an outpatient basis, education as to postoperative expectation is important, especially concerning the amount of bleeding. We routinely inform the patient to expect minimal bleeding or oozing for 1 to 2 days postoperatively. Depending on the procedure, we emphasize whether there will be significant bleeding, when it will commence, and when to expect it to taper off. We routinely check on all outpatients by telephone the following day. They are told that if they soak through one 2×2 mustache dressing every 15 minutes × 3 to contact the office.

The most troublesome bleeding occurs during the first 24 hours. However, it can occur up to 3 days after surgery. Another period of possible bleeding occurs between 10 to 14 days when any clot that has formed liquifies. We have had bleeding requiring active treatment 3 weeks after the procedure. We do not routinely employ nasal packs but do on occasion use internal splints to avoid synechiae. If any untoward bleeding occurs they should be removed. If bleeding persists it is best, if possible, not to pack the nose as this may compromise the reduction that has been performed and can lead to a residual deformity. Cocaine pledgets can be placed in the nose for use as an anesthetic and mucosal vasoconstrictor followed by a nasal endoscope inserted to identify the source of bleeding. When found it is controlled with electrocautery or a recent alternative employed by us, the argon beam coagulator. If this is not adequate or a diffuse ooze is encountered, postage stamp-sized pieces of Surgicel can be placed or Gelfoam with topical thrombin used. If bleeding persists, then management follows the usual treatment for persistent epistaxis.

INFECTION

An infection following rhinoplasty is very rare considering the contaminated environment in which the surgery is performed. The rate of infection varies from 0.8% to 1.6% according to various studies. The senior author has had only two dorsal abscesses in 6000 without prophylaxis (Fig. 17–1). If there are any pustules or other signs of infection about the nose or lip, as is frequently the case in adolescents, surgery may be contraindicated depending on the situation but not dogmatically. Routine prophylactic antibiotics are given according to the dictates of the surgeon but are generally not necessary in primary uncomplicated rhinoplasties when grafts or implants are not used. If signs of infection do occur, then appropriate treatment should ensue in light of the serious processes reported such as meningitis, cerebral abscess,[10] cerebritis,[11] subdural empyema,[12] septic cavernous sinus thrombosis,[13] and endocarditis.[14]

Another uncommon process that necessitates early diagnosis and aggressive treatment is toxic shock syndrome. Early symptoms include nausea, vomiting, diarrhea, erythroderma and hypertension. If this should occur, any packs or splints must be removed, a culture taken, and antistaphylococcal therapy begun.[15-17]

EDEMA AND ECCHYMOSIS

Swelling and bruising to some extent are inevitable in rhinoplasty surgery. Equally inevitable is their resolution with time. The best treatment is prevention with elevation, atraumatic surgery, alacrity, and avoiding packs.[18] Steroids and other nonsteroidal anti-inflammatory agents may be of some use in lessening their effect. Most swelling and bruising resolve after 2 to 3 weeks; however, residual edema may remain for months with external rhinoplasty and dark circles may also persist for long periods especially in patients with dark complexions. Revision nasal surgery is notorious for compounding the morbidity of edema and ecchymosis.

Traumatic Complications

Traumatic complications may include those of the skin, soft tissues, skeletal framework, or adjacent orbital and intracranial structures. Minor skin complications include atopic allergic reactions in reactive individuals that can be treated with corticosteroid creams. A localized infection with pustules may arise that will generally resolve with drying and local care. Occasionally, a diffuse red blush or telangiectasia may arise, which could be an exacerbation of a preoperative condition. If rosacea is a clinical possibility preoperatively, a trial of tetracycline is indicated. If this diagnosis is precluded and a postoperative red nose develops then electrodesiccation or laser can be utilized.[19]

Necrosis of the skin over the dorsum due to circulatory problems or excess pressure from the dorsal splint may occur, but is very rare (Fig. 17–2). The best treatment is "watch and wait" for the eschar to form and dissipate with healing underneath. The final scar may require excision with full thickness gafting. If a full thickness slough of dorsal skin is evident, with danger that the nasal bones and cartilage will become exposed, the slough can be excised and the defect covered with a local flap. Necrosis of the tip skin can occur probably from excessive dissection of the lip and vascular compromise. This represents a surgical disaster for which little can be done.[20]

Inclusion cysts may occur owing to entrapment of epithelium from the nasal vestibule or lining mucosa. The cysts develop along the path of osteotomies and are treated by local excision.[20-23] Septal perforations, generally the result of overvigorous submucous resection or unrecognized septal hematoma, are less common today owing to improved and less radical techniques, the use of septal whip stitch, and avoiding the routine use of septal splints.

Anosmia may result from a variety of causes including failure of oderiferous substances reaching the olfactory organ (nasal obstruction), injury to the olfactory end organ or tracts, central olfactory dysfunction, or functional problems. In 1966 Champion[24] reported that the prevalence of temporary anosmia lasting from 6 to 18 months was 10%. One patient had permanent anosmia. Goldwyn and Shone[25] investigated

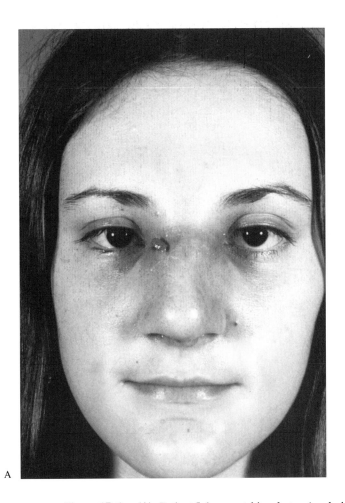
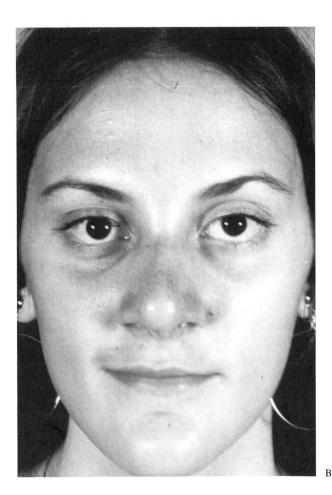

A

B

Figure 17–1. **(A).** Patient 5 days postrhinoplasty. An obvious abscess incision and drainage following splint removal. Wick placed after evacuation. **(B).** Patient 2 weeks postoperative. Drain removal 2 days following the incision and drainage.

by olfactory testing 97 patients who underwent rhinoplasty or septoplasty and found that 80% had a normal sense of smell 2 weeks postoperatively and no patient had anosmia 2 months after surgery. These studies indicate that rhinoplasty has no long-term deleterious effect on olfaction.

Epiphora, although not uncommon in the immediate postoperative course, has not proven to be a long-term complication. Flowers and Anderson,[26] investigating fresh cadavers with anatomic dissection and contrast studies, showed the lacrimal sac to be vulnerable to lateral osteotomies. Of 27 case studies, 21 demonstrated nasolacrimal duct obstruction 2 days postrhinoplasty. This number decreased to 4 at 2 weeks and none after 3 months. Their evaluation of 1000 rhinoplasties revealed none with nasolacrimal obstruction as a long-term complication. Thomas and Griner[27] did lateral osteotomies on fresh cadavers showing no evidence of lacrimal injury on dissection. They advocate low lateral osteotomies without the formation of subperiosteal tunnels. The style of osteotome has little effect and the use of a nasal saw is discouraged. Therefore, although postoperative epiphora may occur, the risk of a permanent problem is highly unlikely. Other much more rare orbital complications include transient lagophthalmus[28] and blindness.[29]

Equally rare are intracranial lesions during rhinoplasty. Cerebrospinal fluid (CSF) rhinorrfiea has been reported by Hallock and Trier[30] to be repaired by temporalis fascia grafting and by Marshall and Slattery[31] to be repaired by dural grafting. Stucker,[18] who routinely fractures the bony septum during septoplasty, reported no cases of CSF rhinorrhea, easily detectable in nonpacked noses.[32] Cavernous sinus thrombosis[31] and carotid cavernous sinus fistula[32] have also been reported as a distinct rarity.

NASAL OBSTRUCTION

Postoperative nasal obstructive symptoms following rhinoplasty are common owing to transient edema, clotted blood, and crusting. These problems generally resolve spontaneously in a few weeks without treatment, although it may take months for the nose to resume its normal physiological function. Perhaps the most common cause of postoperative obstructive symptoms is a persistence or exacerbation of preoperative medical problems. This may be due to allergic or vasomotor rhinitis, rhinitis medicamentosa, or even an overlooked anatomic obstruction or valvular collapse. Nevertheless, these situations should be dealt with or allowed for preoperatively to avoid having a dissatisfied patient.

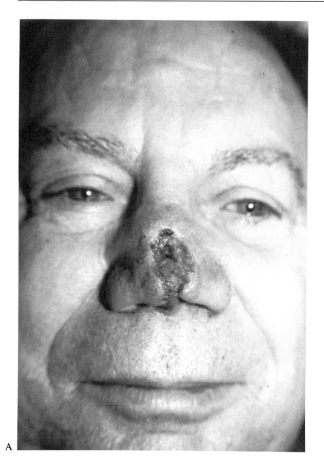

A

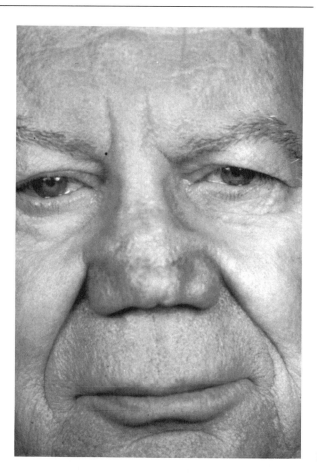

B

Figure 17–2. **(A).** Tip and dorsal necrosis 6 days following surgery. **(B).** Patient 3 months postrhinoplasty with no further surgery.

Nasal obstruction directly attributable to rhinoplasty surgery includes vestibular stenosis due to circumferential contracture along the intercartilaginous or marginal, septal transfixion, and lateral osteotomy incision lines. Minimizing the incisions and using a small 2 to 3-mm osteotome will lessen this risk. Another area of potential scarring is the angle between the upper lateral cartilage and the transfixion incision. This potential area of mucosal blunting can be avoided by intentionally creating a sharp angle at the junction of these incisions and carefully reapproximating the apex of the mucosal flap into the angle[33] (Fig. 17–3).

A depressed tip as well as columellar retraction may develop following excess resection in septoplasty and cause nasal obstruction and deformity. A thickened columella or excessive flaring of the medial crura also can compromise the nasal airway. Methods of compensation include intramural resection of soft tissue, coapting the medial crura with sutures, and very rarely trimming the feet of the medial crura.

The nasal valve area where the caudal portion of the upper lateral cartilage junctures with the nasoseptum can be disrupted during rhinoplasty. This angle, approximating 10 to 15° in the normal state, is freely mobile allowing for variable resistance during respiration. Injudicious or inadvertent removal of the caudal or dorsal aspect of the upper lateral cartilage or transgression of the mucosa at this junction with webbing may allow collapse or cause other obstructive problems.[34]

Perhaps the most disappointing airway complication is the collapse of the lateral bony nasal wall. The inferior bony pyramid of the nasal skeleton is displaced medially, along with the cartilaginous skeleton. This severe cosmetic and functional complication results from completely severing tissues that maintain the base of the skeletal nose in its lateral position (Fig. 17–4). Two important stabilizing structures can be used to prevent this disaster. The first is the investing periosteum. Using a 2-mm chisel for the lateral osteotomy unquestionably increases the likelihood of areas of medial or lateral periosteum remaining attached to the bone. This investing periosteum will then serve as a hinge, permitting the lateral nasal wall to move medially to abut its counterpart at the apex, leaving the base attached laterally. A second and equally important modification of the routine lateral osteotomy is to leave a triangular strut of bone at the piriform aperture. The lateral osteotomy is begun approximately 5 mm superior to the widest point of the piriform aperture. The chisel is directed superolaterally (aimed at the lateral corner of the eye) until it encounters the nasomaxillary groove. Once in this groove, the chisel is directed superiorly in the direction of the traditional lateral osteotomy. This inferior intact triangular strut of bone is the site where the lateral nasalis and nasalis muscles are attached to bone. It is also the region where the aponeurosis and fibrous attachments to the upper lateral cartilages are affixed to bone. This intact strut of bone

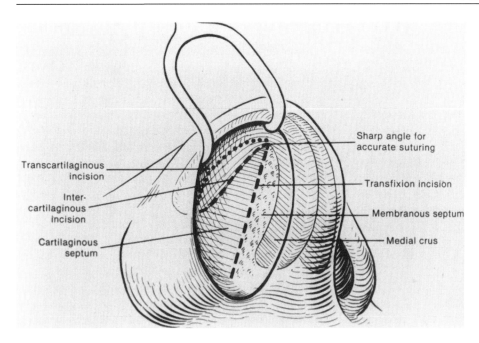

Transcartilaginous incision

Inter-cartilaginous incision

Cartilaginous septum

Sharp angle for accurate suturing

Transfixion incision

Membranous septum

Medial crus

Figure 17–3. Diagram of opening incision to avoid blunting in valve area (from Stucker et al[33]).

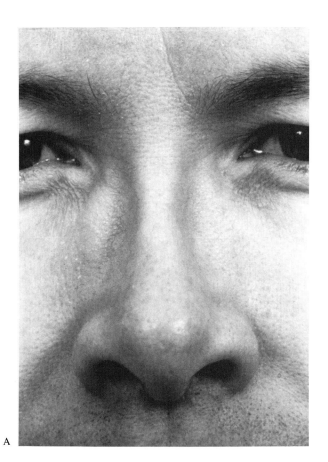

A

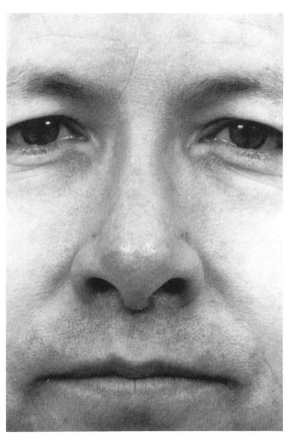

B

Figure 17–4. **(A).** Collapse of lateral support following two previous nasal procedures. **(B).** Four years following correction utilizing a conchal cartilage graft.

restricts medial displacement of the base of the lateral bony skeleton following the lateral osteotomy.[33]

Aesthetic Complications

Residual deformity following rhinoplasty is largely a subjective judgment depending on the viewpoint of the patient and surgeon. According to the literature, the revision rate varies from 5 to 12%.[35] Deformities fall into the following categories: those present but not corrected at the initial surgery, those corrected by the initial surgery, and those that cannot be corrected or lessened, including both those that preexisted and those that were created.[35]

BONY FRAMEWORK

Dorsal bony hump removal is best done conservatively with a chisel and further refinement done with a rasp or shave excision of cartilage. Irregularities of the dorsum can also be rasped if visible; however, those that are only palpable will generally disappear with time and do not necessitate treatment.

Saddle nose deformity can occur owing to excessive hump removal or may result from the osteotomized bones falling into the piriform aperture. The latter may be prevented by preserving as much periosteal integrity of the nasal bones as possible (ie, the use of a small 2-mm osteotome). Correction is best done at the time of surgery by trimming and replacing the excised bony hump or placement of a graft. If the excess hump removal is not noted at the time of surgery, then it is best to wait for complete healing before graft placement is done.

An open nasal deformity or widened dorsum is due to the lateral nasal bones not apposing each other and the septum in the midline. This may be due to a thickened or deviated dorsal septum, thickened bone of the radix, or a greenstick fracture. Treatment is directed at the problem by straightening or debulking the septum, removing a medial triangle of bone at the radix, or redoing the osteotomies. At the other extreme is the overly narrowed dorsum that must be treated with reosteotomies, a spreader graft, or an onlay graft.

"Stair step" deformities occur by placing the lateral osteotomy too high. This can be prevented by placing the osteotomy deep in the nasomaxillary groove and passing through the nasofrontal process of the maxilla. Correction should be attempted by comminuting the ridge with a small osteotome, doing a lower lateral osteotomy, or rasping the ridge. It is critical to mobilize from medial to lateral so as not to compromise subsequent maneuvers.

External bony nasal deviation may be due to a bony septal deformity, incomplete fracture, or asymmetrical nasal bones not corrected by the medial osteotomy. The nasoseptum can be straightened or comminuted. A 2-mm osteotome can be used to complete the osteotomies as can a Quisling chisel and the asymmetrical nasal bones can be corrected with a bone rongeur or very careful rasping.

The shallow nasofrontal angle or overly obtuse angle is a result of hump removal in the patient with a sloping forehead (Fig. 17–5). Correction of the resultant Grecian profile is difficult and limited. Deepening the angle with chisel, rasp, and bone biter is possible, but is limited in degree of correction by accessibility and thickness of bone in this region (Fig. 17–6). Avulsion of the overlying procerus muscle should be avoided because this maneuver results in protracted intercanthal swelling with little ultimate improvement.[36] An apparent deepening of the nasofrontal angle may be accomplished by augmentation of the forehead as described by Foman.[37]

CARTILAGINOUS VAULT

"Polly Beak" deformity or supratip swelling is the most common cause of rhinoplasty revision and can result from excessive scaning, insufficient lowering of septal cartilage, insufficient trimming of upper lateral cartilages, excessive excisions of the lower lateral cartilages, short columella, thick skin, or a combination of these factors. It is often the result of excess hump removal and augmentation may be required for correction.

The key to prevention of "Polly Beak" lies in understanding its causes. There is a certain amount of fibrous tissue in the supratip area of all patients, which if left in place after surgical trauma will thicken with healing. Therefore, some soft tissue should be removed routinely in most primary rhinoplasties. It is imperative that the dead space formed by removal of tissue must be obliterated in the early postoperative period by proper taping and splinting to prevent blood accumulation, granulation formation, and subsequent fibrosis. It may also be possible to improve this deformity when recognized postoperatively by injection of corticosteroids.

Wright[38] has demonstrated the influence of skin thickness on the supratip and recommends allowances be made in lowering the dorsum to achieve an optimal result. There is a tendency for the inexperienced surgeon to err on the side of liberal removal of bony hump and conservatism when lowering the septal cartilage. The performance of tip surgery and a septal transfixion incision routinely produce some postoperative tip ptosis. If not compensated by adequate lowering of the septum, this tip ptosis will result in an apparent supratip prominence.

A cartilaginous saddle deformity is most commonly due to radical septal resection for airway obstruction or disruption of the dorsal cartilaginous support. Correction is carried out by grafting similar to the bony saddle deformity (Fig. 17–7).

Disruption of the upper lateral cartilages caused by surgical trauma severs their attachments to surrounding structures and results in their being free floating. The tendency is to retract laterally and inferiorly in the healing process. If this is not recognized and the cartilages are not aligned and stabilized in a proper position, the not uncommon result is healing in a distorted and angulated position. The end result is a significant concavity or hollowed out appearance on the side of the

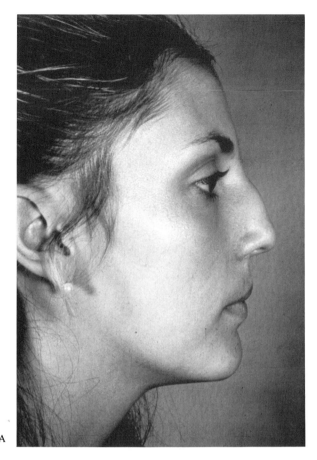
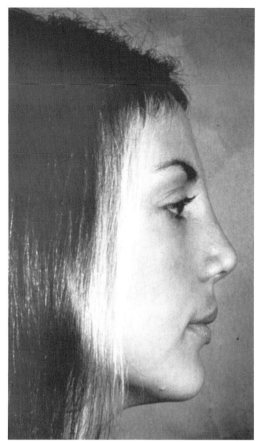

Figure 17–5. **(A).** Preoperative view of patient with a shallow nasofrontal angle. **(B).** Disastrous result when no attempt was made to deepen bony nasofrontal angle.

avulsion which may also cause nasal valve obstruction (Fig. 17–8). Uncorrected cartilaginous septal deviations may cause continued dorsonasal deformity or surgery may unroof a nasal deformity not previously noticed.

THE NASAL TIP

Nasal tip deformities are largely the result of overreduction, underreduction, or asymmetrical reduction of the alar cartilages resulting in a "pinched tip," "ptotic tip," "bifid tip," "pig's snout," under or overprojection, or just lack of definition. Overzealous resection of the lower lateral cartilages is the most common misadventure and will routinely yield an asymmetry or pinched tip with the defect commencing at 6 to 12 months.

Underreduction of the nasal tip may result in excess projection or lack of definition of the tip. Correction is by delivery followed by further cartilage resection either along the cephalad portion and/or the strut, along with debulldng of fibrous tissue and probable suturing of the residual cartilage. Vertical division may be required with reconstruction of the alar arch.

Excessive resection of the alar cartilages and/or discontinuity of the alar cartilages may cause collapse of the tip with a pinched tip defonnity. This not only results in a cosmetic

deformity, but can cause nasal obstruction because of narrowing of the external nares. Correction is difficult and optimally approached via an external rhinoplasty with exposure of the involved structures. Scarring is excised, carved and/or lysed and support cartilage replaced with grafts from the septum or ear concha. Similarly, excess resection of the cephalad alar carfilages may cause over rotation and a pig's snout appearance. Correction employing the external rhinoplasty approach consists of grafting of cartilage or composite grafts of skin and cartilage between the upper and lower lateral cartilages, allowing for a derotation and lengthening of the nose (Fig. 17–8).

A bifid tip is corrected by resection of intercrural fibrofatty tissue and/or suture coapting of the alar domes. A ptotic tip or drooping tip results from failure to reduce or suture the upper or lower lateral cartilages in relation to the shortened caudal septum, allowing the tip to fall away from the septum. Geriatric noses especially have a tendency to droop and must be corrected at rhinoplasty by trimming the upper and/or lower lateral cartilage and suturing the medial crura in proper relationship to the caudal septum (Fig. 17–9).

The boxed tip deformity occurs most commonly in thin-skinned individuals resulting from failure to weaken the alar domes when the excess alar cartilages are reduced. This deformity may appear gradually over several years and is

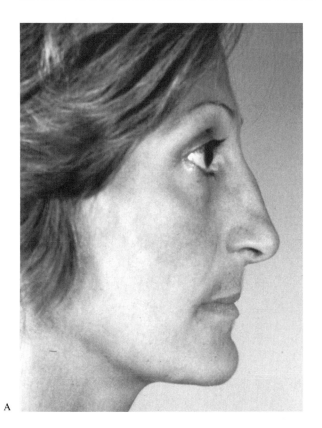

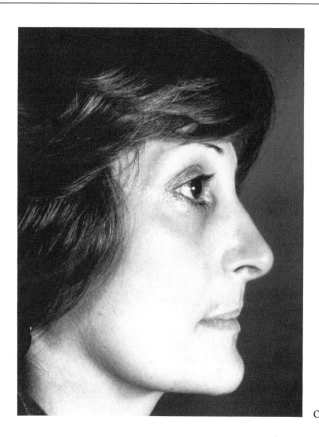

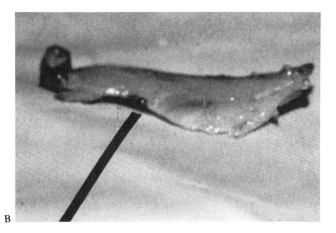

Figure 17–6. **(A).** Another preoperative patient with shallow nasofrontal angle was undertaken. **(B).** Hump and bony angle specimen. Pointer is where routine hump removal is terminated. Curled tissue on left is cartilage hump with rhinion as slight hump to right of pointer. **(C).** Adequately deepened nasofrontal angle 4 years postsurgery.

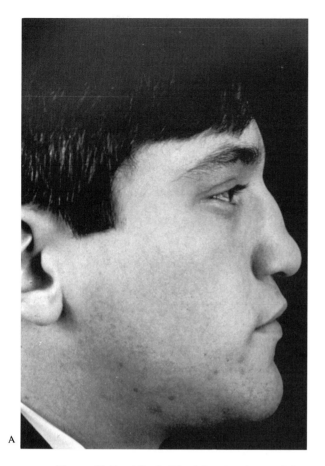
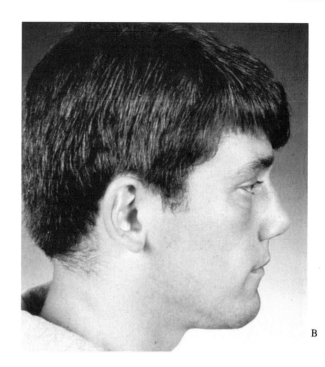

Figure 17–7. (A). Saddle deformity 5 years following septal surgery. **(B).** Three years following correction with conchal cartilage graft.

corrected by resecting the alar domes or weakening by cross-hatching. Asymmetrical nasal tip either iatrogenic or because of failure to correct at initial surgery can be refined by resection or augmentation.[39] Alar rim notching is caused by an inadvertent cut or disruption of the inferior rim of the alar cartilage. Small notches can be corrected by wedge excision and closure whereas larger notches require cartilage grafting.

A hanging columella is caused by overly convex or prominent medial crura or an elongated caudal septum. Repair is best accomplished by elliptical excision of the membranous septum along with caudal septum or a portion of medial crura. The retracted columella is a more difficult situation owing to overaggressive removal of caudal septum, membranous septum, or medial crura. Correction varies from placement of a columellar cartilage strut to a composite graft. Occasionally, rotation flaps from the superior aspect of the lateral alar cartilage are useful.

BLEPHAROPLASTY

A number of complications associated with eyelid surgery can be prevented by careful preoperative assessment of the patient. Preexisting conditions may be aggravated or can precipitate complications and therefore must be screened for by adequate history and physical examination. Surgeons must inquire about ophthamologic conditions such as glaucoma, detached retina, corneal abrasions, epiphora, dry eye, amblyopia, and even visual loss. They must also check for systemic diseases that affect the eyes and adnexal structures such as thyroid and renal disease, hypertension, allergy, diabetes, cardiovascular problems, hormonal effects, and Sjogren's disease.

A thorough physical examination evaluating brow or lid ptosis, skin texture, edema, pigmentation, bony orbit, lagophthalmus, extraocular muscles, and corneal and intraocular lesions must be done. Insipient ectropion and asymmetries, if not noted, can profoundly impact the surgery (Fig. 17–10). Visual acuity of both eyes and gross visual fields must be in the preoperative exam.

Brow ptosis may be accentuated by lid surgery and cosmetic blepharoplasty alone may not correct lid ptosis. Therefore, further surgery needs to be discussed and executed to achieve a satisfactory result. Eyelid edema and/or pigmentation from thyroid disorders, hormonal changes, allergy, etc, should be pointed out and noted that it will probably not be corrected by the planned surgery. Other conditions such as hollow eye, dry eye, lagophthalmus, lid laxity, and fine wrinkles may alter the extent or type of surgery performed.

Cardiac dysrhythmia is a complication that may occur intraoperatively owing to the oculocardiac reflex. A trigeminal vagal reflex arc may induce bradycardia, which can precipitate

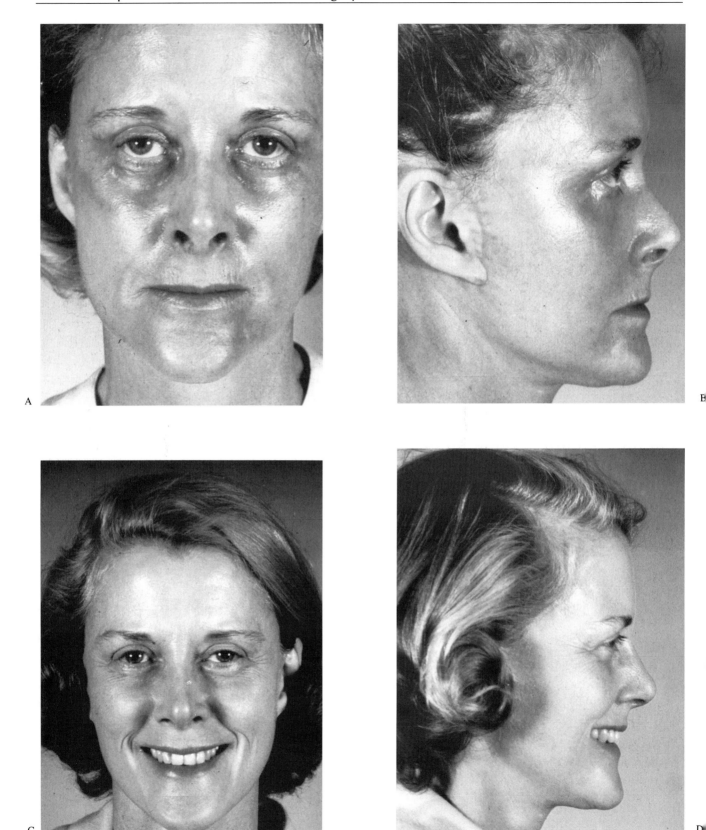

Figure 17–8. **(A).** Full face view of distraught patient 10 days postoperative rhinoplasty, face-lift, and blepharoplasty. **(B).** Lateral view at 10 days postsurgery. **(C).** Full face view of patient 2 years following revision surgery. **(D).** Lateral view 2 years following revision surgery.

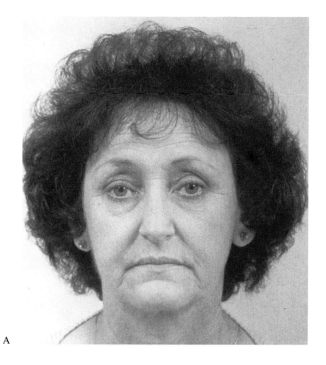
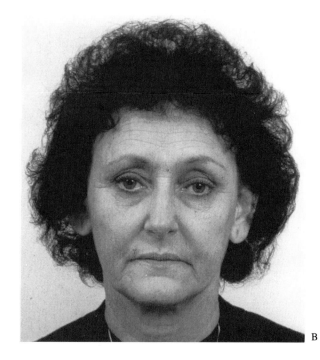
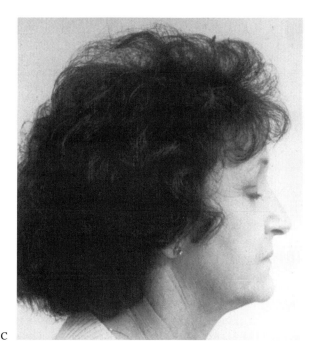
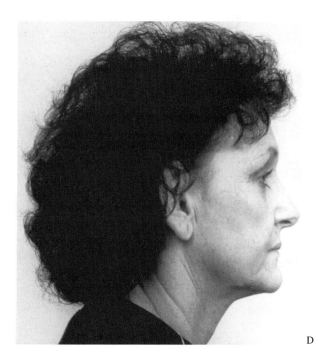

Figure 17–9. **(A).** Full face preoperative geriatric patient. **(B).** Full face 18 months postrhinoplasty. **(C).** Lateral view of patient preoperatively. **(D).** Eighteen months postsurgical latest view.

other cardiac arrythmias. Careful monitoring of vital signs with discontinuation of manipulation in the face of bradycardia and possible intravenous anticholinergic agents is the treatment.[40]

Complications of blepharoplasty may be mild or severe and can be temporary or permanent. Most of the complications develop in the immediate postoperative period and rapid treatment may preclude permanent disability.

Minor Complications

Swelling in the eyelids can at times be quite dramatic, causing total lid closure. The edema gradually resolves over time and can be limited by head elevation and iced saline sponges used for the first 24 to 48 hours. Skin pigmentation may be accentuated by hemosiderin deposition in the tissues, but eventually, gradually resolves.[41]

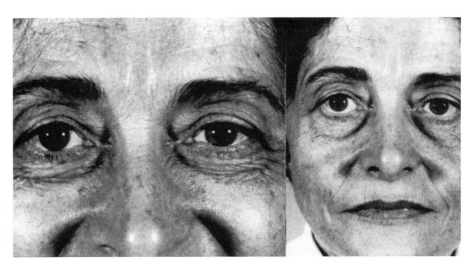

Figure 17–10. Preoperative view on left with incipient ectropion. Rounding and scleral show postoperative on right following a very conservative procedure.

CYSTS AND TUNNELS

Epithelial debris may be trapped in the suture line, causing inclusion cysts or milia. Small cysts can be unroofed using an 18-gauge needle or a no. 11 blade. Larger inclusion cysts may require excision. Epithelial ingowth occurs along the suture tracts, forming tunnels if sutures are left in over 4 days. Treatment is by marsupialization with scissors.

WOUND SEPARATION

Wound separation may occur immediately following removal of sutures or sometime later with rubbing of the eyes, etc. Treatment consists of reapproximation with steri strips or resuturing.

INFECTIONS

Owing to the rich vascular supply, infections are exceedingly rare and generally superficial. On occasions, a periorbital cellulitis or even an orbital abscess may develop, which could be sight threatening.[42,43] Chronic blepharitis of a nonspecific nature can occur, but is distinctly rare.

HYPERTROPHIC SCARS

Scarring occurs especially in fair-skinned individuals; however, keloids have not been reported. Scar hypertrophy is most common medially near the epicanthus and may form a web. Intralesional injection of steroids is the treatment of choice; however, occasionally a Z- or V-plasty may be necessary.

TELANGIECTASIAS

Small preexisting telangiectasias may be intensified in size and number after surgery. These occur mainly along the margins of the upper lid below the incision. This should be discussed prior to surgery. The best treatment is camouflage with cosmetics.

POSTOPERATIVE WRINKLING

Fine crinkling wrinkles cannot be removed with blepharoplasty and this should be pointed out prior to surgery. Postoperatively they become more apparent owing to decreased stretching from fat removal. Chemical peel or dermabrasion should be utilized at a time removed from the blepharoplasty.[44]

LOSS OF EYELASHES

Spontaneous loss of eyelashes, although rare, may occur. The lashes generally regrow without treatment.

CONJUNCTIVAL LYMPHEDEMA

The skin muscle technique of lower eyelid blepharoplasty may disrupt the lymphatics causing conjunctival lymphedema. This is generally short-lived, lasting 6 to 8 weeks and spontaneously resolving.[45]

EPIPHORA

Excess tearing is common following surgery, due to edema distoring or blocking the lacrimal collection system. Long-standing epiphora occurs from ectropion of the puncta or entire lid. Surgical trauma to the collecting system may cause stenosis or obstruction.

CORNEAL INJURY

Intraoperative trauma may result in comeal abrasions or ulcerations. Ulcerations occur owing to electrocauterization, either directly on the comea or the channeling effect with blood or other liquid conducting current to the comea. The use of bipolar or heated filament cautery significantly decreases the risk of electrical trauma. Other sources include rough sponges drawn across the comea, instrumentation, and prolonged exposure during surgery. Postoperatively, the cornea may continue to be exposed owing to edema. Therefore, throughout surgery and the postoperative course the cornea should be protected with lubricant, artificial tears, and/or taping. Pain in the eye may indicate a corneal lesion and should be investigated with fluorescein or rose bengal dye and a slit lamp.

ASYMMETRY

Minor degrees of assymetry occur during the postoperative course and leave little cause for concern as they eventually resolve. Patients should be counseled preoperatively regarding facial assymetry and this should be pointed out to them. Preoperative assymetry should be taken into account when resecting fat, muscle, or skin, and a partial compensation can be accomplished. If excess fat is noted to be missing or has been removed, fat grafts may be helpful.

LAGOPHTHALMUS

Inability to close the lids occurs commonly in the immediate postoperative course and usually resolves in a short period of time. Treatment to prevent dry eye should be instituted and on occasion may be necessary for several weeks. More permanent changes, essentially an ectropion of the upper lid, occur with excess skin removal, fibrous attachment to underlying structures, or suture entrapment. Prolonged corneal exposure may result in keratoconjunctivitis sicca and ulceration if not corrected. Some surgeons bank excised lid tissue to use as a full thickness graft in the event of this occurrence.

Major Complications

ECTROPION

Scleral show postoperatively is so common as to be expected; however, persistent lower lid ectropion gives an unsatisfactory result and can lead to permanent eye damage. The immediate postoperative ectropion caused by chemosis and periorbital edema is a normal wound reaction; ice and elevation will minimize the situation. Ectropion is the most common complication of blepharoplasty and can be prevented in most cases by careful preoperative evaluation and good surgical technique.

Excess skin removal from the lower lid is the primary cause of ectropion and can be caused by overaggressive correction or failure to take into account gravitational changes in the supine position. To avoid excess skin removal, have the patient look up with the mouth open prior to excision. Not uncommonly, postoperative ectropion can occur following fat removal, resulting in concavity of the lid and a relative skin loss. It requires more skin to cover the hollow created following fat removal than was necessary in the preoperative condition. Suture closure of the orbital septum is unnecessary and may result in a downward pull on the lid margin, transmitted through the muscle with resultant ectropion. Also,

unknowing suture of the skin to underlying septum may result in ectropion.

Another common cause of ectropion is the unrecognized senile (insipient ectropion) or overly lax lower lid. This can be assessed preoperatively with the snap test and prevented by a horizontal shortening or lid tightening procedure. Other causes of ectropion include cicatricial scar contracture, paresis, or displacement of the orbicularis muscle, flap hematoma, and scar fixation to the orbital rim.[46]

Ectropion may be graded from I to IV according to degree of severity. Typically, I, II, and III can be treated conservatively and grade IV will require surgery. Conservative treatment should continue for several weeks to months and resolves the majority of problems. This consists of dry eye measures with the use of eye lubricants, tape, and massage. Massage is performed by drawing superolaterally with the ipsilateral index finger several times a day and squinting exercises. The eyes can be taped shut at night and a steri strip used laterally, drawing the lid superolateral giving support during the day. If the ectropion is due to inflammatory changes, injection of corticosteroids may be helpful.

If conservative treatment fails or severe ectropion is present surgical treatment is indicated. If skin loss or scarring is present, release of tissues and full thickness skin graft is necessary. When this is noted in the first few days postoperatively, banked lid skin from the procedure may be used or tissue from excellent donor sites such as the upper lid or postauricular area. If ectropion is due to horizontal lid laxity, a wedge tarsectomy or tarsal strip procedure may be performed. If atony of the lower lid is present a conchal cartilage graft may be placed laterally, for support, during the horizontal tightening procedure. Lower lid tissue expanders have been used, but no long-term follow-up results have been reported.[47,48]

DIPLOPIA

Extraocular muscle disorders with diplopia following blepharoplasty can be divided into temporary functional paresis, resulting from hemorrhage and edema, or permanent paresis due to structural damage to the muscles from instrumentation or accidental incarceration of tissue interfering with normal motility. The inferior rectus muscle, lying superficial between the medial and middle fat compartments of the lower lid, is most susceptible to accidental injury. However, the literature has shown instances of injury to the superior oblique, inferior oblique, superior rectus, and levator muscles.[49]

Either the muscles or the nerves may be traumatized by instrument dissection or electrocauterization. Diplopia generally resolves within 6 weeks. Therefore, no treatment other than observation and possible diplopia fields with lens correction should be performed for at least 6 tissue months. If damage to the muscle is proved and diplopia persists, then resection and recession of the extraocular muscles may be necessary. Another cause of diplopia that is almost always transitory is enophthalmus from excessive fat removal.

PTOSIS

Ptosis may be due to an undiagnosed preexisting condition or result from surgical trauma. Temporary ptosis is not unusual and resolves with the edema. Evaluation for ptosis is a necessary part of the preblepharoplasty workup. A history of eyelid trauma, inflammation, thyroid disorders, recurrent edema, contact lens use, congenital ptosis, or evidence of acquired senile ptosis should be noted. Examination looking for absent eyelid crease and thinning of the upper eyelid as well as degree of ptosis should be done. Eyes are examined in primary, upward, and downward gaze measuring the amount of ptosis. The normal eyelid covers the limbus 1 to 2 mm, mild ptosis would add an additional 1 to 2 mm, moderate 3 mm, and severe ptosis 4 mm or more. Levator muscle function is measured in all patients with lid ptosis by having the patient look upward and downward with finger pressure over the brow to immobilize the frontalis. The distance the eyelid travels between these two points is measured in millimeters: 4 mm, poor function; 5 to 7 mm, fair function; and greater than 8 mm, good function. Normal excursion, approximately 15 mm, is found in acquired senile ptosis. Ptosis and levator muscle dysfunction diagnosed preoperatively can be corrected at the time of surgery, eliminating this potential complication.[50] Ptosis may also result from operative trauma due to instrumentation or electrocautery as well as hematoma, allergy to ointment or sutures, or levator fixation.

KERATOCONJUNCTIVITIS SICCA

Dry eye most commonly results from undiagnosed, preexisting conditions that are aggravated by blepharoplasty. A thorough history and examination needs to be done to evaluate tear production and quality. Postmenopausal patients who are taking certain medications such as tricyclic antidepressants should be particularly scrutinized. When there is a question, ophthalmologic evaluation with special testing is in order to thoroughly inform the patient of the risks of the surgery. It is possible to modify the extent of the surgery to increase the chance of a satisfactory result.[51]

SKIN SLOUGH

Although very rare, the possibility of skin slough exists, generally owing to hematoma formation under the skin flaps. If noted early, the hematoma can be expressed. Once skin necrosis takes place, treatment is conservative with minimal debridement and most often healing will take place without incident. Occasionally, full thickness gafting is necessary.

GLAUCOMA

A preoperative history of migraine-like attack, blurred vision, or halos around lights should arouse suspicion and intraocular pressure should be checked. Although very uncommon, blepharoplasty may precipitate acute closed angle glaucoma and postoperative complaints of eye pain, blurred vision, comeal edema, and dilated pupils warrant an immediate ophthalmologic consultation.[52]

RETROBULBAR HEMATOMA

This is one of the most dreaded complications of eyelid surgery and can lead to blindness if unrecognized and improperly managed. Retrobulbar hemorrhage results from puncture of small vessels during deep injection into the orbit or from tom vessels in the stump of the removed fat pedicle or incised orbital septum. Blood accumulates within the orbit behind the septum causing increasing intraorbital pressure and subsequent elevated intraocular pressure. It is important, therefore, to refrain from deep orbital injection and only inject the fat pads under direct vision prior to excision. The fat pads and other bleeding points need to be cauterized and any undetected bleeding source tamponaded by gentle pressure during surgery. The first indication of retrobulbar blindness may be only eye pain, but this can rapidly progress to proptosis, chemosis, elevated intraocular pressure with decreased retinal pulsations, retinal pallor, and blindness. Any sign of eye pain or decreased vision requires immediate attention.

Treatment consists of immediate reopening of the wounds including the orbital septum. Lateral canthotomy and cantholysis and intravenous mannitol and/or acetazolamide are subsequent steps with orbital decompression the ultimate treatment if blindness ensues. High-dose steroids are indicated in the event of vision loss. Ophthamologic consultation should be sought and may proceed with an anterior chamber paracentesis. Although alarming, retrobulbar hematoma is generally innocuous, promptly resolving with a minimum of difficulty.

VISUAL LOSS

Blindness is a catastrophic but rare complication of blepharoplasty arising from a variety of possible causes. The exact etiology and frequency of occurrence are not well documented but do not bear relation to any particular feature of the operation. However, studies do bear up the importance of preoperative documentation of eye examination.

Retrobulbar hematoma is a possible etiology of blindness due to increased intraorbital and intraocular pressure, choking the ophthalmic vessels. Optic atrophy with visual loss may result from vascular spasm due to orbital fat manipulation. However, this may be completely coincidental and in fact the senior author experienced one such case when a patient developed unilateral spontaneous blindness while spending the preoperative evening in the hospital. Occlusion of the retinal artery following pressure from the anesthetic mask during general anesthesia for another condition has also been reported. Other causes of vision loss during blepharoplasty reported in the literature include retrobulbar optic neuritis, optic nerve trauma, thrombosis of the retinal artery and vein, and unrecognized central nervous system (CNS) disease including multiple sclerosis and toxic amblyopia.

RHYTIDECTOMY

Complications of the face-lift procedure can be psychological or physical, temporary or permanent, and either minor or major in their extent. Psychological complications include an idiopathic postoperative depression that is generally a transient situational reaction resolving with little treatment other than counseling. Dissatisfaction is another problem that depends to some extent on the result obtained, but is more typically the result of inadequate preoperative counseling and unrealistic expectations. Major psychotic episodes can occur in borderline individuals who are missed in the preoperative screen.

Physical complications most often correlate with the extent of surgery involved. As the amount of undermining increases, so does the rate of complications with studies showing a disproportionate degree of improvement.[44] The subplatysmal dissection of a superficial muscular aponeurotic system increases risk of complication with little ultimate improvement over the less extensive SMAS placation type procedure.

The subperiosteal face-lift as recently described,[53] theoretically should give a better result than the conventional lift; however, the actual improvement has been questioned. Moreover, the complication rate especially with facial nerve injury is significant.[54] Modifications of the subperiosteal approach show a decrease in the complication rate and a higher degree of satisfaction.[55] This area is evolving and may represent an advancement yet to be fully realized.

For this discussion, minor physical complications are temporary, less in degree, and although distracting from the final result, do not destroy its value. Major complications threaten the individual or the surgical result to the degree that the purpose of the operative procedure, a better appearance, may be defeated.

Minor Complications
EDEMA AND ECCHYMOSIS

Edema and ecchymosis are inevitable following rhytidectomy and almost always resolve with time. The edema is usually maximum at the third to the fifth postoperative day and resolves to a great extent by the end of the second week. Head elevation, pressure wraps, and steroids all help prevent and treat these problems and the patient can be reassured that this is temporary. Prolonged edema may be due to lymphatic stasis that resolves with the redevelopment of lymphatic channels. Other lumps or surface irregularities may be due to localized fat necrosis or be secondary to the trauma of cauterization, suture ligation, uneven dissection, or bunching from plication. Management consists of reassurance and observation, but massage, pressure wraps, and occasionally an injection of steroid may be helpful.[56]

PAIN

Significant pain is unusual following rhytidectomy. If the pain is localized or unilateral, then a complication such as hematoma should be suspected until examination proves otherwise. Pain following the immediate postoperative period would be distinctly unusual and if localized, may be due to a neuroma or neuritis that can be injected with corticosteroids. A vague feeling of discomfort or tightness in those undergoing a SMAS procedure is usually due to traction on the tissues, which gradually resolves.

HYPESTHESIA AND PARESTHESIA

Sensory nerve abnormalities are very common following rhytidectomy due to direct surgical insult or stretching from edema and manipulation. Sensation almost always returns within several weeks and the patient should be reassured. Prolonged or permanent loss of sensation can result from trauma to the greater auricular nerve or in the case of a brow lift the supraorbital or supratrochlear nerves. If this is noted at the time of surgery every attempt should be made to repair the nerve damage. All patients should be forewarned of the possibilities of nerve damage and must be cautioned as to the potential damage secondary to the use of hair dryers, wearing jewelry, and exposure to cold.

SMALL HEMATOMAS

This is probably the most common complication of rhytidectomy, and the majority, being quite small, will resolve with time. Other small hematomas will liquify between 7 to 14 days postoperatively and can be aspirated or expressed through the suture line. If a localized collection of blood is allowed to remain it may fibrose and eventually even calcify causing skin irregularities. Corticosteroid injections may be helpful during the stage of fibrosis, otherwise reelevating a portion of the flap and excising is the best treatment.

INFECTION

Significant infections are distinctly unusual due to the rich blood supply and are generally the result of some other untoward circumstance such as hematoma, foreign body, flap necrosis, immune compromise, etc. Chondritis may occur if the ear cartilage is exposed, lacerated, or sutured and should be treated promptly when manifested. Minor superficial infections may occur around sutures, hair follicles, or sebaceous glands. The treatment is evacuation and removal of foreign material. The use of Phisohex shampoo and facial wash on the night prior to surgery is recommended. There are surgeons who utilize prophylactic antibiotics.

Local Disfigurements
SCARS

One of the primary keys to a satisfactory rhytidectomy is camouflaging the scar, which is accomplished by proper incision and tension placement (Fig. 17–8b). All necessary tension should be exerted on the temporal and postauricular suture line allowing the periauricular incision lines to simply fall into place with minimal to no tension. Hair-bearing areas, natural creases, and other natural anatomic landmarks should be utilized to camouflage the incision. Avoid permanent hair parting, loss of sideburn, and jagged hairline when working in hair-bearing areas. A natural tragus appearance is maintained by a top tragal incision, pretragal defatting, and reforming the pretragal depression with a deep dermal to cartilaginous canal suture.

The postauricular sulcus can be maintained and a web avoided by incising high on the postauricular pinna and making a V-plasty into the sulcus. Also, deepening the sulcus and placing deep sutures from dermis to the sulcus will help retain the normal configuration. Deep dermal sutures will help to prevent the pulled down earlobe.[57]

Scar hypertrophy is uncommon in areas other than the postauricular sulcus and is probably the result of tension causing a webbing in the sulcus. Keloid should be watched for in darker pigmented individuals and those with a history of such scarring. Prevention is facilitated by proper incision placement and avoidance of tension; as are the widened scars. When hypertrophy is first noted, corticosteroid injection in small doses spaced over 2 to 4 weeks will aide in resolution. Widened scars or dehiscent areas due to excessive tension should be allowed to mature and then excised with wide undermining to relieve any tension.

EARLOBE DEFORMITY

It is of utmost importance in the preoperative evaluation to note the earlobes. They may be too large, too small, webbed or pixie like, also, there may be a crease (as associated with arteriosclerotic cardiovascular disease [ASCVD]). If there appear to be any abnormalities, they should be pointed out to the patient and indication made that the appearance can be improved. The importance of this is that a complication of rhytidectomy is earlobe deformity and preassessment and planned treatment will obviate this problem. Large lobes can be reduced by a number of debulking flaps, small lobes can be enlarged with a lobe-based postauricular flap, webbed earlobes can be reformed by incising proximally on the earlobe toward the canal and reapproximating forming a new lobe. The lobe crease can be removed with a Z-plasty or, as the more common case, removed with a lobe reduction.[58]

DOG EAR

There is always some degree of dog ear in the nape of neck and temporal areas that should be corrected at the time of closure. Care must be taken to align the hairline and any residual deformity is best kept in the hair-bearing area. Most residual irregularities resolve with time, but a minor corrective procedure may be necessary after maturation of the scar.

ALOPECIA

Some hair loss occurs while performing the lift; however, modification of the incision can be accomplished to avoid an unnatural appearance. This is especially important in the male, to prevent loss of sideburn or avoid moving hair-bearing tissue into undesirable locations. Slanting the incisions in the plane of the hair tufts will avoid a permanent part appearance.

Hair loss also results from superficial undermining of the flap that traumatizes or destroys hair follicles. This may also result from excess tension or interruption of the blood supply and is more of a problem with those having thin hair. More commonly, a temporary loss takes place and regrowth occurs in several months.

CONTOUR IRREGULARITIES

Bulging and depressions may occur with SMAS surgery when the transected platysma bunches up or residual muscle remains when dividing platysmal bands in the neck. Also, bunching may occur when plicating the SMAS.

Submental depressions may become apparent where excessive fat removal has taken place in the submental area, allowing the skin to adhere to the muscle. The appearance of jowling can be accentuated by removing triangles of skin adjacent to the submental incision while attempting to tighten the neck. The cobra deformity also results from excess submental fat resection. It is of utmost importance to check for subcutaneous irregularities, both visually and by palpation, prior to closure as edema will hide them in the more immediate postoperative period.

OTHER MINOR SEQUELAE

Telanglectasis present prior to surgery may be exacerbated and become permanent. The smaller ones can be camouflaged with cosmetics and the larger ones can be treated with electrocoagulation or laser coagulation. Occasional hyperpigmentation may occur in areas of prior ecchymosis. This is more common in darker pigmented patients and those with a history of easy bruising.[59] Button holes made inadvertently should be immediately repaired and generally will leave little residual scar. Parotid gland fistulas are very rare and generally are due to parenchymal injury to the gland with subsequent sialocele and fistula. Management is conservative with antisialagogues, pressure dressing, and repeated aspirations as needed. In the authors' experiences all have resolved conservatively however, surgical intervention with oversewing very rarely may be necessary.[6]

Major Complications
HEMATOMA

The most frequent complication in rhytidectomy is hematoma, having an incidence of approximately 10 to 15% with major hematomas requiring surgical intervention averaging

3.7%. Hematomas range in size from those that require no treatment to a massive collection that endangers the skin flap. The incidence of hematoma is more common in men than women (8.7% vs 7.7%).[59] Prevention is the best cure for hematomas. This includes a careful preoperative history for bleeding disorders, abstaining from medication that interferes with coagulation for at least 2 weeks prior to surgery, and laboratory evaluation for hemostasis with prothrombin time (PT), partial thromboplastin time (PTT), and bleeding time.

Hypertension must be well controlled prior to surgery and a markedly labile blood pressure noted early in the procedure may be an indication for aborting the operation. Special care must also be taken in patients with a history of long-term steroid use or Ehlers-Danlos syndrome.[61]

Intraoperatively meticulous hemostasis is fundamental and a second-look type technique is useful to catch any subsequent or missed bleeding.[62] We utilize a variant of the described technique by completing the dissection on one side and packing off to return for hemostasis following completion of dissection on the opposite side. Also, utilizing liposuction to elevate the flaps decreases the amount of bleeding. The greater the undermining, the use of SMAS flap techniques, and resection of platysma, the greater the risk for bleeding. Late bleeding may result from failure to ligate the larger vessels encountered during dissection.[63]

Postoperatively, care must be taken to prevent any untoward coughing or retching that may occur especially with general anesthesia. Also, reactive hypertension may occur in the hours following surgery when the local anesthesia and operative sedation wear off and the patient develops pain and agitation. The prophylactic use of chlorpromazine has been recommended for its tranquilizing, antiemetic, and antihypertensive effects.[64] The authors use ¼-in Penrose drains on the majority of rhytidectomies. These are removed on the first postoperative day with the dressing change and a subsequent pressure dressing is left on for an additional 1 to 2 days. If there is any question regarding hemostasis, drains are definitely recommended.

The majority of major hematomas manifest themselves within the first 12 hours, but can occur up to a few weeks postoperatively, especially if there is some form of trauma or excess activity. Excessive pain, especially unilateral, is uncommon in the uncomplicated facelift and may herald an expanding hematoma. Any untoward pain, ecchymosis, or swelling warrants further investigation with removal of the dressing for direct examination if there is any doubt. Once a major hematoma is diagnosed, this is regarded as a surgical emergency and requires immediate innervation to prevent the loss of the flap. It is strongly recommended that the operating room and general anesthesia be utilized to widely open the flap, evacuate the hematoma, irrigate, and obtain hemostasis. Although the bleeding may be from a localized source, it will generally be diffuse by the time of evacuation requiring time and careful hemostasis.

SKIN SLOUGH

Necrosis of the skin flap is caused by vascular compromise and occurs to some extent in 1% to 3% of rhytidectomies. The most common point of occurrence is in the postauricular areas where the flap is under the most tension, thinnest, and farthest from the blood supply. Skin slough can vary from a superficial peeling to full thickness loss. The initial sign of skin slough is a bluish tinge (due to venous congestion) or an intense pallor (in arteriolar insufficiency) occurring within 48 hours after surgery. In the absence of systemic disease, as diabetes mellitus or cigarette smoking, venous congestion is more common than arteriolar insufficiency.

As is the case in other complications prevention is superior to any subsequent treatment and is achieved by avoiding compromising situations and meticulous surgical technique. The most common cause of skin slough is unrelieved hematoma with vascular compromise of the skin flap. Other causes include undue tension on the flap, excessive pressure from the dressing, rough treatment of tissue and, excessive thinning or undermining of the flap. Systemic disorders including diabetes mellitus, long-term steroid use, and cigarette smoking increase the risk of skin slough. Studies have shown that cigarette smokers have over twice the incidence (2.7% vs 7.5%) of skin slough and many surgeons will not operate unless smoking is discontinued.[65]

Once skin slough has occurred, time is the best treatment. Superficial slough resembles a second-degree burn with blistering and desquamation. Healing is generally satisfactory leaving residual pigmentary changes, coarseness, or superficial scarring (Fig. 17–11). Full thickness loss will develop a black eschar that serves as a biologic dressing. The eschar should be allowed to separate on its own with conservative debriding unless an infection develops. The eschar generally separates completely within 3 to 4 weeks leaving a smaller scar than was expected. Steroid injections and, after an appropriate interval, scar revision will improve the appearance.

FACIAL NERVE INJURY

The incidence of facial nerve injury is less than 1% and generally resolves over weeks to months leaving a residual deficit in approximately 0.1% of patients. Paresis due to injection of local anesthesia resolves by the first postoperative day. If there is residual paresis but not paralysis, chances are good for complete recovery with time. A preoperative evaluation of facial nerve function is extremely important as a previously undetected deficit may be attributed to the surgery.

The most easily damaged branch is the zygomaticofacial nerve and care must be taken where it crosses the zygomatic arch. Other less commonly injured nerves are the buccal and marginal mandibular branches, especially when developing SMAS flaps. Distinctly uncommon is injury to the accessory

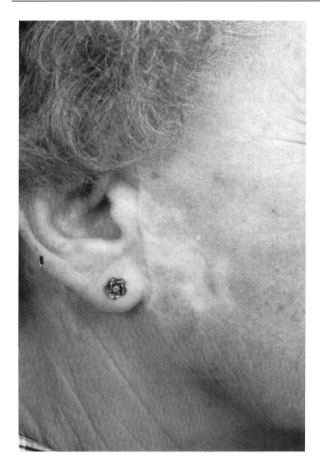

Figure 17–11. Patient 3 years after skin necrosis and slough following neglected postrhytidectomy hematoma. Patient 4 years following face-lift procedure.

nerve if dissection is too deep over the posterior margin of the stemocleidomastoid muscle. We utilize liposuction to dissect out the plane of the flap and have noted a decrease in incidence of even temporary nerve paresis.

The various causes of facial nerve injury include: (1) direct injection of anesthetic agent into the nerve, (2) blunt trauma, (3) stretching, (4) pinching with a clamp or forceps, (5) electrocautery, (6) suture ligation or plication sutures, (7) hematoma, (8) too tight a dressing, and (9) direct transaction of the nerve.[66] Of course, Bell's palsy or other neuropathies can coincidentally occur. If the nerve is noted to be severed at the time of surgery, it is incumbent on the surgeon to reapproximate the nerve endings using microsurgical technique if possible. Transection of the nerve results in only a 15% complete regeneration rate. The remaining 85% heal with some residual deformity that may require surgical correction after a suitable amount of time (at least 1 year).

OTOPLASTY

Otoplasty refers to any surgical procedures that attempt to alter the size and/or shape of the external ear, with or without adjusting its relationship with the head. In the recent literature, the term "otoplasty" has been used to describe procedures that correct prominauris. Otoplasty has been described as early as the 10th century in India.[67] The majority of patients with loop ear deformity have either conchal protrusion or antihelical unfurling.[68]

The fact that many techniques have been described illustrates that no single one is universally applicable. In general, the surgical techniques can be divided into cartilage-cutting or cartilag-sparing types.[69-71] The incidence of complications ranges from 6% to 13% depending on the techniques used.[72]

Early Complications
PAIN

After otoplasty, the normal postoperative course should be relatively pain free. Pain in the first day or two suggests the formation of a hematoma.[73] If associated with fever later on in the postoperative course then infection, that is, chondritis should be ruled out. Small hematomas can be drained in the clinic setting and a pressure dressing applied. We routinely keep the pressure dressing on for 1 week postoperative after the first day postoperative check. Patients with perichondritis should be hospitalized and started on parenteral antibiotics with staphylococcus coverage. Persistent discomfort long after the incisions have completely healed can be related to sensory nerve neuroma in the operated area. If this is pointed out to patients before surgery, the majority of them will tolerate this symptom. The sensation usually recovers in a few months.

HEMATOMA

The incidence of hematoma is 3.0% (range 0.08% to 6%).[74] The most common cause of hematoma is trauma. However, other factors such as bleeding dyscrasias, rebound from vasoconstriction or inadequate hemostasis should be considered. As noted in the previous section, pain is the predominant symptom. If there is any suspicion, the dressing should be removed and the ear examined. Treatment consists of drainage of the hematoma under sterile conditions. To prevent reaccumulation of the hematoma, meticulous hemostasis should be performed, through and through mattress sutures applied and antistaphylococcal antibiotics instituted. The use of a pressure dressing postoperatively cannot be overemphasized.

INFECTION

The organisms involved are *Staphylococcus aureus*, *Escherichia coli*, and *Pseudomonas aeruginosa*. Both cellulitis and chonchitis can result. Infection usually happens around 5 days after the initial surgery. Cellulitis likely results from improper management of the wound such as sloppy sterile techniques. In one study it occurred in about 2% of the cases.[75] The best treatment for this problem is prevention. The absolute observation of sterile technique and the use of a broad spectrum antibiotic are helpful. The immediate evacuation of hematoma will also prevent this problem. We do not find the use of antibiotic ointment helpful in preventing infection; instead, it often precipitates an atopic skin reaction.

Perichondritis is a much more serious infective complication. Fortunately, it occurs in less than 1% of the cases.[75] It may be a consequence of an untreated hematoma or the use of silk sutures for the Mustarde' technique.[76] After perichondritis has developed, the patient should be hospitalized and proper culture obtained. Intravenous antibiotics should be started. Necrotic tissue will have to be debrided and the wound may require repeated irrigation using half-strength hydrogen peroxide. Aggressive treatment is essential because penchondritis may result in resorption of the elastic cartilage resulting in severe ear deformity.

SKIN NECROSIS

This is an uncommon condition owing to the abundant blood supply in the auricular skin flap. Many different incisions have been proposed for exposure of the conchal cartilage, all of which have relatively good success rate without problem with closure. Necrosis could happen with improper or excessively tight suture closure of the wound. Patients with compromised blood supply secondary to systemic problems, such as smokers or diabetics, should be followed closely. When skin accrosis does occur, proper debridement is essential and closure of the exposed cartilage with local flaps is mandatory to preserve the cartilaginous architecture and prevent scar contracture with exposed cartilage. Systemic broad spectrum antibiotics are helpful in treating necrosis.

ALLERGIC REACTIONS

Skin reaction usually manifests by pruritus and/or pain. The ear should be examined to rule out the previously addressed complications. The use of antibiotic ointment is the most common culprit. The only ointment we use postoperatively on the skin incision is A&D ointment. Some suture material such as chromic gut can also cause skin reaction. The treatment for this problem is to identify the offending agent and remove it. Steroids, both topical or systemic, may be required.

Late Complications
SUTURE GRANULOMA OR EXTRUSION

The suture used for otoplasty should be of a color that compliments the patient's skin color. Permanent suture will help to maintain the shape of the correction. The rate of granuloma formation was noted to be 8% postoperative with Mersilene.[77] If granulomas occur, it should be removed postauricularly, usually without cosmetic penalty.

In our experience the braided sutures, although easier to tie, cut and tear the conchal cartilage during passage. Thus, we have been using permanent monofilament sutures. Suture extrusion postoperatively is not a common occurrence. We do not find the use of absorbable sutures reliable in maintaining the shape of the postoperative results.

HYPERTROPHIC SCARS AND KELOIDS

Postauricular skin has a tendency to give a poor incision scar. The lower one-half of the ear is more prone to hypertrophic scar formation. The incidence has been quoted as 0.7%, with keloid formation in the black population postotoplasty as high as 11%.[74]

History of hypertrophic scar and keloid formation should be obtained from the patient prior to surgery. Patients with a positive history should be followed more closely. The basic surgical principle of conservative skin excision and wound closure with no tension should be strongly adhered to. Before closure of the incision in a patient with potential for keloid formation, subcutaneous injections of triamcinolone (Kenalog) have worked well for us. If hypertrophic scar does occur, frequent massage of the incision with injection of triamcinolone and hyaluronidase has been found to be useful. For keloid scars that do not respond to pressure and steroids, we have found carbon dioxide laser excision without wound closure helpful.[78] The old treatment of keloids with radiation therapy should be condemned.

SENSORY DEFICITS

Hypoesthesia behind the auricle is a common complaint postotoplasty. Hyperesthesia, less common, may also occur. In a normal postoperative course, the condition usually improves over the intervening weeks to months. Generally, no special therapy is indicated. Preoperative counseling of the patient is the best approach.

RECURRENCE OF DEFORMITY

The rate of recurrence of the deformity depends on the technique used, which has been reported to range from 4.3% to 6%.[74,79] The compliance of the patient is very important for a good postoperative result. It should be stressed to patients that after the dressing is removed, they are expected to wear a compressive band continuously for 7 days, and at night only for the next 6 weeks. During the first postoperative week, the compressive dressing preserves the shape of the reconstruction and also prevents hematoma formation.

Suture techniques, such as the Mustarde' technique, may be far more successful in children with pliable cartilage. In adults, the stiff cartilage spring has to be broken to achieve a long-lasting result. The use of drills with diamond drillbites may be helpful. In patients with a prominent conchal bowl, we have found lateral conchal resection more helpful than the use of the conchal setback suture.[80]

Any wound complication will of course adversely affect the surgical results. Most deformities will be evident within the first 2 to 8 months after surgery.[81,82] Reassurance is important during the initial presentation of a bad outcome.

A waiting period of 3 to 6 months is indicated for the healing process to occur and scar deformity to settle before reconstruction is considered.

TELEPHONE DEFORMITY

This type of deformity results from overzealous correction of the middle third of the auricle. Any technique utilized for otoplasty can result in this deformity, especially in a large auricle that has a wide scapha. The best way to avoid this deformity is to properly assess the deformity both preoperatively and intraoperatively prior to the permanent placement of any sutures or resection. The correction of this deformity relies on diagnosing its etiology, be it inadequate skin excision in the superior and inferior pole, excessive cartilage or soft tissue excision in the middle pole, or improper placement of conchal mastoid or scapha-conchal sutures during the initial surgery. In revision surgery, the use of a postauricular flap based on the temporal region is helpful to give good exposure for assessing the different components that can contribute to this deformity.

CONCHAL DEFORMITY

Poor preoperative assessment of the prominauris can result in lack of correction. We have found that the lateral cavity resection will usually correct this problem. This will avoid the use of the conchal mastoid suture and at the same time help the unfolding of the scaphoid fossa if Mustarde' sutures are required.[80]

One of the problems with conchal mastoid sutures is the narrowing of the external auditory canal (EAC) in cases where the Webster and Smith[82] or Furnas[70] conchal bowl set back technique is improperly utilized. The ear should be positioned posteriorly and medially to prevent distortion of the EAC when suture set back is done. If narrowing of the EAC results, then redoing the sutures is important.

ANTIHELICAL DEFORMITY

The average distance between the helical rim and the mastoid has been measured to be 15 to 20 mm. A shorter distance is not aesthetically pleasing. The helix also should be 2 to 5 mm lateral to the antihelix. Any overcorrection of the antihelical fold will result in an unnatural appearance. If a suture technique was utilized in the initial surgery, this can be corrected by readjusting the position and tension of the previous sutures. In cases where excessive cartilage has been removed, grafting of the deficient area with autologous or hemologous cartilage may be necessary.

One major detraction to the cartilage-cutting technique for antihelical correction is the appearance of sharp ridges or irregular contours. Correction of this deformity may be difficult. Cartilage grafting in the deformed region followed by the Mustarde' suture technique after allowing time for healing can be tried.

SUCTION LIPECTOMY

This technique has become very popular either as an adjunctive or isolated procedure in the field of facial plastic and reconstructive surgery. Most commonly, this technique is performed in conjunction with rhytidectomy. Any discussion of complications with this procedure has to identify the number and types of different procedures performed simultaneously. The complication rate for dermatolipectomy was noted to be 0.9%.[83] It can be expected that the complication rate for cervicofacial lipectomy will be lower owing to the smaller volume of aspirate removed compared with that of other body areas. Many of the major complications associated with suction lipectomy of other body areas—myocardial infarction, cerebrovascular accident, pulmonary thromboembolism, fat embolism, deep venous thrombosis, and transfusion complication—in general do not apply to the head and neck region. The blood loss per 100 cc aspirate has been calculated to be approximately 37.6 cc for females and 123.2 cc for males. Cervicofacial lipectomy rarely removes more than 50 cc of aspirate.[84]

Infection

The rate of infection with cervicofacial cases was reported to be 0.15%.[85] This low infection rate is due to the good vascularity of the head and neck region. If the lipectomy is carried out as an adjunctive procedure, the rate of infection might increase if foreign bodies are introduced as in chin implantation or in cases such as rhytidectomy in which a higher potential for seroma or hematoma formation exists.

The use of prophylactic antibiotics usually is not necessary in this type of case if no mucosal barrier has been violated. In many instances, the surgeon might choose to prescribe antibiotics owing to the length of the operation or because graft material is involved.

Seroma/Hematoma

The rate of seroma and hematoma formation has been reported to be 0.47% to 2%.[86-88] In isolated cases of ceryicofacial lipectomy, we have been using submandibular regional taping for 24 hours postoperatively together with a rhytidectomy support bandage; no drain is used. If a rhytidectomy is also performed, we routinely use a postauricular drain with heavy circumfacial dressing, our customary rhytidectomy dressing. These precautions have reduced our rate of seroma/hematoma. Signs of this complication usually include pain out of the ordinary. Swelling in the region may be seen after the dressing is removed. Local aspiration of the fluid accumulation together with pressure dressing for another 24 hours is usually all that is required. Depending on the extent of the hematoma, a drain may be reinserted. Large serum/blood collections are rare in isolated lipectomy procedures. If occurring right after surgery, surgical drainage as described in the rhytidectomy section should be undertaken. If these problems are not recognized, infection, skin slough, and airway compromise can occur.

Skin Discoloration

The rate of this complication is reported to be 1%.[89] This problem usually resolves over a period of a few months. Its etiology is related to the deposition of hemosiderin in the dermal layer. The avoidance of trauma during the procedure and the prevention of hematoma formation postoperatively is the best guard against this problem. Bleaching agents may be required if the discoloration persists.

Skin Slough

The incidence of skin slough is reported to be 0.2%.[89] The best way to prevent this problem is to preserve the neurovascular pedicle (subdural plexus) that connects the subdertnal fat with the overlying skin during the procedure. This is especially important if a rhytidectomy is performed simultaneously. Patients with a known history of smoking should be directed to discontinue the habit for at least 6 weeks prior to a flap elevation procedure. The suction port for the cannula should be directed towards the subdural fat to prevent traumatizing the skin. As mentioned before, seroma and hematoma should be detected early and managed appropriately.

Skin Excess

Of all the body areas that are treated with suction lipectomy techniques, the neck area has the highest rate of unsatisfactory results. It has been reported to be as high as 30.5%. This rate, however, does decrese when the surgeon has performed 50 or more of these procedures.[89]

The most common problem is the apparent exaggeration of the neck skin due to a lack of redraping. Interestingly, a recent study showed that isolated suction lipectomy in the neck region seems to eliminate preexisting skin looseness. The result also tends to be longer lasting (up to 10 years) than in other areas of the body.[90] This is especially true in patients in the 30- to 45-year-old age group.

On the face, in contrast, skin retraction is not as easily predictable, thus long-term results without associated rhytidectomy are not as favorable. It seems that the treatment site has a serious impact on the amount of skin retraction seen after suction lipectomy when no other adjunctive procedure is performed.

Nerve Injury

If suction lipectomy is performed in the right surgical plane, no nerve injury should occur. Injuries to the marginal mandibular or greater auricular nerves in the cervical region are rare, and if they occur are usually reversible. If the suction cannula is used for the elevation of the rhytidectomy flap,

the frontal branch of cranial nerve VII can also be damaged. The best way to prevent this is to not use the suction cannula in the temporal region above the zygomatic arch. Use of the suction cannula in this region is mainly for the purpose of dissection. Judicial use of the cannula for this purpose is emphasized. If injury does occur, systemic steriods may be tried; however, the frontal branch deficit may not return.

Hypoesthesia of the skin is an expected sequela of the procedure and should be explained to patients preoperatively. The majority of patients will have return of normal sensation in 6 to 8 months.[91] Most patients with a clear understanding of this consequence tolerate it well.

Irregularities and Scars

Waviness and rippling of the skin are not common complications in the head and neck region after suction lipectomy. The use of suction cannulae that are less than 4 mm in diameter, precludes these problems. Contour irregularities can usually be corrected at the time of operation if meticulous inspection is carried out. Feathering of the adjacent region also helps prevent this problem. If associated rhytidectomy is to be performed, fine tuning of the cervicofacial contour can be done at the end of the procedure by open suction of any area that is noted to be irregular. In situations where excessive fat has been removed, autogenous fat grafts, collagen, other filler material can be reinjected into the area. The long-term result is not uniformly predictable. The underlying structural irregularity may be unmasked after the suction lipectomy. A ptotic submandibular gland, prominent platysmal banding, or ptotic chin should be recognized and corrected at the time of operation. To obtain the optimal profile after suction lipectomy, all the components from skin, fat, platysmal banding, and chin ptosis to the mandibular projection should be thoroughly evaluated and addressed.

Dermal scarring and dimpling result from overly aggessive removal of subcutaneous fat; with scarring of the dermis to the facial musculature. If this occurs, massage during the healing period will be beneficial. Local triamcinolone injection can be used, keeping in mind that overinjection can cause atrophy of the skin and the formation of telangiectasias. In severe situations, surgical dissection may be necessary between the dermal and muscular planes with insertion of a fascial graft. Preexisting facial or cervical scars should be recorded and pointed out to patients. Sometimes deep ice pick type scarring becomes more shallow after suction lipectomy.

CHEMEXFOLIATION

This procedure involves the application of a chemically caustic agent to the skin to produce a partial thickness burn to the epidermal and dermal layers under controlled conditions. The histology of the healed skin after chemical peel has been studied and at the epidermal level, it is noted to have less cellular atypia with uniform thickness of the basement membrane. In the dermal layer, the papillary dermis is thickened with new horizontally striated normally staining collagen and also shows an increase of elastic tissue.[92]

Many indications for chemical peel have been identified. Peels with different depths of penetration have been developed over the years, each with its specific application (trichloroacetic acid [TCA] 10% to 25%, TCA 35% with Jessner solution, Baker's solution). Ideal patients for chemexfoliation are females with a fair complexion and nonoily skin. They tend to have less problems postpeel. Patients with Fitzpatrick skin types III and IV should be peeled with caution. Trichloroacetic acid peel can be used in those patients; a phenol peel, however, gives more problems. In our experience, black patients have a very high risk of pigmentary problems postpeel and usually are not good candidates for any type of peeling agents.

Systemic Complications

Phenol has a number of systemic toxicities that the surgeon must understand prior to using it. On the other hand, TCA and other superficial to medium depth peeling agents are relatively devoid of systemic problems. Phenol is rapidly absorbed into the circulation after application to the skin.[93] Sixty-five percent of the absorbed phenol is conjugated with sulfates and glucuronides in the liver, 25% is oxidized to carbon dioxide and water, and 10% exists as free phenol. The free phenol and conjugates are excreted through the kidney.[94] From the pharmacokinetics above, it is obvious that renal and hepatic dysfunction can adversely enhance the toxicity of phenol.

Cardiotoxicity is the most common and dramatic systemic complication of the phenol peel. Arrhythmias reported include bigeminy, ventricular tachycardia, and paroxysmal atrial tachycardia.[95] Hydration with intravenous fluid is very important before the peeling procedure. To avoid arrhythmia, no more than 50% of the face should be treated during a 30-minute interval.[94,96] The incidence of arrhythmia is much lower if any aesthetic subunit is treated in a longer period of time. The facial aesthetic subunit is painted separately with 10 to 15 minutes to each subunit. Cardiac monitoring is required during this procedure. If arrhythmia is noted, lidocaine bolus intravenously should be given. The rhythm disorder should resolve and after 15 minutes of normal sinus rhythm the procedure can be continued at a much slower rate.

Pigmentation Changes

Proper patient selection is the best way to avoid this problem. Fitzpatrick skin types I and II tend to have good results after the peel. Pigmentation problems are most common with phenol peels, especially among dark-skinned patients. Demarcation effects can be improved by feathering the peel with the surrounding region, that is, along the border of the mandible if a regional peel is performed. Hypopigmentation is a common postphenol peel appearance. The porcelain doll appearance should be pointed out to the patient preoperatively, this can be altered with makeup.

The blotchy pigmentation that complicates this procedure is more common in dark-skinned individuals, especially those who have unprotected sun exposure during the first 6 months after the peel. Hormonal changes, either physiological or pharmacological can enhance any pigmentary changes. Hyperpigmentation is helped with the use of a combination of hydroquinone, retinoic acid, and triamcinolone cream 0.1% (Kligman's formula) as soon as reepithelialization is complete.[97] The replacement of triamcinolone with a nonfluorinated steroid has been found to cause less atrophy and telangiectasias. This formula should be used for 3 months together with the daily use of sunblock if going outdoors. If no improvement is noted 6 months after the treatment, a re-peel should be considered. Hypopigmentation in small areas can be appropriately treated with makeup or repigmentation with microtattooing techniques.[98] Erythema can persist beyond 3 weeks post-peel. Daily application of topical hydrocortisone cream can help with its resolution. Reassurance of the patient during this period is important.

SCARRING

Scarring is reported to have an incidence of 21% using phenol and taping.[99] High-concentration TCA also is very caustic and can produce severe scarring. The lip, chin, perioral, and jawline are areas most commonly associated with scarring. Skin areas that have been undermined will have a compromised vascular supply, therefore, these areas have a higher chance of skin slough and scar formation. We do not recommend concomitant rhytidectomy with chemical peels. Regional peels in areas away from the undermined skin are acceptable. We usually allow a time lapse of at least 3 months after any type of skin undermining before a peel procedure is performed. Taping or occlusive dressings (even a shower cap) after the peel also increase the risk of skin slough and scar formation.[100] Hair dye or other hair chemicals will affect the depth of peel penetration and should be avoided for 2 weeks before the peel.

Ectropion has been reported as a complication of peels.[101] The risk is higher after a lower lid blepharoplasty. Extreme caution when considering chemical peels in patients with previous lower lid blepharoplasty.

The earliest sign of scarring is usually erythema. A conservative approach involving massage and compression along with the use of topical corticosteroids is initiated as soon as possible. Intralesional steroids will be necessary if the above measure does not improve the scar. Most likely, time and reassurance rather than scar revision are necessary.

The depth of peel is related to the potential for scarring, however, there are no good predictive factors for identifying patients who will scar. History of keloid formation is not an absolute contraindication to chemical peels. A judicial approach to other surgical procedures at the same time as chemexfoliation is the key.

Scarring and delayed healing are noted in patients that use Acutane (isotretinoin). We usually would not perform any peeling in patients who have used this topical ointment within 12 months of the peel.

Infection

Infection is not a common problem, probably owing to the excellent blood supply to the face. The most common bacterial pathogens are staphylococcus and streptococcus. With meticulous wound management after the procedure, infection usually can be avoided. We instruct our patients to wash their face four times a day with water and apply moisturizing cream. We like Eucerin on the face in between the face washing. They are instructed to continue this regime for 7 days. We see our postpeel patients on the first postoperative day and then on the seventh day.

With a compliant patient, epithelialization should be completed within 5 to 7 days. We do not feel prophylactic antibiotics are helpful. There are reports of toxic shock syndrome in the literature after chemical peels.[102,103] This is due to the exotoxin produced by *S. aureus*. There may not be signs of wound infection and blood culture may be negative. The major signs are fever, rash, skin desquamation, and hypotension. Treatment should be started with parenteral β-lactamase-resistant antibiotics, along with aggressive symptomatic therapy with fluids and renal and cardiac support if necessary.

The most common viral infection after this procedure is caused by the herpes simplex virus (HSV). Previous history of herpetic infection in the head and neck region should be obtained because chemical peeling reactivates the virus. Patients with previous herpetic infections are started on a prophylactic regimen of acyclovir. We start the medication 2 days prior to the procedure and continue it for 7 days. The dosage is 200 mg five times a day by mouth. In patients with no previous history of infection, the first symptom is usually intense pain, superficial ulceration on the skin can also be seen. This usually occurs on the fourth or fifth day postpeel. Culture of the skin should be done to ascertain the causative organism. Prior to culture results we start our patients on acyclovir and also antistaphylococcal medication. Topical cleansing with water every 2 hours with the use of Eucerin cream is recommended. We do not find the use of antibiotic ointment helpful, except to induce an atopic reaction. Chemical peeling should be postponed if at the time of surgery the patient has ulceration on the face or signs of bacterial or viral infection.

Skin Abnormalities

Patients should be forewarned that the deep rhytids in the perioral and periorbital areas can be only moderately improved with chemical peels. Total eradication of these deep rhytids is not to be expected.

Existing nevi may become darker after chemical peel. Telangiectasias can also become more numerous. These side effects of chemical peel are beyond technical control. If the patient is dissatisfied with any of the above-mentioned accentuations of preexisting skin conditions, follow-up correction such as the use of laser for the telangiectasias or excision of nevi can be accomplished.

Milias are epidermal inclusion cysts not uncommon after chemical peel. With time, they ususally disappear. If they remain a persistent problem, they can be unroofed with an 18-gauge needle. In patients prone to form milias, starting them on tretinoin after epithelialization has occurred seems to decrease the incidence of this problem.

DERMABRASION

The best way to avoid complications with this procedure is to have proper patient selection. Dermabrasion is contraindicated in patients who have certain medical conditions such as chronic radiodermatitis, pyoderma, active herpes simplex, infection, psychosis, severe psychoneurosis, alcoholism, xeroderma pigmentosum, verrucae Planae, and burn scars.[104]

Patients with Fitzpatrick skin type IV to VI in general also are poor candidates for this procedure. Among different ethnic groups, Orientals seem to have more problems with pigmentary changes postoperatively. The psychological makeup of the patient should undergo the same kind of scrutiny as is done for any other facial plastic surgery patient. The likely compliance of the patient in terms of long-term postoperative instruction should be assessed.

Milia and Skin Texture Changes

This is the most common complication of dermabrasion. It usually appears 3 to 4 weeks postoperatively. Often it may resemble acne whiteheads. Patients should be forewarned of this problem. This complication is seen more often in females. Pre and posttreatment of the skin with tretinoin has markedly reduced the incidence of this problem.[105]

Enlargement of pore size in central facial areas is a possible side effect of dermabrasion. It is likely due to lowering the surface of the skin to the level where the diameter of the follicles may be larger. This problem is difficult to correct, and should be understood by the patient before the surgery.

Pigmentary Changes

Hyperpigmentation is a common complication of this procedure. It is likely related to the inflammatory response secondary to the surgery. It usually happens in darker skin individuals. Areas over bony prominences such as the malar prominence and along the border of the mandible are more susceptible. It is also more common in cases where spot dermabrasion is done. Sun avoidance should be strongly followed for 6 months as the sun will aggravate the condition. Early aggressive therapy with morning applicafion of tretinoin cream (0.025%) followed with an opaque makeup and then hydroquinone lotion (2 to 4%) in the evening is indicated.[106] Resolution is common and usually takes 3 to 4 months.

Hypopigmentation is a result of melanotic injury and is seen in deeper-level dermabrasion.[107] Alt[113] believes that this complication is overemphasized. It is common in dark-skinned white or Asian patients. Normal pigmentation usually will resume within 12 to 24 months. Actinic damage will enhance the color contrast. Hypopigmentation, unlike hyperpigmentation, can be permanent. The best treatment for this complication is reassurance and time. After proper epithelialization and expectant treatment a superficial peel with TCA (20%) can be used.

Scarring

The best way to prevent scarring is to perform the dermabrasion to the correct level of skin depth. The papillary dermis should be the deepest level entered. While performing the procedure, no pressure should be applied to the wire brush. Avoidance of back and forth or circular movements may prevent gouging of the skin. Wounding that penetrates beyond the reticular dermis will produce a scar. Bony prominences as noted in the previous section are also more susceptible to hypertrophic scar. The choice of refrigerants can potentiate the depth of tissue destruction and thus, must be used with caution.

Topical steroids (eg, Cordran [flurandrenolide] tape) should be applied to areas suspected of early scar formation. In most cases, this will prevent the hypertrophic scar/keloid formation. If scarring occurs, intralesional steroids (triamcinolone 40 mg/mL and hyaluronidase 150 U/mL mixture) should be used. The lesions can be reinjected in a 4-week interval.

Patients using Acutane for acne have been noted to have delayed healing and subsequent scarring after the procedure.[108,109] We generally like to have the patient discontinue Acutane for more than 12 months and preferably longer before we perform the dermabrasion. Patients with a history of hypertrophic scars or keloids or those who are black or Oriental should be forewarned of this complication; alternative procedures may be necessary.

Thermal Injury

The literature has multiple examples of skin injury resulting in scarring after the use of certain types of refrigerants.[110-112] Areas that have been dermabraded must be protected from further thermal injury by refrigerants with proper covering. Certain mixtures have been shown to cause deeper skin damage. Freon 11 and freon 12 produced maximal cooling to the temperature of −52°C. They should not be used.[111] Fluroethyl (ethylchloride-dichlorotetrafluoroethane) and Frigiderm (dichlorotetrafluoroethane) are two products that have been shown to be effective over time.[113]

Pigmentary changes (either hyper or hypo) can also occur with the refrigerant. Hyperpigmentation is related to inflammation and hypopigmentation is due to melanotic damage secondary to the freezing. Their management has been outlined before.

Infections

Bacterial infection is rare during the healing phase. The most common bacterial organism is *S. aureus*. When it occurs, it presents itself about 2 to 3 days postoperatively. Aggressive wound management including cleansing and moisturizing together with antistaphylococcal systemic antibiotics should be initiated. We do not routinely start our patients on prophylactic antibiotics if there is no sign of infection.

Patients with a previous history of HSV infection are started on acyclovir capsules preoperatively and the regimen continues after the dermabrasion. In patients with no prior HSV infection who develop the condition, prompt administration of both systemic and topical acyclovir usually controls the infection and prevents any scarring.

Yarborough and Beeson[114] have recommended that in patients with a prior history of frequent herpetic infection, the dermabrasion be performed in two stages. We find that with the prophylactic acyclovir regimen we can dermabrade the trigger area without activation of the HSV infection.

Candida infection occurs at 5 to 7 days postoperatively and results in delayed healing. Exudation and facial swelling are noted. Proper culture should be obtained to identify the organism. Topical ketoconazole is the treatment.

Side Effects on Skin

Persistent erythema for more than 8 weeks after surgery, especially with texture change, represents potential scar formation. Topical steroid cream or flurandrenolide can be used in these areas.

An acne flare can occur if the patient has active acne. If this occurs, starting the patient on tetracycline usually can help with the resolution of the problem. Telangiectasias can be aggravated postdermabrasion. If this becomes aesthetically unacceptable, laser treatment may be necessary.

TISSUE EXPANDER

Since Radovan's[115] early attempt, tissue expansion has been gaining popularity as a technique of reconstruction. The complications with this procedure can be divided into major and minor types. Major complications are defined as those that abort the expansion and prevent the intended outcome. Minor complications are those that require treatment but do not effect the final result.[116] The complication rate varies widely depending on the surgeon, the amount of experience, the anatomic site of expansion, and the local tissue condition. The complication rates are variable in the literature, ranging from 10% to 60%.[117,118]

Antonyshy et al[119] noted a 48% complication rate in the head and neck, but 70% of the patients had successful completion of their planned reconstruction. Sasaki[120] reported an initial complication rate of 40%, but this decreased to 3% over the next 7 years.

The complication rate is highest for tissue expansion in the head and neck. Within these anatomic regions, the cheek and neck have the highest rate (69%) followed by the forehead (50%).[119] The scalp has the lowest risk (17%). The key to prevention of complication is proper patient selection.

Implant Exposure

This is the most common type of complication, occurring in 30% of cases.[119] Several factors contribute to this problem, one being incision too close to the area of expansion.[121] The use of permanent sutures also is necessary to close the deeper layers of the incision, which helps to prevent incision disruption during inflation of the expander. Adequate dissection and the selection of a proper size implant will also prevent this complication. Prior to wound closure, any persistent fold in the expander requires adjustment because the fold can produce increased pressure in the overlying skin. Excessively rapid and overzealous inflation is another common cause of implant exposure.[122] A progressive thinning of the dermis and subsequent dissipation of the overlying skin and capsule are common; these are more frequent when there is inadequate tissue coverage of the expander during implant placement and/or with expansion of previously irradiated skin.[123] Preventive measures include allowing a period of 2 weeks between creation of the pocket and the beginning of expansion, slow expansion, and taping or supporting the overlying skin with external wrappings.[123,123]

Treatment of implant exposure depends on the degree of exposure and the amount of expansion that has been accomplished. Early in the course of expansion, the implant is best removed and the procedure repeated 3 to 4 months later.[122] If an adequate amount of expansion has occurred, it is best to proceed with expander removal and the reconstruction undertaken. In a situation with inadequate expansion and minimal exposure, the implant may be left in position for a limited time while expansion continues.[123] A&D ointment application and frequent washing of the exposed area are performed. Antibiotic ointment has not been helpful and can result in atopic reactions. Use of perioperative antibiotics is routine with tissue expansion; systemic antibiotics are not required in implant exposure if no sign of infection is noticed. The amount of inflation should be smaller and the interval more frequent. The patient should be followed very closely for overt signs of infection.

Implant Failure

Implant failure is not common with the latest generation of implants. Most prostheses are able to tolerate inflation up to three to five times their intended volume. The most common error is in faulty assembly of the connection device that joins the stem of the injection port with that of the silicone balloon.[121] Most recent expanders are available in a single unit. Leakage is an iatrogenic complication that results from puncture of the balloon or the tubing during inflation. Spontaneous leakage from the inflation reservoir is uncommon and if minor, does not necessitate implant replacement.

If the prosthesis is deflating, replacement is indicated. There is no significant loss of tissue volume from the expansion if the expander is removed within a few days. If replacement of the expander is necessary, the implant can be filled to the volume that local tissue allows. One to 2 weeks should be allowed before further inflation is undertaken to allow for maturation of the incision.

Infections

Infection with implants is not common in the head and neck region. Meticulous surgical technique is the best way to avoid infection. Perioperative antibiotics are routinely used. The antibiotic of choice should be broad spectrum with antistaphylococcal coverage. Seroma and hematoma, if detected, should be drained immediately and the implant cavity irrigated. If the implant is placed near the vicinity of hemangiomas, there will be an increase in the chance of hematoma formation. Closed suction drainage at the time of implant placement is necessary if the potential for hematoma is high. Partial inflation of the implant to compress the surrounding tissue also seems to help. Infections that do not respond to drainage and antibiotics should be treated with removal of the implant and packing of the cavity.

Psychological Intolerance

Patients should have an understanding of the temporary disfigurement that occurs while the implant is in place. The distortion of body image may in some patients rekindle emotions they associated with the previous trauma or surgery.[125] Psychological maladjustment is an uncommon complication despite the significant physical deformity that occurs with tissue expansion.[126]

Ischemia or Necrosis

Previous tissue insults such as irradiation and compromised tissue perfusion with peripheral vascular disease or diabetes can predispose to flap necrosis. If expansion is too vigorous or too prolonged, ischemia can occur. Pain usually prevents this from happening. Excess saline should be removed from the implant in cases where overexpansion occurs.

Tissue expansion has the same effect on the flap as a delay procedure. Epinephrine has an adverse effect on delayed flaps.[127] Several cases of expanded flap death have been reported, all associated with the use of epinephrine solution injected during the insetting of previously expanded flaps.[125] The pathophysiology of this phenomenon is poorly understood. Epinephrine, however, should be avoided during reconstruction at the time of removal of the expander.

Pain

Pain during tissue expansion occurs in association with the tenseness of expanded skin at the limit of expansion when the lack of capillary refill signals the need to withdraw a few milliliters of saline.[123,128] In the head and neck region, the temporal area and the posterior occiput are the most common sites where pain occurs with expansion.[126] Pain usually decreases 4 to 6 hours after expansion with reduced tenseness of the expanded skin 8 to 12 hours after expansion.[129]

Compromise of Adjacent Structures

Impairment of nerve function in the area adjacent to the expansion is uncommon. Successful expansion has been carried out over the facial nerve. Large volume or rapid expansion can produce nerve compression. If neuropraxia occurs, the prosthesis should be deflated and more gradual expansion undertaken.[122] If it recurs, the implant should be removed.

Expansion adjacent to the great vessels of the neck has been undertaken without erosion or cerebral ischemia. In patients who have undergone a previous radical neck dissection and had radiation treatment, the vessel wall can be compromised. Tissue expansion should be avoided in these situations.

Bone resorption during scalp and forehead skin expansion has been observed on occasion.[130,131] This is associated with prolonged implant placement with large volume expanders (400 mL or greater). The outer cortex of the calvarium is resorbed. The use of a scalp expander in the pediatric age group should be avoided until the fontanelles are closed.[131] The depression on the underlying bone created by the implant resolves with time.

IMPLANTS AND FILLER AGENTS

Multiple implants and filler materials have been developed over the years, both alloplastic and autologous, none of which is universally applicable. Most of these materials will provide adequate short-term results; however, resorption is a common fate after a period of more than 6 months. Complication rates for this procedure have been relatively low. Each individual compound has its own inherent adverse effects.

Autologous Materials

Common autologous materials employed in facial plastic surgery are fat, fascia, muscle, dermal gaft, cartilage, bone, and recently autologous collagen (Autogenesis Technologies, Inc). All can be used as either implant or filler. For facial augmentation, the benefit of these materials is the absence of allergic reaction from the body. Many of the materials can be used with a vascular pedicle, therefore increasing survival, for example, temporalis fascia flaps or free pedicle bone grafts.

The most common complication after gafting is hematoma and wound infection. The incidence has been reported as 5% to 14%.[132] The use of prophylactic antibiotics is helpful with any of these materials. Resorption is a common observation with free nonvascularized grafts (Fig. 17–12). The long-term results for free autologous grafts have been disappointing. The long-term survival rate for fat obtained with atraumatic techniques is 50% and this decreased to 20% if the fat had been manipulated.[133] With dermal grafts there is the possibility of epidermoid cyst formation which can lead to the formation of a sinus tract. Careful de-epithelialization of the graft can be undertaken with the carbon dioxide laser.[134] If a sinus tract occurs, excision is indicated. Survival for free septal or conchal cartilage grafts has been excellent with minimal resorption over time.[135,136]

Extrusion is not a common problem with any of the autologous materials; however, if there is a sign of infection with or without hematoma, the nonvascularized graft should be removed.

Malposition of any of the gaft material is possible. Careful preoperative aesthetic evaluation and meticulous surgical technique can avoid this problem. If this occurs, removal or readjustment of the gafting material will be indicated.

Within the past year, autologous collagen has been popularized.[137] Initial studies indicate a favorable result, with less overcorrecting. Longer-term follow-up will be necessary.

Alloplastic Materials

Many different alloplastic materials have been developed for maxillofacial augmentation. This group can be divided into metals such as titanium, polymers such as silicone, ceramics such as hydroxyapatite, and biologic materials such as collagen. The implants are usually made up of the materials from the first three groups and filler materials from the last group. In facial plastic surgery the majority of implants are derivatives of polydimethylsiloxane (silicone). The use of injectable silicone is no longer approved by the Federal Drug Administration (FDA) and will not be discussed.

The complications of facial augmentation include displacement, misalignment, infection, and hematoma formation. Misalignment occurs in 15% to 20% of patients.[137] This is due to either a misaligned pocket in the subcutaneous or subperiosteal plane or the size of the initial pocket being too large. Treatment for this problem is realignment. Perioperative antibiotics markedly decrease the incidence of infection. Meticulous hemostasis will avoid the formation of hematoma. If this occurs, incision and drainage will be necessary. Implants in the malar and chin region have the potential of injuring the infraorbital branch of the trigeminal nerve and the mental nerve, respectively. This can lead to hyper- or hypoesthesia of the specific region. With neuropraxia, the offending implant should be removed and an appropriate sized one reinserted without irritation of the nerve.[138]

The most popular filler material since 1978 has been bovine collagen. A few types Zyderm I, Zyderm II, and Zyplast have been developed. Zyplast is a glutaraldehyde cross-linked collagen, which makes it less susceptible to collagenase degradation and therefore is longer-lasting.[139] The most frequent adverse reaction to collagen injection is an allergic response. Skin testing is used to detect both humoral and cellular immunity to the bovine collagen. The incidence of a treatment site reaction after a single negative skin test ranged from 1%

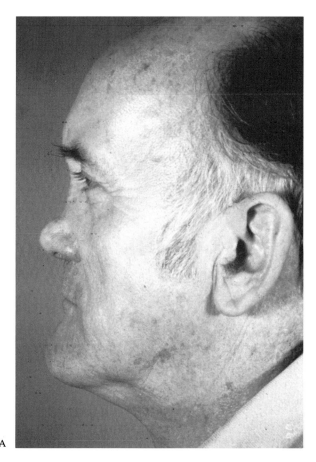 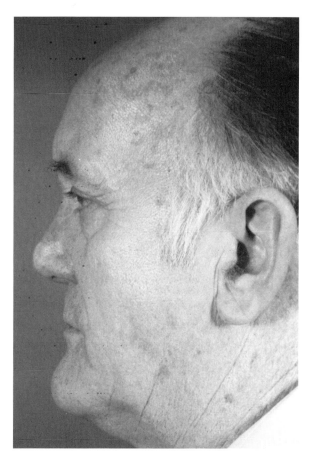

Figure 17–12. **(A).** Patient postoperative two previous augmentation procedures of iliac bone graft and septal cartilage. **(B).** Patient 3 years postoperative augmentation with mesh material previously implanted over mastoid area.

to 5%.[140] All allergic reactions to collagen are manifested by erythema and induration, with or without pruritus. Usually, all the treatment sites will react, but sometimes only one site may show a reaction.[141] This may be related to the development of delayed hypersensitivity.[142] The induration may require several months before resolution. Systemic symptoms such as arthralgia, arthritis, fever, and urticaria rarely occur, and usually are a manifestation of the immune response, which is usually self-limiting and managed symptomatically.[143] The potential for autoimmune cross-reactivity to human collagen has not been substantiated.[144] To detect the development of a reaction from exposure to the initial skin test dose, a second (double) skin test may be done. This will detect the development of a reaction from exposure to the initial skin test dose. Although double skin testing is not required, it has become routine for many practitioners.[145] The best treatment for skin reactions is reassurance, allowing them to naturally resolve. Antipruritic and antiinflammatory regimens, either steroid or nonsteroidal, may be helpful for short-term relief.

A second type of reaction is characterized by intermittent swelling limited to only some of the treatment sites. This response is not accompanied by an elevation of anti-Zyderm antibodies. This reaction occurs in 1% of patients. The swelling is precipitated by exercise, sun exposure, menstruation, or intake of alcohol. No treatment is necessary for this problem; however, the patient should be informed that the swelling can recur and last as long as a few months.[146]

One episode of unilateral partial blindness has been reported with injection of collagen for correction of glabellar creases.[145] Occlusion of the retinal artery after injection of the implant material into a communicating vessel in the glabellar region was the proposed etiology. Careful intradermal placement of collagen, especially in the glabellar region, cannot be overemphasized.

Overcorrection of the facial defects is due to excessive injection of the collagen. This is more common with Zyderm II and Zyplast. The patient should be reassured that with time this will gradually settle. If the collagen is not injected into the proper plane, that is, the dermis, it can lead to compression of skin vascular supply and necrosis at the injection site. Scarring can result with unfavorable results.

Angioedema has been reported in a patient after her third collagen injection.[146] The symptom subsided with time. The causal relationship between the collagen injection and this reaction is difficult to ascertain.

REFERENCES

1. Aarstad RF, Hoasjoe DK, Stucker FJ. A comparison of blood loss during aesthetic facial surgery using local vs general anesthesia. In press.

2. Cruse PJ. Prospective study of 20,105 surgical wounds with emphasis on use of topical antibiotics and prophylactic antibiotics. Presented at the 4th Symposium on Control of Surgical Infections; November 10, 1972; Washington, DC.

3. Serepian R, Reynolds BM. Wound infections after preoperative depilatory versus razor preparation. *Am J Surg.* 1971: 121–251.

4. Burge TF. The effective period of preventive antibiotic action in experimental incisions and dermal lesions. *Surgery.* 1961;50:161–168.

5. Johnson JT, Myers EN, Sigler BA, Thearle PB, Schramm VL. Antimicrobial prophylaxis for contaminated head and neck surgery. *Laryngoscope.* 1984;94:46–51.

6. Piccart M, Dar P, Klostersky J. Antimicrobial prophylaxis of infections in head and neck cancer surgery. *Scand J Infect Dis.* 1983;39(suppl):92–96.

7. Churukian MM, Zempleny J, Sterner M, Kamer FM, Cahen A. Post-rhinoplasty epistaxis. *Arch Otolaryngol Head Neck Surg.* 1988;114:748–750.

8. Klabunde EH, Falces E. Incidence of complications in cosmetic rhinoplasties. *Plast Reconstr Surg.* 1964,34:192.

9. Flowers RS, Anderson R. Injury to the lacrimal apparatus during rhinoplasty. *Plast Reconstr Surg.* 1968;42:577.

10. Lacy GM, Conway H. Recovery after meningitis with convulsions and paralysis: cause for pause. *Plast Reconstr Surg.* 1965;36:254.

11. Lewin ML, Argamaso RV, Friedman S. Localized cerebritis following an esthetic rhinoplasty. *Plast Reconstr Surg.* 1979;64:720–723.

12. Kubik CS, Adams RD. Subdural empyema. *Brain.* 1943;66:18.

13. Casaubon JM, Dion MA, Larbrisseau A. Septic cavernous sinus thrombosis after rhinoplasty: case report. *Plast Reconstr Surg.* 1977;59:119–123.

14. Coursey DL. Staphylococcal endocarditis following septorhinoplasty. *Arch Otolaryngol Head Neck Surg.* 1974;99:454.

15. Toback J, Fayerman J. Toxic shock syndrome following septorhinoplasty. *Arch Otolaryngol Head Neck Surg.* 1983;109:627–629.

16. Jacobson JA, Kasworm EM. Toxic shock syndrome after nasal surgery. *Arch Otolaryngol Head Neck Surg.* 1986;112:329–332.

17. Wagner R, Toback J. Toxic shock syndrome following septoplasty using plastic septal splints. *Laryngoscope.* 1986;96:609–610.

18. Stucker FJ. Prevention of post-rhinoplasty edema. *Laryngoscope.* 1976;84:536–541.

19. Noe JM, Finley J, Rosen S, Arndt K. Post-rhinoplasty "red nose": differential diagnosis and treatment by laser. *Plast Reconstr Surg.* 1981;67:661–664.

20. Rees TD, Wood-Smith D. *Cosmetic Facial Surgery.* Philadelphia, Pa: WB Saunders Co; 1973.

21. Grocutt M, Chir B, Fatah MF. Recurrent multiple epidermal inclusion cysts following rhinoplasty—an unusual complication. *J Laryngol Otol.* 1989;103:1214–1216.

22. Shulman Y, Westreich M. Post-rhinoplasty mucous cyst of the nose. *Plast Reconstr Surg.* 1983;71:421–422.

23. Harley Eh, Erdman JP. Dorsal nasal cyst formation. *Arch Otolaryngol Head Neck Surg.* 1990;116:105–106.

24. Champion R. Anosmia associated with corrective rhinoplasty. *Br J Plast Surg.* 1966;19:182–185.

25. Goldwyn RM, Shone S. The effects of submucous resection and rhinoplsty on the sense of smell. *Plast Reconstr Surg.* 1968;41:427–432.

26. Flowers RS, Anderson R. Injury to the lacrimal apparatus during rhinoplasty. *Plast Reconstr Surg.* 1968;42:577–581.

27. Thomas JR, Griner N. The relationship of lateral osteotomies in rhinoplasty to the lacrimal drainage system. *Otolaryngol Head Neck Surg.* 1986;94:362–367.

28. Lawson W, Kessler S, Biller HF. Unusual and fatal complications of rhinoplasty. *Arch Otolaryngol* 1983;109:164–169.

29. Chevey ML, Blair PA. Blindness as a complication of rhinoplasty. *Arch Otolaryngol Head Neck Surg.* 1987;113:768, 769.

30. Hallock GG, Trier WC. Cerebrospinal fluid rhinorrhea following rhinoplsty. *Plast Reconstr Surg.* 1983;71:109–113.

31. Marshall DR, Slattery PG. Intracranial complications of rhinoplsty. *Br J Plast Surg.* 1983;36:342–344.

32. Song IC, Bromberg BE. Carotid cavernous sinus fistula occurring after a rhinoplasty. *Plast Reconstr Surg.* 1975;55:92–96.

33. Stucker FJ, Bryarly RC, Shockley WW. *Plastic and Reconstructive Surgery of the Head and Neck.* Vol. 1. St Louis, Mo: CV Mosby Co; 156–160.

34. Sacks ME. Post-rhinoplastic nasal obstruction. *Otolaryngol Clin. North Am.* 1989;22:319–332.

35. Keith JD, Bytell DE. Revision in unsuccessful rhinoplasty. *Otolaryngol Clin North Am.* 1974;7:1:65–74.

36. Stucker, FJ, Smith TE. The nasal bony dorsum and cartilaginous vault. *Arch Otolaryngol Head Neck Surg.* 1976;102:695–698.

37. Forman S. *Cosmetic Surgery, Principles, and Practice.* Philadelphia, Pa: JB Lippincott, Co; 1960.

38. Wright WK. Study on hump removal in rhinoplasty. *Laryngoscope.* 1967;77:508–517.

39. Kamer FM, Churukian MM, Hansen L. The nasal bossa: a complication of rhinoplasty. *Laryngoscope.* 1986;96:303–307.

40. Matarasso A. The oculocardiac reflex in blepharoplasty surgery. *Plast Reconstr Surg.* 83:243–248.

41. Beeson, WH, McCollough EG. *Aesthetic Surgery of the Aging Face.* St Louis, Mo: CV Mosby Co; 1986.

42. Allen MV, Cohen KL, Grimson BS. Orbital cellulitis secondary to dacrocystitis following blepharoplasty. *Ann Ophthalmol.* 1985;17:498, 499.

43. Rees TD, Craig SM, Fisher, Y. Orbital abscess following blepharoplasty. *Plast Reconstr Surg.* 1984;73:126, 127.

44. Conley JJ. *Complications of Head and Neck Surgery.* Philadelphia, Pa: WB Saunders Co; 1979.

45. Levine MR. Prevention and management of complications of blepharoplasty. *Facial Plast Surg.* 1984;4:311–321.

46. Edgarton MT. Causes and prevention of lower lid ectropion following blepharoplasty. *Plast Reconstr Surg.* 1972;49:367–373.

47. McGraw BL, Adamson PA. Post-blepharoplasty ectropion. *Arch Otolaryngol Head Neck Surg.* 1991;117:852–856.

48. Carraway JH, Mellow CG. The prevention and treatment of lower lid ectropion following blepharoplasty. *Plast Reconstr Surg.* 1990;85:971–981.

48. Hanley RD, Nelson LB, Flanagan JC, Calhoun JH. Ocular motility disturbances following cosmetic blepharoplasty. *Arch Ophthalmol.* 1986;104:542–544.

50. Millay DJ, Larrabee WF. Ptosis and blepharoplasty surgery. *Arch Otolaryngol Head Neck Surg.* 1989;115:198–201.

51. Jelks GW, McCord CD. Dry eye syndrome and other tear film abnormalities. *Clin Plast Surg.* 1981;8:803–810.

52. Green MF, Kadri SWM. Acute closed-angle glaucoma, a complication of blepharoplasty: report of a case. *Br J Plast Surg.* 1974;27:25.

53. Tessier P. Facelifting and frontal rhytidectomy. In: Ely JF, ed. *Transactions of the Seventh International Congress of Plastic and Reconstructive Surgery.* 1980.

54. Psillakis JM, Rumley TO, Camargos A. Subperiosteal approach, an improved concept for correction of the aging face. *Plast Reconstr Surg.* 1988;82:383.

55. Ramirez OM, Maillard GF, Musolas A. The extended subperiosteal facelift: a definitive soft tissue remodeling for facial rejuvenation. *Plast Reconstr Surg.* 1991;88:227–236.

56. Berman WE, Monell CM. Complications in blepharoplastics and facelift operations, *Otolaryngol Clin North Am.* 1974;7:87–105.

57. Ellenbogan R. Avoiding visual tipoffs to facelift surgery. *Clin Plast Surg.* 1992;19:447–454.

58. Lindgren VV. Problems and complications related to the earlobes. In: Gradinger K, ed. *Symposium on Problems and Complications in Aesthetic Plastic Surgery of the Face.* St. Louis, Mo: CV Mosby Co; 1984:295–304.

59. Rees TD, Aston SJ. Complications of rhytidectomy. *Clin Plast Surg.* 1978;5:109–119.

60. Bansberg SF, Krugman ME. Parotid salivary fistula following rhytidectomy. *Ann Plast Surg.* 1990;24:61, 62.

61. Guerrerosantos J, Dicksheet S. Cervicofacial rhytidoplasty in Ehler-Danlos syndrome: hazards on healing. *Plast Reconstr Surg.* 1985;75:100–103.

62. Schanur PL, Burkhardt BR, Tofield, JJ. The second-look technique in facelifts—does it work? *Plast Reconstr Surg.* 1980;65:298–301.

63. Goldwyn RM. Late bleeding after rhytidectomy from injury to the superficial temporal vessels. *Plast Reconstr Surg.* 1991;88:443–445.

64. Berner RE, Morain WD, Noe JM. Postoperative hypertension as an etiological factor in hematoma after rhytidectomy. *Plast Reconstr Surg.* 1976;57:314–319.

65. Rees TM, Liveretl DM, Guy CL. The effect of cigarette smoking on skin-flap survival on the facelift. *Plast Reconstr Surg.* 1984;73:911–915.

66. Castanares S. Facial nerve paralysis coincidental with/or subsequent to rhytidectomy. *Plast Reconstr Surg.* 1974;54:637.

67. Appaix A, Pech A, Garcin M, Rouvies P. La Chirurgie des oreilles duollees. *J Fr Orl Audiophol Chir Maxillo Fac.* 1968;17:385.

68. Adamson PA, McGraw BL, Troppin GJ. Otoplasty: critical review of clinical reslts. *Laryngoscope.* 1991;101:883–888.

69. Farrior RT. A method of otoplasty. *Arch Otolaryngol Head Neck Surg.* 1959;69:400.

70. Furnas DW. Correction of prominent ears by concha-mastoid sutures. *Plast Reconstr Surg.* 1968;42:189.

71. Mustarde' JC. The correction of prominent ears using simple mattress sutures. *Br J Plast Surg.* 1963;16:170.

72. Goode RL, Proffitt SD, Rafaty FM. Complications of otoplasty. *Arch Otolaryngol* 1970;91:352–355.

73. Elliott RA. Complications in the treatment of prominent ear. *Clin Plast Surg.* 1978;5:479.

74. Baker DC, Converse JM. Otoplasty: a twenty year retrospective. *Aesthetic Plast Surg.* 1979;2:36.

75. Adamson PA. Complications of otoplasty. *Ear Nose Throat J.* 1985;64:568–574.

76. Zohan T. Otoplasty (ett). *Arch Otolaryngol Head Neck Surg.* 1972;96:187.

77. Rigg BM. Suture materials in otoplasty. *Plast Reconstr Surg.* 1979;63:409–440.

78. Stucker FJ, Shaw GY. Management of keloids and hypetrophic scars. In: Papel I, ed. *Plast Surgery of the Face.* Chicago, Ill: Year Book Medical Publishers; 1992.

79. Spiva M. Reduction otoplasty. In: Goldwyn RM, ed. *The Unfavorable Results in Plastic Surgery: Avoidance and Treatment.* Boston, Mass: Little Brown & Co; 1984:307.

80. Stucker FJ, Christianse TA. The lateral conchal resection otoplasty, *Laryngoscope.* 1977;87:58–62.

81. Fenerstein SS. Revision techniques in otoplasty: evaluation and management, symposium on revision surgery in otorhinolaryngology. *Otolaryngol Clin North Am.* 1974;7:133.

82. Webster RC, Smith RC. Otoplasty for prominent ears. In: Goldwyn RM, ed. *Long-Term Results in Plastic and Reconstructive Surgery.* Boston, Mass: Little Brown & Co; 1980:146.

83. Teimourian B, Rogers WB. A national survey of complications associated with suction lipectomy: a comparative study. *Plast Reconstr Surg.* 1989;84:628–631.

84. Dolsky RL. Blood loss during liposuction. *Dermatol Clin.* 1990;8:463–468.

85. Newman J, Dolsky RL. Evaluation of 5,458 cases of liposuction surgery. *Am J Cosmetic Surg.* 1984;1:25.

86. Hanke WC, Lee MW, Bernstein G. The safety of dermatologic liposuction surgery. *Dermatol Clin.* 1990;8:563–568.

87. Pitman GH, Teimourian B. Suction lipectomy: complications and results by survey. *Plast Reconstr Surg.* 1985;76:65.

88. Teimourian B. Complications associated with suction lipectomy. *Clin Plast Surg.* 1989;16:385.

89. Pitman GH, Teimourian B. Suction lipectomy: complications and results by survey. *Plast Reconstr Surg.* 1985;76:65–69.

90. Goddio AS. Skin retraction follow-up suction lipectomy by treatment site: a study of 500 procedures in 458 selected subjects. *Plast Reconstr Surgb.* 1991;87:66–75.

91. Courtiss EH, Donelan MS. Skin sensation after suction lipectomy: a prospective study of 50 consecutive patients. *Plast Reconstr Surg.* 1988;81:550.

92. Stegman SJ. A comparative histologic study of the effects of three peeling agents and dermabrasion on normal and sun damaged skin. *Aesthetic Plast Surg.* 1982;6:123.

93. Wexler, MR, Halon DA, Teitelbaum A, et al. The prevention of cardiac arrhymthmias produced in an animal model by the topical application of a phenol prepartion in common use for face peeling. *Plast Reconstr Surg.* 1984;73:595.

94. Litton C, Szachowicy EH, Trinidad GP. Present day status of the chemical peel. *Aesthetic Plast Surg.* 1986;10:1.

95. Matarasso SL, Glogan RG. Chemical face peels. *Dermatol Clin.* 1991;9:131–150.

96. Truppman ES, Ellenby JD. Major electrocardiographic changes during chemical face peeling. *Plast Reconstr Surg.* 1979;63:44.

97. Kligman A, Willis I. A new formula for depigmenting human skin. *Arch Dermatol.* 1975;111:40.

98. Mandy SH, Landsman L. Dermabrasion and chemical peel. In: Papel ID, Nachalas NE, eds. *Facial Plastic and Reconstructive Surgery.* St Louis, Mo: Mosby Year Book; 1992.

99. Litton C, Trinidad G. Complications of chemical face peeling as evaluated by a questionnaire. *Plast Reconstr Surg.* 1981;67:738.

100. McCollough EG, Beeson WH. Chemical peel. In: Beeson WH, McCollough EG, eds. *Aesthetic Surgery of the Aging Face.* St Louis, Mo: CV Mosby Co; 1986:182.

101. Wojno T, Tenzel RR. Lower eyelid ectropion following chemical face peeling. *Ophthalmic Surg.* 1984;15:596, 597.

102. LoVerne WE, Drapkin MS, Courtiss EH. et al. Toxic shock syndrome after chemical face peel. *Plast Reconstr Surg.* 1987;80:115–118.

103. Dmytryshyn JR, Gribble MJ, Kassen BO. Chemical face peel complicated by toxic shock syndrome. *Arch Otolaryngol.* 1983;109:179.

104. Roenick HH Jr. Dermabrasion: state of the art. *J Dermatol Surg Oncol.* 1985;11:306–314.

105. Mandy SH. Tretinoin in the pre and postoperative management of dermabrasion. *J Am Acad Dermatol.* 1986;15:878.

106. Fulton JE, Jr. The prevention and management of post-dermabrasion complications. *J Dermatol Surg Oncol.* 1991;17:431–437.

107. Stegman SJ. A study of dermabrasion and chemical peels in animal model. *J Dermatol Surg Oncol.* 1986;6:490.

108. Moy R, Zitelli J, Vitto J. Effect of 13 cisretrinoic on dermal wound healing. *J Invest Dermatol.* 1987;88:508.

109. Rubenstein R, Roenigk HH, Jr. Atypical keloids after dermabrasion of patients taking isotretinoin. *J Am Acad Dermatol.* 1986;15:280.

110. Hanke CW, O'Brien JJ. A histologic evaluation of the effects of skin refrigerant on animal model. *J Dermatol Surg Oncol.* 1987;13:644.

111. Hanke CW, O'Brien JJ, Solow Eb. Laboratory evaluation of skin refrigerants used in dermabrasion. *J Dermatol Surg Oncol.* 1985;11:45.

112. Hanke CW, Roenigk HH, Pinske JB. Complications of dermabrasion resulting from excessive cold skin refrigerants. *J Dermatol Surg Oncol.* 1985;11:896.

113. Alt TH. Dermabrasion. In Krause CJ, Mangat DS, Pastorek N, eds. *Aesthetic Facial Surgery.* Philadelphia, Pa: JB Lippincott Co; 1991.

114. Yarborough JM, Jr, Beeson WH. Dermabrasion. In: Beeson WH, McCollough EG, eds. *Aesthetic Surgery of the Aging Face.* St Louis, Mo: CV Mosby Co; 1986:142.

115. Radovan C. Adjacent flap development using expandible silastic implant. Presented at the annual meeting of the American Society of Plastic and Reconstructive Surgeons; 1976; Boston, Mass.

116. Masser, MR. Tissue expansion: a reconstructive revolution or a cornucopia of complications? *Br J Plast Surg.* 1990;43:344–348.

117. Mander EK, Oask TE, An VK, et al: Soft tissue expansion in the lower extremities. *Plast Reconstr Surg.* 1988;81:208.

118. Buhrer, DP, Huang, TT, Yee HW, Blackwell, SJ. Treatment of burn alopecia with tissue expanders in children. *Plast Reconstr Surg.* 1988;81:512.

119. Antonyshyn O, Grass JS, Zuken R, Mackinnon SE. Tissue expansion in head and neck reconstruction. *Plast Reconstr Surg.* 1988;82:58–68.

120. Sasaki G. Complications in tissue expansion. Presented at the annual meeting of The American Society of Plastic and Reconstructive Surgeons; October 1986; Los Angeles, Calif.

121. Baker SR, Swanson NA. Tissue expansion of the head and neck: indications, technique, and complications, *Arch Otolaryngol Head Neck Surg.* 1990;116:1147–1153.

122. Argenta LC, Aaustad ED. Principles and techniques of tissue expansion. In McCarthy JG, ed. *Plastic Surgery 1.* Philadelphia, Pa: WB Saunders Co; 1990.

123. Manders EK, Schenden MJ, Funey JA, et al. Soft tissue expansion: concepts and complications. *Reconstr Surg.* 1984;74:493–507.

124. Argenta LC, Marks MW, Pasyk, KA. Effects of rate of tissue expansion on the creation of new tissue. *Surg Forum Plast Surg.* 1987;38:591–593.

125. Austad ED. Complications in tissue expansion. *Clin Plast Surg.* 14:549–550.

126. Argenta LC, Marks MW, Pasyk KA. 1985;12:159–171.

127. Reinisch J, Myers B. The effect of local anesthesia with epinephrine on skin flap survival. *Plast Reconstr Surg.* 1974;54:324.

128. Dickson WA, Sharpe DT, Jackson IT. Experience with an external valve in small volume tissue expanders. *Br J Plast Surg.* 1988;41:373–377.

129. Marcus J, Horan DB, Robinson JK. Tissue expansion: past, present, and future. *J Am Acad Dermatol.* 1990;12: 813–825.

130. Leighton WD, Johnson ML, Friedland JA. Use of the temporary soft tissue expander in post-traumatic alopecia. *Plast Reconstr Surg.* 1986;77:737–742.

131. Maves MD, Lusk RP. Tissue expansion in the treatment of giant congenital melanocytic nevi. *Arch Otolaryngol Head Neck Surg.* 1987;113:987–991.

132. Vihlein A, Jr. Use of the cutis graft in plastic operations. *Arch Surg.* 1939;38:118.

133. Churukian MM. Autologous fat injection. In: Papel ID, Nachalas NE, eds. *Facial Plastic and Reconstructive Surgery.* St Louis, Mo: CV Mosby Co; 1991.

134. Shockley WW, Stucker FJ. Dermal grafts and flaps in facial augmentation. *Facial Plast Surg.* 1986;3:75–80.

135. Sheer JH. *Aesthetic Rhinoplasty.* 2nd ed. St. Louis, Mo: CV Mosby Co; 1987.

136. Brent B. Auricular repair with a cochal cartilage graft. In: Brent B, ed. *The Artistry of Reconstructive Surgery.* St Louis, Mo: CV Mosby Co; 1987.

137. Fagien S. Soft tissue augmentation with autologous injectable dermis. Presented at American Academy of Facial Plastic and Reconstructive Surgery Winter Meeting; January 1993; Boca Raton, Fla.

138. Schoenrock LD. Malarplasty. In: Krause CJ, Pastorek N, Magort DS, eds. *Aesthetic Facial Surgery.* Philadelphia, Pa: JB Lippincott Co; 1991.

139. Kligman AM, Armstrong RC. Histologic response to intradermal zyderm and zyplast (glutaldehyde cross-linked) collagen in humans. *J Dermatol Surg Oncol.* 1986;12:351.

140. McCoy JP, Schade WJ, Siegle RJ, et al. Characterization of the humoral immune response to bovine collagen implants. *Arch Dermatol.* 1985;121:990.

141. Stegman SJ, Tromovitch TA, Hogan RF. Filling agents. In: Stegman SJ, Tromovitch TA, Hogan RG, eds. *Cosmetic Dermatologic Surgery.* Chicago, Ill: Year Book Medical Publishers; 1990.

142. Cooperman L, Michael D. The immunogenicity of injectable collagen. I. A one year prospective study. *J Am Acad Dermatol.* 1984;10:638.

143. Baker TJ, Stuyin JM. Chemical peeling and dermabrasion. In: McCarthy, ed. *Plastic Surgery.* Philadelphia, Pa: WB Saunders Co; 1990.

144. Cohen IK, Peacock EE, Chapil M. Zyderm (letter). *Plast Reconstr Surg.* 1984;73:857.

145. Sleonge JW, Divan RV. Soft tissue augmentation with injectable collagen. In: Papel ID, Nachalas NE, eds. *Facial Plastic and Reconstructive Surgery.* St Louis, Mo: Mosby Year Book; 1992.

146. Kamer FM, Churukian MM. Clinical use of injectable collagen: a three year retrospective review. *Arch Otolaryngol Head Neck Surg.* 1984;110:93–98.

18 Complications of Reconstructive Flaps

Richard F. Debo, M.D., Paul A. Levine, M.D.

Advances in tissue transfer now permit us to reconstruct defects from large soft tissue resections with vascularized, multicomponent tissue. Closure of these complex defects requires the transfer of tissue from other regions of the body to resurface skin or mucosal defects, to restore function, to protect major vascular structures, and to augment the appearance and restore bone support of regional deficiencies. The choices of wound closure are based on the functional, cosmetic, and oncologic requirements of the defect created.

A variety of reconstructive techniques are available to the head and neck surgeon ranging from simple split thickness skin grafting to complex microvascular tissue transfer. Careful analysis of the advantages versus the potential complications and morbidity of each repair must be considered before selecting the best method of reconstruction in each particular patient. Factors influencing this decision include the knowledge and technical skills of the surgeon, the anatomic and cosmetic necessity of the defect, oncologic considerations, and the intrinsic and extrinsic factors that affect wound healing. Complications from reconstruction are related to factors that adversely affect wound healing or compromise blood flow to the flap. Although some complications may be related to the recipient tissue bed of the host and his general medical condition, most can be avoided by careful preoperative planning and surgical technique.

OPERATIVE PLANNING

The unique characteristics of each patient and defect are important when planning the reconstruction. A myriad of patient factors such as age, gender, occupation, functional and cosmetic needs, medical condition, nutrition, previous irradiation, skin type, and psychological makeup must be considered in addition to the physical characteristics of the defect.

Facial appearance and body image are important; however, patients' age, sex, and psychosocial background may strongly influence their perception of a successful repair. What may be cosmetically and functionally acceptable for one patient may be unacceptable for another. Particularly in the facial region, appearance should be given appropriate recognition.

The flap should be carefully planned to minimize scarring. Incisions should be placed in relaxed skin tension lines, tissue should (when possible) be replaced with tissue of similar color, bulk, and texture, and cosmetic units should be respected. Adequate preoperative education of the patient about the anticipated results and potential complications of the repair are important to ensure that a satisfactory result is appreciated by both the patient and the surgeon.

The defect to be closed must be evaluated for bulk, size, type of tissue needed (ie, skin, muscle, or bone), and coverage required. It is also important to know the type and quality of the tissue in the recipient bed because, for example, closure of a mucosally lined surface is associated with a higher complication rate owing to bacterial contamination.

Many factors contribute to flap complications and are divided by Kerrigan[1] into two groups, extrinsic and intrinsic. The extrinsic factors include systemic conditions that might adversely affect wound healing and local conditions or mechanical factors that predispose to complications. These include reversible hematologic disorders, medical problems that predispose to delayed wound healing (such as diabetes, malnutrition, or atherosclerosis), or a history suggestive of microvascular injury or spasm (such as previous high-dose radiation therapy or recent smoking history). Most head and neck cancer patients are ardent smokers, and this is associated with increased flap complications.[2] The intrinsic factor responsible for flap complications is inadequate nutrient blood flow.

Any past medical history or family history suggestive of a bleeding diathesis should be evaluated preoperatively. The best single screening test to evaluate whether a bleeding disorder exists is a bleeding time. Additional testing will depend on the outcome of the medical history or an abnormal bleeding time. When taking a medical history one must not forget to inquire about over-the-counter medications. Excessive bleeding can create a hematoma that can apply pressure to the vascular pedicle, create a nidus for infection, and result in flap ischemia and wound breakdown. Patients with hypercoagulable states such as polycythemia may also jeopardize the arterial supply.

Malnutrition

Malnutrition is a common cause of delayed wound healing and increased complications because of the body's reduced reserve for protein synthesis and immunologic protection. Excessive alcohol ingestion and poor alimentation, related to the local and systemic effects of the tumor, place head and neck cancer patients at high risk. Adding these factors to the resection of the contaminated pharynx creates a significant potential for infection and wound breakdown.

Prevention of this begins with recognition of the patient in need of aggressive nutritional support. Clinical data such as excessive weight loss, severe dysphagia, and decreased energy level obtained from the patient's history, along with physical findings such as temporal wasting, loss of tissue turgor, and interdigital wasting will frequently indicate which patients are in need of more complete evaluation. A nutritional workup includes assessment of the patients' clinical, anthropomorphic, biochemical, and immunologic parameters. If there is a 10% weight loss or more these patients deserve a nutritional evaluation. Although a 20% decrease in weight has been associated with an increased risk of postoperative mortality, weight loss itself is one of the least reliable factors for predicting nutritional status because of the wide fluctuations that can occur from fluid shifts. Despite this, it is still a useful, easily obtainable indicator of the need for a more indepth evaluation.

Anthropomorphic measurements estimate the patients' fat stores and skeletal muscle mass providing an indication of nutritional status. Standard measurements include the triceps skinfold test and the midarm muscle circumference. Visceral proteins can be estimated by measuring serum albumin, prealbumin, and transferrin levels. Although the value serum albumin is more commonly used, it has a half-life of 20 days and responds slowly to changes in nutritional status. Patients with a serum albumin value of 3.5 mg/dL or higher have a decreased surgical mortality and fewer postoperative complications.[3] Serum transferrin has a half-life of 8 days and prealbumin has a half-life of 2 days, making them more sensitive indicators of nutritional status. Downward changes in the concentrations of these proteins are seen with severe or prolonged malnutrition but also are affected by age, hepatic and renal disease, iron status, total body water, and stress. Prealbumin, because of its short half-life and small pool size, is more susceptible to early changes in nutrition.[4]

Studies by Slade et al[5] and Daly et al[6] demonstrated the relationship between malnutrition and immunocompetence. Total lymphocyte counts of less than 1200-MM[3] are associated with an impaired immune response. This can be further defined by delayed hypersensitivity testing with recall antigens such as *Candida*, *Trichophyton*, streptokinase-streptodornase, and purified protein derivative (PPD). Meakins et al[7] and Christou and Meakins[8] showed an increased risk of infectious complications and mortality in anergic surgical patients. However, patients who were anergic but became reactive during therapy showed reduced mortality rates.[9]

Radiation Effects on Wound Healing

Patients who have undergone radiation therapy at tumoricidal doses (ie, 60 to 75 Gy) are more likely to have delayed healing and increased complications. The effects of radiation therapy on wound healing are directly related to the dose of radiation administered, treatment frequency, and inversely related to vessel size. As the vessel caliber decreases, the effects of the radiation become more pronounced owing endothelial fibrosis. These changes are dose dependent with little effect being observed below 10 Gy in divided doses.[10]

Acute and chronic skin changes occur after exposure to radiation therapy. The acute effects are observed during and for several weeks after the administration of radiation therapy. The capillaries, small arterioles, and, at times, the venules and lymphatics, exhibit dilation and congestion. As the radiation dosage increases, the injury becomes more severe, and endothelial cells swell and cause capillary obstruction. Some capillaries remain dilated and allow increased leakage of fluid to the interstitium, which becomes edematous and infiltrated by erythrocytes and leukocytes.[11] It is for this reason that it is best to wait 4 to 6 weeks before surgery in a patient who has received planned preoperative radiotherapy.

On completion of radiation therapy the acute inflammatory reaction subsides, the vascular and connective tissue injuries persist, and there is a continuum of change. About 4 to 6 months after completion of radiation, the small vessels demonstrate a progressive and irreversible obliteration and decrease in the number of capillaries.[11] Arterioles and arteries also undergo progressive vascular sclerosis and even large arteries have accelerated development of atherosclerosis.[12] Because of this, operating on a patient 4 to 6 months after a curative radiation dose is frought with substantial healing complications. A gradual increase in the amount of fibrosis in the irradiated tissues develops resulting in decreased compliance and tissue ischemia. The wound edges may suffer ischemic necrosis, particularly when under tension. These fibrotic changes may stabilize after many months, but the tissues remain poorly vascularized and ischemic.

Although preoperative radiation therapy may have a deleterious tissue effect, it can be controlled. The period of least effect appears to be dose dependent. For moderate doses of radiation, the delay in healing probably reaches a plateau with a radiation to surgery interval of 2 to 3 weeks. The 5-4-4 rule is a good guideline for the delivery of preoperative radiation therapy for head and neck cancer patients. The radiation should be delivered in a divided dose schedule to the patient over a 5-week period, followed by a 4-week rest period to allow the acute effects of the radiation to subside, but before the onset of decreased vascularity from the endothelial fibrosis. There then follows a 4-week window of opportunity for surgery.

The effects of radiation play a more significant role in the healing of flaps whose blood supply is dependent on the delicate microvasculature of the dermal-subdermal plexus.[13] Flaps with an axial blood supply are more resistant to the effects of radiation therapy. Faucher et al[14] reviewed their series of 311 flaps and demonstrated no difference in healing between axial cutaneous versus myocutaneous flaps. They did report a 87.5 versus 65.2% complete healing rate for flap repairs without and with radiation therapy, respectively. Not surprisingly, radiation doses greater than 60 Gy and surgery performed more than 2 months after completion of radiotherapy demonstrated a significantly higher incidence of complications.[14,15] Some controversy persists, however, as other studies have noted no increased incidence of complications with preoperative radiotherapy and the use of pectoralis musculocutaneous flaps.[16-20]

Mechanical Factors

Mechanical factors that adversely affect wound healing include tension across the suture line, gravity, poor placement of incisions, and inappropriate flap design. Tension of the wound closure has a complex relationship with wound healing. Generally, flaps used in reconstruction should be designed to be large enough and have a long enough pedicle to close the defect without excessive stress. This reduces the risk of wound dehiscence, widening of the scar,[21] and, especially for longer flaps, distal flap necrosis.[22] Planning should consider the location of incisions so that they are situated in skin creases to camouflage the scar. Avoid placing the pedicle in a position where it requires an extreme arc of rotation that may result in kinking of the pedicle and compromise of the vascular supply. Flaps with a vascular pedicle higher than their distal tip after rotation (ie, nasolabial and forehead flaps) may develop venous congestion and lymphedema because of their dependent position. Without proper support, gravity may cause increased tension on the superior wound edge of larger flaps.

INTRINSIC FACTORS AFFECTING FLAP HEALING

"Flaps survive by virtue of their blood supply."[23] Therefore, a thorough knowledge of the anatomy of the flap is required. This includes its vascular pedicle, the proper tissue plane of elevation to avoid injury to the blood supply, and a familiarity with potential anatomic pitfalls. The basis for the blood supply to a majority of the head and neck reconstructive flaps is either directly from cutaneous arteries or from perforating vessels arising from the underlying musculature.

FLAP VIABILITY

Skin flap failure represents the culmination of a number of interrelated ischemic events that result in arteriolar insufficiency and loss of nutrient capillary perfusion.[24] A variety of techniques have been tried to improve flap viability and resuscitate failing flaps. These methods include cooling, pharmacological manipulation of the flap blood flow, hyperbaric

oxygen, and flap delay. The efficacy of these manipulations remains controversial.

Delay Phenomena

Of the many methods that have been tried to improve flap viability, surgical delay is the most effective means of increasing survival for random or axially based skin flaps. This does not have much benefit for hardier flaps such as the pectoralis major myocutaneous flap, which carries with it a more robust vascular pedicle and its muscular perforating branches to supply the skin. Delay of a flap involves its elevation prior to transfer then returning it to its original bed. The initial elevation of the flap disrupts the sympathetic innervation to the skin, opening arteriovenous shunts and decreasing nutrient blood supply to the distal flap.[25] In 14 to 21 days spontaneous closure of these shunts occurs, leading to improved perfusion and flap viability. Although a number of investigators have questioned the advantages of flap delay,[25-28] clinically it has proven to be helpful in those patients with potentially poor small vessel tissue perfusion.

Pharmacological Manipulation

The importance of the vascular pedicle to flap survival has prompted considerable interest in pharmacological manipulation of flap perfusion. Kerrigan and Daniel[29] viewed the data regarding these studies. They divided the medications studied into four groups: sympatholytics, direct vasodilators, agents that alter blood flow characteristics, and medications that increase flap tolerance to ischemia (Table 18-1). The benefit of these pharmacological manipulations remains controversial. Additional work with these agents must be done to determine dosages, schedules, duration of therapy, and efficacy before they can be of reliable clinical benefit.

Cooling

Kiehn and Desprez[30,31] demonstrated in the early 1960s that cooling of pedicled skin flaps in a rabbit model enhanced viability by delaying the onset and reducing the severity of necrosis. This is accomplished by the effects of the local hypothermia alter skin circulation, reduce lymphatic flow, and reduce cellular metabolism. Local cooling of wounds for

Table 18-1. Methods to Improve Flap Survival

Sympatholytics	Phenoxybenzamine, reserpine, 6-OH dopa, propanolol, guanethidine
Direct vasodilators	Topical dimethylsulfoxide, histamine, hydralazine, isoxsuprine, prostaglandin inhibitors
Blood flow alteration	Pentoxifylline, heparin, dextran, induced anemia, protein depletion
Improved ischemia tolerance	Steroids, hyperbaric oxygen, topical flamazine

From Kerrigan and Daniel.[29]

72 hours does not appear to have a detrimental effect on the early or acute phase of wound healing but does inhibit epithelial repair and collagen deposition for the duration of its application.[32] This a rapidly reversible effect. The chronic inflammatory reaction of later wound healing cleans up the edges of the wound preparing it for repair. This cleansing action can potentially destroy more than is necessary[33] and adversely affect wound healing. Cooling delays this late inflammatory phase enhancing the early phase of wound healing.[32]

RANDOM PATTERN FLAPS

Smaller facial defects are often reconstructed by local flaps because of their ease of application, defect proximity, and ability to provide skin of similar color, texture, and thickness. The viability of these flaps is dependent on the dermal-subdermal vascular plexus. The blood supply of random flaps is not derived from a finite vessel, but rather from the extensive vascular network of the head and neck skin. Mechanical factors such as tension, gravity, and pedicle location are important considerations. Pressure on the pedicle from excessive rotation of the flap, tight dressings, hematoma, and infections can lead to vascular compromise, resulting in partial or full thickness necrosis of the flap secondary to ischemia or venous congestion.

The physical properties of the dermal-subdermal plexus limit random flap dimensions to a length to width ratio of no greater than 2:1. Longer flaps are more susceptible to the effects of high-tension closure than are shorter, more well-vascularized flaps.[22,34,35] A simplified explanation for this is that the hydrostatic pressure in the small dermal-subdermal vessels cannot overcome the hemodynamic resistance of longer flap.[36] Moderate undermining can help reduce this tension but wide undermining can injure the delicate vasculature.

Numerous techniques have been utilized to assess vascular perfusion of flaps. Clinical assessment of color, temperature, and capillary refill are the most reliable indicators of flap viability. A cool, pale flap suggests ischemia whereas a dark blue or purple color suggests venous congestion. If gentle dermal pressure shows good capillary refill within 5 seconds and the cut edges bleed freely, then the flap is probably viable. Another simple and clinically useful test of viability is dermal bleeding, which can be assessed by pricking the flap with a needle and observing the bleeding. Fluorescein dye injection and evaluation of the flap with a Woods lamp, as well as Laser doppler velocimetry, correlate well with flap survival[22,35] but are technically more complex and require special testing equipment.

AXIAL PATTERN FLAPS

Skin flap survival depends on adequate surface perfusion. Reconstruction of large defects of the head and neck frequently require transfer of greater amounts of tissue than can be adequately perfused by simply the dermal-subdermal plexus. Axial pattern flaps have a finite artery and vein preserved in the fascia beneath the skin, and the size of the flaps is not defined by the length to width ratio but by the length of the single axial vessel on which the flap is based. The axial pattern flap can also be extended for a short distance by relying on random pattern blood flow to supply the distal tip of the flap, so the ultimate surviving length of the flap is determined by the equilibrium between perfusion pressure and intravascular resistance. The line of demarcation of a flap may represent the point at which perfusion pressure drops below the critical closing pressure of the dermal arterioles.[37]

The blood supply must be recognized and preserved on flap elevation. Stretching or twisting of the pedicle can cause vascular spasm and ischemia. Factors that increase the likelihood of vascular spasm include debulking the proximal vascular pedicle of muscle or fat to create an island flap and transposing the unit in a direction 180° from the entrance of the vascular pedicle to the flap. Further, compression of the vascular pedicle by traction over a fixed bone, passage through a tight tunnel, or with pressure from a tight dressing or tracheotomy tube tie may lead to a cycle of venous congestion and flap edema leading to more pressure on the pedicle and flap failure. Hemostasis and drainage are needed to prevent the development of a hematoma, which could lead to increased pressure on the flap pedicle.

Deltopectoral Flap

The medially based deltopectoral flap, as originally described by Bakamijian in 1965,[38] is a cutaneous flap with an axial blood supply based on the first four intercostal A perforating branches of the internal mammary artery. This flap has proven to be a reliable method of transferring a large amount of chest wall skin for reconstruction of the head and neck and for years had been the reconstructive flap of choice for large defects. It has even been described as a cutaneous free flap based on the second intercostal perforating artery by Harii et al.[39] Distally, additional length can be obtained by extending the flap onto the lateral deltoid region; however, this portion of the flap relies on random blood supply for its survival. Because of the more tenuous blood supply to the distal flap, it may be advisable to delay the flap first. Delay should also be considered when the flap will be transferred into a recipient bed that is at risk for delayed healing. Several studies suggest that patients with severe metabolic disorders such as diabetes, atherosclerosis, or malnutrition, and poor tissue turgor, or previous high-dose irradiation to the recipient bed are at an increased risk for complications.[38,40-44] Disadvantages of the flap include the large defect at the donor site, which usually must be covered by a split thickness skin graft, and the requirement for a multistage reconstruction, especially if delay is required.

Major complications in which there is a loss of a significant portion of the flap are reported to occur in 9.5 to 18%[38,40-44] of these flaps. Comparison of results with these flaps is somewhat confusing because of variability in definitions and reporting of major and minor complications. Some studies that have also looked at minor complication rates have demonstrated rates as high as 40%,[40] but these have included complications such as fistulae, wound infection, and partial flap necrosis in which the flap still fulfilled its intended function.

Flap failure can occur during the initial raising of the flap (rare), between elevation of the flap and transaction of its pedicle, and after transaction of its pedicle. Early failure typically occurs because of compromise of the vascular pedicle. Common causes of this include constriction of the pedicle from passage through a tight tunnel, tracheotomy ties constricting the pedicle of the flap, and by kinking the flap over the mandibular rim to cover the floor of the mouth. Transversely folding the tip of the flap on itself or over a mandibular bar increases the risk of ischemic necrosis because of the random blood supply to this part of the flap.

Traction on the flap from a short pedicle or patient head movement can lead to separation of the wound edges, ischemic necrosis, or both. This increases the risk for contamination with oral or skin flora and may result in infection or fistula formation and is a common cause of delayed flap failure. Postoperatively the patient's head should be immobilized in a neutral position for a few days to prevent traction on the suture line. Gravity also contributes to traction on the wound edges, especially in women with large pendulous breasts.[42] Care must be taken that the flap is well supported.

Delayed wound healing secondary to previous heavy irradiation, malnutrition, severe diabetes, or atherosclerosis can result in failure of the flap at the time of division of the proximal pedicle. The metabolic derangement results in delayed wound healing impairs the neovascularization to the flap, which would allow division of the pedicle. These high-risk patients should also be considered for delay of the flap and tested by temporary occlusion of the base of the pedicle prior to its division.

MUSCULOCUTANEOUS FLAPS

Pectoralis Major Myocutaneous Flap

There are numerous musculocutaneous flaps available for head and neck reconstruction but, because of its versatility, reliability, and the ability to raise this flap without altering the patient's position, the pectoralis major myocutaneous flap has become the "work horse" of head and neck reconstruction. Since Ariyan's first description,[45] it has been demonstrated to be a hardy and versatile flap with many applications for single-staged reconstruction of the head and neck. Its long vascular pedicle allows transfer of a generous muscle or skin muscle paddle to most areas of the head and neck without a significant increase in operative time. The muscular component can be used to cover and protect important vascular structures in the neck and the pedicle can also be tailored to provide variable amounts of bulk for the reconstruction. This flap in conjunction with changes in the

delivery of radiation therapy has significantly reduced the incidence of carotid "blow out."

The skin incision for creating a pectoralis muscle flap should be designed to permit the secondary elevation of a deltopectoral flap, if possible. This requires that the skin island be incised to the level of the pectoralis fascia and then laterally extended to the anterior axillary fold. It is important to avoid shearing forces on the muscular perforating vessels to the skin by anchoring the skin to the underlying muscle as the dissection proceeds. After the free lateral edge of the pectoralis muscle is identified, the pectoralis is elevated from the chest wall with blunt dissection in the bloodless areolar plane between the muscle and the chest wall. The vascular pedicle from the thoracoacromial artery is identified laterally and preserved with flap elevation. Once the entire flap is elevated and the origin is freed from the ribs and the clavicle, the insertion to the humerus is divided. The flap can be tailored to the muscular male or full-breasted female to fit under the neck flaps by removing muscle medial and lateral to the vascular pedicle. The pectoralis muscle around the vessels should not be reduced too much, because the muscle protects the vessels from undue trauma. The pectoral nerve should also be divided to prevent constricting of the vascular pedicle and flap compromise.

Complications

The rate of total flap necrosis is low in most series, occurring between 0 to 14%, less than for the deltopectoral flap (Table 18–2) Wilson et al[46] reported a 93% success rate addressing only partial and total necrosis of the flap. Several larger series performed more comprehensive analyses and reported total complication rates between 20 and 63%.[2,47–49] It is accepted that minor complications such as partial flap necrosis, fistula, and wound separation will occur between 10 and 20% of the time. As is true for all reconstructive techniques, closure of a mucosal defect is associated with a higher incidence of complications than repair of a skin defect,[2] caused by contamination of the wound with oral flora, which increases the risk for wound infection. A "spit tight" mucosal closure, as advocated by Conley,[50] must be accomplished.

Technical factors in design, elevation, and transfer of the these flaps appear to play a larger role in the development of complications than do systemic factors. Larger tumors have been noted by both Shah et al[2] and Kroll et al[49] to be associated with a higher incidence of flap complications. Contraction of the dermal elastic fibers from the skin island of the flap in combination with the weight of the flap can produce excessive tension on the wound edges and lead to wound dehiscence.[19] This is one of the more common problems occurring in 5 to 6% of flaps.[2,16,19,20,47,49] Often one patient will have multiple complications. In the series of Shah et al,[2] 79% of the patients who developed wound dehiscence, also developed other complications. It is easy to imagine that separation of the flap margins could lead to contamination of the wound by saliva and result in a wound infection. Wound

Table 18–2. Results of Pectoralis Major Myocutaneous Flap Reconstruction

	# FLAPS/ # PATIENTS	TOTAL COMPLICATIONS (%)	NECROSIS TOTAL (%)	PART (%)	DEHISCENCE (%)	FISTULA (%)	INFECT (%)	DONOR (%)	REOPERATIVE (%)
Schuller[46]	15/14		0	1(7)	1(7)			3(20)	
Biller et al[16]	42/42		0	3(7)	2(5)	4(9.5)	13(31)	4(9.5)	
Baek et al[47]	133/126	58(43)	2(1.5)	9(7)	17(13)	18(13.5)	7(5)	5(3.8)	11(8.3)
Maisel[81]	14/14	2(14)				4*		2(14)	
Mehrhof[82]	73/67	36(49.3)	3(4.1)	9(12)	9(12)	12(16.4)	2(3)		24(36)
Ossoff et al[20]	95/86	19(20)	1(1)	4(4)	10(11)	5(5.3)	1(1)	3(3.2)	
Wilson et al[45]	112/102	18(16.1)	8(7.1)	10(9)					
Kroll et al[48]	168/168	106(63)	2(2.4)	29(17)	43(25.6)	35(20.8)	22(13.1)		
Shah et al[2]	214/211	135(63)	7(3)	62(29)	56(26)	61(29)	51(24)		35(26)
Huang et al[18]	44/45	26(58)	7(16)	16(36)		16(36)	8(18)	2(4)	
Keidan and Kusiak[17]	40/40	16(40)	1(2.5)	8(20)	1(2.5)	2(5)	6(15)	1(2.5)	

*Complications reported together.

infections occur in 15% of flaps, the range being from 1 to 31%.[2,20,49] The use of perioperative antibiotics helps to decrease postoperative wound infection when the pharynx is involved.[50]

Compromise of the vascular pedicle is a frequent cause of significant complications. Several reports of flap failure have been attributed to constriction of the flap pedicle by tight dressings, tight tracheotomy ties, or kinking of the pedicle by improper head position. Sewing the tracheotomy in position, loose or no dressing on the flap, and immobilization of the patient's head in a neutral position for a few days after surgery help to minimize these complications.

The use of a metal prosthesis for mandibular reconstruction in combination with a pectoralis major myocutaneous flap is also associated with a higher incidence of complications,[18,47] in particular total and partial necrosis of the flap. Most of these complications have been associated with compression of the vascular pedicle by the prosthesis or from the metal plate eroding the flap.

The role of systemic factors in producing complications remains somewhat obscure. Partial necrosis of the flap is frequently related to loss of the skin island. The underlying muscle is much hardier. Because the skin relies on the musculocutaneous perforators for nourishment, traversing the fat and subcutaneous tissues, obesity contributes to increased complications with this flap. The two largest series investigating flap complications are at odds about this. Kroll et al[49] found no increased complications with flaps performed on obese patients,[48] whereas Shah et al,[2] using nomogram tables to define overweight patients, found a significantly increased incidence of complications in overweight patients. The increased thickness and weight of the flap produced by obesity or female breast tissue increase tension on the closure and wound complications. Transfer of only the muscular portion of the flap with good support to surrounding tissues, such as the prevertebral fascia, etc., will decrease these complications.[49]

Most complications can be managed conservatively, only occasionally requiring revision surgery and rarely requiring additional flaps for closure. In the series of Shah et al[2] only 35 of 214 flaps required reoperation and only 2 required a second flap.

Sternocleidomastoid Flap

The sternocleidomastoid myocutaneous flap has been employed to reconstruct the oral cavity and oropharynx. The sternomastoid vascular supply has three components: superiorly from the occipital artery, inferiorly from the inferior thyroid artery, and in the middle from the superior thyroid artery. Because of this, the skin paddle may be located superiorly near the mastoid tip or inferiorly near the clavicle. It is recommended that two arteries be preserved when raising the flap to improve flap viability.

There is a 50% incidence of partial loss of the skin paddle reported in series by Ariyan[45] and Sasaki[52] when using this flap for intraoral reconstruction. Total flap loss is unusual, the surviving muscle remucosalizes effecting adequate closure of the wound. Charles et al[53] and Marx and McDonald[54] suggest that preservation of the platysma over the entire muscle would decrease the incidence of skin loss.

Trapezius Myocutaneous Flap

The trapezius myocutaneous flap has had significant usages for reconstruction of major head and neck defects. Although two arteries supply this flap, the dominant artery is the superficial branch of the transverse cervical artery. The upper portion of the flap derives its blood supply from the occipital artery. Disadvantages of this flap include the variability of its vascular supply and the special positioning required to harvest this flap. Despite its short arch of rotation, Panje has employed this flap to transfer scapular bone for mandibular reconstruction.[55] In his series he had an 87% success rate and noted that failures occurred in patients who required more than a 6-cm segment of bone for reconstruction and patients who developed intraoral bone exposure. The patients who failed also lost the skin and muscle of the flap. Significant shoulder dysfunction can occur in patients who have required a trapezius flap on the same side as a previous pectoralis major flap.

Latissimus Dorsi Myocutaneous Flap

This flap can provide a large amount of skin for coverage of major head and neck defects. Its blood supply is from the thoracodorsal artery and it is innervated by the thoracodorsal nerve. This flap also requires repositioning after completion of the resection to raise the flap for head and neck reconstruction. Despite the long tunnel required, the total flap failure rate is only 5% from venous thrombosis or pedicle strangulation. The partial necrosis rate is 11%.[56,57] There have been reports of injury to the brachial plexus and transient radial nerve weakness.

MICROVASCULAR FREE TISSUE TRANSFER

Inadequacies of major defect repair with local and regional flaps, such as difficulty reaching areas of the head because of limited arc of rotation, cosmetic defect of the donor site, and inability to tailor tissue bulk to suit the defect, have encouraged the continued development of the microvascular technique for free tissue transfer. The technique was first introduced by Jacobson and Suarez in 1960,[58] but it wasn't until 1974 when the first successful transplant of skin was accomplished by Hari et al.[59] Since then it has become an increasingly more popular method of reconstruction of head and neck defects. It is limited by the special training required to perform the anastomoses and, in many instances, the length of time it adds to the operative procedure. There is also a steep learning curve for these procedures. Carlson and Coleman[60] published a comparison of their early experience during 1977 to 1982 with their later experience during 1983 to 1987. They found a flap failure rate of 28.6% for their early group as compared with 9.1% for their later series. Currently it is accepted that there is a 90% or better success rate at major centers performing these types of reconstruction.

Early experience with free flaps was primarily concerned with free skin flaps from the scalp, groin, and dorsum of the foot (Table 18–3). As experience increased, it was found that compound musculocutaneous, osteocutaneous, and osteomusculocutaneous flaps could be reliably transferred for use in head and neck reconstruction.

Patient Selection

Although, theoretically, any tissue with a closed arteriovenous vascular circuit can be transferred as a free flap, practically, a flap must have at least one artery and one vein of greater than 0.8 mm in external diameter to enable a microvascular

Table 18–3. Microvascular Free Flaps

Cutaneous and fascio-cutaneous flaps	Radial forearm Lateral arm Deltopectoral Superficial groin Lateral thigh flap
Muscle and musculo-cutaneous flaps	Serratus anterior Rectus abdominis gracilis
Osteocutaneous flaps	Scapula Radial forearm Dorsalis pedis fibula
Osteomusculo-cutaneous flaps	Deep circumflex illiac crest Internal oblique iliac crest
Grafts	Gastroomental Olmentum Jejunum

anastomosis. Although advanced age is frequently associated with diabetes, hypercholesterolemia, hypertension, and atherosclerosis, it should not be considered an absolute contraindication to free flap reconstruction. Arteriosclerotic plaque deposition is common in the branches of the external carotid system, and it can reduce blood flow or act as a nidus for thrombus formation. Minor twisting or kinking of these atherosclerotic vessels can further compromise blood flow resulting in thrombosis. In spite of these factors, free tissue transfer can often be successfully accomplished in this patient group. Patients with blood coagulopathies, collagen vascular diseases, sickle cell disease, and polycythemia are not considered candidates for microvascular surgery.

As mentioned earlier, malnourished patients are at risk for wound healing problems and other postoperative complications, including free flap failure. Obesity also may influence the surgical result, particularly when direct cutaneous flaps are transferred from the groin or chest area. The increased adipose tissue can make the dissection of the vascular pedicle difficult and may make the flap too bulky, yet defatting aggressively during the inital transfer can injure the blood supply. For this reason groin and chest flaps should be avoided for oral cavity reconstruction. One must be very conservative in defatting any flap during the inital transfer. When these flaps are transferred into an irradiated field, there is not any increased risk of thrombosis of the anastomosed vessels.

Technique

Technique has been identified to be the single most important factor influencing the success or failure of a free flap. The technical aspects of effecting a microvascular anastomosis have been widely published,[61] but a few points deserve special emphasis. Prior to flap transfer, the recipient bed must be prepared. The reconstruction can be expedited if a second team harvests the flap while the recipient vessels are identified and dissected free of adjacent tissue and elongated by ligating extraneous branches. The size of the flap and the length of the donor vessels should not be committed until the tumor resection bed has been determined clear by frozen section, and the recipient vessels have been prepared. The recipient artery must be trimmed back until good pulsating flow is observed even if it requires interposition of a vein graft. Placement of a vein graft is preferable to creation of an anastomosis under tension as this may result in vasospasm and thrombosis. The vein graft must be reversed to prevent obstruction of flow by venous valves. Two percent lidocaine (Xylocaine) can also be dripped onto the vessel to help reduce vasospasm. The donor and the recipient vessels should be of similar diameter. When the recipient site is ready, the donor vessels are then divided. The stumps are irrigated with heparinized saline solution (10 U/mL saline), and the adventitia near the vessel ends is gently removed to prevent blood exposure to this thrombogenic tissue. The deeper vessels are then attached first with an end-to-end anastomosis, and when the anastomosis is complete, the vascular clamps are removed from the venous side first. Although a small amount of initial leakage of blood is typical, pulsatile bleeding must be controlled. The flap should be checked for color, and the vessels should be observed for patency. Expansile pulsations signal a patent vessel but longitudinal pulsations signal partial or complete occlusion of the anastomosis. Doppler can assist in confirming good patency of the anastomosis. The flicker test and the strip test are not clinically appropriate because they are traumatic to the vessels and should be reserved for laboratory use.[62] Other methods have been employed to assess vascular patency including transcutaneous doppler, laser doppler velocimetry, nuclear medicine isotope uptake scans, skin transillumination and transcutaneous oxygen tension monitoring. Once the flap is successfully reperfused, the remainder of the defect can be closed with the flap. Care should be taken to assure that the anastomosis is not placed under tension and the vascular pedicle is not kinked or twisted.

Postoperatively it is important that the patient be watched closely for evidence of flap failure. The most common cause of flap failure is venous thrombosis, although it occurs later than arterial thrombosis, which is more likely to occur during the first 72 hours, making frequent flap monitoring necessary. It is important to recognize flap failure early because ischemia longer than 6 hours may jeopardize flap survival.

The earliest signs of arterial thrombosis can frequently be observed at the bedside and include: cutaneous pallor, loss of capillary refill, a decrease in temperature, and loss of flap turgor. Venous occlusion results in a rapid increase in swelling, a change in color first to pink-red, and as engorgement of the flap occurs, the development of diffuse petechiae. The flap then becomes thick and tense, and puncture results in rapid bleeding of dark red blood. At this stage the flap can still be salvaged by exploration and venous thrombectomy. If it appears the flap is failing, reexploration should be performed immediately because there is a direct relationship between increasing periods of ischemia and increased peripheral resistance to blood flow after flap reperfusion. In a study by May et al,[63] 100% survival of flaps was demonstrated if the flaps were reperfused in 1 to 4 hours. There was an 80%

survival rate if reperfusion was established by 8 hours, and there was a 100% failure rate if blood flow to the flap was not reestablished by 12 hours of ischemia time. This "no-reflow" phenomenon is believed to be caused by ischemia-induced dysfunction of the sodium-potassium membrane pump, which leads to swelling of the endothelial cells and sludging of the intravascular blood flow. If intervention is not prompt, severe flap engorgement and cyanosis occur.

The use of aspirin 650 mg twice per day for 2 weeks reduces platelet aggregation and prevents venous thrombosis. Heparin and sodium warfarin (Coumadin) are not routinely recommended postoperatively owing to the risk of postoperative bleeding and hematoma formation. However, when an early venous thrombosis occurs in a patient who is unable to be reexplored, heparin can be utilized to prevent further thrombosis and may result in flap salvage.

CUTANEOUS AND FASCIOCUTANEOUS FLAPS

Radial Forearm Flap

This is an extremely reliable and highly versatile cutaneous flap that is based on the radial artery and its venae comitantes or a superficial forearm vein. It can provide a pedicle of 10 to 18 cm in length with the diameter of the vessels of 2 to 4 mm. The thin pliable character of this flap makes it valuable for reconstruction of the oral cavity, pharynx, and esophagus, and it has even been tubed to reconstruct circumferential defects of the pharyngoesophagus.[64,65] The potential for sensory reinnervation through the antebrachial nerves can enhance the functional result of the reconstruction leading to improved speech, oral competence, mastication, and swallowing.[66] A superficial branch of the radial nerve can be included for use as a vascularized nerve graft and has been successfully employed by Urken et al[66] in the reconstruction of the facial nerve. A portion of the radius may also be harvested along with the soft tissue for bone reconstruction.

Disadvantages of this flap include the severe cosmetic defect at the donor site on the forearm that often requires skin grafting to cover. This area remains insensate as will the dorsum of the hand if the superficial branch of the radial nerve is harvested. Transection of the sensory nerves of the flap can result in painful neuromas but the likelihood of this occurring can be reduced by burying the cut nerve end in deeper muscle tissue.[66] Poor healing of the skin graft that covers the donor site can impair hand function and there have also been reports of fractures of the radius when a section of it has been incorporated in the flap.[65,67]

Lateral Forearm Flap

This is a fasciocutaneous flap that derives its blood supply from the posterior branch of the profunda brachii artery. This flap can also potentially provide sensory innervation from the lateral antebrachial cutaneous nerve of the arm. It too is thin, hairless, and supple and has a vascular pedicle of 8 to 10 cm in length with vessels 1 to 2 mm in diameter.[68] The flap is commonly used for reconstruction of facial and intraoral defects.

Disadvantages include the long linear scar created on the lateral forearm and the potential sensory disturbance over the volar aspect of the forearm from sacrifice of the posterior antebrachial cutaneous nerve.[68]

MUSCLE AND MUSCULOCUTANEOUS FLAPS
Latissimus Dorsi Flap

The latissimus dorsi was first described as a free flap in 1978. Its main blood supply is derived from the thoracodorsal artery and the 9th through the 11th intercostal arteries. It can provide a vascular pedicle of 8 to 15 cm in length and it is usually reserved for reconstruction of extensive defects of the head and neck.

Studies by Harii et al,[69] Maxwell et al,[70] and Baker[71] report few complications in reconstructions using this flap. Others have reported a high incidence of postoperative hematoma and seroma formation,[72] so meticulous hemostasis should be insured and active drains placed before closure of the skin. The use of this muscle for reconstruction can create problems with weakness for patients who like to perform some athletic activities such as weight lifting, cross country skiing and swimming. A small series by Laitung and Peck,[73] however, noted no significant loss in power or shoulder mobility in these patients, unless they had developed a scar contracture.

Rectus Abdominis

The rectus abdominis free flap is advocated by Urken to be one of the most versatile soft tissue flaps for head and neck reconstruction. It provides a very large skin paddle based on a long vascular pedicle from the large diameter deep inferior epigastric vessels. This flap is very reliable and particularly useful for repair of defects that require substantial soft tissue bulk for contouring. The flap, however, removes major support from the anterior abdominal wall predisposing to development of a ventral hernia. Meland et al[74] and Urken et al[75] showed a 0 to 1.3% incidence of hernia formation demonstrating that careful reconstruction of the anterior rectus sheath can avoid this problem. Seromas and infections were also seen,[74] supporting the need for drainage of the donor site and prophylactic antibiotic therapy.

OSTEOCUTANEOUS FLAPS
Scapula

The scapular free flap is a reliable source of bone for mandibular reconstruction. It is based on the circumflex scapular artery and can provide a vascular pedicle 6 to 8 cm in length and 3 to 4 mm in diameter. It can be harvested as a fasciocutaneous or osseocutaneous flap with transfer of a large amount of hairless skin along with 10 to 14 cm of bone.

The head and neck resection must be accomplished before the flap is harvested because of the need for positioning in the lateral decubitus position. Although the skin approaches the color of facial skin, the skin flap is quite thick. Sullivan et al[76] in his series of 17 patients reported only one failed mandibular reconstruction. There is also a considerable decrease in shoulder strength and range of motion when scapular bone is harvested with the flap, and these patients require physical therapy postoperatively to improve shoulder function.[76]

OSTEOMUSCULOCUTANEOUS FLAPS
Internal Oblique Iliac Crest

This flap provides the largest amount of bone that has a natural contour for reconstruction of the mandible and is capable of accepting osseointegrated implants for dental restoration,[77] which may be placed in the bone at the time of flap transfer. A large amount of thin pliable skin can be harvested along with this flap, which is 6 to 8 cm in length and 1 to 2 mm in diameter. The vascular anatomy is very consistent.

Because of the division of many abdominal muscles and inguinal ligaments patients who undergo this flap are at high risk for developing subsequent groin hernias. The bony donor site may also bleed significantly and should be drained adequately.[78]

GRAFTS
Jejunum

The jejunum has been a popular method of pharyngoesophageal reconstruction because of its mucosal lining and intrinsic peristaltic contractions. These contractions are not however functional in swallowing and may actually contribute to some dysphagia. The graft tolerates pre and postoperative radiotherapy well.[79] However, because of its inability to develop neovascularization through its serosa, its survival is perpetually linked to maintenance of its vascular pedicle.

Gluckman et al[80] reported a 90.3% overall success rate with this graft and a 7.6% graft failure rate. Stenosis of the pharyngeal or esophageal anastomosis occurs 10% of the time and can cause persistent dysphagia. Other disadvantages include the requirement of a laparotomy with all of the associated complications from abdominal surgery, including postoperative ileus, peritonitis, abcess, bowel stenosis, and postoperative bowel adhesions that may prolong the hospitalization.

CONCLUSION

The need for reconstructing progressively more complex defects of the head and neck and improved understanding of wound healing have led to the development of a variety of alternative flaps. The reconstruction must be carefully planned preoperatively, and the increasing armamentarium provides the head and neck surgeon with options for each procedure. Knowledge of anatomy, wound healing, and surgical technique provides the head and neck surgeon with the best defense against flap complications.

REFERENCES

1. Kerrigan CL. Skin flap failure: pathophysiology. *Plast Reconstr Surg*, 1983;72:766,777.
2. Shah JP, et al. Complications of the pectoralis major myocutaneous flap in head and neck reconstruction. *Am J Surg*. 1990;160:352–355.
3. Mullen JL. Consequences of malnutrition in the surgical patient. *Surg Clin North Am*. 1981;5:465–487.
4. Winkler MF, et al. Use of retinol-binding protein and prealbumin as indicators of the response to nutrition therapy. *J Am Diet Assoc*. 1989;5:684–687.
5. Slade MS, et al. Immunodepression after major surgery in patients. *Surgery*. 1975;78:363–372.
6. Daly JM, et al. Effects of protein depletion and repletion on cell mediated immunity in experimental animals. *Ann Surg*. 188:791–796.
7. Meakins JL, et al. Delayed hypersensitivity: indicator of acquired failure of host defenses in sepsis and trauma. *Ann Surg*. 1977;186:241–250.
8. Christou NV, Meakins JL. Neutrophil function in surgical patients: two inhibitors of granulocyte chemotaxis associated with sepsis. *J Surg Res*. 1979;137:536–542.
9. Copeland EM III, et al. Nutritional concepts in the treatment of head and neck malignancies. *Head Neck*. 1979;1:350–363.
10. Moore MJ. The effect or radiation on connective tissue. *Otolaryngol. Clin North Am*. 1984;17:389–399.
11. Naryan K, Cliff WJ. Morphology of irradiated microvasculator. *Am J Pathol*. 1982;106:47–62.
12. McGuirt WF, et al. Irradiation-induced atherosclerosis: a factor in therapeutic planning. *Ann Otol Rhinol Laryngol*. 1992;101:222–228.
13. Baker DG, Krochak RJ. The response of the microvascular system to radiation: a review. *Cancer Invest*. 1989;7:287–294.
14. Faucher A, et al. Cutaneous versus myocutaneous flaps in the repair of major defects in head and neck cancer: a study of 331 flaps. *Head Neck*. 1984;7:104–109.
15. Joseph DL, Shumrick DL. Risks of head and neck surgery in previously irradiated patients. *Arch Otolaryngol Head Neck Surg*. 1973;97:381–384.
16. Biller HF, et al. Pectoralis major myocutaneous flap in head and neck reconstruction analysis of complications in 42 cases. *Arch Otolaryngol Head Neck Surg*. 1981;107:23–26.
17. Keidan RD, Kusiak JF. Complications following reconstruction with the pectoralis major myocutaneous flap: the effect of prior radiation therapy. *Laryngoscope*. 1992,102:521–524.
18. Huang RD, et al. Pectoralis major myocutaneous flap: analysis of complications in a VA population. *Head Neck*. 1992;14:102–106.
19. Baek SM, et al. Reconstruction of the hypopharynx and cervical esophagus with pectoralis major island myocutaneous flap. *Ann Plast Sug*. 1981;7:18–23.
20. Ossoff RH, et al. Complications after pectoralis major myocutaneous flap reconstruction of head and neck defects. *Arch Otolaryngol Head Neck Surg*. 1983;109:812–814.
21. Burgess LP, et al. Wound healing relationship of wound closing tension to scar width in rats. *Laryngoscope*. 1989;99:783–788.
22. Larrabee WF, et al. Wound tension and blood flow in skin flaps. *Ann Oto Rhinol Laryngol*. 1984;93:112–115.
23. McCraw JB, Vasconez LO. Musculocutaneous flaps: principles. *Clin Plast Surg*. 1980;7:1:9–13.
24. Pellitteri PK, et al. The influence of hyperbaric oxygen therapy on skin flap survival in a swine model. *Arch Otolaryngol Head Neck Surg*. 1992;118:1050–1054.
25. Reinsch JF. The pathophysiology of skin flap circulation: the delay phenomena. *Plast Reconstr Surg*. 1974;54:585–598.
26. McFarlane RM, et al. A study of the delay phenomenon in experimental pedicle flaps. *Plast Reconstr Surg*. 1965;35:245–262.
27. Milton SH. Experimental studies on island flaps. *Plast Reconstr Surg*. 1972;49:444–447.
28. Meyers MB, Cherry G. Mechanism of the delay phenomenon. *Plast Reconstr Surg*. 1969;44:52–57.
29. Kerrigan CL, Daniel RK. Pharmacologic treatment of the failing skin flap. *Plast Reconstr Surg*. 1982;70:541–548.
30. Kiehn CL, Desprez JD. The effects of local hypothermia on pedicle flap tissue I: enhancement of survival of experimental flaps. *Plast Reconstr Surg*. 1960;25:349–359.
31. Desprez JD, Kiehn CL. The effects of local hypothermia on pedicle flap tissue II: hemodynamic changes. *Plast Reconstr Surg*. 1962;29:539–550.
32. Esclamado RM, et al. The effect of local hypothermia on early wound repair. *Arch Otolaryngol Head Neck Surg*. 1990;116:803–808.
33. Abramson M, et al. Inflammation induced connective tissue breakdown following injury. *Otolaryngol Clin North Am*. 1984;17:353–359.
34. Myers MB, et al. Wound tension and wound slough: a negative correlation. *Am J Surg*. 1965;109:711–714.
35. Larrabee WF, et al. Skin flap tension and would slough: correlation with laser doppler velocimetry. *Otolaryngol Head Neck Surg*. 1982;90:185–187.
36. Panje WR. Musculocutaneous and free flaps: physiology and practical considerations. *Otolaryngol Clin North Am*. 1984;17:401–412.
37. Gullane PJ, Heeneman H. Regional flaps of the head and neck. *SIPAC* AAOHNS, 1982.
38. Bakamijian VY: A two staged method for pharyngoesophageal reconstruction with a primary pectoral skin flap. *Plast Reconstr Surg*. 1965;36:173–184.
39. Harii K, et al. Free deltopectoral skin flaps. *Br J Plast Surg*. 1974;27:231–239.
40. Mendelson BC, et al. Experience with the deltopectoral flap. *Plast Reconstr Surg*. 1977;59:360–365.
41. Gingrass RP, et al. Complications with the deltopectoral flap. *Plast Reconstr Surg*. 1972;49:501–507.
42. Krizek TJ, Robson MC. Potential pitfalls in the use of the deltopectoral flap. *Plast Reconstr Surg*. 1972;50:326–331.
43. Park JS, et al. Reconstructive experience with the medially based deltopectoral flap. *Am J Surg*. 1974;128:548–552.
44. Lore JM, Zingapan EG. Delto-pectoral flap. *Arch Otolaryngol Head Neck Surg*. 1971;94:13–18.
45. Ariyan S. One-stage reconstruction for defects of the mouth using a sternomastoid myocutaneous flap. *Plast Reconstr Surg*. 1979;63:618–625.
46. Wilson JSP, et al. Some observations on 112 pectoralis major myocutaneous flaps. *Am J Surg*. 1984;147:273–279.
47. Schuller DE. Limitations of the pectoralis major myocutaneous flap in head and neck cancer reconstruction. *Arch Otolaryngol Head Neck Surg*. 1980;106:709–714.
48. Baek SM, et al. An analysis of 133 pectoralis major myocutaneous flaps. *Plast Reconstr Surg*. 1982;69:460–467.
49. Kroll SS, et at. Analysis of complications in 168 pectoralis major myocutaneous flaps used for head and neck reconstruction. *Ann Plast Surg*. 1990;25:93–97.
50. Conley JJ. Skin flap and skin graft complications. In: Conley JJ, ed. *Complications of Head and Neck Surgery*. Philadelphia, PA: WB Saunders Co; 1979.

51. Goode RL, et al. Effect of prophylactic antibiotics in radical head and neck surgery. *Laryngoscope.* 1979;89:601–608.

52. Sasaki CT. The sternocleidomastoid myocutaneous flap. *Arch Otolaryngol Head Neck Surg.* 1980;106:74–76.

53. Charles GA, et al. Sternocleidomastoid myocutaneous flap. *Laryngoscope.* 1987;97:970–974.

54. Marx RE, McDonald DK. The sternocleidomastoid muscle as a muscular or a myocutaneous flap for oral and facial reconstruction. *J Oral Maxillofac Surg.* 1985;43:155–162.

55. Panje WR. Mandible reconstruction with the trapezius osteomusculocutaneous flap. *Arch Otolaryngol Head Neck Surg.* 1985;111:223–229.

56. Sabatier RE, Bakamjian VY. Transaxillary latissimus dorsi flap reconstruction in head and neck cancer. *Am J. Surg.* 1985;150:427–434.

57. Barton FE, et al. Head and neck reconstruction with the latissimus dorsi myocutaneous flap: anatomic observations and report of 60 cases. *Plast Reconstr Surg.* 1983;p71:199–204.

58. Jacobson JH, Suarez EL. Microsurgery in anastomosis of small vessels. *Surg Forum.* 1960;11:243–245.

59. Harii K, Ohmori K, Ohmori S. Hair transplantation with free scalp flaps. *Plast Reconstr Surg.* 1974;53:410–413.

60. Carlson GW, Coleman JJ III. Microvascular free-tissue transfer. *Arch Surg.* 1989;124:438–440.

61. Baker SR (ed). *Microsurgical Reconstruction of the Head and Neck.* New York, NY: Churchill Livingstone; 1989.

62. Sullivan MJ. Microvascular surgical technique. In: Baker SR, ed. *Microsurgical Reconstruction of the Head and Neck.* New York, NY: Churchill Livingstone; 1989:15.

63. May JW Jr, et al. The no-reflow phenomenon in experimental free flaps. *Plast Reconstr Surg.* 1978;61:256–267.

64. Hayden RE. Microvascular free flaps for soft-tissue defects. *Otolaryngol Clin North Am.* 1991;24:1343–1366.

65. Soutar DS. Radial forearm flap in head and neck reconstruction. In: March JL, ed. *Current Therapy in Plastic and Reconstructive Surgery.* Toronto: BC Decker; 1989.

66. Urken ML, et al. The neurofaciocutaneous radial forearm flap in head and neck reconstruction: a preliminary report. *Laryngoscope.* 1990;100:161–173.

67. Sullivan MJ. Head and neck reconstruction by free tissue transfer. In: Cummings CW, et al, eds. *Otolaryngology Head and Neck Surgery.* 2nd ed. St Louis, MO: CV Mosby Yearbook; 1993.

68. Sullivan MJ, et al. Lateral arm free flap in head and neck reconstruction. *Arch Otolaryngol HeadNeck Surg.* 1992;118:1095–1101.

69. Harii K, et al. The free lateral thoracic flap. *Plast Reconstr Surg.* 1978;62:212–222.

70. Maxwell P, et al. Experience with thirteen latissimus dorsi myocutaneous free flaps. *Plast Reconstr Surg.* 1979,64:1–8.

71. Baker S. Free lateral thoracic flap in head and neck reconstruction. *Arch Otolaryngol Head Neck Surg.* 1981;107:409–413.

72. Slavin S. Drainage of seromas after latissimus dorsi myocutaneous flap breast reconstruction. *Plast Reconstr Surg.* 1989;83:925–926.

73. Laitung JKG, Peck F. Shoulder function following the loss of the latissimus dorsi muscle. *Br J Plast Surg.* 1985;38:375–379.

74. Meland B, et al. Experience with 80 rectus abdominis free-tissue transfers. *Plast Reconstsr Surg.* 1989;83:481–487.

75. Urken M, et al. The rectus abdominis free flap in head and neck reconstruction. *Arch Otolaryngol Head Neck Surg.* 1991;117:857–866.

76. Sullivan M, et al. Free scapular osteocutaneous flap for mandibular reconstruction. *Arch Otolaryngol Head Neck Surg.* 1989;115:1334–1340.

77. Urken M, et al. Primary placement of osseointegrated implants in microvascular mandibular reconstruction. *Otolaryngol Head Neck Surg.* 1989;101:56–73.

78. Phillips SD, Mattox DE. Complication of microvascular surgery. In: Eisele DW, ed. *Complications in Head and Neck Surgery.* St Louis, MO: CV Mosby Yearbook; 1993.

79. Beil MA, Maisel RH. Postoperative radiation—Associated changes in free jejunal autografts. *Arch Otolaryngol Head Neck Surg.* 1992;118:1037–1041.

80. Gluckman JL, et al. Complications associated with free jejunal graft reconstruction of the pharyngoesophagus—a multi-institutional experience with 52 cases. *Head Neck.* 1985;7:200–205.

81. Maisel RH, et al. Complications of pectoralis myocutaneous flaps. *Laryngoscope.* 1983;93:928–930.

82. Mehrhof Al, et al. The pectoralis major myocutaneous flap in head and neck reconstruction: analysis of complications. *Am J Surg.* 1983;146:478–482.

19 Complications of Surgery for Facial Fractures

Robert H. Mathog, M.D.

Individuals who sustain facial fractures are at risk for a complication of the fracture and/or from the treatment to correct the injury. Often times it is difficult to determine whether the unfortunate sequelae have occurred as a result of the intervention or the injury. Not all repairs will return the patient to normal and occasionally some dysfunction and/or deformity can be expected.

GENERAL
Respiratory Obstruction

Facial fractures can be associated with respiratory distress and early intervention should be directed to either correct or prevent this problem. Mandibular fractures, especially those with comminution or involvement of multiple sites, can cause relaxation of the tongue and oropharyngeal obstruction. The respiratory difficulty can be made worse by blood and secretions that further obstruct the airway. In such a situation it is important to suction the patient, reduce the fracture(s), and if necessary, apply an intraoral airway. In obtunded patients nasotracheal (or orotracheal) intubation must be considered. Tracheotomy may be indicated if there are associated injuries involving the midfacial region.

Respiratory distress can also occur with direct injury to the pharynx and/or larynx. Tissues of the upper airway can swell or there can be a dislocation of the cartilaginous framework of the larynx obstructing the air passageway. Vocal cord paralysis may also complicate the problem. The diagnosis of airway obstruction can be made on the basis of neck swelling and/or dislocation of laryngeal cartilages associated with respiratory difficulties. These upper airway injuries must be recognized immediately and measures taken to relieve the distress. If the patient is cooperative, it may be possible to perform an indirect or fiberoptic laryngeal examination. The airway, however, must be secured, and this is usually best performed by oral or nasal intubation or tracheotomy. If there is insufficient time to conduct a formal tracheotomy, then a cricothyrotomy is performed followed within 24 hours by a tracheotomy.

Cervical Spine Injury

All patients with facial fractures should be suspected of also having injury to the cervical spine. The potential devastation

of this complication mandates that initial efforts be directed to an evaluation of this possibility. If patients are responsive, they can be asked about neck pain. Palpation may elicit tenderness along the vertebral column. In general patients should be moved cautiously, and in suspected cases, the neck should not be moved until the cervical spine is examined with x-ray analysis.

Aspiration

Patients with maxillofacial trauma usually will have nasal or oral bleeding and accumulate secretions in the upper aerodigestive tract. If there is a neural injury, especially of the pharyngeal plexus, then there may be swallowing difficulty with aspiration of food or secretions into the lower respiratory system. The obtunded patient is especially prone to such a complication. The problem can be avoided by control of bleeding, suction, and use of alternative airways. Should aspiration occur, then there should be precautions to prevent the possibility of pneumonia.

Other Injuries

Soft tissue and skeletal trauma is not necessarily confined to the craniofacial region and the patient must be carefully examined for other potential injuries. A careful checking of vital signs in conjunction with a complete physical examination should be carried out soon after the diagnosis of the facial injury. Unexplained problems dealing with blood pressure and respiration should direct attention to the chest or abdomen. The patient's level of consciousness should be evaluated and if there is any question of cranial injury, appropriate neurosurgical consultation should be obtained.

SOFT TISSUE INJURIES
Lacerations and Abrasions

Frequently, facial fractures are associated with skin injury that must be evaluated before or during the repair of the facial fracture. It is not unusual to find lacerations on the prominences of the facial skeleton, and if this laceration is appropriate for exploration and reduction-fixation of the fracture, then it can and should be used for access to injury. If the plan is to wait before repair of the fracture, then the facial injury must be repaired immediately.The longer the time for the repair, the greater the chance of infection, more skin injury, and subsequent scar formation.

Abrasions of the skin should also be evaluated, cleaned and treated early to prevent infection, deeper injury, and unnecessary scarring. Foreign bodies embedded in the abraded tissues must be removed, or else, there will be permanent tattooing of that area of skin.

The preferred treatment of skin injury is to first get a history of toxoid immunization. If the patient has not had a recent booster, then toxoid should be administered. Prophylactic antibiotics, although somewhat controversial, are indicated, especially when one is trying to prevent a potential infection from spreading to the orbit or intracranial areas.

All wounds should be cleaned of foreign material with copious irrigations of normal saline, but if this is not sufficient, a scrubbing with a surgical scrub brush is necessary. The lacerated areas should be prepared with antiseptic solution and draped out for a surgical repair. Surgical debridement should be kept to a minimum, and irregular edges should be retained for camouflage purposes. In general the skin is undermined in a subcutaneous plane and the deeper muscles and fascia are closed with chromic sutures. The dermis is approximated with 4-0 chromic or 5-0 white Merseline suture and the skin closed with 5-0 or 6-0 nylon suture. In the eyelid skin, a running subcuticular nylon or Prolene suture is desirable.

Essentially the scars that develop as a result of the injury are treated in a similar fashion as in the acute situation.[1] A new laceration is created with beveled edges (Fig. 19–1). The skin is then undermined and closed in layers.

If the scar is long and across crease lines, the scar should be excised in a zig-zag fashion, placing the cross-lines in the direction of the least tension lines (Fig. 19–2). This approach will help to avoid contraction and also confound the observer by providing a camouflaged effect. A final stage of dermabrasion is desirable.

In cases where the scar crosses crease lines, the scar can be rotated with a Z-plasty technique to the improved orientation. In designing these repairs, the diagonal of the Z will rotate usually in a line parallel to a line drawn through the tips of the arms of the Z. In general a diagonal of a 60° Z-plasty (which is the most common type) will rotate about 90°.

Scar contraction can also be a problem and sometimes can be released by excision and undermining. On the other hand if there is a significant distortion of facial features, then the surgeon should consider either a Z-plasty or a full or split thickness skin graft. Rotation of the flaps with Z-plasty will theoretically bring more tissue into the area of the diagonal, and if the diagonal is placed along the line of contraction, release of these tension lines will be affected. Large wide scars may require split thickness grafts. Lower eyelid contraction (ectropion) is traditionally treated with a full thickness skin graft usually obtained from the postauricular area.

In cases where tattooing occurs, the affected area can either be excised or treated with dermabrasion. Usually small areas of tatoo are better excised whereas large areas of tatoo, such as on the cheek or forehead, will require a dermabrasion technique. Serial dermabrasions carried out at 6-month intervals may be necessary to obtain a satisfactory result.

Facial Nerve Injury

Facial paralysis can occur as a result of injury at any site along the course of the facial nerve. Before one can think of repair, the exact location must be determined. Most injuries will be located in the soft tissues of the face or within the temporal bone.

The diagnosis of the location and of the facial nerve injury is important. Stab wounds in the face may cut through one or several branches. If the inj:ury is anterior to the masseter muscle, the neural lacerations are probably too small to repair; moreover, there are usually sufficient neural anastomoses assuring satisfactory long-term results. Injuries to the facial nerve between the stylomastoid foramen and the anterior border of the masseter must be explored or repaired by microsurgical techniques.[2-4] Temporal bone injury of the nerve, often associated with hearing loss and/or dizziness and bloody discharge within the external auditory canal usually, is explored and either decompressed or repaired if the paralysis is of immediate onset. The exact site of injury is determined by computer tomograph (CT) scan imaging studies.

Exposure of the extratemporal facial nerve will usually require a superficial parotidectomy (Fig. 19–3). Once the laceration is found, the edges should be sharpened with a knife blade, and the epineurium approximated (under the microscope) with 7-0 nylon sutures. These sutures should be placed at least in one thirds or one fourths around the circumference of the nerve.

If a segment of the nerve is missing, then the ends should be identified and the missing segment replaced with a microscopic anastomosis of the greater auricular nerve (Fig. 19–3B). Knowing the the marginal branch passes over the posterior facial vein and that the buccal branch passes near the parotid duct is helpful in identifying these branches of the nerve. The frontal branch lies about midway between the tragus and lateral canthus at the level of the zygomatic arch.

If the injury occurs in the temporal bone, then a mastoidectomy and/or middle fossa exploration is indicated. Suture neurorrhaphy is not usually possible. In these cases the nerve ends are approximated and held together with gel foam and fibrin glue. The removal of bone spicules and decompression of the nerve should also be considered.

Parotid Duct Injury

Sharp penetrating wounds anterior to the masseter should be evaluated for parotid duct injury.[3] In suspected cases clear fluid will usually be flowing from the wound. First, a small cannula is inserted into the parotid duct orifice and passed

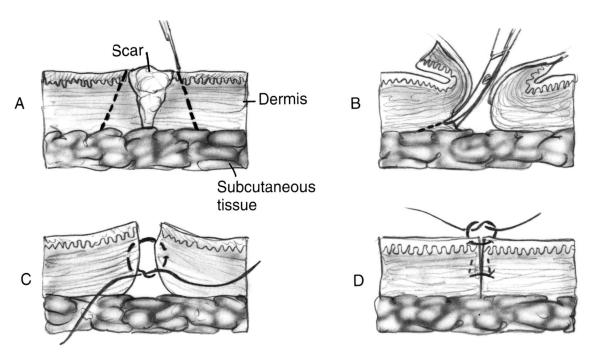

Figure 19–1. Techniques of skin incision and closure. **(A).** Beveling of the incision. **(B).** Undermining of subcutaneous tissues. **(C).** Closure of the dermis (subcuticular sutures). **(D).** Closure of the skin (from Mathog[1]).

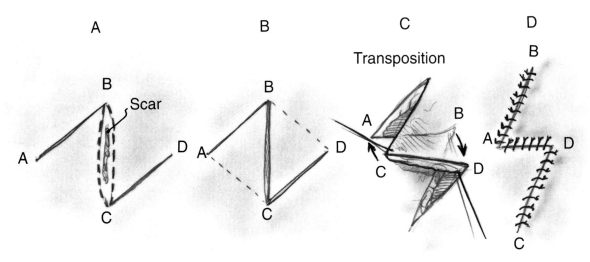

Figure 19–2. Z-plasty. Lines A, B, C, and D define a Z-plasty. The dotted lines help to describe a parallelogram with a diagonal B, C. On transposition of the flaps B to D and C to A, a lengthening is noted in B to C at the expense of A to D. The difference between the two diagonals is the amount of relaxation (from Mathog[1]).

through the area of injury (Fig. 19–4A). Using a microscope and appropriate retraction, the cannula is passed through both proximal and distal segments of the duct. The edges of the duct are then sutured over the catheter with 7-0 nylon suture. The cannula is left in place by securing it to the cheek for 5 to 7 days and used as a stent for healing of the duct. If injury to the duct is near the duct orifice, then it is practical to just close the subcutaneous tissues and skin and establish drainage internally.

Canalicular Injury with Epiphora

Lacerations of the eyelids near the medial can thus can be associated with injury to the lacrimal canaliculi as they traverse the area from the puncta to the lacrimal sac. Because most lacrimal flow is through the inferior canaliculus, it is important that the damage be recognized and that the canaliculus be repaired early after injury. The superior canaliculus may also be repaired, but a functioning lower canaliculus will probably suffice.

The procedure for repair is carried out with the operating microscope (Fig. 19–4B). The laceration is irrigated with normal saline and the edges examined for the ends of the severed canaliculus. The proximal segment (near the puncta) is easy to identify because the surgeon can dilate the puncta with lacrimal dilators and pass the probe through the canaliculus into the laceration. The probe will then point to the severed

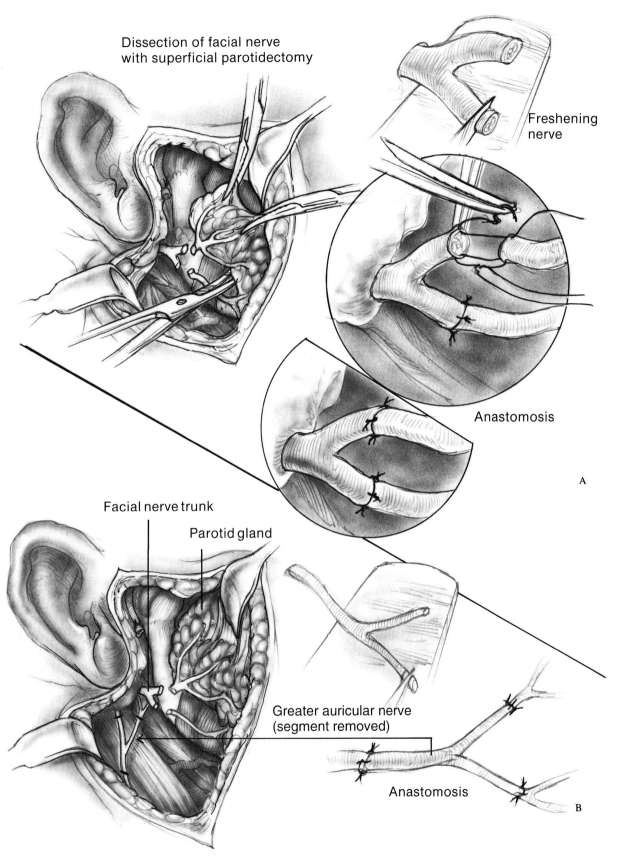

Dissection of facial nerve with superficial parotidectomy

Freshening nerve

Anastomosis

A

Facial nerve trunk

Parotid gland

Greater auricular nerve (segment removed)

Anastomosis

B

Figure 19–3. **(A).** Neurorraphy of facial nerve using superficial parotidectomy and epineural approximation (from Mathog[35]). **(B).** Neurorraphy of facial nerve using superficial parotidectomy and greater auricular nerve graft (from Mathog[35]).

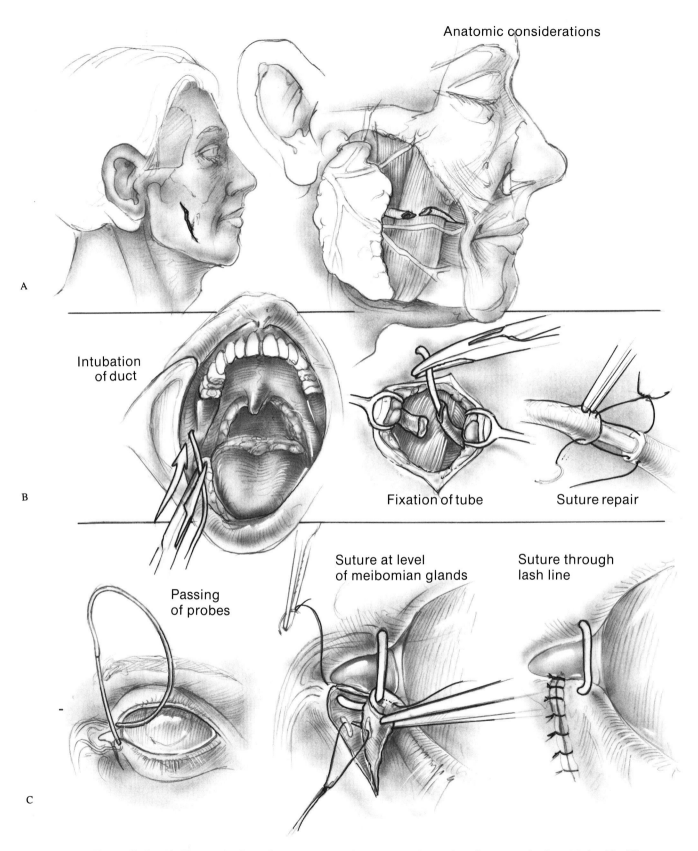

Anatomic considerations

A

Intubation
of duct

B

Fixation of tube

Suture repair

Passing
of probes

Suture at level
of meibomian glands

Suture through
lash line

C

Figure 19–4.   (A, B). Repair of parotid duct by exploration and cannula stenting of anastomosis (from Mathog[35]). **(C).** Canalicular repair using Crawford tube and layered eyelid closure (from Mathog[35]).

canaliculus of the opposite side. If the distal end still cannot be seen, the surgeon can then irrigate the superior canaliculus, press on the sac, and force the fluid retrograde through the inferior canaliculus. Following identification of the ends of the canaliculus a silastic tube swaged on a flexible probe (Crawford tube) is passed through the canalicular system into the sac and out through the nasal lacrimal duct. The other swaged end is passed through the superior canaliculus to follow a similar route to the nose. The tubing is then tied in the nose and the metal probes are cut from the tubing. The eyelid is closed with special techniques in which sutures are placed along the tarsal border, at the level of the meibomian gland orifices and at the junction of skin and conjunctiva.[5] An anteriorly placed suture is used to secure the skin and tie down the ends of the other sutures. The Crawford tube is left in place for 2 to 3 weeks.

Hematoma
CHONDRITIS OF THE EAR

Trauma to the pinna can commonly be associated with a subperichondrial accumulation of fluid. This hematoma is dangerous because it can cause pressure necrosis of the underlying cartilage and interfere with blood supply that is necessary for survival of the tissues. Such injuries commonly occur in wrestlers and can be prevented by appropriate headgear.

Treatment of the auricular hematoma consists of immediate diagnosis and application of pressure dressings. For this procedure the ear is prepared with an antiseptic solution and an incision of 3 to 4 cm made in appropriate creases (ie, between the helix and antihelix). The clot is removed and a rubber band or small penrose drain is inserted and secured to the skin edges. Compression dressings consisting of cotton balls soaked in Betadine and fluffs are placed over the ear. The drains are removed in 24 to 48 hours and a dressing reapplied for 5 to 7 days. Reaccumulation of fluid should be drained immediately. Antibiotic coverage is mandatory.

If the hematoma is not adequately treated then the patient will develop a deformity of the cartilage of the ear. Thickened areas of cartilage will have to be trimmed and deficient areas replaced with standard microtia techniques. The results of such surgery are limited, although improvement can be expected.

CHONDRITIS OF THE SEPTUM

Hematoma developing along the septum has a pathophysiology similar to the auricular hematoma and one can also expect necrosis and loss of tissue if it is not treated immediately. Because the septum helps to support the dorsum of the nose, loss of the septum can cause a saddling and compromise of the nasal airway. These patients also develop a retraction of the columella.

The initial hematoma should be immediately drained by placing a vertical incision along the septum, suctioning out clots from the subperichondrial pocket. A small Penrose or rubber band drain is inserted into the pocket and secured with a suture to the edge of the mucosa. The nose is then packed bilaterally with 1/2-in gauze treated with bacitracin ointment. Antibiotics are provided. Packing is removed in 3 days and the nose inspected regularly for proper healing.

Should a saddling and columella retraction develop, then the surgeon must consider reconstructive surgery. The procedures, however, should not be performed until the nose has stabilized and this will take 4 to 6 months. Most procedures require that a subcutaneous pocket be developed along the cartilaginous dorsum and that grafts of septal or auricular cartilage be placed into the defect. Additional implants are placed into the columella. The nose is then stabilized with a tape and plaster dressing for 7 to 10 days.

FACIAL SKELETON INJURIES
Mandible Fractures
NONUNION

This complication is often a result of infection and usually associated with pain and abnormal mobility of the jaw.[6,7] The infection can be caused by contamination of retained foreign bodies or failure to immobilize and reduce the fracture. Other contributing factors include an impaired blood supply and malnourishment, conditions that ultimately affect the healing of bone. Nonunion of the mandible can occur in a variety of locations but is often found in the unfavorable angle or parasymphyseal fracture, or in a fracture of an area of an edentulous atrophic body. Nonunion of the ramus, condyle, or coronoid process can also develop, but in these locations, it does not pose a functional problem.

A stepwise progression of medical and surgical treatment is necessary. The goal is to obtain a clean, vascularized, and mobilized jaw. In the dentulous patient maxillary fixation can be used to stabilize the jaw whereas in the edentulous patient, the biphase with bicortical pins placed away from the fracture can be helpful. Essential to both techniques is the local treatment of the wound with debridement and irrigation. Sometimes the immobilization during this "clean-up period" will allow for new bone to bridge the gap.

Following conservative measures the patient's jaw should be analyzed for stability. Any abnormal movement of the jaw (with or without pain) should indicate a problem with healing and the need for bone graft technique. To optimize conditions for surgery the infection should be brought under control and there should be a period of 4 to 6 months in which there is no evidence of soft tissue infection or osteomyelitis.

There are many methods for bone grafting and stabilization, but the reconstruction plate has become the most popular (Fig. 19–5). This technique has the advantage of rigid fixation with early mobility and function of the jaw. Bone grafts can be harvested from a variety of sites, but the ilium is preferred. Iliac bone is easy to obtain and easy to shape and fit into the nonunion defect. Other options, especially when there is an atrophic mandible, include using a titanium mesh to bridge the defect and filling the mesh with cancellous bone chips. For these cases the mesh is also strong enough to provide rigid fixation and early mobility of the jaw.

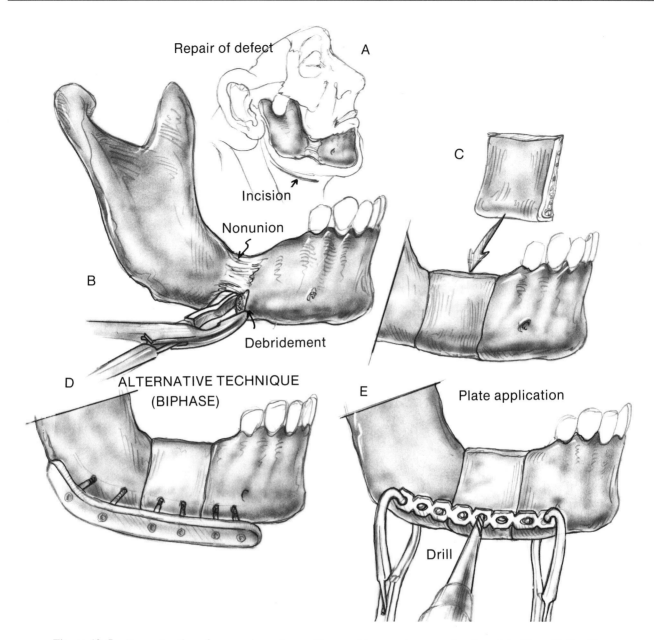

Figure 19–5. Reconstruction of a nonunion using an iliac crest bone and a reconstruction plate (from Mathog[35]).

MALUNION

Malunion of the mandible can occur following mandibular fracture when there is imperfect reduction, inadequate fixation and stabilization, and periods of infection and reabsorption of bone. The degree of malalignment dictates the degree of deformity and dysfunction. Correction should be considered for patients with malocclusion, temporomandibular joint disorders, and facial asymmetry.[8,9]

Minor discrepancies of occlusion can often be managed by conservative occlusal adjustments. For moderate occlusal problems, orthodontic therapy will be required. Sometimes, when a single tooth, or several teeth, are a problem, extraction may be a simple and effective approach. In the edentulous patient discrepancies can be corrected by denture modification.

For the more serious malunion, the jaw will have to be refractured with surgical osteotomies. Occlusal relationships

will have to be reestablished with appropriate methods of fixation. Surgical planning requires a careful evaluation of the preexisting occlusal relationships (models and/or dental records), up-to-date radiography, and a set of impressions with dental casts. In general the dental cast is osteomized and fractured segments are placed on an articulator and mobilized into anatomic and functional relationships. This procedure gives the surgeon the "plan" and suggests whether bone grafting will be necessary and what means of fixation will be required to hold the segments in the desired position. Occasionally lingual or interocclusal splints are used as a guide during the surgical procedure to correctly place the fragments.

The incision and approach will depend on the site of fracture. The osteotomy is performed with Lindeman burrs, oscillating saws, or with fine sharp osteotomes. Care is taken not to further injure the inferior alveolar nerve. Occlusion is adjusted and maintained with intermaxillary fixation or splints. If there is a defect in the bone, then this should be filled with a cortical or cancellous bone graft. The segments of the mandible are then held in fixation with plates or mesh as described in the treatment of nonunion. Fixation is maintained for 6 to 8 weeks. Prophylactic antibiotics are administered for 5 to 7 days or longer if bone grafts are used.

ANKYLOSIS OF THE TEMPOROMANDIBULAR JOINT

Immobility of the jaw secondary to temporomandibular joint ankylosis is an unfortunate sequela following injury to the head of the condyle and/or joint area. Failure to open the jaw can be associated with pain, poor nutrition, and dysarthria. In children there can be retardation of mandibular growth and serious secondary deformities.

The diagnosis and condition of the patient will dictate therapeutic options. Dynamic radiographs and CT scans are important. From a diagnostic standpoint it is essential to determine whether the patient's inability to open the mouth is secondary to scarring and contraction of soft tissues or a true fibro-osseous union between the condyle and glenoid fossa.

If the dysfunction is caused by scarring then steroid injections and jaw opening exercises should be instituted. If there is a bony fusion of the joint, then a more aggressive surgical approach is required.[10-12] In the elderly patient an osteotomy through the neck of the condyle with a soft tissue interposition may be all that is necessary. In the younger patient, it may be judicious to resect the condyle and reconstruct the condyle with an alloplastic implant or autogenous bone graft. In most adults, however, a rib graft is ideal and provides autologous nonreactive tissues. This technique has the advantage of a cartilage end for mobility and bone-to-bone union for restoration of strength of the mandible.

There are several approaches that can be used for condylar surgery (Fig. 19–6). Direct exposure is probably best obtained through a preauricular incision with a dissection inferiorly from the zygomatic arch to the joint capsule. Care must be taken to avoid injury to the facial nerve. Once the condyle and neck of the mandible is exposed, the bone can be removed

with cutting burrs and/or rongeurs. The glenoid fossa is also carved to receive the head of the implant.

To reconstruct the condyle a rib graft is harvested from the seventh rib. The cartilage portion is retained and smoothed out to fit into the glenoid fossa. The periosteum of the mandible is then elevated, and to help with this exposure, a separate incision is made beneath the angle of the mandible. The rib is then inserted beneath the periosteum into the new glenoid fossa and secured to the mandible with wires or lag screws. Some form of intermaxillary fixation is employed for 4 weeks. Opening and closing exercises are initiated as soon as intermaxillary wires and elastic bands are removed.

TOOTH INJURIES

Damage to the dentition commonly occurs with facial fractures. Treatment of this injury depends on whether the tooth involved is deciduous or permanent, the severity of injury (including number of teeth affected), the health of the injured tooth, and the cost-effectiveness of the repair.[13] Consultation with dentists, endodontists, orthodontists, and oral surgeons is desirable.

Tooth fractures are classified according to whether there is injury to the dentition and/or pulp (Fig. 19–7). Those injuries confined to the enamel can often be treated by smoothing the edge of the tooth with an abrading disk. When the injury involves both enamel and dentine, the edges are abraded and a dressing of calcium hydroxide (or zinc oxide) is placed followed by a stainless steel or acrylic crown. The definitive restoration can be permanently placed sometime later.

Complicated dental injuries that involve the pulp are treated differently depending on the timing of the repair. If the injury is seen early, it is possible to cap the pulp with calcium hydroxide and then apply a temporary acrylic crown. At 6 to 24 hours after injury, the pulp should be exitrpated, a calcium hydrdoxide dressing should be placed, and a temporary crown fabricated. For repairs requiring at a later time, a complete endodontic procedure should be performed (Fig. 19–8).

The treatment of root injuries will depend on the level of injury (Fig. 19–9). For the more apical fracture, the tooth

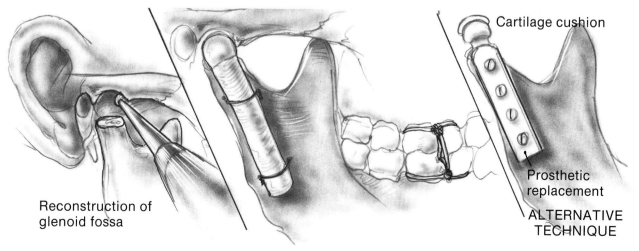

Figure 19–6. Reconstruction of glenoid fossa with autogenous rib graft (from Mathog[35]).

ENAMEL INJURY

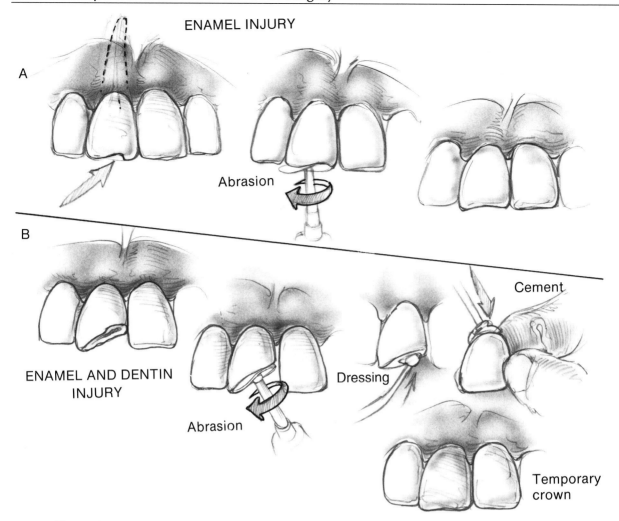

Figure 19-7. Repair of tooth injuries involving enamel and/or dentition. **(A).** Abrasion. **(B).** Temporary crown techniques (from Mathog[35]).

often can be salvaged with acrylic or composite splints. For fractures in the middle or coronal third, extraction is usually the treatment of choice. It is however possible to splint the tooth, and if pulp disease ensues, perform endodontic therapy or formal extraction of the tooth.

For teeth that are partially avulsed, the tooth is placed into a normal anatomic position and then stabilized with a splint or orthodontic appliance. If the tooth is avulsed, and it is less than 2 hours from the time of injury, then the tooth can be reset and stabilized accordingly. For these cases the tooth socket should be debrided and the apex of the tooth amputated.

Maxillary Fractures

MALUNION

Malposition of maxillary factures can cause multiple dysfunctions and deformities. The face can be elongated and/or retruded; there can be masticatory, temporomandibular, and speech problems. Psychological changes may eventually occur. The evaluation of maxillary malunion should include photographic, radiographic, and clinical assessment of the functional and aesthetic imbalance. Information should be obtained regarding anosmia, cerebral spinal fluid leaks loss

of vision, diplopia, epistaxis, loss of facial sensation, and nasal obstruction. Facial fractures should be analyzed for flattening in the anteroposterior direction, loss of projection of nose, and depression of the malar eminences. Intercanthal distances and changes in height of the palpebral fissures should be recorded. Globe position in the anteroposterior and vertical directions should also be determined. Mandibular occlusal relationships should be noted.

To help in this evaluation the patient should have cephalometric analyses, facial bone films, dental films, and CT scans. Three-dimensional CT scan reconstructions are desirable. Dental occlusion should be recorded and quantitated on dental models. Orthodontic and prosthodontic consultations are valuable. Interocclusal acrylic wafers made from dental models should be manufactured and available for orientation of the occlusion in the operating room.

The type of procedure that is performed will depend on the site and extent of fractures.[14-16] Usually the malunions can be classified in such a way that osteotomies created along the Le Fort fractures will obtain the desired results.

In most cases anesthesia is provided by nasotracheal intubation. The face and neck are scrubbed and draped as sterile fields. Arch bars or Ivy loops are then applied to the upper

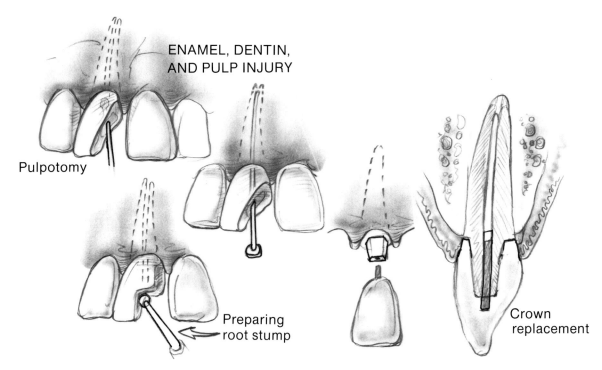

Figure 19–8. Endodontia repair of tooth injury involving enamel, dentin, and pulp (from Mathog[35]).

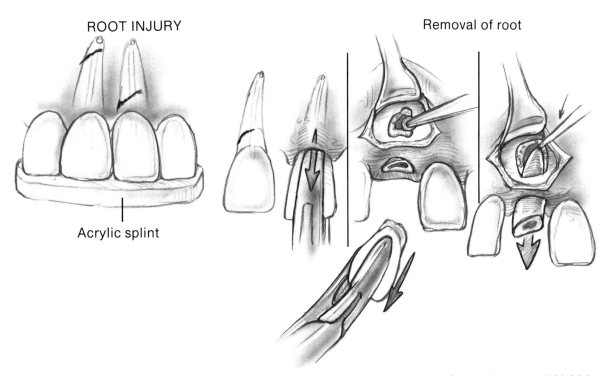

Figure 19–9. Treatment of root injury. Acrylic splinting of high apical injury (left). Extraction for middle or coronal third injury (right) (from Mathog[35]).

and lower dentition. Incisional lines are subsequently marked and infiltrated with 1% lidocaine containing 1:100,000 epinephrine. The nasal mucus membranes are treated with 4% cocaine containing epinephrine.

Le Fort I osteotomies are generally used for low maxillary retrusion (Fig. 19–10). For this procedure, the surgeon makes

an incision in the gingival labial sulcus and elevates the periosteum off the lower portion of the maxilla. The septum is separated from the columella and floor incisions are made to help elevate the soft tissues upward over the entire maxilla. Mucoperiosteal tunnels are then made along the septum to free the mucoperichondrium from the quadrilateral plate

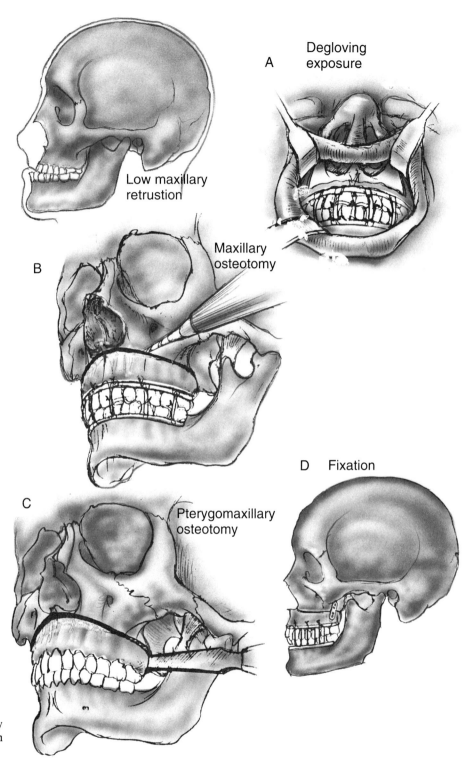

Figure 19–10. Le Fort I osteotomy for low maxillary retrusion (from Mathog[35]).

and mucoperiosteum from the vomer and perpendicular plate of the ethmoid. The mucoperiosteum is then elevated off the floor and onto the lateral walls of the nose.

Using Lindeman burrs, electric saws, or mallet and chisels, horizontal cuts are made through the lateral rim of the pyriform apertures at a level of at least 5 mm above the apices of the dental roots. Osteotomies are then made along the lateral walls of the nose trying to avoid injury to the floor flaps and sinus mucosa. The cartilaginous and bony septum

is separated from the palate with sharp septal chisels. Exteriorly the maxilla is loosened from the pterygoid plates with a curved osteotome directed into the pterygomaxillary grooves. After all osteotomies are carried out, the maxilla is downfractured and mobilized forward. The palatine vessels should be visualized and care taken to avoid injury to them. The jaws are then placed into occlusion (with the help of the interocclusal wafer) and fixed to each other with 26-gauge stainless steel wire. Miniplates are used to stabilize the fracture at the zygomatico-maxillary buttresses. Postoperatively the inter-maxillary fixation can be released and the patient placed on a soft diet. The progress of the patient should be monitored with standard radiographs, cephalometric films, and photographs.

For the patient having retrusion of the midface and lengthening of the face, a Le Fort II osteotomy procedure must be considered. These patients usually have normal projection of the malar eminences but depression of the nasal maxillary complex. Open bite deformities are common.

The osteotomies for the Le Fort II procedures require gingival labial sulcus, medial canthi, and infraciliary incisions (Fig. 19–11). The gingival labial incision exposes the lateral maxillary, retromaxillary, and lower portion of the nose. The medial canthal incision allows exploration for the attachment of the nasal bones to the frontal processes of the maxilla and the frontomaxillary buttresses. The infraciliary incisions promote access to the inferior rims and floors of the orbits.

The exposure of the lower maxilla is identical to that performed for the Le Fort I osteotomy. Working through the medial canthal incisions, the periosteum is elevated off of the nasoglabellar angle and medial walls of the orbits. Care is taken not to injure the medial canthal ligaments and lacrimal collecting systems. Using Lindeman burrs, chisels, or osteotomes, cuts are made across the bridge of the nose, beneath the nasofrontal suture line, across the frontal processes of the maxilla, and then along the medial aspects of the orbit. Working through the infraciliary incisions, the floors of the orbits and inferior orbital nerves are exposed, and osteotomies are made just lateral to the neurovascular bundles. Using the gingival labial exposures, the osteotomies are completed through the zygomaticomaxillary buttresses. The pterygomaxillary spaces are then entered with a curved chisel and the maxilla separated from the pterygoid plates. The final osteotomy is done with a fine chisel directed from the nasofrontal angle diagonally to the junction of the septum and palate. Using a Rowe disimpaction forceps, the maxilla is rotated forward and positioned in appropriate occlusal relationships with the mandible. As in the Le Fort I procedures, fixation is achieved with miniplates across the zygomatico-maxillary buttresses. Bone grafts should be placed into the defects caused by the osteotomies. Postoperative care is similar to that used in the Le Fort I procedure.

Le Fort III osteotomies are primarily used for midfacial retrusion associated with inadequate malar and infraorbital rim projection. Such patients have concave facial profiles and a lengthening of the face. The maxillary arch is usually retruded and there can be an open bite deformity.

In these cases a tracheostomy is a preferred method of anesthesia. Arch bars or Ivy loops are applied. Gingival labial, infraciliary, and coronal incisions are used for appropriate exposure. Gingival labial exposure is used for access for the pterygomaxillary osteotomies. The infraciliary incision is used to explore the floors of the orbits and the coronal incision is used for access to the bridge of the nose and the zygomas.

The procedure begins with the coronal incision (Fig. 19–12). A plane is developed between the galea and periosteum of the frontal bone and the dissection proceeds to the nasofrontal region. The periosteum is elevated off the superior orbital rims and frontal processes of the zygomas, and if necessary, bone is removed from around the supraorbital artery and nerve to give additional exposure. An osteotomy is made with Lindeman burrs just beneath the nasofrontal angle and with sharp narrow chisels, osteotomies are carried through the frontal processes of the maxilla and down along the medial walls of the orbit. Osteotomies are also made along the frontozygomatic sutures and along the zygomatic arches. Additional cuts are extended along the lateral walls of the orbit to the floor regions. The orbital floor osteotomies are completed through the infraciliary exposures. The pterygomaxillary osteotomies are then performed to allow the entire maxilla to be rocked forward with Rowe disimpaction forceps. Occlusion is obtained through intermaxillary fixation and an interocclusal wafer. The osteotomy sites are stabilized with miniplates and small bone grafts. Intermaxillary fixation is best continued for 6 weeks. Stability of dental occlusion is monitored clinically and radiographically. Long-term follow-up is necessary to evaluate or halt regression.

Malar Fractures
MALUNION

Malar fractures that are displaced and malunited pose significant problems of deformity and possible dysfunction. Depression of the cheek can be associated with enophthalmos, hypophthalmos, and limitation of mastication and conjugate gaze. In the early stages of healing, osteotomies and repositioning of the malar bones is a reasonable approach. However, if the processes of the zygoma have undergone resorption, then the bone will be unstable following osteotomy and adjunctive bone grafts become important.

Exposure for malar osteotomies can be made through either a coronal or brow incision combined with an infraciliary incision (Fig. 19–13). The frontozygomatic suture line should be exposed and periosteum elevated off the lateral wall of the orbit. During this dissection the zygomaticosphenoid suture line and inferior orbital fissure are exposed. The infraciliary incision should at first separate the eyelid skin and orbicularis muscle from the orbital septum. The dissection is then continued to the anterior wall of the maxilla where the periosteum is incised and elevated off the inferior orbital rim. The floor of the orbit is subsequently elevated as well as the periosteum of the zygomaticomaxillary buttress.

In general the osteotomies follow the fracture lines. The initial cut is started at the zygomaticofrontal suture and continued along the lateral wall of the orbit to the inferior orbital fissure. The next cut starts at the inferior orbital rim and follows the fractures laterally to the inferior orbital fissure. The osteotome is then turned downward along the lateral face of the maxilla through the zygomaticomaxillary buttress. A heavy clamp is then inserted underneath the zygomatic arch, and with an elevator directed through the inferior orbital rim osteotomy, the malar bone is rocked and directed into the preferred position. The bone is then fixed at the zygomaticofrontal buttress and inferior orbital rim with small plates (or wires).

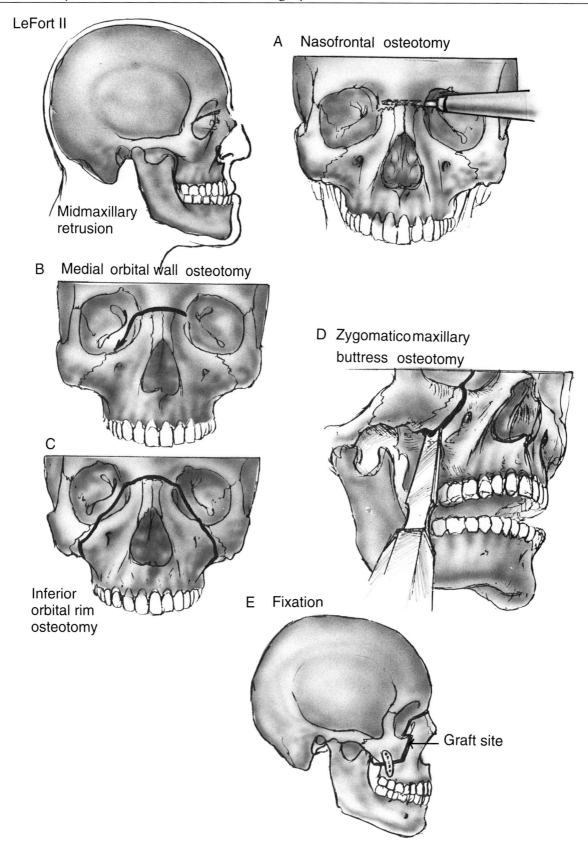

Figure 19–11. Le Fort II osteotomies for retrusion of the midface. Osteotomies are performed through medial canthal, infraciliary, and gingival labial incisions (from Mathog[35]).

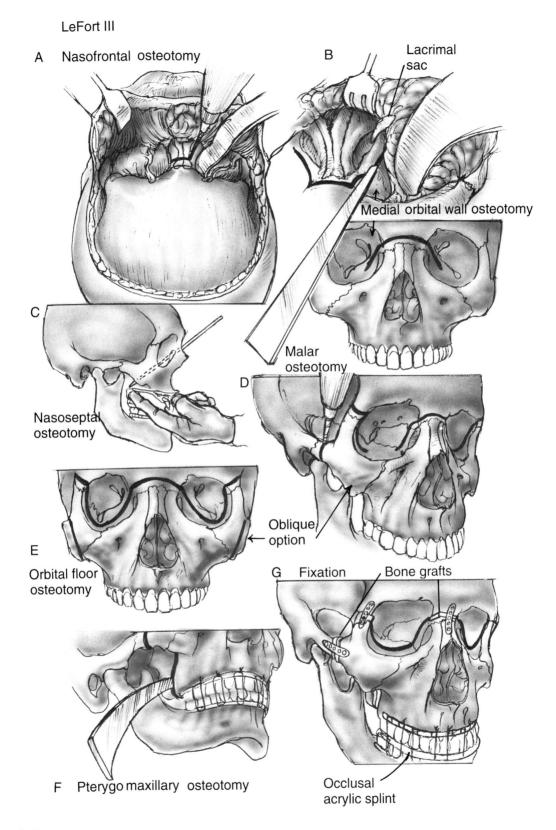

LeFort III

A Nasofrontal osteotomy

B Lacrimal sac

Medial orbital wall osteotomy

C

Nasoseptal osteotomy

Malar osteotomy

D

Oblique option

E

Orbital floor osteotomy

G Fixation   Bone grafts

F Pterygo maxillary osteotomy

Occlusal acrylic splint

Figure 19–12.   Le Fort III osteotomies for midfacial deformities. Osteotomies are performed through coronal, infraciliary, and gingival labial incisions. The newly positioned maxilla is stabilized with miniplates, bone grafts, and a temporary occlusal splint (from Mathog[35]).

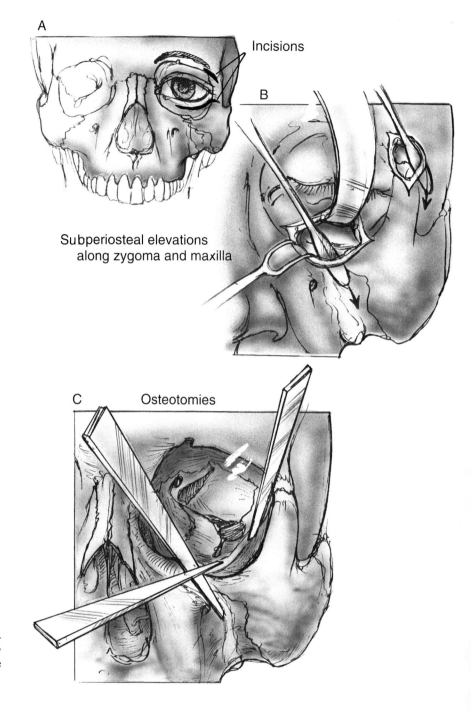

A   Incisions

B

Subperiosteal elevations
along zygoma and maxilla

C   Osteotomies

Figure 19–13. Osteotomies performed through brow and infraciliary incisions for malunion of malar bone (from Mathog[35]).

If the malpositioned malar bone has completely healed, it is probably best treated with onlay grafts. The procedure, however, will not help alleviate associated trismus or difficulty in mastication resulting from the malar bone impinging on the coronoid process. For this problem, osteotomy and/or intraoral coronoidectomy should be considered.

To correct the resorbed malunited malar bone, a bone graft is usually obtained from the hip, cranium, or rib. The hip is ideal if it is a major deformity and there is a need to use multiple pieces of bone. Rib has an excellent contour but unfortunately it is unpredictable regarding reabsorption. Cranial grafts are excellent because of their long-term stability, but they are difficult to carve and bend to appropriate position.

The exposure for the malar implant is usually obtained through a brow and extended infraciliary incision (Fig. 19-14). For this procedure an infraciliary incision is carried to the lateral canthus and then laterally in the crow's foot crease onto the cheek. The brow incision is used to expose the frontal process of the zygoma and the lateral wall of the orbit, whereas the infraciliary incision is used for the infraorbital rim, anterior maxillary wall, and body of the zygoma. A bone graft is then shaped to fit over the maxilla and malar bone and adjusted to the desired level in relation to the orbital rim. Several small pieces of bone are then placed on the surface of the frontal process of the zygoma and the anterior floor of the orbit. The bones are fixed with wire or, preferably,

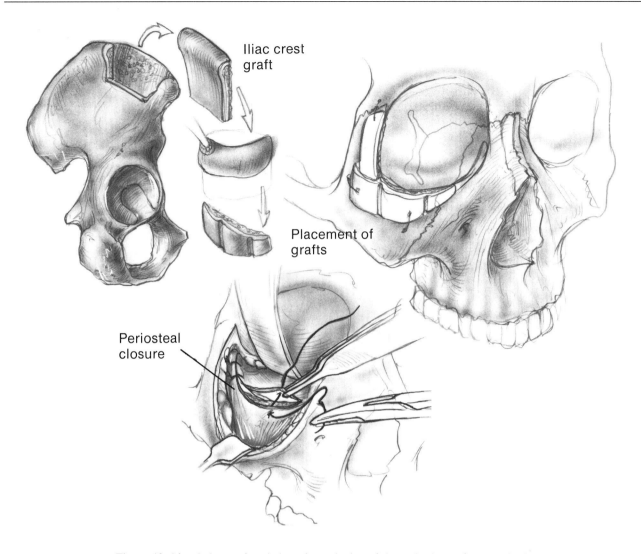

Iliac crest
graft

Placement of
grafts

Periosteal
closure

Figure 19–14.   Onlay graft technique for malunion of the malar bone (from Mathog[35]).

the lag screw technique. The periosteum, which was elevated off the malar-maxillary complex, is then brought over the bones and secured with 2-0 chromic sutures. The infraciliary and brow incisions are then closed followed by application of a light pressure dressing. Patients should be followed closely for reabsorption of the implants. Usually the lateral canthal ligament will adjust upward and obtain a normal anatomic position, but if this has not occurred, then a lateral canthoplasty must be considered.

INFRAORBITAL NERVE COMPRESSION

Fracture of the malar bone is often associated with loss of sensation over the cheek and upper dentition. The return of sensation is variable and occasionally the patient develops pain and paresthesia. A fracture near the infraorbital canal is usually evident on CT scan. Injection of 2% lidocaine at the infraorbital foramen should alleviate the pain. Long-term correction requires either an alcohol block or decompression of the infraorbital nerve.

The procedure is carried out through an infraciliary incision. A skin muscle flap is developed and the orbital septum is followed to the anterior wall of the maxilla. The periosteum is then elevated to expose the orbital rim, orbital floor, and infraorbital foramen. Fragments of bone are subsequently elevated from the orbital floor. The foramen is enlarged with rongeurs or cutting burrs. The wound is closed in layers. Although pain can be expected to be lessened or disappear, hypesthesia will return and often be permanent.

CORONOID IMPINGEMENT

A malunited depressed zygoma can sometimes fuse to the coronoid process causing limitation in opening the jaws and occasionally frank ankylosis. The preferred treatment is a refracturing of the malar bone (with or without osteotomies), but if bony union has taken place then alternative measures should be considered. Onlay grafts as described above can be used to correct the malar deformity; functional restoration of the jaw is best managed by a coronoidectomy.

The procedure is usually carried out through an intraoral approach (Fig. 19–15). An interocclusal bite block is placed on the side opposite fixation. The coronoid can usually be palpated and incisions made over the prominence of the process and the adjoining ramus. The periosteum and temporalis muscle insertion is then elevated off of the coronoid process.

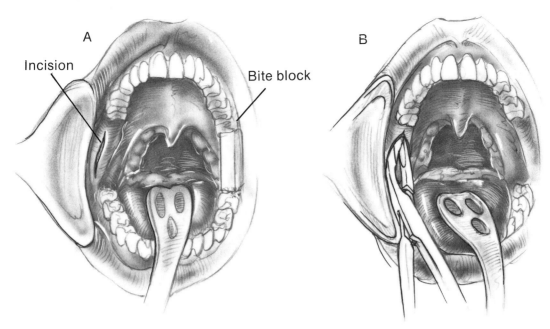

Figure 19–15. Intraoral coronoidectomy for impingement on malar bone (from Mathog[35]).

The coronoid is subsequently removed piecemeal with bone-cutting rongeurs. Jaw opening exercises and steroid injections into the area of surgery are helpful in the postoperative period.

Orbital Fractures

ENOPHTHALMOS, HYPOPHTHALMOS, AND DIPLOPIA

Complex orbital injuries, even when adequately treated, can sometimes develop sequelae of enophthalmos, hypophthalmos, and/or diplopia. The enophthalmos occurs as a result of expansion of the orbital wall, reduction of space occupied by intraorbital tissues, or a shift of fat behind the globe to a more peripheral position. Other causes are dislocation of the superior oblique muscle, cicatricial contractions of retrobulbar tissues, or rupture of the orbital ligaments. The hypophthalmos occurs from the lack of support of the globe, and the diplopia develops as a result of muscle imbalance from entrapment of fibrous septae around the muscle, neuromuscular injury or displacement of the axis of the globe. On the floor, the inferior rectus is often involved whereas on the medial wall there can be injury to the medial rectus muscle.

Treatment of these sequelae secondary to orbital injury depend on the site, timing, and degree of injury. Most blowout fractures can be repaired early by elevation of the floor fragments and reenforcing the floor with marlex mesh.[18,19] If the wall (or floor) is severely comminuted, then repair may require reconstruction with a carved piece of parietal bone. When the injury is noted later, there is often cicatrization, malposition, and reabsorption of an orbital wall and/or atrophy with loss of soft tissues. In these situations reconstruction must be considered. The muscles and their attachments will have to be freed and the walls of the orbit will have to be rebuilt by osteotomy or onlay grafts. The soft tissues are replaced or augmented by implant materials.

Reconstructive techniques are designed to reduce the size of the orbit and increase the size of intraorbital contents.[20]

Bone may be harvested from the ilium or parietal regions and for limited reconstructions cranial bone grafts work well.

The procedures are carried out under general anesthesia (Fig. 19–16). With the patient in the supine position the enophthalmos is measured, comparing one side to the other. Forced duction tests are repeated to evaluate the location of "entrapped" muscle. Computed tomograph scans in horizontal and coronal planes are important to evaluate the areas of deficit that will receive the graft(s).

The surgical approaches are usually through three incisions; the lower eyelid, the lateral eyebrow, and medial canthus. The lower eyelid or infraciliary incision is used to explore the floor region. Usually the dissection continues posteriorly to the junction of the inferior orbital fissure and infraorbital canal. It is also extended laterally to the lateral wall and medially to the medial wall of the orbit. The medial canthal incision is used to release the trochlea and the periosteum off of the medial wall of the orbit. This dissection continues behind the lacrimal collecting system and medial canthal ligament to join the pocket created on the floor. The anterior ethmoidal vessel is usually cauterized or ligated with vascular clips to control bleeding. The lateral eyebrow incision exposes the lateral wall of the orbit down to the floor region. The dissection also is extended posteriorly and superiorly behind the globe to the level of the pupil. The subperiosteal dissections should ultimately release all the soft tissues, carefully sparing the annulus tendinous and medial quadrant containing the ophthalmic artery and optic nerve.

The implantation is initiated with a shield-shaped implant along the floor region. If this implant does not raise the globe sufficiently, then additional layers of bone can be added. A curvilinear-shaped implant is placed through the brow incision behind the globe and a pyramidal-shaped implant is placed along the medial wall. The ultimate effect of these implants is to push the eye upward and outward without

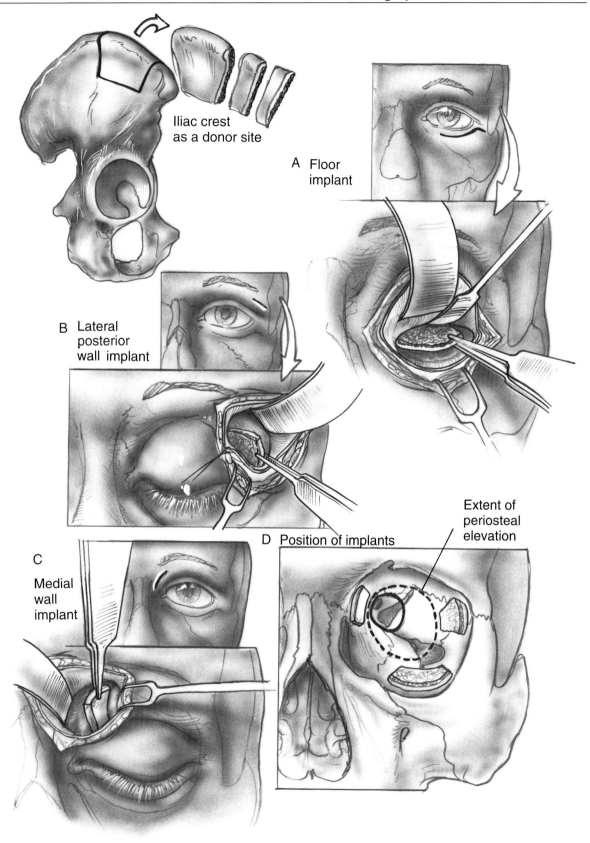

Iliac crest
as a donor site

A Floor
implant

B Lateral
posterior
wall implant

C
Medial
wall
implant

D Position of implants

Extent of
periosteal
elevation

Figure 19–16.   Strategic implantation of bone grafts to the orbit to correct enophthalmos, hypophthalmos, and diplopia. Grafts are harvested from the iliac crest and inserted through infraciliary and brow incisions (from Mathog[35]).

medial or lateral displacement. Ideally the surgeon should be aiming at an overcorrection of the hypophthalmos and enophthalmos by about 1 to 2 mm. Tension on the globe should be checked and forced duction tests are carried out to assure relaxation of the muscles. The periosteum is closed around the orbit and the wound closed in layers. The patient's vision should be evaluated in the recovery room and if there is any loss, then one or several implants should be removed. Usually a successful implantation will correct position of the eye and diplopia. The implants do not generally reabsorb and the results are stable over a long period of time.

When the patient has a combination of a floor and malar fracture, a more severe degree of deformity and dysfunction can be expected. With the floor fracture, the loss of the floor leads to failure and support of the globe and hypophthalmos. With the malar fracture, the suspensory ligament of Lockwood is displaced inferiorly, contributing more to the support problem. The floor fracture, when depressed, causes an increase in the volume of the orbit. This may be associated with some atrophy or necrosis of tissues. The malar fracture causes an even greater depression and lateralization of the walls adding to the discrepancy. When these conditions occur, then it is prudent to combine procedures. The orbital wall deformity is treated with strategic implantation of bone; the malar deformity, with onlay grafts. For these procedures cranial graft is somewhat limited whereas iliac bone is abundant and easily carved to the correct size and contour of the defects.

Nasal Fractures

Most nasal fractures are easily treated with closed reduction techniques. These procedures are best carried out within 7 to 10 days of the injury. If the nasal fracture is not treated early and adequately, then there can be malunion of the nasal bones and/or septum resulting in nasal obstruction and/or deformity.

A variety of deformities can be described alone or in combination: dorsal hump; c- or s-shaped deviation of the septum; depression of the dorsum; saddle deformity; deviation of the tip; fallen tip; retracted columella; asymmetry of the nasal bones; and asymmetry of the lower lateral cartilages. In addition, the septum can be displaced to one side or another and buckling can occur in the caudal-cephalad or supero-inferior direction. Once these deformities occur, then rhinoplasty and septoplasty techniques are indicated. When to perform these procedures is somewhat controversial, but in general, if there is severe deformity or dysfunction then they should be performed early. On the other hand, there is an advantage to allow the bones to heal solidly before surgery and this will usually take 3 to 6 months after the injury.

There are many procedures to fix the deformed nose.[21,22] Some are more logical than others depending on the location and severity of the deformity. The surgeon's experience and techniques will also be factors. For most deformities a transfixion incision using either an intercartilaginous or intra-cartilaginous incision is satisfactory. For those patients requiring dorsal implants and/or repair of the tip, delivery through a rim incision is helpful. Septoplasty alone can be approached with a septal-columella or septal incision.

The septorhinoplasty is traditionally approached through an inter or intracartilaginous incision. The dorsal skin and subcutaneous tissues are elevated off the cartilages and nasal bones. The incision is brought through the membranous septum to complete the transfixion. A septoplasty is then carried out. A mucoperichondrial flap is elevated off of the concave side of the septum. The dissection proceeds to further elevate the mucoperiosteum of the perpendicular plate of the ethmoid and vomer. A cut is generally made in front of the deflection and the mucus membrane elevated off of the opposite side of the septum. Deformed bone is removed. Some cartilage may be removed but it is generally scored and bent back to a straight position. Dorsal and caudal struts must be retained. Large maxillary crest spurs can be managed by floor tunnels combined with septal tunnels with removal of the projecting bone and cartilage.

If the tip is bulbous, the cephalic borders of the lower lateral cartilages are removed. The cartilaginous hump is trimmed with a sharp knife or scissors. The bony hump is taken down with rasps, osteotomes, or saws. Osteotomies are then completed with osteotomes directed toward the glabella on each side of the septum. Lateral osteotomies are carried out with osteotomes or saws and the nasal bones narrowed to close the dorsal defect. Internal and external splints are applied. A light nasal packing or tampons are used for 24 to 48 hours to control bleeding and prevent hematoma formation.

Severely deformed noses can also be treated with an open rhinoplasty technique. In this procedure an incision is made at the junction of the upper and lower middle thirds of the columella. The lateral portions of the incision are brought just beneath the rim. The dissection proceeds along the superior surface of the nasal cartilages and bone to expose these structures. The formal rhinoplasty is then carried out. The advantage of this approach is a direct visualization of the anatomy while osteotomies and resections are conducted.

Deficits of the nasal bones and cartilages are best treated with onlay grafts (Fig. 19–17). For these procedures, septal cartilage or bone or conchal cartilage can be used. For the saddle nose deformities these grafts can be layered on each other and held together with a chromic suture. The graft(s) can then be inserted through an intracartilaginous, intercartilaginous, or a rim incision into a pocket along the dorsum. Columella implants can be placed through a small incision through the medial crura and into a pocket between the crura. Tip and lower lateral implants can also be added through appropriate incisions.

Nasal Orbital/Ethmoid Fractures
TELECANTHUS AND EPIPHORA

Injuries to the frontal process of the maxilla, lacrimal, and ethmoid bones are usually classified as nasal orbital injuries. They are commonly associated with medial canthus deformities and dysfunctions. In many cases there is a change in appearance of the palpebral fissure accompanied by tearing and failure of the lacrimal collecting system.

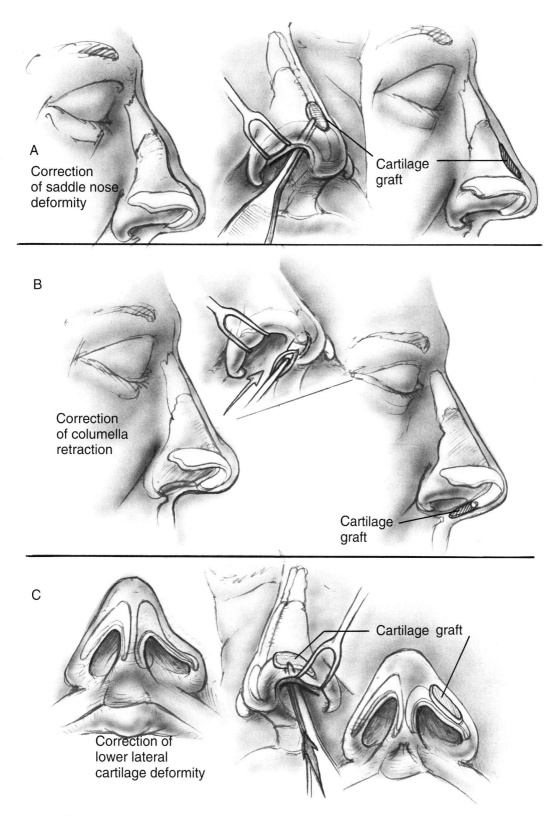

Figure 19–17. Repair of nasal deformities with cartilage onlay grafts (from Mathog[35]).

The pathophysiology is derived from the skeletal and soft tissues that are disrupted by the injury. The medial canthal ligament is important in defining the palpebral opening. The medial canthal ligament is an extension of the tarsal plates, which in turn inserts into the lateral wall of the orbit. The tarsal plates and ligaments receive insertions of the orbicularis oculi muscle. If the medial canthus is displaced, then the eyelids become lax and the palpebral fissure narrows. The medial caruncle moves laterally and the medial aspect of the eyelid takes on a rounded appearance. Usually the palpebral fissure width equals the palpebral fissure of the opposite side and this is the same as the intercanthal distance. When the medial canthus is displaced these relationships are changed.

Another aspect of the injury is the effect on the lacrimal collecting system. Tears normally enter the puncta at the medial free edge of the upper and lower eyelids. The eyelids are usually in contact with the globe and this abutment is important for the capillary action of the tears on the surface of the globe. However, if the eyelid is lax, the puncta will evert and not collect these tears. Horner's muscle, which pulls the eyelids against the globe, will also not be able to function.

Another factor is the pump mechanism. The orbicularis oculi, which surrounds the sac, also may become lax. When this occurs there will be a weakness in opening and closing of the eyelids and a loss of positive and negative pressures on the sac. Failure of this pumping action as a result of trauma will also result in epiphora.

The nasal orbital injury can be classified into three types based on the degree of injury and type of repair.[23,24] Type I injury indicates that the medial canthal ligament has been displaced with a small piece of attached lacrimal bone or that the ligament has been severed completely. The patient presents with telecanthus, epiphora, blunting of the inner angle, and a narrowing of the palpebral fissure. A type II injury implies that the medial wall of the orbit is comminuted and displaced. In addition to the signs and symptoms associated with a type I injury, there can be entrapment of the medial rectus muscle, cerebrospinal fluid leakage, and damage to the optic nerve. In the type III injury, the medial walls of the orbits are fractured. This implies also a fracture of the nasal ethmoid complex in which patients demonstrate a flattening and widening of the nasal dorsum, nasal obstruction and epistaxis, bilateral telecanthus, blunting of the inner angles, narrowing of the palpebral openings, and epiphora. Intracranial damage and cerebrospinal fluid leak often occur.

The type I telecanthus is best treated through a medial canthal incision combined with a lateral brow incision for exposure and relaxation of the lateral canthus. Once the periosteum is lifted off the frontal process of the maxilla, the trochlea attachment is released and elevation continued along the medial wall of the orbit. Additional exposure can be obtained by ligating the anterior ethmoidal artery. The lacrimal sac is then elevated from the lacrimal fossa and evaluated for damage. The dissection along the lateral wall of the orbit should be sufficient to release the lateral canthal ligament. The medial canthal ligament is identified in a subcuticular plane and affixed with a strong nonabsorbable suture to the posterior lacrimal crest (Fig. 19–18). This upward and backward pull is essential for proper placement of the lower eyelid against the globe. Once correction is achieved, the wound is closed in layers.

In the type II repair a transnasal technique is desirable (Fig. 19–19). For these patients medial and lateral canthal exposures identical to those performed for the type I repair are performed. In addition another medial canthal incision is made on the opposite side to expose the lacrimal fossa and crest of the intact orbit. The displaced ligament is subsequently secured with 30-gauge wire that is then carried by a large trocar needle to the opposite side. The other end of the wire is passed in a similar way so that the wire can be tied down on the intact anterior lacrimal crest. Wounds are closed appropriately.

In a type III repair, essentially both medial and lateral orbital walls are explored (Fig. 19–20). The lateral canthi are released and the medial canthal ligaments are identified bilaterally. The medial canthal ligament of one side is then secured with a 30-gauge wire that is passed transnasally and affixed to the medial canthal ligament of the opposite side. The passage of the wire through the septum should be high enough so that the medial canthi are tightened on each other and slightly elevated as they are pulled toward the midline. An alternative technique is to pass wires transnasally to the frontal processes of the maxilla. In this repair the wires are crossed diagonally and individually tightened to position the canthi.

In those patients who have undergone healing, there may be new bone formation along the medial orbital wall and scarring that extends along the periorbita. To correct the medial canthal ligaments under these conditions, it will be necessary to cut away the bone along the medial orbital wall with cutting burrs and elevate the periorbita along the floor region. Passage of the wires intranasally may require drill holes; the wires are then passed through catheters that are inserted into these holes. The catheters are subsequently removed leaving the wires, which are then secured to their appropriate positions.

TELECANTHUS AND DACRYOCYSTITIS

If tear collection is inadequate or obstructed, epiphora will occur. Stasis of secretions potentially causes a dacryocystitis. Sometimes this may be treated adequately with topical antibiotic drops but if obstruction is not relieved, then infection will continue to recur. In those cases in which the etiology is a kinking and twisting of the lower part of the collecting system, surgery must be considered.

The diagnosis of the level and degree of obstruction is important. The fluorescein dye test will determine if the system is functioning normally. If the puncta and canaliculi must be irrigated to pass the dye, then there must be some obstruction, usually in the lower part of the system. Failure to irrigate the dye suggests a high obstruction, supposedly within the canaliculi.

For chronic obstructions of the lacrimal collecting system involving the sac or nasolacrimal duct, a dacryocystorhinostomy should be performed (Fig. 19–21). In this procedure, the lacrimal fossa is exposed through a medial canthal or Iliff incision and an osteotomy made near the junction of the lacrimal and maxillary (frontal process) bone. The lacrimal sac is then identified and cut lengthwise. The nasal mucosa is incised in the form of an I. The posterior and anterior flaps are secured with fine chromic sutures. In cases complicated by scarring and disruption of the anatomy, Crawford tubes are desirable.

A

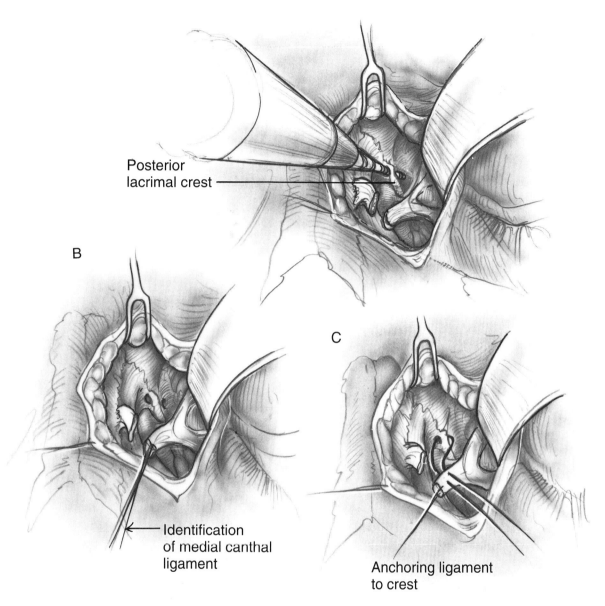

Posterior
lacrimal crest

B

C

Identification
of medial canthal
ligament

Anchoring ligament
to crest

Figure 19–18.   Type I repair of nasal orbital injury. The medial canthal ligament is secured to the posterior lacrimal crest (from Mathog[35]).

In patients who have obstruction of the canaliculi, other measures must be considered.[25,26] Older individuals who have reduced secretions may be treated conservatively. On the other hand, if the patient has symptomatic epiphora, then a conjunctivorhinostomy should be used (Fig. 19–22). For this procedure flaps are created from the conjunctiva and nasal mucosa. These flaps are then passed toward each other, and with exposure obtained through a medial canthal incision, the mucosal flaps are sutured together. Jones or Crawford tubes are optional.

CEREBROSPINAL FLUID LEAKS

Nasal orbital injuries that involve the ethmoid bone are often associated with anosmia and cerebrospinal fluid leaks.

Several pathologic processes can take place. If the dura is torn, pressure differences will force fluid into the upper respiratory system. If the dura is partially torn, constant intracranial arterial and respiratory pressures can slowly separate the dural fibers and cause a delayed presentation leak. Alternatively, a hematoma may form over the area of injury, and as it dissolves, the fluid becomes noted.

Many dural tears heal spontaneously. The main problem with cerebrospinal fluid leak is that there is no way to predict which leak will stop and which one will be associated with intracranial infection. In many patients the leak will stop with reduction of the facial fractures; but for those in whom the leak persists, it is important to localize the site and prepare for a surgical exploration and repair.

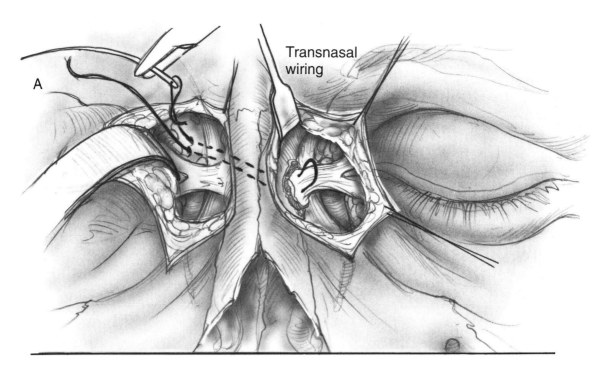

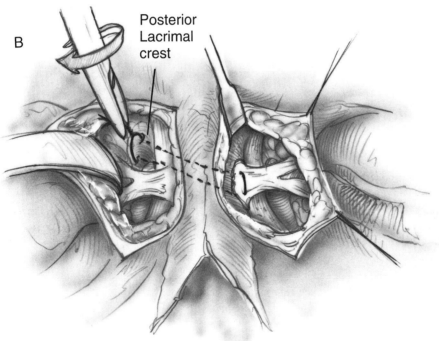

Figure 19–19.   Type II repair of nasal orbital injury. The medial canthal incision is secured transnasally to the posterior lacrimal crest of the opposite side (from Mathog[35]).

For most cerebrospinal fluid leaks in the nasal orbital region the diagnosis will be established by a gushing of clear fluid from the nose. For more occult leaks, the prescence of B_2-transferrin in the fluid has been shown to be specific for cerebrospinal fluid. This may be associated with anosmia. If visualized, the leakage will be coming through the superior vault or middle meatus. Imaging studies should help localize the fracture cand accumulation of fluid, but if there is still difficulty in determining the site, then the patient should undergo specific dye studies (metrizimide, radioactive materials, and fluorescein)[27,28] (Fig. 19–23).

Fractures associated with persistent cerebrospinal fluid leak along the cribriform plate are best treated with exploration and direct repair. For this procedure a frontoethmoidectomy is performed with removal of the floor of the frontal sinus, frontal process of the maxilla and a portion of nasal bones. A complete ethmoidectomy is then carried out to expose the floor of the anterior fossa. The cribriform plate and sphenoid

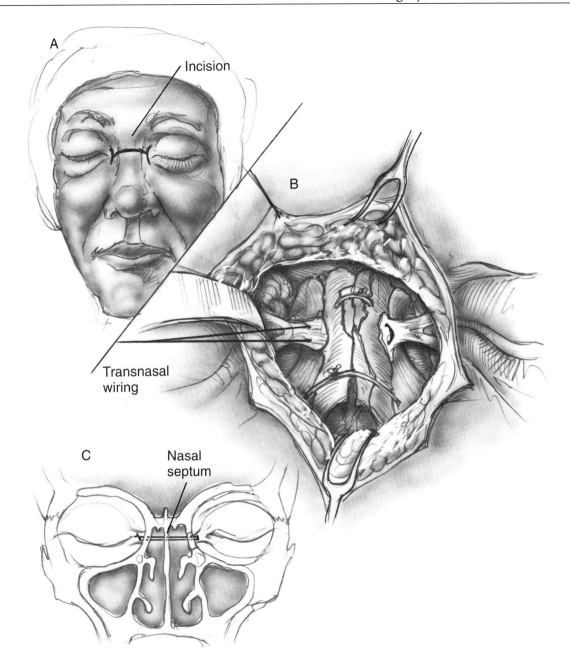

Figure 19–20. Type III repair of nasal orbital injury. The medial canthal ligaments are secured transnasally through the septum to each other (from Mathog[35]).

sinus are identified. To find the fistula a microscope is useful. The opening in the bone is then cleared of mucosa and packed with temporalis fascia. If possible a small flap of mucosa is rotated over the defect. Layers of 1/2-in gauze treated with Bacitracin ointment are used to hold the tissues in position.

Frontal Bone Fractures
CEREBROSPINAL FLUID LEAK

In the frontal bone region the dura is tightly adherent to bone and often lacerated with fractures of the posterior table. When this occurs there can be clear fluid leaking from the wounds of the forehead or through the nose. The patient often has associated cranial injury and there is usually evidence

of air (pneumocephalus) within the anterior fossa. Because of the possibility of persistence of the leakage and contamination of the leakage leading to meningitis, exploration and repair are desirable.[29,30] Confirmation of the site should be obtained by appropriate imaging studies.

The standard surgical approach is through a coronal incision (Fig. 19–24). A plane is developed between the galea and periosteum and elevation continued to the orbital rim. Care is taken to preserve the supraorbital vessels and nerves. Using a template of the frontal sinus made from a 6-foot Caldwell x-ray, an outline of the sinuses is made on the periosteum. Osteotomies are placed just within the markings with oscillating saws and osteotomes. The anterior wall of the frontal sinus is elevated and fractured at the level of the

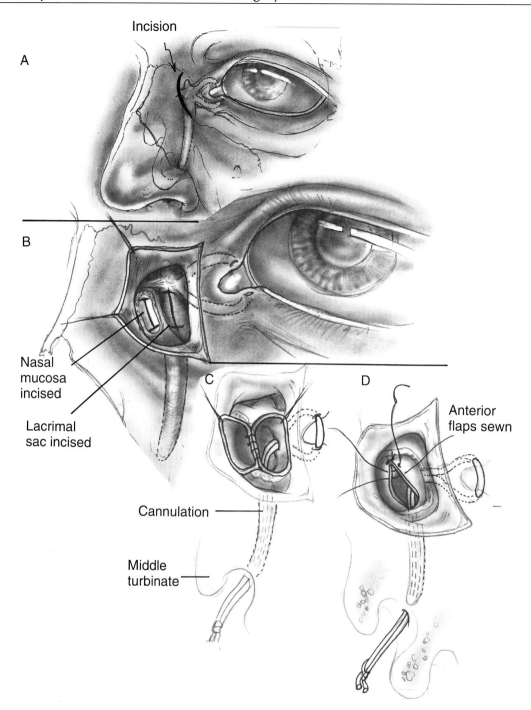

Figure 19–21. Dacryocystorhinostomy with Crawford tubes (from Mathog[35]).

superior orbital rim. The mucosa is removed and the leak is identified. Pieces of bone are then removed from around the leak to expose the dura. A small tear can be packed with fascia, whereas larger tears require more exposure and direct closure of the laceration with nonabsorbable suture. The sinus is subsequently packed with fat harvested from the abdomen after meticulously removing all mucosa from the sinus. The anterior wall is rotated into place and the periosteum secured with chromic sutures. The forehead flap is replaced and closed in layers. A light compression dressing is applied.

MUCOCELE

If the frontal sinus fracture involves the nasofrontal duct, it is possible for the opening to become obstructed and affect the function of the sinus.[31] This can ultimately lead to a large cyst or sinus mucocele that can expand and erode adjacent bone. These mucoceles can also be infected and in turn infect the orbit and areas of the anterior fossa. The patient in the early stages may complain of pain and fullness of the frontal region. Later, as the mucocele erodes into the orbit, there may be proptosis and displacement of the globe.

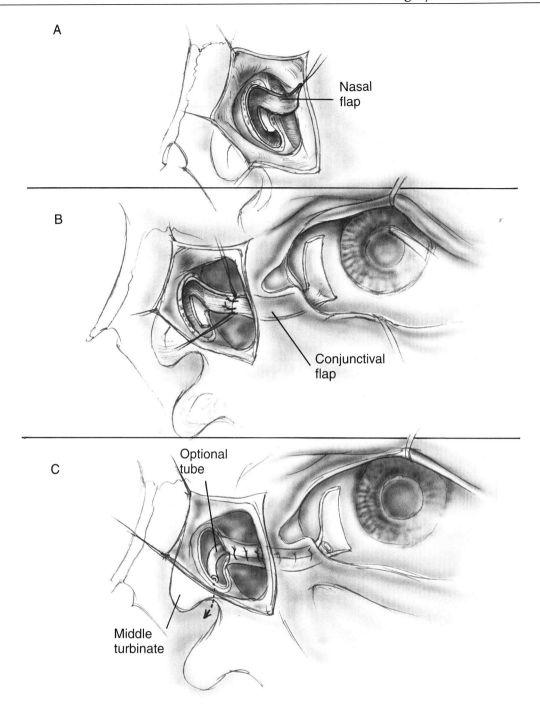

A

Nasal flap

B

Conjunctival flap

C

Optional tube

Middle turbinate

Figure 19–22. Conjunctivorhinostomy using conjunctival and nasal mucosal flaps (from Mathog[35]).

Intracranial extension is silent and usually realized by appropriate imaging studies.

Mucocele is a surgical disease. Oncethe diagnosis is established the frontal sinus should be explored, the mucocele removed, and the sinus obliterated with fat. The usual approach is through a coronal incision and osteoplastic flap (Fig. 19–24). The procedure is similar to that performed for the correction of the posterior wall fracture with cerebrospinal fluid leakage. All mucous membranes must be removed. The walls of the sinus are usually cleaned further with cutting burrs and the sinuses obliterated with fat. The patient should be followed closely for the possibility of reoccurrence.

MALUNION

The malunited frontal sinus fracture usually appears as a deformity of forehead and/or brow region. This condition is caused by inadequate reduction or absorption of bone. The defect is usually not noticeable early after repair, but the affected patient will often return years later complaining of a depression of the forehead or brow region. For small defects, recontouring the forehead with cutting burrs and application of onlay split grafts is desirable.

For most patients, a coronal incision with elevation of the forehead flap will provide optimal exposure. The dissection

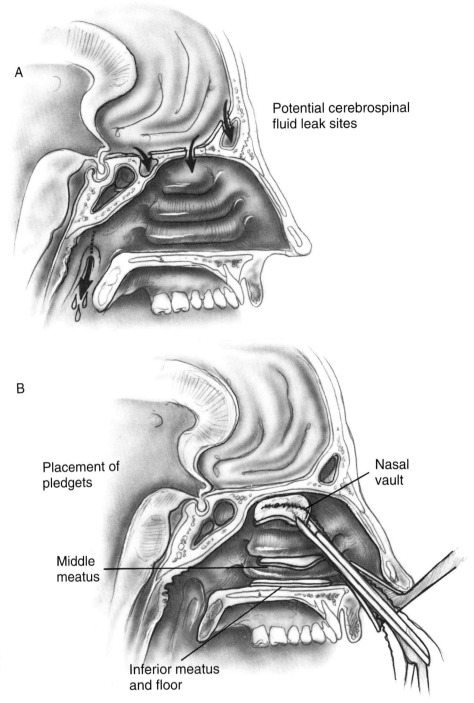

Potential cerebrospinal
fluid leak sites

Placement of
pledgets

Nasal
vault

Middle
meatus

Inferior meatus
and floor

Figure 19–23. Pledget placement for intrathecal dye test (from Mathog[35]).

is carried out in a plane between the galea and periosteum. At the level of the defect the periosteum is elevated as a separate flap. The deformity is subsequently measured and a piece of bone is obtained from the parietal region to fill this defect. The graft is contoured and placed under the periosteum. It is secured with miniplates or a tight closure of the periosteum. The forehead flap is returned and the incisions are closed in layers. A light pressure dressing will prevent edema and help hold the graft in place.

Sphenoid Bone Fractures

CEREBROSPINAL FLUID LEAKS

Considering that facial fractures can be associated with a dural tear anywhere within the anterior fossa, there is also a possibility that the cerebrospinal fluid leak is coming through the walls of the sphenoid sinus. These sinus injuries are generally found with fractures of other facial bones.[32] Because the fractures involve the base of the skull,

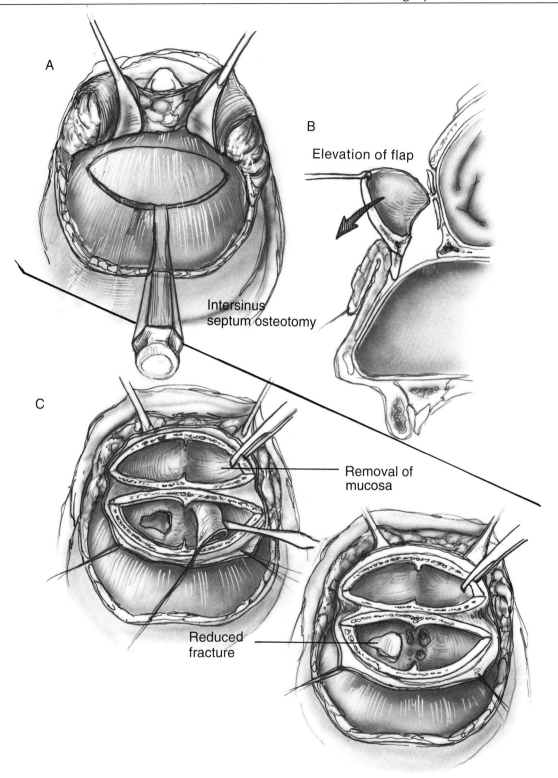

Figure 19–24. Frontal sinus exploration with osteoplastic flap and obliteration with abdominal fat (from Mathog[35]).

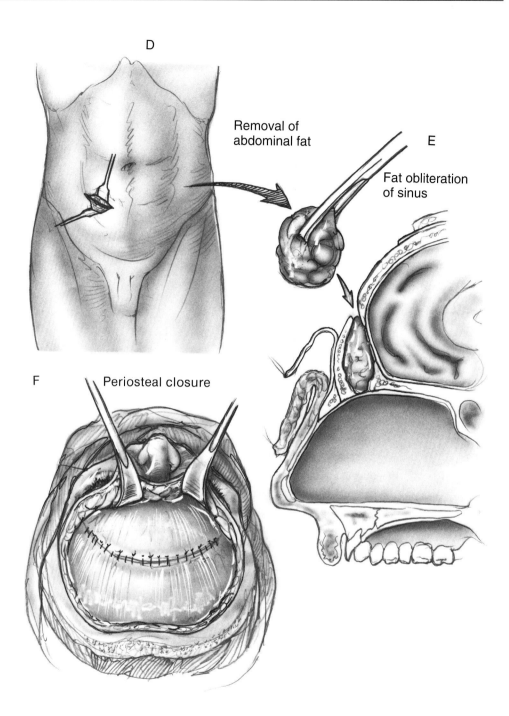

Figure 19–24   (continued).

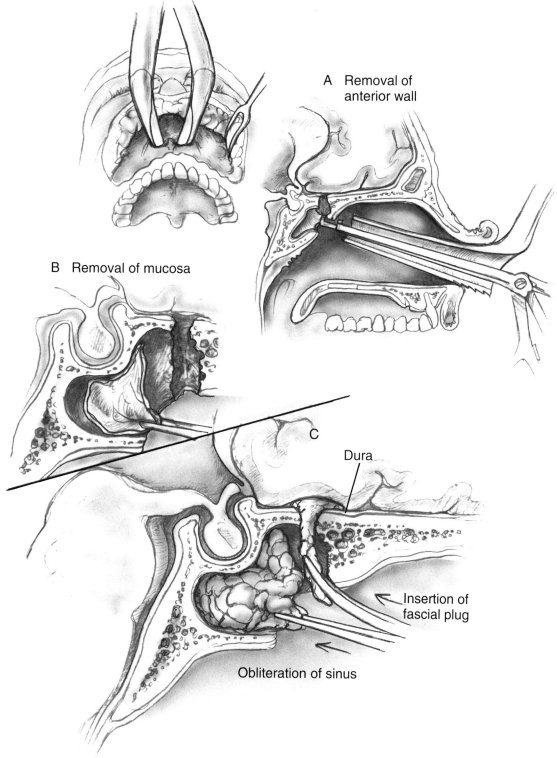

A   Removal of
    anterior wall

B   Removal of mucosa

C

Dura

Insertion of
fascial plug

Obliteration of sinus

Figure 19–25.   Transphenoidal repair of cerebrospinal fluid leak (from Mathog[35]).

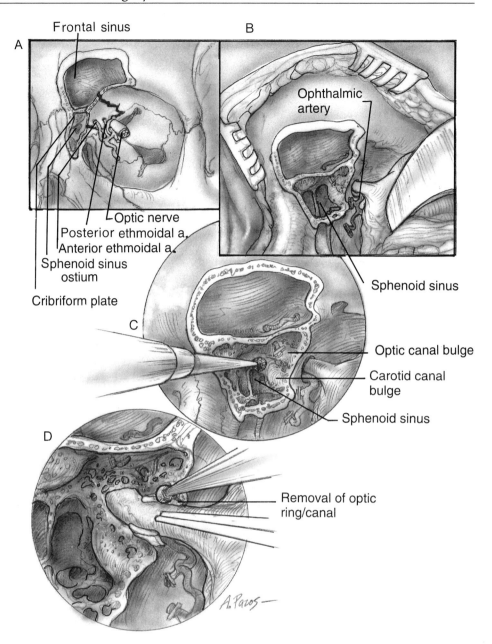

Figure 19–26. Transethmoidal decompression of optic nerve (from Mathog[35]).

there are often multiple neuropathies as well as intracranial damage.

The location and extent of the leak is best evaluated by a combination of plain radiographs, tomographs, and CT. Dye studies may be carried out. In most cases expectant waiting will be appropriate. Antibiotic prophylactic therapy is indicated. If the leak does not stop, then surgical exploration and repair should be performed.

Of the several generally accepted approaches for correction of cerebrospinal fluid leaks of the sphenoid sinus, probably the transseptal repair is the most common (Fig. 19–25). For this procedure a sublabial incision provides excellent exposure. The periosteum is elevated off of the premaxilla and incisions are made between the columella and septum and carried to the floor of the nose. Subperiosteal and subperichondrial tunnels are then performed and the septum

rotated to one side of the nose. Special refractors are placed to expose the face of the sphenoid sinus. Usually the sphenoid ostea can be used as a guide and the anterior wall of the sphenoid sinus removed. A microscope can be set up for better lighting and visualization. The mucosa is then removed from the sinus. A fascia plug is inserted into the leak and the sinus packed with abdominal fat. The tissues are held in place for 7 to 10 days with 1 1/2-in gauze treated with Bacitracin ointment.

Another approach is through a frontoethmoidectomy. This technique, similar to that described for the cribriform plate leak, exposes and removes the anterior wall of the sphenoid sinus. Under microscopic visualization the mucosa is removed from the sinus. The leak is identified and plugged with fascia. The sinus is obliterated with fat, which is held in position by Bacitracin-treated gauze packing.

TRAUMATIC OPTIC NEUROPATHY

Sudden progressive loss of vision following craniofacial trauma may indicate optic nerve damage. In such situations the patient usually demonstrates a Marcus Gunn pupil (afferent pupillary defect). Visual potentials are often markedly diminished or absent.

A variety of mechanisms have been used to describe optic nerve damage. The optic nerve may be mechanically impacted by displacement of adjacent bone fragments or it may be contused or compressed by blood clots or swelling within the optic canal. There is also a possibility that the nerve has been lacerated and severed from its attachment. Immediate loss of vision suggests a laceration or cutting whereas a gradual loss is more consistent with a compression phenomenon.

Imaging studies are important to determine whether there are displaced fractures in the area of the optic nerve. Patients are started on 100 mg of dexamethasone followed by 50 mg every 6 hours for three doses. If the patient responds, the steroids are tapered. If the patient does not respond or if there is a relapse after gradual improvement, then the steroids are stopped (or tapered) and a surgical decompression is considered.[32-24]

The transethmoidal approach is direct and relatively easy to perform (Fig. 19–26). The patient is put in a Trendelenburg position. The surgeon sits at the head of the table. A fronto-ethmoidectomy is then performed exposing the posterior wall of the frontal sinus and cribriform plate region. Additional exposure is obtained by ligating the anterior ethmoidal artery and removing the medial wall of the orbit. The posterior ethmoidal vessel is identified and clipped to control bleeding. The anterior wall of the sphenoid sinus is then removed and the surgeon can subsequently visualize the optic nerve bulge within the sinus and the optic nerve within the orbit transversing the optic canal. The optic canal can be removed with cutting burrs and rongeurs to decompress the nerve. The procedure has the advantage of a direct approach. On the other hand removing the medial wall of the orbit will cause enophthalmos.

SUMMARY

Complications developing from facial fractures can cause major functional and cosmetic problems. Early diagnosis and repair of the craniofacial injury can often prevent the undesirable sequelae. Present day approaches call for wide exposure, accurate reduction, and rigid stable fixation of the fragments. Soft tissue injuries should be carefully evaluated and treated appropriately.

Once a complication has developed it is important to evaluate its cause and pinpoint the site and extent of the problem. Modern imaging studies are essential for this analysis. It is also important to determine the best timing and management of the problem. Often times a carefully planned and executed surgical procedure will provide an optimal result. Although perfection in all patients is desirable, many will be left with variable degrees of dysfunction and/or deformity.

REFERENCES

1. Mathog RH. Scar revision. *Minn Med.* 1974;57:31–36.
2. Fisch U. Facial nerve grafting. *Otolaryngol Clin North Am.* 1974;7:517–529.
3. Mathog RH. Large facial wounds. In: Gates GA, ed: *Current Therapy in Otolaryngology-Head and Neck Surgery.* Philadelphia, Pa: BC Decker; 1987;3:73–77.
4. Hagan WE. Microneural techniques for nerve grafting. *Laryngoscope.* 1981;191:1759–1766.
5. Smith BC, Nesi F. *Practical Techniques in Ophthalmic Plastic Surgery.* St Louis, Mo: CV Mosby Co; 1981:44–46.
6. Mathog RH, Boies LR Jr. Non union of the mandible. *Laryngoscope.* 1976;86:908–920.
7. Rowe N. Nonunion of the mandible. In: Mathog RH, ed. *Maxillofacial Trauma.* Baltimore, Md: Williams & Wilkins Co; 1984:177–185.
8. Walker RV. Delayed occlusal and maxillofacial deformities after trauma. *JAMA.* 1977;85:858–861.
9. Macintosh RB. Malunion and malocclusion of mandibular fractures. In: Mathog RH, ed. *Maxillofacial Trauma.* Baltimore, Md: Williams & Wilkins Co; 1984:186–207.
10. Dingman RO, Grabb WC. Reconstruction of both mandibular condyles with metatarsal bone grafts. *Plast Reconstr Surg.* 1964;34:441–451.
11. Macintosh RB, Henny FA. A spectrum of application of autogenous, costochondral grafts. *J Maxillofac Surg.* 1977;5:257–267.
12. Mathog RH, Leonard MS. Reconstruction of the hemimandible with rib autograft. In: Bernstein L, ed. *Plastic and Reconstructive Surgery of the Head and Neck.* New York, NY: Grune and Stratton; 1981;2:198–206.
13. Andreason JO. *Traumatic Injuries of the Teeth.* 2nd ed. Philadelphia, Pa: WB Saunders Co, 1981:71–237.
14. Nikura K, Hasuite T, Nikura K, et al. Occlusal rehabilitation combining LeFort I osteotomy and prosthetic techniques in a case of maxillary fractures. *Josai Shika Daisaku Kiyo.* 1984;13:448–454.
15. Tessier P. Total osteotomy of the middle third of the face for faciostenosis or for sequelae of LeFort III fractures. *Plast Reconstr Surg.* 1971;48:533–541.
16. Newman H. Nonunion and Post-traumatic deformity of the maxilla. In: Mathog RH. ed. *Maxillofacial Trauma.* Baltimore, Md: Williams & Wilkins Co. 1984:245–256.
17. Stanley RB, Mathog RH. Evaluation and correction of combined orbital trauma syndrome. *Laryngoscope.* 1983;93:856–865.
18. Burres S, Cohn AM, Mathog RH. Repair of orbital blow-out fractures with marlex mesh. *Laryngoscope.* 1981;91:1881–1886.
19. Scapini D, Mathog RH. Repair of orbital floor fractures with marlex mesh. *Laryngoscope.* 1989;99:697–701.
20. Mathog RH, Hillstrom R, Nesi FA. Surgical correction of enophthalmos and diploplia: a report of 38 cases. *Arch Otolaryngol Head Neck Surg.* 1989;115:169–178.
21. Courtiss EH. Septorhinoplasty of the traumatically deformed nose. *Ann Plast Surg.* 1978;1:443–449.
22. Farrior RT. Corrective and reconstructive surgery of the external nose. In: Naumann HH, ed. *Head and Neck Surgery,* Stuttgart; Georg Thieme; 1980;1:173–277.
23. Mathog RH, Bauer W. Post-traumatic pseudohypertelorism (telecanthus). *Arch Otolaryngol.* 1979;105:81–85.
24. Stranc MF. The pattern of lacrimal injuries in naso-ethmoid fractures. *Br J Plast Surg.* 1970;23:335–346.
25. Jones LT. The cure of epiphora due to canalicular disorders; trauma and surgical failure on the lacrimal passages. *Trans Am Acad Ophthal Otol.* 1962;66:506–524.
26. Arden R, Mathog RH, Nesi FA. Flap reconstruction techniques in conjunctivorhinostomy. *Otolarynol Head Neck Surg.* 1990;02:150–155.

27. Dukert LG, Mathog RH. Diagnosis in persistent cerebrospinal fluid fistulas. *Laryngoscope.* 1977;87:18–25.
28. Kirchner FR, Proud GO. Method for identification and localization of cerebrospinal fluid rhinorrhea and otorrhea. *Laryngoscope.* 1960;70:921–930.
29. Mathog RH. Frontoethmoid fractures. In: Gates FA, ed. *Current Therapy in Otolaryngology-Head and Neck Surgery.* Philadelphia, Pa: BC Decker; 1984–1985:100–104.
30. Montgomery WW. *Surgery of the Upper Respiratory System.* Philadelphia, Pa: Lea and Febiger; 1979;1:115–l25, 142, 143, 163, 164.
31. May M, Ogura JH, Schramm V. Nasofrontal duct in frontal sinus fractures. *Arch Otolaryngol Head Neck Surg.* 1970;92:534–538.
32. Ghobrial W, Amstatz S, Mathog RH. Fractures of the sphenoid bone. *Head Neck Surg.* 1986;8:447–455.
33. Sofferman RA. Sphenoethmoid approach to the optic nerve. *Laryngoscope.* 1981;91:184–l96.
34. Spoor TC, Mathog RH. Restoration of vision after optic nerve decompression. *Arch Ophththalmol.* 1986;104:804–805.
35. Mathog RH. *Atlas of Craniofacial Trauma.* Philadelphia, Pa: WB Saunders Co; 1992.

20 Complications of Middle Ear and Mastoid Surgery

Thomas L. Eby, M.D., F.A.C.S.

COMPLICATIONS FROM PRESSURE EQUALIZING TUBES

Insertion of pressure equalizing tubes for eustachian tube dysfunction with resultant middle ear pathology is probably the most common surgical procedure performed in this country. Although the majority of patients with tubes have no problems with them, some complications are likely to be seen by every otolaryngologist.

Intraoperative complications of pressure equalizing tube placement are rare. Potentially the most serious are anesthetic complications when general anesthesia is required, particularly in children.[1] Cardiac arrhytlimias, airway obstruction, and hyperthermia are all potentially lethal complications and are independent from procedure risks.

Difficulty in placement of the pressure equalizing tube may lead to tears in the tympanic membrane or loss of the tube in the middle ear. In most cases the consequences are negligible, however chronic tympanic membrane perforation and chronic otitis media may result. If a tube is lost in the middle ear and cannot be retrieved easily, it should be left and the patient so informed. Persistent conductive hearing loss, otorrhea, or tympanic membrane retraction or thickening are indications for later tympanotomy to retrieve the lost tube. Significant hemorrhage from incision into a high-riding jugular bulb or even anomalous carotid artery can rarely complicate myringotomy.[2] Suspicious pulsatile masses found at the time of myringotomy should not be opened nor should biopsies be performed until angiography can be performed to determine their origin and nature. It has been suggested that placement of the myringotomy incision in the posteroinferior quadrant will avoid injury to an aberrant carotid artery,[3] however an aberrant carotid artery has been reported posteriorly displaced. Damage to the ossicular chain by tube insertion should be averted by avoiding the posterosuperior quadrant of the tympanic membrane as a site for tube insertion (Fig. 20–1).

The most common postoperative complication of pressure equalizing tube insertion is persistent otorrhea. The incidence of this complication in reported studies varies and can be more usefully divided into simple and chronic otorrhea. Simple otorrhea, a single episode that cleared within 3 weeks, occurred in 20% of one large study whereas chronic or recurrent otorrhea occurred in 3.6% of this group.[4] Otorrhea in the immediate postoperative period appears to be related to the pathogens already present in the middle ear fluid at the time of the procedure. A significantly higher risk of postoperative otorrhea has been found in patients having a mucoid rather than serous effusion[5] and in those growing a pathogen from the middle ear fluid.[6] Tubes placed for recurrent acute otitis media have a higher incidence of postoperative otorrhea than those placed for hearing loss from otitis media with effusion.[7] In ears with a history of spontaneous rupture from acute otitis media, the incidence of postoperative otorrhea reaches 25%. The age of the patient also seems to influence the incidence of postoperative tube otorrhea, with children younger than 2 years having more than twice the rate as those over 6 years of age. Likewise the bacteriology of otorrhea from tympanotomy tubes differs with age. In patients younger than 3 years, *Haemophilus influenza* and *Diplococcus pneumoniae* are found in more than one half of cultures whereas *Staphylococcus aureus* and *Pseudomonas aeruginosa* are the two most common pathogens found in children older than 3 years.[8] To reduce the incidence of postoperative otorrhea, several procedures have been tried. Because an increased risk of otorrhea is seen when pathogens are cultured from the external ear canal at the time of myringotomy,[6] some surgeons have suggested preoperative canal irrigation with antimicrobial solution. Controlled studies of external canal irrigation with antimicrobial solution prior to tube insertion show that the irrigation is not effective in sterilizing the canal and does not reduce the incidence of postoperative otorrhea.[6,9,10] Prophylactic treatment with either gentamicin drops, sulfacetamide/prednisolone drops, or a solution of polymyxin B sulfate, neomycin sulfate, sulfonamide and hydrocortisone at the time of tube insertion also fail to significantly reduce postoperative otorrhea in controlled trials.[5,11,12] Others have suggested that irrigation of the middle ear at the time of tube insertion[13] or systemic antimicrobial treatment in the perioperative period[6] may reduce the incidence of postoperative otorrhea, however, definitive studies have not be done. The type of tube used is

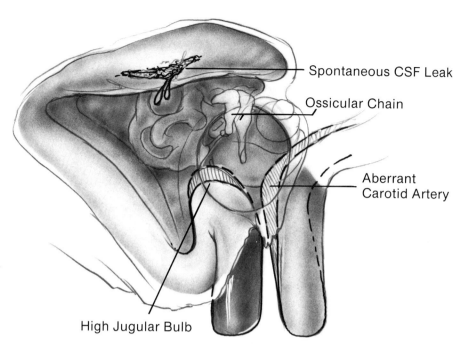

Figure 20–1. Potential hazards of pressure equalizing tube insertion include ossicular chain damage, perforation of an aberrant jugular bulb or carotid artery, and cerebrospinal fluid otorrhea from a spontaneous leak.

Spontaneous CSF Leak

Ossicular Chain

Aberrant Carotid Artery

High Jugular Bulb

also important to the incidence of this complication.[14] Postoperative otorrhea as well as perforation are more likely with the long-term tubes.

Postoperative otorrhea has usually been treated with oral antibiotics and/or topical drops. There has been some controversy surrounding the use of topical preparations since reports of ototoxicity with their use in experimental animals. One study showed ototoxic effects of topical bacitracin zinc, polymyxin B sulfate, neomycin sulfate, and hydrocortisone suspension (Cortisporin) when placed in the ear canals of chinchillas with tympanotomy tubes in place.[15] Although these reports have caused concern, no clinical evidence of ototoxicity has emerged despite their widespread use. For treatment of *P. aeruginosa* and other sensitive organisms, the use of gentamicin and tobramycin ophthalmic solutions has been advocated. Topical treatment in these cases may be the only appropriate outpatient treatment because to date the only effective oral agent, ciprofloxacin hydrochloride, is contraindicated in patients younger than 18 years. In refractory cases, intravenous antibiotics based on culture and sensitivities may be required. In some cases the otorrhea will persist until the tubes are removed.

Cerebrospinal otorrhea is a rare but important complication of myringotomy tube placement. Early recognition and repair of the cerebrospinal fluid (CSF) leak is essential to prevent the potentially catastrophic consequences of meningitis.

Continuous clear otorrhea from a tube in a patient with a history of head trauma, particularly temporal bone fracture, should raise suspicions of CSF otorrhea. However, CSF otorrhea may occur from spontaneous leakage of CSF into the middle ear. This may occur in either children or adults and tend to have separate etiologies. Three types of spontaneous middle ear CSF leak have been classified by Neely.[16]

The most common type of spontaneous CSF leak to the middle ear occurs through a perforation of the stapes footplate in children with unilateral profound congenital hearing loss. These children usually also have loss of vestibular function in the ear and may have recurrent bouts of meningitis. A Mondini malformation of the cochlea may be found on radiological investigation. A second type also occurs in children, but is much more uncommon. These children have a conductive hearing loss and normal vestibular function associated with spontaneous CSF middle ear fluid. Radiological studies of the inner ear are normal. In these patients the leak of CSF is through a patent Hyrtl's fissure or fallopian canal and recurrent meningitis can occur. The third type of spontaneous CSF leak to the middle ear is more common in adults although it has been reported as a complication of myringotomy tube placement in a child.[17] These patients also have a conductive hearing loss and normal vestibular function. It is caused by fluid leak from a meningoencephalocele through a defect in the mastoid tegmen. This type of leak has been ascribed to slow erosion by arachnoid granulations.[18]

The incidence of tympanic membrane perforation after pressure equalizing tube extrusion or removal is about 2%.[4] This includes only perforations that persist for 6 months because spontaneous closure is significant even after 6 weeks. The type of tube markedly influences the incidence of this complication. Tubes designed for longer retention in the tympanic membrane have the highest rate of associated perforations. Per-Lee[19] reported a 25% incidence of perforations using his wide-flanged long-term middle ear ventilation tubes. The T tube, another widely used long-term tube, results in a 17% rate of perforation.[20] Because tympanoplasty is usually required to repair these perforations, some surgeons have advocated myringoplasty using fat, paper, or Gelfilm at the time of removal of long-term tubes.

Cholesteatoma as a result of tube placement is rare, representing less than 1/2% incidence in large series.[4] In some cases cholesteatoma may be coincidental, but when the process begins beneath the drum surface adjacent to the tube insertion site, there must be a high suspicion of cause and effect. The seriousness of this potential complication warrants routine follow-up otoscopy after tube insertion.

Complications involving the tympanic membrane such as retraction or atelectasis have been reported in a small percentage (1 to 2%) of cases. It may be difficult to determine if these conditions are complications of tube placement or a progression of disease despite their placement. Likewise, the incidence and significance of tympanosclerosis after pressure equalizing tube placement has been controversial. Tympanosclerosis was found in over one half of tympanic membranes after tube placement compared with 13% in the nonintubated opposite ear in one study.[21] However, long-term observation of hearing failed to demonstrate any significant difference between ears.

TYMPANIC MEMBRANE AND MIDDLE EAR SURGERY

Surgery on the tympanic membrane and middle ear can result in intraoperative and postoperative complications. Intraoperatively, malformations and anatomic variations may rarely cause difficulties.[22] As with tympanotomy tubes, an anomalous high-riding jugular vein may cause bleeding if not recognized. Persistence of the stapedial artery or superficial petrosal branch of the middle meningeal artery near the posterior oval window niche may complicate surgery on the stapes. If disrupted, hemorrhage can be brisk enough to obscure the operative field and terminate the procedure. Although frightening to the surgeon, blood loss is not excessive and stops spontaneously with pressure. Markedly aberrant facial nerve position in the middle ear is very rare, and usually only reported with other anomalies of the branchial arch derivatives. The facial nerve can be found inferior to or overlapping the oval window, complicating stapedectomy or ossiculoplasty. Dehiscence of the bony facial canal is most common over the oval window. The normal nerve may bulge out of the opening slightly, making it vulnerable to injury. Biopsy of this region in asymptomatic patients should be performed with caution if at all. Sacrifice of the chorda tympani nerve may be required in some middle ear surgery and the resultant loss of taste sensation to the ipsilateral two thirds of the tongue may be expected. Intraoperative manipulation of the chorda may cause postoperative dysgeusia, which may be troublesome in certain patients for several months. Intraoperative dislocation of the malleus or incus may result in conductive hearing loss. Sensorineural hearing loss including complete cochlear loss has been reported from tympanoplasty and ossiculoplasty. The incidence is low, however, about 1.5% in one experienced surgeon's hands.[23] The hearing loss can be the result of either transmission of excessive vibration from surgical manipulations or exposure of the inner ear with labyrinthitis a result. Excessive vibration of the ossicles can occur with even momentary contact with the surgical drill bit. The con-

sequences of burr contact have been documented in experimental animals.[24] However, excessive energy can be transmitted to the inner ear by manipulation of the ossicles, which can occur with disarticulation of the incus from stapes, positioning prostheses and tissue grafts, or removing diseased tissue from the middle ear structures. This may be the result of nonphysiological changes in perilymph fluid pressure in the scala tympani by the plungerlike action of the stapes or from a serous labyrinthitis caused by surgical trauma. In one report,[23] complete hearing loss in seven cases followed removal of tympanosclerosis, cholesteatoma, or thick granulation tissue from the ossicles and round and oval window niches. The perilymphatic spaces can be exposed during tympanoplasty either by an inadvertent surgical maneuver or by removal of tissue that invades the labyrinthine capsule. Inadvertent stapes extraction or footplate fracture is likely to cause sensorineural hearing loss unless the resultant perilymph leak is recognized and sealed. Rarely, complete hearing loss may occur after tympanoplasty for no apparent reason. Tears in the tympanic membrane can usually be repaired with a piece of fascia, perichondrium, or fat and do not cause any permanent sequelae. Local anesthetic use will occasionally cause facial paralysis or vertigo that may last up to 4 to 6 hours. This is uncomfortable for the patient and surgeon alike but causes no permanent problems.

Postoperative complications include residual or recurrent tympanic membrane perforation after tympanoplasty. Reported success rates after tympanoplasty using a variety of techniques have been 90% or higher.[25,26] However, longer follow-up results indicate there is a siginficant delayed reperforation rate.[27] Survival life tables show late perforations to continue at least to 11 years after surgery. Factors that increase failure rates are conditions that may affect neovascularization of the graft, including corticosteroids and tobacco use, as well as some disease conditions.

Late complications of tympanoplasty also include recurrent conductive hearing loss. This may be due to blunting of the normal angle between the tympanic membrane and the external auditory canal (Fig. 20-2). Blunting is more likely to occur after repair of anterior perforations where it is difficult to reconstruct the annulus. The thick fibrous tissue that forms in the grafted region is a poor transmitter of sound and causes a conductive hearing loss. A more severe hearing loss results when the entire tympanic graft lateralizes, usually after total tympanic membrane replacement. If the graft is not adequately anchored to the bony annulus and malleus, it may heal in a position in the external canal lateral to the normal tympanic membrane. This results in a severe conductive hearing loss and loss of normal landmarks on otoscopy. Several authors have suggested ways to prevent this complication.[25,28,29] These include creating a deepened anterior annulus with a diamond drill and perforating the fascia to better anchor the graft in the proper position or tucking the anterior graft into an annular pocket after elevating the fibrous annulus. Skin grafting over the graft at the anterior annulus may also help promote early epithelialization and prevent fibrotic blunting. Other causes of conductive hearing loss

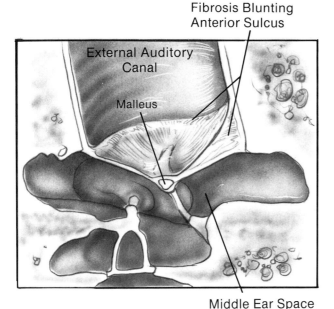

Figure 20–2. Blunting of the anterior tympanic annulus is a complication of tympanoplasty in this region.

include graft thickening and adhesions to the promontory and middle ear structures. These healing results may be unavoidable, although use of a thin fascial graft and middle ear Silastic or Gelfilm has been suggested to prevent these complications. Severe atelectasis of the grafted tympanic membrane can also be considered a complication leading to conductive hearing loss. One technique to prevent this complication is the use of multiple small strips of cartilage to give structural support to the reconstructed tympanic membrane (cartilage palisade technique). Recurrence of negative middle ear pressure or effusion might better be considered unavoidable consequences of underlying eustachian tube dysfunction. This only serves to highlight the limited success clinicians have had in preoperative prediction of eustachian tube function using current tests. This is especially true in children in whom it has been suggested that waiting until after age 8 years will lead to fewer tympanoplasty failures.[30]

The introduction of a prosthesis for ossiculoplasty also brings potential complications both early and late. A myriad of prostheses have been introduced to replace the function of one or more ossicles. The merits of one versus the other may be debated but all must be accurately placed and sufficiently stabilized to achieve good hearing results. If the prosthesis leans against the bony annulus or falls out of position, an early postoperative conductive hearing loss will result. Late complications can occur from prosthesis extrusion, resorption, as well as displacement. Extrusion of a prosthesis after months or years has been reported and is most common with manmade materials. Plastapore prostheses have enjoyed the most widespread usage since their introduction, but have been associated with delayed extrusions in up to 15% of cases. To prevent this, surgeons have advocated the use of cartilage between the prosthesis and the tympanic membrane. This has reduced the incidence of extrusion to about 3%. The most popular emerging manmade material for use in middle ear prostheses is hydroxyapatite. The prostheses made of this material have been used without interposed cartilage with a very low extrusion rate, presumably because of its similarity to bone and therefore improved biocompatability.[32] Some other manmade materials introduced for middle ear prostheses have been largely abandoned because of complications. Ceravital and bioglass were found to have significant long-term resorption in clinical studies, causing worsened hearing over time. Autologous and homologous cartilage were also found to resorb with time, and be often unsatisfactory for long-term middle ear reconstruction.[33] On the other hand, when autologous or homologous bone is used for middle ear reconstruction, resorption has not been a problem over the long term, even though it appears that viable osteocytes do not exist in the prosthesis.[34] Another artificial material often used in middle ear reconstruction is Silastic. A sheet of Silastic is often left in the middle ear over the promontory to prevent adhesions and ensure an adequate airspace.

COMPLICATIONS FROM MASTOID SURGERY

In addition to the risks for tympanoplasty, mastoid surgery entails other risks because of the pathology treated and the techniques to remove it. At risk are the structures within and bordering the temporal bone. These include vascular injury to the sigmoid sinus, dural laceration with CSF leak, injury to the labyrinth with perilymph leak, and/or labyrinthitis with loss of hearing or balance function and facial nerve injury. Persistent or recurrent symptoms of ear disease such as hearing loss, otorrhea, vertigo, or recurrent cholesteatoma may occur as late complications.

The sigmoid sinus is at risk from the cutting burr especially if it is more anterior or superior than usual. Bleeding from the sinus can be brisk but is usually readily controlled by gentle pressure. Often absorbable material such as Surgicel or Gelfoam can be left as a patch over the laceration after initial tamponade and gives excellent hemostasis for the rest of the surgery. The low pressure of this vein allows this thin patch technique to work. It is advisable to leave a thin shell of bone over the sigmoid sinus during mastoid surgery to protect this delicate structure. An island of bone will allow the sigmoid to be safely compressed for better exposure when deep dissection of the temporal bone is required. Difficult venous bleeding may also be encountered from the inferior or superior petrosal veins. These structures are not encountered during routine mastoid surgery, but may be troublesome during temporal bone dissection for acoustic neuromas, glomus jugulare tumors, or other deep tumors of the temporal bone. To stop bleeding from these vessels, occlusion by Surgicel, avitene, muscle, or other materials may be required.

Arterial bleeding is rarely a problem in mastoid surgery. Small vessels bleeding from the bone can be controlled by using a diamond burr. The carotid artery is exposed to potential injury in the anterior tympanum adjacent to the eustachian tube. Drilling in this area to remove diseased mucosa can cause inadvertent injury to the carotid. Study of temporal bone histology shows that the arterial wall is significantly thinner in its intratemporal course, which may increase the risk. Injury to the carotid artery may require more than pressure with packing to control. Although pressure may control the bleeding initially, balloon occlusion of the carotid artery using angiographic embolization techniques may be needed.

The middle fossa and less often the posterior fossa dura may be exposed during mastoid surgery. This may be done by the surgeon or by chronic granulation tissue, which erodes the bone overlying the dura. With few exceptions, small exposure of the dura does not cause complications and may help provide landmarks in a diseased mastoid. However, as a result of contact with a burr or sharp instruments, the surgeon may create a hole in the dura with subsequent CSF leak. Tiny CSF leaks may stop spontaneously or with placement of Gelfoam or Surgicel. Larger leaks require repair with temporalis fascia held in place with sutures or packing. Delayed or unrecognized CSF leaks may occur after surgery on the mastoid, usually clinically manifest as clear otorrhea or rhinorrhea. If small, these can sometimes be managed conservatively with bedrest and observation. Use of antibiotics has been controversial but is usually not advised in the absence of signs of meningitis unless a specific pathogen from mastoid infection is targeted. Surgical reexploration will be required to repair the leak if conservative measures fail. This requires location of the leak in the mastoid followed by coverage with fascia. To keep the fascia patch in place, a few sutures may be helpful. Often however, sutures will be difficult to place and the fascia should be reinforced by a thin piece of conchal cartilage or calvarial bone, which can be placed under the edges of the bone surrounding the defect.

Occasionally a dural leak will lead to pneumocephalus with headache, meningisimus, or other neurological deficits including hemiplegia, seizures, and coma sometimes without overt signs of CSF leak.[35] This may occur because of a ball valve like effect in the dura with increased middle ear pressure from a Valsalva maneuver or from the "Coke-bottle effect" when the continuous loss of CSF results in relatively negative intracranial pressure allowing air to replace the lost fluid. The resultant intracranial air may enter any of a number of spaces: most commonly the subdural or subarachnoid space near the temporal lobe. This air may be under pressure and a potentially dangerous tension pneumocephalus may result. Factors that reduce intracranial pressure such as use of hyperosmotic agents, intrathecal catheter drainage, or even head elevation may contribute to this complication. When this complication occurs as a result of middle ear or mastoid disease or surgery the treatment is surgical repair. This usually can be performed via a mastoid approach to identify the defect and then covering the dural leak with temporalis fascia with cartilage support or a temporalis muscle-fascia flap. Failure to recognize and treat this complication may lead to meningitis or neurological deficits caused by increased intracranial pressure from a tension pneumocephalus.

Large exposure of the middle fossa dura may cause late complications from menigoencephalocele. Although not seen at the time of the surgery, a herniation of dura and brain tissue can occur later into the mastoidectomy defect. This may present as a pulsatile mass in the mastoid bowl or as a spontaneous CSF leak. A coronal CT scan will demonstrate the defect in the mastoid tegmen and herniation of intracranial contents. This complication can be repaired either through the mastoid or middle fossa. Usually the middle fossa approach is reserved for patients who have failed the mastoid approach. The dura and brain tissue hernia must be reduced and the defect in the tegmen closed. Usually autologous fascia and bone or cartilage are placed through the defect to close it and create adaquate support. The herniated brain expands into the available mastoid space and is difficult to completely loosen and reduce through the bony defect in the tegmen. A portion of this nonfunctioning brain tissue may have to be excised to complete the repair.

Injury to hearing because of ossicular manipulation or contact with the surgical drill has been discussed for tympanoplasty surgery but also apply to mastoidectomy. In addition, there is the risk of hearing loss and vestibular dysfunction from opening the labyrinth. Both cholesteatoma and chronic granulation tissue may thin the labyrinthine bone making it vulnerable to fistula formation during surgical removal. This occurs most often with attempts to remove cholesteatoma, which has eroded labyrinthine bone. Removal of the thin matrix may create a fistula and the risk of damage to the delicate membranous labyrinth either by mechanical trauma or labyrinthitis. The most common location for iatrogenic or pathologic fistula formation is in the lateral semicircular canal. It is vulnerable to injury especially when the normal landmarks of the antrum and short process of the incus are obscured by a disease process. Opening a labyrinthine fistula in this location may cause vestibular dysfunction and postoperative vertigo, but the long-term prognosis remains good if the fistula is identified immediately and covered. As soon as a labyrinthine fistula is recognized, it should be covered with Gelfoam or similar available material until a tissue seal can be obtained. This will minimize exposure of the perilymph to blood or bacterial pathogens that may cause labyrinthitis and its associated hearing loss and vertigo. It will also protect the fistula from further surgical manipulation especially suctioning during the remainder of the procedure. If not immediately recognized, even momentary suctioning over an open fistula may cause collapse of the membranous labyrinth with severe impairment to hearing and balance or a dead ear. A series of patients with surgically injured lateral semicircular canals including disruption of the membranous canal showed only mild sensorineural hearing loss and vestibular dysfuction after 1 year.[36] In all these patients the fistula was covered by fascia or other tissue seal as soon as the injury was recognized. This emphasizes that disability from this complication can often be minimized by early recognition and management. The difficulty managing fistulas and potential for hearing loss and vertigo have led to a debate about cholesteatoma management when labyrinthine fistula is suspected. Labyrinthine fistulas complicate about 4 to 10% of cholesteatomas and the lateral semicircular canal is the most common site found in about three fourths of the cases.[37,38] Some otologists advocate leaving the thin epithelial matrix over the fistula after removing the bulk of the cholesteatoma and surrounding granulation tissue. This site can then be exteriorized in the mastoid cavity, or a second-look operation can be planned in 6 months and any recurrent cholesteatoma can be removed more safely at this time. This approach is advocated for large fistulas when the matrix is adherent to inner ear structures and in elderly patients or when the affected ear is the only hearing one to avoid the risk of postoperative sensorineural hearing loss and dizziness. Alternatively, some otologists maintain that cholesteatoma should be completely removed including the matrix to prevent future recurrence and that this can be accomplished safely in skilled hands. Clearly cholesteatoma in some locations in the temporal bone such as in the supralabyrinthine and infralabyrinthine cell tracts may prevent complete removal without substantial risk of formation of a fistula that cannot be sealed. The surgeon must choose between two possible complications: a higher risk of recurrent disease or the risk of hearing loss and disequilibrium from injury to the labyrinth. In rare cases an alternative approach to cholesteatoma in the supralabyrinthine region or petrous apex through the middle fossa should be considered to provide better exposure and solve the dilemma.

Facial nerve injury is probably the surgeon's most feared complication of mastoidectomy. Even though the incidence of this complication is low, the devastating consequences of a severe facial nerve injury with very visible disfigurement and limited prospects for recovery make it mandatory to avoid. The most commonly injured portion of the facial nerve during mastoid surgery is near the second genu, as the nerve curves inferior and slightly lateral to the horizontal semicircular canal into its mastoid segment. The nerve may course more lateral than expected, and may be dehiscent and covered with granulation tissue making identification difficult. In cases of known congenital malformation of the ear such as congenital aural atresia, the chances of an anomalous facial nerve course are much greater and so too is the potential for facial nerve injury. Experience of the surgeon and thorough knowledge of temporal bone anatomy are most valuable to avoid facial nerve injury but some guidelines may be helpful. Most of the time it is best to positively identify the facial nerve in at least one segment of its temporal bone course (Fig. 20–3). The tympanic portion of the facial nerve can be identified in the middle ear as it runs above the stapes or oval window. The cochleariform process is a useful landmark for finding the nerve. At the second genu, the nerve can also be found inferior to the lateral semicircular canal and medial to the short process of the incus by 1.4 to 3.0 mm.[39] The safest approach to this portion of the nerve is to locate the level of the middle fossa dura, and thinning the bone covering it starting at the sinodural angle, and working anteriorly and medially until the antrum is identified. The short process of the incus lying over the dome of the lateral semicircular canal will aid identification of the facial nerve just inferior and medial to it. It is sometimes difficult or impossible to identify the facial nerve in these locations because of extensive disease and loss of the ossicles and other normal landmarks. In that situation the facial nerve may be first found distally near the stylomastoid foramen. The sigmoid sinus is skeletonized inferiorly as it leads toward the jugular bulb. In the mastoid tip region, the groove for the digastric tendon is found as it indents the mastoid running inferior and medial towards the stylomastoid foramen. The facial nerve with surrounding fibrous tissue can be found there and traced up to its more proximal portions. Once the facial nerve is positively identified in one portion of the temporal bone, it can be traced to other segments to avoid injury while performing the mastoidectomy. Drilling should always follow the expected

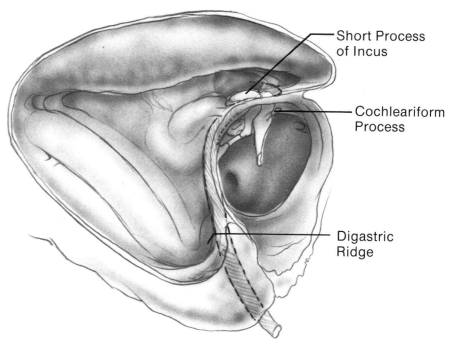

Figure 20–3. Injury to the facial nerve during mastoidectomy can be avoided by locating it using anatomic landmarks along its course: the cochleariform process, the short process of incus, and the digastric ridge.

Short Process of Incus

Cochleariform Process

Digastric Ridge

course of the facial nerve and bone should be removed in broad layers so that if encountered unexpectedly, the nerve may be unroofed but not transacted. Diamond burrs will do less injury than cutting burrs if contact is made with the nerve and should be used when dissecting in its, immediate vicinity. Adequate irrigation while drilling is essential because complete loss of function of the facial nerve from thermal injury by the burr may occur even if the nerve is not exposed.

If an injury to the facial nerve is noted during the course of a mastoidectomy, it should be assessed and repaired immediately. Complete transaction of the nerve will require freshening of the ends by sharp dissection back to healthy tissue and primary reanastomosis if possible. If there is a gap where injured nerve is missing, a cable graft is used to reestablish nerve continuity. The best graft donor site is the greater auricular nerve because of its proximity and ease of harvesting. The greater auricular nerve call be found coursing over the sternocleidomastoid muscle in a line bisecting the line between the mastoid tip and angle of the mandible. Partial nerve injury with continuity of at least a portion of the nerve is more difficult to assess. If one half the nerve remains intact, reapproximation of the remaining nerve and regional decompression will probably give the best result. When more than one half of the nerve is severed, especially if there is questionable viability of the rest, it may be better to remove the injured segment and perform a nerve graft as if it were a complete transection.

Recurrent cholesteatoma can be considered a complication of mastoid surgery and has spawned a controversy about the best management of this disease. The debate has centered around the merits of canal wall up or combined approach mastoidectomy versus canal wall down mastoidectomy often modified by some procedure to partially obliterate the mastoid cavity. Evaluation of the success of these procedures has centered on not only the primary goal of eliminating cholesteatoma and preventing recurrence, but also on the secondary goals of maximizing hearing gain and minimizing long-term postoperative care. Advocates of the canal wall up procedures point to better hearing results and preserved normal external auditory canal without the mastoid bowl, which requires regular cleaning.[40] The disadvantage of leaving the canal wall up is lack of exposure to the anterior epitympanum, sinus tympani, and facial recess that may hide residual cholesteatoma. Moreover, Smyth[41] concluded after a lifetime of study that the high rate of recurrent cholesteatoma with the canal wall up combined approach makes it undesirable in cholesteatoma surgery. Comparative studies of postoperative hearing results using the canal wall up procedure have not shown significant advantages over canal wall down procedures. The other major disadvantage cited about the canal wall down mastoidectomy has been addressed by several techniques that partially obliterate the mastoid cavity to reduce postoperative care. The use of muscle pedicles, bone plate, or other subtances has been advocated and concerns about hiding potential recurrent cholesteatoma have not proven to be a problem.

When mastoidectomy is performed for chronic otitis media without cholesteatoma, recurrent chronic otorrhea can be a complication. Treatment is guided by culture and sensitivities of the causative organism and by frequent suctioning and cleaning of the mastoid cavity. Appropriate oral as well as topical antibiotic treatment should be instituted. Frequently the otorrhea is from a gram-negative bacteria most commonly *P. aeruginosa* or *Proteus* in which case ciprofloxacin may prove useful. Ophthalmic topical medications have also been advocated for use in the ear to treat chronic otitis media because they are available in a much wider variety than otic preparations and are generally well tolerated in the ear. In addition to antibiotic solutions and powders, other antimicrobials such as boric acid or even acetic acid irrigation may be helpful. Failure of mastoid bowl epithelialization with granulation tissue sometimes responds to frequent cleaning and selective cauterization with silver nitrate as well as topical antibiotics based on culture of the otorrhea. A persistent problem area may require skin grafting. Split thickness skin grafting is an established and successful technique for treating minor mastoid bowl problems where failure of epithelialization in one area may cause persistent otorrhea. For successful grafting, a thin skin thickness must be obtained. Skin that is thick enough to curl along the edges is too thick for grafting in the ear. Because the amount of skin needed is small, graft harvesting by hand with a straight razor blade is easiest. The thin supple hairless skin of the upper inner arm is an excellent donor site. The split thickness skin is placed with the epithelial surface down on a piece of sterile silk or synthetic cloth with antibiotic ointment to form a backing. This call then be cut to the appropriate size and shape and placed in the mastoid bowl. Overlapping skin grafts are not a problem because any excess will slough. The grafts are held in place by packing for 1 to 2 weeks, after which all packing as well as the cloth backing is removed. Some surgeons advise this grafting as a primary procedure on every mastoid patient with an open cavity to prevent potential complications.

Often, however, the treatment of recurrent suppurative chronic otitis will require revision mastoidectomy. In cases of mastoid surgery failure without recurrent cholesteatoma, the causes include persistent suppurative disease in unexenterated air cells and technical factors such as a high facial ridge or meatal stenosis, which cause retention of debris in the mastoid cavity (Fig. 20–4). Nadol[42] found the factors most likely to be found on revision mastoidectomy were persistent suppurative disease in the air cells of the sinodural angle and along the tegmem and a high facial ridge. Other frequently found problems were neglected suppurative cells in the mastoid tip, facial recess, and hypotympanum and meatal stenosis. The reason that the sinodural angle, the facial ridge, and the tegmen are less well explored may well be from a concern about injuring normal structures such as the facial nerve, middle fossa dura, and sigmoid sinus in these areas. Unfortunately, concerns for the safety of these structures may lead to inadequate removal of diseased air cell tracts and a higher rate of mastoidectomy failure in the hands of less experienced ear surgeons.

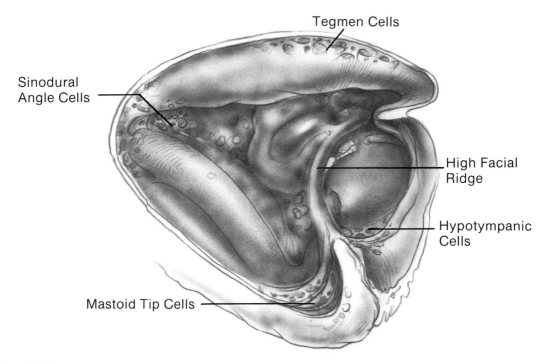

Tegmen Cells

Sinodural
Angle Cells

High Facial
Ridge

Hypotympanic
Cells

Mastoid Tip Cells

Figure 20–4.   Recurrent suppurative chronic otitis media is usually caused by failure to remove disease adequately in the sinodural angle, tegmen, and facial ridge. Less frequently it may be from cells in the mastoid tip or hypotympanum.

COMPLICATIONS OF STAPEDECTOMY SURGERY

Without a doubt, one of the triumphs of modern otology has been the development and refinement of stapedectomy procedures to improve hearing for patients with otosclerosis. These have enjoyed enormous success and restored hearing to thousands, but as with any surgical procedure, complications have had an important in shaping its development.

Although a variety of stapedectomy procedures remain in use, the most serious intraoperative complications will all occur as a result of surgical manipulation of the footplate. Common to all stapedectomy procedures is creating all opening into the vestibule prior to prosthesis placement. During this part of the procedure a part or all of the footplate may become mobile and dislodged. Often fragments can be retrieved using small angled picks. In some patients the downward pressure on the stapes arch to fracture the crura may cause the entire footplate to become mobile. When the entire footplate is mobile and freely floating in the oval window, Schuknecht has advocated the use of a marginal burr hole so that a small hook can be inserted under the footplate to remove it. To avoid this problem, Fisch[28] and others fenestrate the stapes footplate before removing the stapes arch. This creates a control hole through which an instrument can be placed to remove the footplate if necessary (Fig. 20–5). Alternatively the laser has been used to minimize the manipulation at the footplate. If a bone fragment or the entire stapes footplate is lost in the vestibule, it is probably not wise to try to retrieve it. The potential for damage to the saccule and utricle is greater from further surgical measures than from the bone fragments themselves. There is evidence that stapedotomy utilizing a small fenestra, with less need for footplate bone removal, results in fewer complications from surgical manipulation of the footplate and better long-term hearing results in the higher frequencies.[43,44]

The rapid release of perilymph after fenestrating the stapes footplate or the "perilymph gusher" is a rare but difficult intraoperative problem. This complication is more likely to occur in a patient with congenital stapes fixation and a patent cochlear aqueduct and represents pressure and fluid from the CSF compartment vented through the inner ear. The rapid flow of fluid may require the surgeon to apply pressure to the fistula site with packing in the ear and abort the procedure until the CSF pressure call be reduced. This can be accomplished by osmotic agents such as mannitol and sometimes also a lumbar drain. The goal is to reduce CSF pressure sufficiently to allow the surgeon enough exposure to seal the leak. A tissue seal over the oval window fistula using fascia, perichondrum, or fat is performed. The stapes prosthesis is helpful in keeping the patch in place. If the footplate opening is small, piston type prostheses will hold pressure on the oval window graft after it is crimped onto the incus. If the entire footplate is absent, a large fat wire prosthesis may plug the leak of perilymph. Postoperative hospitalization and continued reduction in the CSF pressure is advisable to ensure that the perilymph leak will not persist. Postoperative vertigo is expected and hearing results may be poor after perilymph gusher repair.

Other technical problems during surgery may complicate the stapedectomy procedure. As with other middle ear procedures, anatomic anomalies such as a persistent stapedial

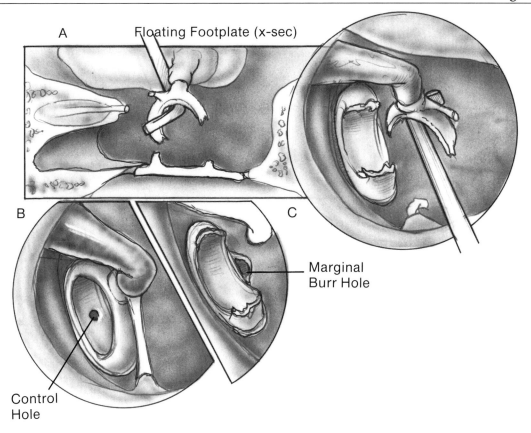

A   Floating Footplate (x-sec)

B

C

Marginal
Burr Hole

Control
Hole

Figure 20–5. A floating footplate **(A)** may complicate stapes arch removal during stapedectomy. This can be avoided by using a control hole prior to removing the stapes arch **(B).** Alternatively, a marginal burr hole **(C)** will allow a hook to be inserted under the footplate.

artery or facial nerve, which is dehiscent and overhanging the oval window, may prevent completion of the procedure. Transcanal exposure of the stapes footplate can be limited by a narrow external auditory canal or by the position of the posterior bony annulus. The cartilaginous canal can be widened using an endaural incision superiorly and spreading with a mastoid retractor or large ear speculum. The posterosuperior bony canal usually must be curetted and occasionally the chorda tympani nerve must be sacrificed for adequate exposure. Placement of a piston prosthesis will cause vertigo if it is too long and protrudes far enough into the vestibule to stimulate the saccule or utricle. When the stapedectomy is performed under local anesthesia, the patient can notify the surgeon of this problem and the prosthesis call be shortened. It is for this reason that the procedure is more safely performed under local anesthesia; any surgical manipulation that causes vertigo can be recognized and complications avoided. The wire of the piston type prosthesis must be adequately crimped and tightened around the long process of the incus for a good hearing result. A loose or poorly shaped wire that does not conform to the incus circumference will cause persistent conductive hearing loss that may fluctuate and cause distortion of some sounds. Stapedectomy techniques that use other types of prostheses, such as the Robinson bucket handle prosthesis, avoid this problem. If the long process of the incus is eroded or absent so that a prosthesis cannot be attached, reconstruction must be made to the malleus or tympanic membrane directly. A malleus to

oval window piston prosthesis can be positioned so that the wire will wrap around the neck of the malleus and the end will fit into an oval window fenestra usually covered by a tissue seal (Fig. 20–6). Alternatively, a total ossicular replacement prosthesis may be used to create a columella directly to the tympanic membrane. Rents in the tympanic membrane occasionally occur when elevating the fibrous annulus and should be repaired. These small holes are repaired by reapproximating the edges and supporting them with a small piece of earlobe fat, perichondrium, or other connective tissue on the medial surface of the perforation.

Delayed complications of stapedectomy may occur within days or not for years (Fig. 20–7). Immediately after stapedectomy vertigo and tinnitus may complicate the patient's recovery. Usually this is self-limited and inproves rapidly. Atraumatic surgical technique, especially around the stapes footplate, will minimize but not eliminate this problem. In some patients a serous labyrinthitis develops as a result of surgical manipulation or containination of the vestibule. The effects of tinnitus, sensorineural hearing loss, and vertigo are most often mild and limited to the first few days after surgery. However, in a small percentage, less than 1%, the process will continue to worsen resulting in the loss of all inner ear function. The reason for this severe reaction in a few individuals is not known and cannot be predicted preoperatively.

Severe postoperative vertigo and sensorineural hearing loss can also be the result of a more severe complication, suppurative labyrinthitis and meningitis. This complication is

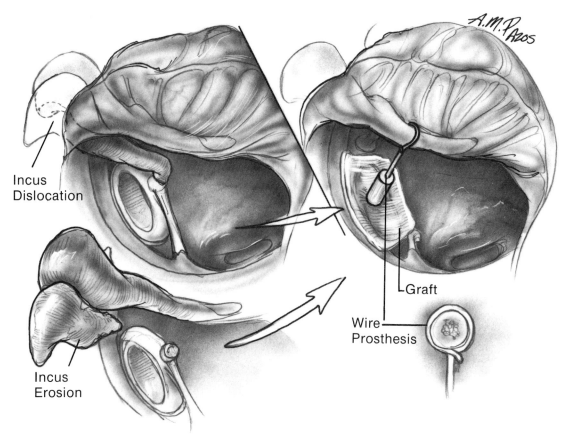

Figure 20–6.   Incus erosion or dislocation may complicate stapedectomy surgery. A malleus to oval window prosthesis
will solve this problem. The wire must be tightly wrapped around the malleus.

extremely rare but fatalities have been reported.[45] Bacterial
contamination of the perilymph during stapedectomy leads
to a rapidly progressive infection that spreads through the
labyrinth to involve the meninges. Strict aseptic operative
technique and prophylactic antibiotics are routinely used to
prevent this complication.

Progressive sensorineural hearing loss and vertigo beginning several days after surgery are suggestive of postoperative
granuloma formation with associated serous labyrinthitis. This
complication usually is diagnosed about 10 days after
stapedectomy. The presence of a poststapedectomy granuloma
is important to recognize because the effects on hearing and
balance are potentially reversible. The treatment of this complication is surgical reexploration and removal of the abnormal tissue that usually surrounds the prosthesis and may extend into the vestibule. The prosthesis is removed along with
the granuloma in most cases and a new prosthesis placed with
tissue seal over the oval window.

Poststapedectomy perilymph fistulas may occur either early
or late, and are suspected by symptoms of episodic vertigo
especially with exertion, sensorineural hearing loss, or loss
of speech discrimination. The symptoms of perilymph fistula
may be intermittent and variable and can mimic those of
Meniere's disease, which also may follow surgery for
otosclerosis. Suspicion should always be high for fistula in
a patient with these symptoms following stapedectomy, The
fistula sign of eye deviation or nystagmus with changes of

air pressure on the tympanic membrane may be documented
by electronystagmography, but is not always positive when
a fistula is present. Fistulas were more common with the initial polyethylene prostheses and later gel wire prostheses,
which are no longer used.[46] Currently most stapedectomy
techniques use some type of tissue seal at the oval window
around the prosthesis to try to prevent fistula formation. In
large fenestra techniques a layer of connective tissue covers
the fenestra before the prosthesis is placed. The same may
be done in small feinstra stapedectomy but often fat, connective tissue, fibrin glue, or even blood is placed around
the prosthesis to achieve a seal and prevent a perilymph
fistula. Suspected fistulas require exploratory tympanotomy
and repair of the leak using connective tissue. Perichondrium
and fascia have proven more effective than adipose tissue.
The patch is usually held in place with Gelfoam packing and
the patient told to avoid flying for 2 weeks and strenuous activities for 2 to 4 weeks.

Persistent or recurrent conductive hearing loss after
stapedectomy may occur as a result of technical factors during the surgery, missed diagnosis, or postoperative changes
in the middle ear or prosthesis position. Malleus fixation can
cause a hearing loss very similar to otosclerosis and should
be obvious to the surgeon by palpation of the ossicles at the
time of surgery. If the malleus is fixed but incus and stapes
are mobile, stapedectomy will not improve hearing. Mobilization of the malleus rarely gives lasting hearing improvement.

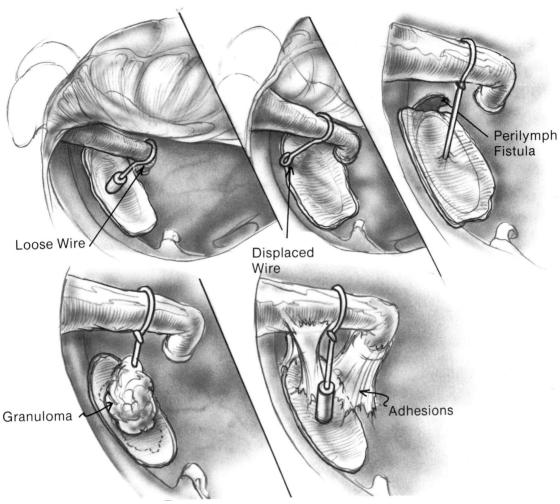

Figure 20–7. Postoperative stapedectomy complications that affect hearing include a loose wire on the incus, displaced wire in a Gelfoam or tissue graft in the oval window, perilymph fistula, granuloma around the prosthesis, and adhesions.

A better solution to this problem is to sever the head of the malleus where the fixation occurs and perform an incus interposition between stapes head and manubrium. (Fig. 20–8).

If both malleus and stapes are fixed, a stapedectomy and removal of malleus head are required, followed by reconstruction from oval window to malleus as described previously.

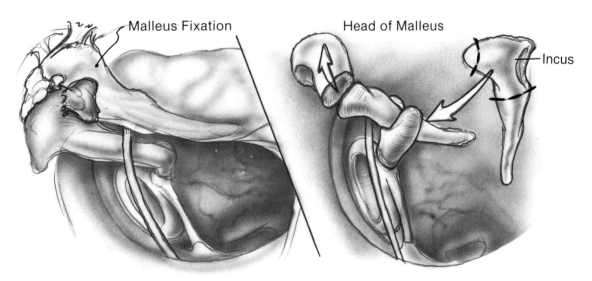

Figure 20–8. Malleus fixation causing conductive hearing loss can be treated by removing the head of malleus and interposing the sculpted incus between the manubrium and stapes head.

The round window niche should always be examined for the possibility of obliterative otosclerosis, which will prevent hearing gain after stapedectomy. Because the round window membrane is not readily visible, a small drop of saline can be placed in the niche and movement of the round window will be seen as a change in the light reflection on the meniscus when the prosthesis is gently palpated. A conductive hearing loss may occur if the stapes prosthesis is displaced either by head trauma or a large change middle ear pressure. Other causes include necrosis of the long process of the incus, fibrosis that may tether the incus or the prosthesis, or migration of the prosthesis in the oval window. The latter occurs most often with gel wire or tissue wire prosthesis when the wire becomes drawn to the edge of the oval window over time.[47] All of these are indications for reexploration and revision stapedectomy. Revision stapedectomy carries a higher risk of complications and lessened chance of hearing improvement than the primary procedure.[46–48] When possible the portion of the prosthesis that enters the vestibule should be left and a second fenestra and prosthesis placed. This side steps the problem of injury to the utricle or saccule by adhesions to the prosthesis from the first surgery.

REFERENCES

1. Markowitz-Spence L, Brodsky L, Naseera S, Stanievich J, Volk M. Anesthetic complications of tympanotomy tube placement in children. *Arch Otolaryngol Head Neck Surg.* 1990;116: 809–812.

2. Campbell G, Renner G, Estrem SA. Bilateral aberrant internal carotid arteries. *Otolaryngology Head Neck Surg.* 1992; 107:124–128.

3. Glasscock ME III, Dickins JRF, Jackson CG, Weit RJ. Vascular anomalies of the middle ear. *Laryngoscope.* 1980;90:77–88.

4. McLelland CA. Incidence of complications from use of tympanostomy tubes. *Arch Otolaryngol.* 1980;106:97–99.

5. Scott BA, Strunk CL. Post-tympanostomy otorrhea: a randomized clinical trial of topical prophlaxis. *Otolaryngol Head Neck Surg.* 1992;106:34–41.

6. Giebink GS, Daly K, Buran DJ, Satz M, Ayre T. Predictors for postoperative otorrhea following tympanostomy tube insertion. *Arch Otolaryngol Head Neck Surq.* 1992;118:491–494.

7. Debruyne F, Jorissen M, Poelmans J. Otorrhea during transtympanal ventilation. *Am J Otol.* 1988;9:316–317.

8. Schneider ML. Bacteriology of otorrhea from tympanostomy tubes. *Arch Otolaryngol Head Neck Surg.* 1989;115:1225, 1226.

9. Aland JW Jr, Baldwin RL. Effect of povidone-iodine preparation on the incidence of post-tympanostomy otorrhea. In: Lim DJ, ed. *Recent Advances in Otitis Media.* Burlington, Ontario: BC Decker Inc; 1988:263–265.

10. Scott BA, Strunk CL. Posttympanotomy otorrhea; the effecacy of canal preparation. *Laryngoscope.* 1992;102:1103–1107.

11. Ramadan HH, Tarazi T, Zaytoun GM. Use of prophylactic otic drops after tympanostomy tube insertion. *Arch Otolaryngol Head Neck Surg.* 1991;117:537.

12. Epstein JS, Beane J, Hubble R. Prevention of early otorrhea in ventilation tubes. *Otolaryngol Head Neck Surg.* 1992;107(pt 1):758–762.

13. Balkany TJ, Arenberg IK, Steenerson RL. Ventilation tube surgery and middle ear irrigation. *Laryngoscope.* 1986;96: 529–532.

14. Bulkley WJ, Bowes AK, Marlowe JF. Complications following ventilation of the middle ear using Goode T tubes. *Arch Otolaryngol Head Neck Surg.* 1991;117:895–898.

15. Meyerhoff WL, Morizono T, Shaddock LC, Wright CG, Shea DA, Kikora MA. Tympanostomy tubes and otic drops. *Laryngoscope.* 1983;93:1022–1027.

16. Neely JG. Classification of spontaneous cerebrospinal fluid middle ear effusion: review of forty-nine cases. *Otolaryngol Head Neck Surg.* 1985;93:625–634.

17. Jones NS. Cerebrospinal fluid otorrhea at myringotomy. A meningocele through a defect in the tegmen. *Int J Ped Otorhinolaryngol.* 1991;21:79–83.

18. Gacek RR. Arachnoid granulation cerebrospinal fluid otorrhea. *Ann Otol Rhinol Laryngol.* 1990;99:854–862.

19. Per-Lee JH. Long-term middle ear ventilation. *Laryngoscope.* 1981;91:1063–1072.

20. Matt BH, Miller RP, Myers RM, Campbell JM, Cotton RT. Incidence of perforation with Goode T-tube. *Int J Pediatr Otorhinolaryngol.* 1991;21:1–6.

21. Tos M, Stangerup SE. Hearing loss in tympanosclerosis caused by grommets. *Arch Otolaryngol Head Neck Surq.* 1989;115: 931–935.

22. Hough JVD. Malformations and anatomical variations seen in the middle ear during operations on the stapes. *Am Acad Ophthalmol Otolaryngol.* 1961;17–39.

23. Bellucci RJ. Cochlear hearing loss in tympanoplasty. *Otolaryngol Head Neck Surg.* 1985;93:482–485.

24. Paparella M. Acoustic trauma from the bone cutting burr. *Laryngoscope.* 1962;72:116.

25. Sheehy JL, Glasscock ME. Tympanic membrane grafting with temporalis fascia. *Arch Otolaryngol.* 1967;86:391–402.

26. Pappas DJ, Simpson C. Annular wedge tympanoplasty. *Laryngoscope.* 1992;102:1192–1197.

27. Halik JJ, Smyth GDL. Long-term results of tympanic membrane repair. *Otolaryngol Head Neck Surg.* 1988;98:162–169.

28. Fisch, U. *Tympanoplasty and Stapedectomy: A Manual of Techniques.* New York, NY: Thieme-Stratton Inc; 1980:8–19.

29. Farrior JB. The anterior tympanomeatal angle in tympanoplasty: surgical techniques for the prevention of blunting. *Laryngoscope.* 1983;93:992–996.

30. Koch WM, Friedman EM, McGill TJI, Healy GB. Tympanoplasty in children; the Boston Children's Hospital. *Arch Otolaryngol Head Neck Surg.* 1990;116:35–40.

31. Emmett JR, Shea JJ, Moretz WH. Long-term experience with biocompatible ossicular implants. *Otolaryngol Head Neck Surg.* 1986;94:611–616.

32. Grote JJ. Reconstruction of the ossicular chain with hydroxyapatite implants. *Ann Otol Rhinol Laryngol Suppl.* 1986;123:10–12.

33. Smyth GDL. *Chronic Ear Disease.* New York, NY: Churchill Livingstone; 1980:162–167.

34. Lang J, Kerr AG, Smyth GDL. Long-term viability of transplanted ossicles. *J Laryngol Otol.* 1986;100:741–747.

35. Andrews JC, Canalis RF. Otogenic pneumocephalus. *Laryngoscope.* 1986;96:521–528.

36. Canalis RF, Gussen R, Abemayor E, Andrews J. Surgical trauma to the lateral semicircular canal with preservation of hearing. *Laryngoscope.* 1987;97:575–581.

37. Palva T, Konja J, Palva A. Openings of the labyrinth during chronic ear surgery. *Arch Otolaryngol Head Neck Surg.* 1971;93:75–78.

38. Parisier SC, Elelstein DR, Han JC, Weiss MH. Management of labyrinthine fistulas caused by cholesteatoma. *Otolaryngol Head Neck Surg.* 1991;104:110–115.

39. Anson BJ, Donaldson JA. *The Surgical Anatomy of the Temporal Bone and Ear.* Philadelphia, Pa: WB Saunders Co; 1967:91.

40. Sheehy JL, Patterson ME. Intact canal wall tympanoplasty with mastoidectomy. A review of eight years' experience. *Laryngoscope*. 1967;77:1502–1542.

41. Smyth GDL. Cholesteatoma surgery: the influence of the canal wall. *Laryngoscope*. 1985;95:92–96.

42. Nadol JB. Causes of failure of mastoidectomy for chronic otitis media. *Laryngoscope*. 1985;95:410–413.

43. Fisch U: Stapedotomy versus stapedectomy. *Am J Otol*. 1982;4:112–117.

44. Pedersen CB. The use of a small fenestra technique with the Fisch piston in the treatment of otosclerosis. *J Laryngol Otol*. 1987;101:542–547.

45. Jablokow VR, Kathuria S. Fatal meningitis due to Serratia marcescens after stapedectomy. *Arch Otolaryngol Head Neck Surg*. 1982;108:34, 35.

46. Sheehy JL, Nelson RA, House HP. Revision stapedectomy: a review of 258 cases. *Laryngoscope*. 1981;91:43–51.

47. Derlacki EL. Revision stapes surgery: problems with some solutions. *Laryngoscope*. 1985;95:1047–1053.

48. Crabtree JA, Britton BH, Powers WH. An evaluation of revision stapes surgery. *Laryngoscope*. 1980;90:224–227.

21 Complications of Cranial Base Surgery

Jeffrey L. Wilson, M.D., Dan G. Deschler, M.D., Michael J. Kaplan, M.D.,
Harold C. Pillsbury III, M.D.

Cranial base surgery has seen important developments in the past decade that have led to a better understanding of this complicated field. Several factors have led to more clearly defined patient selection criteria, indications, contraindications, and choices of surgical approaches. The concept of a team approach among otolaryngologists, neurosurgeons, plastic surgeons, radiotherapists, and interventional radiologists has had perhaps the greatest impact on this field. This approach combined with advances in computed tomography (CT), magnetic resonance imaging (MRI), interventional radiology, and microsurgical techniques, has given physicians many options for the treatment of skull base pathology. Along with these advances has come the realization that the decision to operate must be made keeping in mind factors such as the patient's overall health, age, life expectancy, morbidity, natural history of the disease, and tumor location. The decision not to operate is made on an individual basis, but general guidelines include involvement of the sphenoid sinus with a malignant process, involvement of both orbits or both optic nerves with a malignant process, invasion of the cavernous sinus, complete destruction of the clivus, involvement of the carotid artery near the sphenoid sinus or petrous apex, and distant metastasis. Often, postoperative complications are a predictable sequela of tumor extirpation and should be used to guide treatment options before surgery.

Intraoperative monitoring has also seen advances in recent years. Techniques such as electromyography (EMG) of the ocular, facial, trapezius, and tongue muscles with direct nerve stimulation, auditory brain evoked responses (ABR), and direct nerve action potential monitoring of the eighth nerve have all proven useful. Other monitoring techniques include cochlear action potentials, sound-activated monitoring of vocal cord motion, visual evoked responses, and direct optic nerve potential recordings. Although these techniques are helpful, there are still unresolved issues regarding cost and benefit. Furthermore, intraoperative monitoring is no substitute for the basic knowledge of principles of surgery such as adequate exposure, mastery of anatomy, meticulous hemostasis, debridement of devitalized tissue, obliteration of any dead space, and the avoidance of foreign bodies in the wound.

In this chapter, we will discuss complications of cranial base surgery as they relate to disease location and operative approach. Obviously the location and histology of a particular tumor will determine the approach used, and often a combination of approaches will be necessary for treatment. A partial listing of tumors often involving the skull base includes: esthesioneuroblastoma, adenocarcinoma, squamous cell carcinoma, sinonasal undifferentiated carcinoma, juvenile nasopharyngeal angiofibroma, chordoma, glomus jugulare, vagale, and carotid body tumor, acoustic neuroma, salivary gland neoplasms, petrous apex cholesteatomas and meningiomas. The best way to treat complications is to avoid them. Prevention, recognition, and management will all be stressed.

ANTERIOR CRANIAL BASE

The modification and extension of standard otolaryngological surgical approaches to the sinuses and orbits combined with an appropriate craniotomy have facilitated marked advances in en bloc tumor resection at the anterior and anterolateral skull base. The defects created with this approach violate the sterile barrier separating the brain from the aerodigestive tract. It is not surprising that early efforts at craniofacial resection were hampered by severe intracranial infections. Yet with advances in operative techniques and postoperative intensive care and rehabilitation, craniofacial resection as part of a multidisciplinary approach to tumors of the anterior skull base provides clearly improved survival with acceptable mortality and morbidity, as well as likely improved palliation.

Improved preoperative MRI, CT, and angiography with balloon test occlusion and embolization permit far more accurate and thorough planning of surgical ablation and reconstruction. Advances in reconstruction techniques using dependable and well-vascularized tissue flaps significantly decrease the complications associated with thorough resection. Improved broad-spectrum antibiotics with excellent cerebrospinal fluid (CSF) penetration have reduced infections. Radiation therapy has become more versatile and less morbid: charged particles, gamma-knife radiosurgery, and implants supplement conventional three-dimensional planning. As we have learned to integrate and advance these techniques, cases previously thought incurable have been treated with improved preservation of function and cosmesis, allowing a potential for cure.

The potential for complication is great with the extensive surgery required in skull base resections. Since the publication of Ketcham et al's[1] first series in 1963 and the review of subsequent series, the operative complication rate has steadily decreased from nearly 80% to 30 to 40% in current large series.[2-6] Likewise, mortality has decreased from 7 to 11% to 0 to 4%.[2,3,5-8]

The indications for craniofacial resection include intracranial extension by tumors of the sinuses, orbits, and floor of the anterior cranial fossa. Although the majority of cases are malignant, locally aggressive benign paranasal sinus or orbital lesions in this critical region may warrant such an approach as well. For example, extensive juvenile nasopharyngeal angiofibromas with intracranial extension may often be successfully treated. At times, other benign neoplasia such as pleomorphic adenomas, osteomas, fibrous dysplasia, and inverting papillomas have been reported warranting craniofacial resection. A second common indication for anterior or anterolateral skull base resection is the extension of intracranial disease inferiorly to the skull base, orbit, paranasal sinuses, or infratemporal fossa. The most common histology is meningioma, although occasional cranial nerve neuromas or other histologies are seen. Finally, selected CSF leaks as well as unusually difficult mucoceles may best be addressed with skull base approaches.

Anatomy

The anterior cranial base is defined as the portion of the skull base bounded anteriorly by the frontal bone, superiorly by the frontal, ethmoid, and sphenoid bones, and posterioly by the anterior clinoid processes and the sphenoid wings. The frontal bone contains the frontal sinus that must be managed in most anterior cranial base operations. Additionally, the supraorbital foramina transmit the supraorbital nerves and vessels, which must be preserved if the galea and pericranium are to be used in reconstruction of the surgical defect.

Intracranial landmarks include the foramen cecum, located anteriorly, which provides venous communication between the superior sagittal sinus and the veins of the nasal cavity. The crista galli protrudes superiorly in the midline between the openings of the cribriform plate which transmit the olfactory nerves. Just posterior to the cribriform plate lies the planum sphenoidale which is the roof of the sphenoid sinus. The anterior clinoid processes and lesser sphenoid wings delineate the most posterior limit of the anterior cranial base.

Extracranial structures of the anterior cranial base include the nasal cavity, ethmoid and sphenoid sinuses, and orbits. Important landmarks and relationships exist in this region. Specifically, the anterior and posterior ethmoid foramina transmit the anterior and posterior ethmoid arteries. Ligation of these vessels is often performed to decrease bleeding

in the nasal cavity. Additionally, these foramina indicate the position of the frontoethmoid suture line, which helps the surgeon know the level of the ethmoid roof and anterior fossa floor in this region. The superior orbital fissure transmits the oculomotor, trochlear, ophthalmic, and abducens cranial nerves (III, IV, and VI) as well as the ophthalmic vein. The inferior orbital fissure contains the maxillary nerve (V-2) and communicates with the pterygopalatine fossa. The optic canal transmits the optic nerve and ophthalmic artery.

Prognostic Factors

The most reliable prognostic factors for long-term survival following successful craniofacial tumor resection are tumor histology and extent of intracranial and dural involvement. Shah et al[6] described an overall 5-year survival rate of 56% in a review of 71 patients. Those with high-grade carcinomas, sarcomas, and melanomas had significantly worse survival compared with patients with less aggressive tumors such as esthesioneuroblastomas and adenoid cystic carcinomas. Likewise, tumors invading the dura, brain, and orbit fared poorly. There appears to be a significant difference in survival rate between dural and brain involvement. Van Tuyl and Gussack[3] reported a 22% 3-year survival rate for patients with dural involvement compared with 83% for those with no dural involvement. Patients requiring orbital exenteration similarly had poorer prognosis.

Specific contraindications to surgery have been suggested by various authors. Some believe tumor extension through the dura into the frontal lobes, posterior sphenoid sinus extension, optic nerve involvement, and cavernous sinus involvement, or extremely high-grade malignancies preclude surgical therapy.[9] These parameters may, and often do, clearly affect both prognosis or the ability to achieve either an en bloc resection or even gross total removal. Prior radiation therapy or surgery may limit current surgical or irradiation options, although neither has appeared to increase perioperative complications in either the experience of Shah et al[6] or our own. As is true with any decision regarding cranial base surgery, the treatment must be individualized after considering the patient's wishes, the surgical risks in that patient, expected natural course of disease, likelihood of achieving significant palliation or cure, and the degree of likely success for surgical and nonsurgical alternatives.

Surgical Approach

Prior to selection of the surgical approach to lesions of the anterior cranial base, preoperative assessment by a multidisplinary team and radiographic definition of tumor extent must be performed. A complete general, neurological, and ophthalmologic history and physical exam, with special attention to impaired or at-risk cranial nerve function, will best anticipate the patient's likely perioperative and postoperative needs. Assessment will also include the patient's social history and available family or other support available to help cope with the postoperative course and possible dysfunction associated with treatment. Radiographic modalities include MRI with gadolinium contrast which provides multiplanar images, necessary for the three-dimensional planning required of the physician performing the skull base surgery. Soft tissue definition is excellent with MRI as is the ability to differentiate tumor from inflamed mucosa, dura, and brain. Computed tomography, with standard axial as well as coronal cuts, may selectively augment the assessment of bony involvement and disruption. Finally, angiography of both carotid arteries is indicated for tumors in the region that appear to abut or displace an internal carotid artery.

Once the tumor extent has been assessed, different approaches to the skull base may be necessary. The requisite neurosurgical exposure usually consists of a bifrontal craniotomy, which may be extended to the orbitozygomatic region. Some authors use a minifrontal craniotomy, suggesting this decreases potential complications, but it also may sacrifice essential exposure for resection and reconstruction. Care is taken with the craniotomy to preserve the galeal and pericranial tissue flaps for later reconstruction.[10-15] The bone flap may be completely removed or pedicled on pericranium and temporalis. If a galeal or pericranial flap is to be used, it is crucial that any frontal sinus within the bone flap be stripped of all mucosa and burred down to avoid subsequent mucocele formation. The frontal sinus may be formally cranialized or obliterated; if remaining inferior frontal sinus is uninvolved and previously drained normally into the ethmoids without prior infection, then it may be left alone. A lumbar subarachnoid drain (LSAD) is often placed preoperatively both to reduce the extent of brain retraction and to assist in the prevention of potential CSF leaks. This is especially helpful if an extradural repair is anticipated. Appropriate intravenous antibiotics with excellent CSF penetration and coverage of aerodigestive tract organisms are administered. Ceftizoxime, with or without vancomycin, is a reasonable choice once the craniotomy has been performed. The frontal lobe is gently retracted as the dural attachments to the cribriform plate are divided and the anterior skull base is exposed. The paranasal sinus exposure usually requires a transfacial approach, using any of a variety of techniques selected to accommodate the particular resection. When the tumor is limited to the ethmoids and sphenoid sinus, exposure via the craniotomy often suffices. When more exposure is needed (as in the antrum, pterygomaxillary space, or inferior orbit), a lateral rhinotomy approach with medial maxillectomy is sufficient in most cases.[16] This may be extended to a full Weber-Ferguson approach if needed. A midfacial degloving approach, with the elimination of facial skin incisions, may be selectively used.[17]

Following resection, the goals of anterior skull base reconstruction are to (1) provide dural repair to avoid CSF leak, (2) place a barrier between the sterile intracranial cavity and the colonized aerodigestive tract, and if necessary, (3) provide sufficient support to prevent brain herniation. Reconstruction must protect the brain not only in the immediate postoperative period but also during and after subsequent irradiation and other adjuvant therapy. As infections

are the most frequent complication following anterior skull base surgery, successful reconstructive efforts are crucial to the success of such resection.

Most skull base reconstructions use well-vascularized tissue placed in the defect. For extradural lining and support, the pericranial flap is favored at our institution, especially for smaller defects.[13-15] It provides a dependable and versatile tissue flap that is easily harvested, maintained, and placed. The vascular supply from the supraorbital and supratrochlear vessels is excellent. We strongly advocate the use of a split thickness skin graft to line the sinus surface. If dura has been removed, it is usually necessary to replace this prior to placing the subsequent pericranial flap. We usually use fascia lata; other alternatives are temporalis fascia (in small defects), cadaveric dura, or the pericranium (as an intradural repair). The galeal and scalp flaps also provide durable reconstructions but can have added morbidity due to their thickness.

For larger defects, myogenous, myocutaneous, and free vascular flaps are usually employed. The temporalis flap is versatile but limited by its small size and short rotational arc; we have occasionally found it helpful after orbitozygomatic approaches. Large pedicled flaps such as the pectoralis major, trapezius and latissimus dorsi flaps have been described with success, but the applicability of these flaps is limited by the superior location of the skull base defect. The advances in microvascular expertise have provided many versatile and dependable flaps that cannot only be used for primary reconstruction but also for addressing potential complications.[18] For larger defects, especially when orbital exenteration has been necessary, we commonly use the rectus abdominis flap based on the inferior epigastric vessels; this may be harvested with limited morbidity as a myocutaneous or solely myogenous free flap.

Nasal and paranasal packing is placed below the reconstruction and antibiotics are maintained for the duration of packing placement, usually 6 to 7 days. Airway diversion may be initially maintained with intubation or tracheotomy to reduce potential pneumocephalus, although pneumocephalus more commonly is the result of a CSF leak. Patients are monitored carefully in a neurointensive care unit. Lumbar subarachnoid drainage is closely monitored and the CSF is allowed to equilibrate with brain reexpansion into remaining intracranial dead space. Dexamethasone, as well as antiseizure agents, is often used in the postoperative period.

Complications

Although the following is a list of complications of anterior cranial base surgery, it should be kept in mind that expected postoperative sequelae will be inevitable. The patient should be counseled in detail on these expected outcomes before the decision is made to operate. Table 21–1 lists the most commonly occurring complications of craniofacial resection.

CSF LEAK

Cerebrospinal fluid leaks are the single most common complication following anterior skull base surgery with reported

Table 21-1. Complications of Craniofacial Resection

TYPE	INCIDENCE
CSF leak	3–20%
Pneumocephalus	5–12%
Infection	14–21%
Meningitis	<1–9%
Osteomyelitis	<1–21%
Cerebral abscess	<1%
Epidural abscess	<1%
Sinusitis	<1%
Periorbital cellulitis	<1%
Flap necrosis	<1%
Intracranial and neurological	Each usually <1%
Hemorrhage	
Cerebral edema	
Venous infarction	
Frontal lobe affect	
Frontal lobe infarct	
Seizure	
Diabetes insipidus	

rates of occurrence between 3 and 20%.[3-7] They are a constant concern in any skull base operation and may manifest as rhinorrhea, pneumocephalus, and meningitis. Anterior cranial base surgery differs from middle cranial base surgery in that the dural defect can be closed under direct vision. In resection of large acoustic neuromas via the translabyrinthine approach, the dural defect is usually closed by laying in strips of fat. Anterior cranial base surgical defects can be reconstructed in a multilayered closure. Preventing CSF leaks starts with predicting the extent of dural defect preoperatively with the aid of CT, MRI, and angiography where indicated. Appropriate consultation with neurosurgeons and plastic surgeons should be done at this stage.

The choice of reconstructive technique depends on tumor location, size, and degree of invasion. Johnson et al[19] have used temporalis fascia covered with a rectus abdominis microvascular free flap with good success in large skull base tumors that invade the cranial cavity. A pericranial flap rotated through the bottom of the craniotomy defect and sewn to the dura near the planum sphenoidale is probably the most commonly used reconstruction technique. Certain authors have advocated adding bone or cartilage on the nasal side of the defect[20] while Snyderman et al[15] have determined that solid reconstruction along with skin graft and nasal packing may not be necessary. Although they observed good mucosalization of the nasal surface with no increase in the incidence of meningitis or CSF leak, this has not been our experience.

Another way of preventing CSF leaks is to check for leakage at the end of the procedure. This can be accomplished by either positioning the patient's head lower than their heart, or by having the anesthesiologist hold an inspiration thereby effecting a Valsalva maneuver. Even if no CSF leak is witnessed at this time, a lumbar drain should be left in place 5 to 7 days after the operation if the risk for CSF leak is believed to be high.

Despite the best efforts at prevention, a CSF leak may manifest itself postoperatively. The presentation of a CSF leak after anterior cranial base surgery may become evident by rhinorrhea, pneumocephalus, or meningitis. Any cranial base operation that results in a leak into the middle ear or mastoid cavity may also present as rhinorrhea as the CSF will drain into the nasopharynx from the eustachian tube. Fluid draining from the nose may be differentiated from CSF by several methods. At the bedside, if CSF is mixed with blood it may exhibit the classic ring shape if placed on any surface that exposes the liquid to capillary action such as filter paper or bed linens. This fluid will also reveal a significant amount of glucose as normal CSF contains approximately two thirds of the glucose concentration of serum. Cerebrospinal fluid also contains about 124 mEq/L of chloride whereas nasal secretions do not contain chloride. These methods for checking the presence of CSF are subject to error owing contamination, dilution, or meningitis, which can alter glucose levels. Tau transferrin is another entity only found in CSF and may be detected by electrophoresis, immunofixation, and silver staining.[21,22]

Once the diagnosis of CSF leak has been made the surgeon must determine the location of the leak if this is not obvious. Attempts to localize the site of leak may include injecting a dye into the CSF and watching for its appearance in the nose or wound. Indigo carmine, methylene blue, and fluorescein have all been used; however, methylene blue has caused neurological sequelae and should be avoided.[23] Fluorescein can also cause an arachnoiditis and should be used in low concentration (<1%).[24] Neuropatties are placed in the decongested nose after injection of the dyes and direct visualization and staining of the neuropatties may lead to localization of the fistula. An ultraviolet light can be used to help look for the fluorescein both in the nose and on the neuropatties. Once the dye is in, the patient may be subjected to a Valsalva maneuver or the head may be placed lower than the heart to encourage leakage of the dye. The same technique can be used with radioactive tracers such as technetium Tc 99m DTPA and albumin labeled with iodine-131; however, the localization in this particular case is less accurate and requires a gamma counter. The advantage of this technique is minimal chance of meningeal irritation. Conversely, one disadvantage is the absorption of the isotope into the blood with subsequent secretion into the nasal secretions, causing a false-positive result. Third, contrast radiography using iodophendolate intrathecally can be used. After the contrast is injected into the intrathecal space, the patient is once again placed in the head down position and a CT scan is obtained to try to locate the leak. Iodophendolate is quite viscous and has a high incidence of meningeal irritation. Metrizamide is to be avoided owing to the potential for arachnoiditis, headaches, nausea and vomiting, and seizures. If the contrast study is negative but there is strong suspicion of CSF leak, an overpressure contrast study can be obtained. This technique involves raising the intrathecal pressure via a lumbar catheter to 40 to 50 cm H_2O for approximately 15 minutes utilizing a Harvard pump and artificial CSF (Elliot's solution) to promote leakage and subsequent visualization. The CT gantry is placed at the area most suspicious for a leak and repeated films are taken every 2 minutes. Radioactive tracers may also be used at the same time.

Initial treatment of a CSF leak may simply involve placement of a lumbar drain and observation for several days. Coverage with antibiotic therapy is controversial with views both supporting and opposing it.[25] In general, if the leak is into a contaminated area such as the nose, then concomitant antibiotic coverage should be strongly considered. The same paradigm would apply to the temporal bone where if mastoiditis was present prior to the leak, antibiotics would be recommended.

If the leak does not stop with an adequate trial of a lumbar drain, repair must be undertaken. The technique to be used depends on location of the leak. If the leak is near the cribriform plate, a septal mucoperichondrial flap may be used. If it is in the sphenoid sinus, a fascia graft followed by filling the sinus with fat is recommended. For large defects, the same techniques should be used as for intraoperative repair at the time of the original cranial base surgery, including water tight closure using pericranium, temporalis fascia, fascia lata, or cadaver dura. A regional myocutaneous or free myofascial flap may also be considered. The technique of repair is usually tailored to the site and size of the leak.[26] Success in operative repair of CSF leaks is not assured. Even experienced surgeons have a failure rate of approximately 20%.[25] The lumbar drain must be continued at least 5 days postoperatively to allow maximal chance for success.

PNEUMOCEPHALUS

Clinically significant persistent pneumocephalus is reported in 5 to 12% of postoperative craniofacial patients.[3,5,6,8] (There is always a mild degree of pneumocephalus postoperatively until intracranial expansion is complete.) Some advocate obtaining lateral skull films as baseline studies immediately postoperatively. Pneumocephalus usually presents as altered mental status with deterioration of neurological function. Diagnosis may be made with conventional lateral skull films, but CT scan better defines its extent for subsequent serial comparisons and assists in the differential diagnosis of obtundation. Brain edema, infarct, and intracerebral or subarachnoid hemorrhage may all initially present similarly. A preventable cause of pneumocephalus is overly aggressive drainage of CSF via a lumbar drain thus preventing normal intracranial expansion and favoring the persistence and accumulation of intracranial air. Tension pneumocephalus with significant cerebral compression may result from a ball-valve action of the flaps used to reconstruct the skull base. Treatment consists of emergently draining the accumulated air in a controlled fashion with needle aspiration, usually through one of the craniotomy burr hole sites.[27] In some cases, further operative intervention is required whereas others with stable neurological exams and decreasing air

collections may be followed expectantly. Airway diversion and nasal repacking may be adjunctive measures. Diffusion of nitrous oxide has been postulated as an etiology of pneumocephalus, but controlled studies did not support this hypothesis. Prophylactic tracheotomy to divert the airway in an effort to avoid pneumocephalus may be considered, depending on the debility of the patient (Fig. 21–1).

MENINGITIS

Meningitis is a rare but serious complication of cranial base surgery. During anterior cranial base surgery there is usually only a pericranial flap and skin graft or other thin barrier separating the aerodigestive tract from what is usually a large exposure of meninges.

There are many predisposing factors to meningitis, probably the most significant of which is a residual CSF leak from the time of surgery. Indeed, infection rates range from 9 to 36% when CSF leakage persists beyond two weeks.[28] Other factors that predispose to infection include procedures that last longer than 12 hours during which many people come in and out of the operating room. Measures to reduce the chance of meningitis include standard surgical techniques that prevent infection including the use of perioperative antibiotics, obliteration of dead space, and meticulous hemostasis, debridement of any devitalized tissue, avoidance of any foreign material in the wound, and irrigating the wound with antibiotic solutions.[29] Computed tomographic imaging should be used when meningitis is suspected to rule out specific intracranial sources such as abscess, osteomyelitis, or CSF leak. Sinusitis, resulting from impaired drainage of the remaining sinuses secondary to postoperative scarring and edema, may also be a source of intracranial infection either by direct or hemotogenous spread. Wound cellulitis, of course, may be readily observed and usually responds rapidly to intravenous antibiotic therapy.

If meningitis developed, the clinical signs are usually headache, fever, and a stiff neck. Laboratory values show CSF leukocytosis with a preponderance of neutrophils, a glucose level that is usually less than one half of the simultaneous serum glucose, and an elevated CSF protein concentration. Culture and sensitivity should direct the antibiotic therapy of an appropriate drug with adequate central nervous system penetration.

Another possibility includes aseptic meningitis in which the clinical picture is one of bacterial meningitis; however, no organisms are cultured from the CSF. Although not well understood, the etiology has been suggested to be the presence of blood breakdown products in the CSF. It is sometimes difficult to differentiate between aseptic meningitis and a partially treated bacterial meningitis, in which case, the safest course is to treat the patient as if it was initially a case of bacterial meningistis.[29]

Other infectious compliciations may also occur. Rates range from 14 to 21% in published series.[5–8] Epidural abscess constitutes a major and potentially morbid complication. Diagnosis may be confirmed by CT scan and culture of

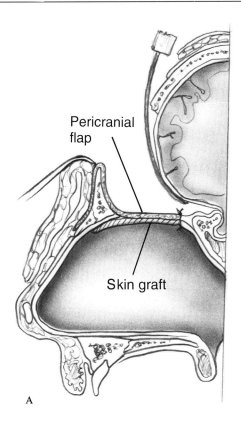

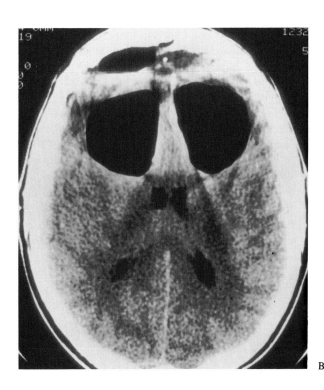

A   B

Figure 21–1. **(A).** Placement of pericranial flap for reconstruction of craniofacial resection. The pericranial flap is spiculed, with the skin graft on the nasal surface being demonstrated using interrupted lines. Failure of this flap can lead to many complications including pneumocephalus as seen in the CT scan **(B).**

exudate. Treatment requires drainage and debridement with directed antibiotic coverage. As the bone is extremely susceptible to infection and osteomyelitis, persistent abscess may indicate bone flap involvement. Such progression may require bone flap removal and possible placement of a vascularized tissue flap. Van Tuyl and Gussack[3] reported a 29% occurrence of bone flap osteomyelitis necessitating removal in two thirds of cases. Similarly, the University of San Francisco reports the removal of bone flaps in 10% of its cases.[30] The rate at the University of North Carolina is 4% and is strongly linked to antecedent administration of radiotherapy. It is plausible that increased use of myogenous flaps may reduce this incidence.

HEMORRHAGE

Hemorrhage is a frequent and serious complication of cranial base surgery, especially with certain tumors encountered in anterior cranial base surgery such as juvenile nasopharyngeal angiofibroma. Tumors that are located in areas requiring a middle cranial or anterolateral cranial base approach are also often quite vascular and include carotid body, glomus jugulare, and glomus vagale tumors. The venous drainage of these tumors can involve the dural sinuses. Back bleeding and difficulty in exposing these structures can lead to significant blood loss. In addition, surgery of the skull base often involves drilling away bone and exposing marrow,

which can be a significant source of blood loss as well as a possible source of air embolism. (See "Air Embolization," later in this chapter). In the case of juvenile nasopharyngeal angiofibroma, preoperative embolization of the vascular supply was first performed in the early 1970s by Dr Roberson and his colleagues, Drs Biller, Sessions, and Ogura.[31] Following this in 1975, Pletcher et al[32] published their series of 7 embolized juvenile nasopharyngeal angiofibromas compared with 16 historical controls. These patients were embolized using Gelfoam and the authors noted that the average amount of blood lost in the embolized group was one half that of the control group. Later follow-up series of juvenile nasopharyngeal angiofibroma resection by Economou et al[33] as well as the experience of Spector[34] confirm that preoperative embolization decreases the amount of blood loss during these cases.

With the groundwork of preoperative embolization laid, the next technique to come into use was super selective embolization. In the series by Ward et al,[35] 11 cases were resected without embolization with an estimated blood loss of greater than 1000 mL per case. In six cases in which preoperative embolization with polyvinyl ethanol was used, the estimated blood loss was 400 mL. Additionally, total operative time was decreased and fewer postoperative cranial nerve deficits were noted in the embolized cases. Similar results have been noted in cases of glomus jugulare tumors.[36,37]

It should be noted that not all published series have shown such promising results. Indeed, Duvall and Moreano[38] in their series from the University of Minnesota noted that the last five patients of their series had been embolized using Gelfoam. They did not notice a large decrease in bleeding and in fact failed to show the presence of Gelfoam or histological tumor infarction on microscopic exam. This does bring to light the fact that technique is important during embolization of skull base tumors. In general, the resection should occur within 24 hours of the embolization as collateral circulation occurs rapidly. The complications of embolization can be devastating and include stroke and cranial nerve palsies secondary either to tumor swelling or embolization of the vasa nervorum.[36,39] The decision to use preoperative embolization should be based on the availability of an experienced neuroradiologist. These procedures are both complex and rare and neuroradiologists with experience in these techniques are also rare.

When the resection of a vascular tumor is scheduled on an elective basis rather than emergently, consideration should be given to autologous blood donation. By this method, the risk of transmissible disease via blood products is minimized.

OCULAR COMPLICATIONS

Ocular complications are a rare and potentially devastating complication of surgery of the anterior cranial base. The most serious complication is blindness. Blindness can result from a number of different causes. If orbital exenteration due to tumor extension is planned, this is an obvious cause of blindness. In this case, the patient should be informed preoperatively. Previous indications for orbital exenteration are being reevaluated in cases of sinus malignancy.[40] Trauma at the skull base can cause either an orbital hematoma or direct trauma to the optic nerve resulting in visual loss. If the loss of vision does not respond to medical therapy, optic nerve decompression may be indicated.[41,42] Corneal damage can result if destruction of the ophthalmic division of the trigeminal nerve results in corneal anesthesia. In addition, damage to the facial nerve can compound corneal injury secondary to exposure. A retrobulbar hematoma such as may occur if an ethmoid artery retracts into the orbit or venous bleeding accumulates within the periorbita can also cause blindness. The mechanism for this is not entirely clear although high pressure causing venous outflow obstruction and subsequent hypoxia in the retina and optic nerve has been postulated.[43] Treatment includes ophthalmologic consultation if not already obtained, eye massage, 1 to 2 g/kg of mannitol IV, and lateral canthotomy and cantholysis. If this does not relieve the pressure, a Lynch medial orbital decompression of the orbit with or without decompression of the optic nerve is indicated.[43] Sympathetic uveitis may also occur if an injured eye is not removed.[44]

Less devastating complications include enophthalmus, diplopia, and epiphora. Diplopia can occur if cranial nerves III, IV, or VI are involved with the tumor or in the resection. If the tumor involves the cavernous sinus, this is often the case. If the resection must involve the periorbita, resultant scarring and contraction of the extraocular muscles can occur, causing diplopia. Diplopia can also occur if the medial canthus is not reattached medially.[5,45] This can be done with a transnasal wire secured to a medial canthal button or a permanent suture from the medial canthal tendon to the bony remnant of the medial orbit.[5] Epiphora can occur if the lacrimal drainage system is interrupted and is treated with a dacryocystorhinostomy. Enophthalmos may occur if the periorbita is resected when a total maxillectomy is performed. Suspension of the orbital contents with a lateral temporalis muscle-fascial flap may help, but this is not ideal.

MIDDLE AND ANTEROLATERAL CRANIAL BASE

Anatomy

The middle cranial base is the site of tumors that arise primarily in the temporal bone. The intracranial extent is bounded anteriorly by the posterior edge of the lesser sphenoid wing and posteriorly by the posterosuperior edge of the petrous part of the temporal bone. The extracranial extent is bounded by the posterolateral walls of the maxillary sinuses anteriorly and the petro-occipital sutures posteriorly. The osseus underpinning, which comprises the middle cranial base, includes the greater wing and body of the sphenoid, and the petrous and squamous portions of the temporal bone. This region is complex and contains numerous foramina that conduct neural and vascular structures. Surgically important structures in this area include the carotid canal, superior orbital fissure, optic canal, and foramen rotundum. The origin of the internal jugular vein, from the transverse sinus, with its tributary of the superior petrosal sinus, and the sigmoid sinus, with its tributary of the inferior petrosal sinus, is located in this region. The foramen ovale transmits the mandibular nerve (V-3) and the foramen spinosum transmits the middle meningeal artery.

The anterolateral cranial base can be thought of as the lateral extension of the anterior cranial base and consists of the infratemporal and pterygomaxillary fossae. The roof of the infratemporal fossa consists of the flattened inferior surface of the greater wing of the sphenoid and as a result is contiguous with the middle cranial base. In this area the foramen ovale and foramen spinosum are located. The infratemporal fossa is bounded laterally by the ramus of the mandible. The posterior boundary is the carotid artery and the cartilaginous eustachean tube forms the posteromedial boundary. Anteriorly the posterior wall of the maxillary sinus forms the boundary. The lateral pterygoid lamina and fissure are located at the anteromedial boundary of the infratemporal fossa. The pterygoid fossa is the concavity between the medial and lateral pterygoid plates. The pterygopalatine fossa is that area bounded by the maxilla and the pterygoid portion of the sphenoid bone and the perpendicular lamina of the palatine bone. The internal maxillary artery courses through this region. Its branches include the middle meningeal branch that passes through the infratemporal fossa and the inferior alveolar artery that passes into the mandible. The nerves include the mandibular branch of the trigeminal nerve after it exits the foramen ovale and the maxillary branch after passing through the foramen rotundum into the pterygopalatine fossa.

Operative Approaches

The surgical approaches to the middle and anterolateral cranial base are numerous and reflect the complex anatomy of this region. It is beyond the scope of this chapter to detail all the approaches to this region but a brief review will be included. Krespi and Sisson[46] divide the middle cranial base approaches into those procedures that provide exposure to the central and lateral compartments. These compartments are defined as follows: The central compartment is that area between two parasagittal lines drawn from the medial pterygoid plate to the occipital condyle as seen from the bottom of the skull. This area includes the pituitary fossa, the sphenoid rostrum and lower sphenoid sinus, the nasopharynx, the pterygopalatine fossa, and the lower portion of the clivus. The lateral compartment includes the infratemporal fossa, the parapharyngeal space, and the petrous portion of the temporal bone. Of course, the location of the lesion may exclude such division and a combination of approaches may be necessary.

Approaches to the central compartment include the transeptal and transethmoidal sphenoidotomy routes to the sphenoid and parasellar areas. These approaches are safer than more lateral approaches because they avoid the neurovascular structures located there. However, these approaches have the disadvantage of limited exposure and for more extensive lesions other approaches are indicated. The lateral rhinotomy and transantral approaches also avoid laterally located structures and offer more exposure. When even more exposure is required, a midfacial degloving either by itself or in combination with a Le Fort I osteotomy will offer even greater acces to the oropharynx and nasopharynx. A mandibulotomy approach provides access to lower areas in this region including the craniovertebral junction. This approach can be used in combination with exposure of the parapharyngeal space allowing proximal dissection and control of the carotid artery and internal jugular vein. Other approaches for extensive clival and craniovertebral junction lesions include the extended maxillotomy[47] and the midfacial split approach.[48]

Operative approaches to the lateral compartment include the transtemporal approaches more commonly associated with lesions in the posterior cranial fossa such as the transcochlear[49] and translabyrinthine approaches.[50,51] These approaches can be combined with craniotomy, infratemporal, or transfacial approaches for access to the middle cranial base. The infratemporal approach as described by Fisch and Pillsbury[52,53] provides exposure to large lesions involving the clivus and parasellar regions. The exact operation performed is determined by the anterior extension of the disease. The type A approach is used primarily for glomus tumors and lesions in the infralabyrinthine and labyrinthine parts of the temporal bone. The type B approach is used for lesions of the clivus and nasopharynx and is used for more anteriorly based tumors. The type C approach is used for removal of tumors in the parasellar areas. All three of these approaches involve facial nerve dissection and transposition. If the facial nerve is involved in a tumor, it is resected and reconstructed with a suitable graft. These approaches also involve dissection and control of the internal carotid artery in the petrous bone. For lesions located more inferiorly in the infratemporal fossa, a transparotid or extended rhytidectomy approach may be used. Intracranial approaches to the middle cranial base have also been used. In particular the middle fossa approach of House[54] provides access to the internal auditory canal (IAC) by drilling bone superiorly along the petrous portion of the temporal bone.

Complications
CAROTID ARTERY

The internal carotid artery is often involved in the middle cranial base by glomus jugulare tumors. Other tumors that may involve the carotid artery include carotid body tumors as well as glomus vagale tumors. Squamous cell carcinoma located high in the neck may also involve the carotid, however this is often regarded as a relative contraindication for resection as this has not led to increased survival.[55]

If the extent of a benign cranial base lesion is such that removal is impossible without sacrificing the carotid artery, preoperative assessment must determine if the carotid can be removed without resulting in stroke and whether an attempt at bypass should be made. Early attempts at prediction included the Matas test. This involved carotid occlusion in the neck with subsequent neurological exams.[56] Other methods evolved including measurement of carotid stump pressure and ocular pneumoplethysmography. These methods reflect the blood pressure in the distal internal carotid artery, but give no information regarding blood flow in the anterior and middle cerebral arteries. Work has also been done with transcranial Doppler ultrasound, radioactive washout techniques, and monitoring of evoked potentials.[57-59] The temporary balloon occlusion test of the internal carotid artery with subsequent xenon cerebral blood flow studies has become the most important diagnostic method to determine whether carotid artery resection with reconstruction is feasible.[60-62] This involves occlusion of the internal carotid artery through the transfemoral route and repeated neurological examination during a 10 to 15-minute period. If there is development of a neurological deficit the test is terminated immediately. If the patient tolerates the test, a xenon CT scan is performed to quantify cerebral blood flow. Normal cerebral blood flow to the brain is approximately 55 mL/100 g/min with the lower limit of normal defined as 35 mL/100 g/min (2 SD below average flow). If there is no change in cerebral blood flow the patient will likely tolerate permanent internal carotid occlusion. Patients usually do not develop neurological symptoms until the cerebral blood flow is less than 20 mL/100 g/min.[62] It is assumed that patients who develop neurological deficits during carotid occlusion have flow below 20 mL/100 g/min. This leaves the group with cerebral blood flow between 35 and 20 mL/g/min as those at intermediate risk. The authors predict that these patients will tolerate temporary internal carotid artery occlusion and if the artery is excised an interposition vein graft is preferred. If the decision is made to excise the artery in the high-risk group, an extracranial-intracranial bypass may be considered but this has not been studied well. In the study by de Vries et al,[61] 136 patients were studied in the above fashion. Eleven failed carotid occlusion, 96 had minimal to no change in cerebral blood flow, and 13 were in the intermediate-risk group. This group tended to tolerate temporary occlusion but the authors believed they had inadequate reserves for further compromise in flow (ie, hypotension or anemia) or were at risk for stroke with sacrifice of the internal carotid artery.

If the decision is made to bypass the internal carotid artery, generally a reversed saphenous vein graft is used. Venous grafts have the potential to thrombose and there is a risk of stroke by either thrombus propagation or distal embolization. This risk can be minimized by choosing a vein of similar diameter, meticulous handling of the graft and anastamotic technique, and keeping the patient on antiplatelet and steroid therapy perioperatively. The risk of carotid blowout and hemorrhage is significantly increased if there is a wound infection. Consideration of a vascularized flap should be given if the upper aerodigestive tract is entered during the procedure.[63]

When the carotid is injured inadvertently during a procedure, intraoperative reconstruction should be attempted. A small hole should be simply closed with direct suturing of the carotid artery wall during temporary arterial occlusion with clips. If a segment of the artery is significantly damaged or if the artery must be resected, a vein graft should be considered. Some authors recommend excision and occlusion in patients who tolerate the xenon CT perfusion test and who have malignant tumors and relatively short life expectancies.[61] They also point out if the common carotid or the internal cartotid is occluded low in the neck, a long thrombus may form within the internal carotid which can propagate distally into the middle cerebral artery or anterior communicating artery. Small emboli can then form. This is less likely to occur if the internal carotid artery is occluded close to the ophthalmic or posterior communicating artery.[61]

AIR EMBOLIZATION

Although the topic of air embolism is included in this section, this complication can occur with any surgery of the head and neck. Cranial base surgery is unique in that the venous structures include the dural venous sinuses that do not collapse in the way the internal jugular and other large veins in the neck do. Additionally, air can enter the venous system through diploic bone, which must be sealed with bone wax at the time of injury to prevent air embolism. Air embolism is a risk during head and neck surgery because the head is often placed above the heart to decrease venous bleeding. This can lead to a situation where the pressure in the right heart is less than the pressure at the level of the open vein.

Once air enters the vein it follows the venous circulation to the right atrium, through the right ventricle, and into the pulmonary arterial circulation. A very small amount of air will diffuse into the alveoli and be expelled during ventilation. If greater than 50 mL of air is embolized into the venous system intensive pulmonary arterial vasoconstriction occurs, which can lead to cor pulmonale and pulmonary edema.[64] Larger amounts of air can actually lodge in the right atrium and ventricle, causing an air lock, with subsequent absence of cardiac output. Severe hypotension and hypoxia then immediately occur. A venous air embolism of greater than 200 mL is said to be fatal. Also, in approximately 20% of people, the foramen ovale, although closed with high left-sided heart pressures, can become functionally open to allow air to pass from the right atrium into the left atrium. This air can then embolize in the cerebral or coronary circulation with obvious disastrous effects.[65] Also, nitrous oxide is more soluble in blood than in air. If an air embolism occurs while nitrous oxide is being used, there will be a concentration gradient favoring the diffusion of nitrous oxide out of the blood and into the air embolism.

Communication between the anesthesiologist and surgeon is essential in diagnosing and treating air embolism. The first indication of an air embolism may be an audible sucking sound at the site of entry. If a chest Doppler has been placed, it will immediately detect the presence of as little as 1 mL of air in the circulation,[66] although it can also miss certain episodes.[67] A "mill wheel" or machinelike cardiac murmur may be heard and any number of cardiac dysrhythmias may also occur. If a large air embolus is present and an air lock occurs in the right ventricle, sudden systemic hypotension will ensue. Also, because the lungs are not being perfused with blood, the end expiratory CO_2 will drop. The central venous pressure will acutely rise because the venous return to the heart has been cut off by the air lock in the right ventricle.

Treatment of an air embolism starts with immediate packing of the wound with saline-soaked sponges and occluding the open vein. Additionally, the jugular veins in the neck should also be compressed to prevent further entrance of air. If the patient has a previously placed right atrial catheter, it should be used to aspirate the air, although this sometimes proves difficult.[67] If the patient does not have a right atrial catheter placed, a needle may be inserted into the right ventricle from a subxiphoid approach to aspirate the air. Ventilation should immediately be switched to 100% oxygen and any nitrous oxide should be discontinued. Vasopressors may be used in the case of severe hypotension to help ensure adequate perfusion to vital organs. The patient should be placed in the left lateral Trendelenburg position to attempt to trap the air in the right side of the heart and prevent it from embolizing to the pulmonary arterial circulation.

The prevention of an air embolism is the best management. Meticulous hemostasis and surgical care when operating near large veins are very important. Rapid application of bone wax to exposed diploic bone is also helpful. A right atrial catheter should be used in any major cranial base surgery and a chest Doppler may also be used to help detect air embolism early. End tidal CO_2 should also be continsouly monitored during these cases.

CERVICAL SYMPATHETIC TRUCK

Located in close approximation to the internal carotid artery is the cervical sympathetic trunk. This structure consists of two to four ganglia generally referred to as superior, middle, vertebral, and inferior with an interconnecting trunk. The fibers consist largely of ascending preganglionic sympathetic fibers that have emerged through the ventral roots of the upper thoracic nerves, entering the cervical sympathetic trunk via the white rami communicantes and passing upward to synapse in the higher ganglia. The superior cervical ganglion lies somewhat posteromedial to the first portion of the internal carotid artery and just anterior to the inferior (nodose) ganglion of the vagus. Postganglionic fibers leave the superior cervical ganglion to form the internal carotid plexus and course upward with the internal carotid artery to supply sympathetic innervation to the face, nose, and eye.[68] Interruption of the cervical sympathetic chain results in Horner's syndrome, which includes ptosis, anhydrosis, and myosis. Ptosis is due to lack of innervation of Müller's muscle, which holds up the eyelid. Anhydrosis of the unilateral face results from disruption of the sympathetic innervation to the sweat glands on the skin. Myosis results owing to lack of sympathetic innervation to the pupil. To date, there is no good way to reverse these symptoms after section of the cervical sympathetic plexus (Table 21-2).

POSTERIOR CRANIAL BASE
Anatomy

The posterior cranial base extends from the posterosuperior edge of the petrous ridge anteriorly to the occipital bones posteriorly. Important foramina and structures located here include the IAC, which contains the seventh and eighth cranial nerves, the foramen magnum, the hypoglossal canal, which transmits the hypoglossal nerve, and the jugular foramen, which transmits cranial nerves IX, X, and XI along with the jugular vein and posterior meningeal artery.

OPERATIVE APPROACHES

The operative approaches to the posterior cranial base include those techniques designed to expose the cerebellopontine angle (CPA). Additionally, lesions located in the anterior and middle cranial base that affect neurovascular structures located in the posterior cranial base may be approached with these techniques as well. The choice of approach depends on tumor size, histology, and preoperative cranial nerve function. The translabyrinthine

Table 21-2. Complications of Glomus Jugulare Removal

TYPE	INCIDENCE
CSF leak	12–22%
Aspiration	5–58%
Cranial nerve palsy	Incidence varies widely with tumor size and location
X	
IX	
VII	
XII	
Infection	3–6%
Other complications	
Stroke	
Cholesteatoma	
Tympanic membrane perforation	
Internal carotid injury	

approach is often used for medium and large CPA tumors usually associated with hearing loss, as well as small CPA tumors in which there is no serviceable hearing. This approach obviously results in total hearing loss. The retrosigmoid and suboccipital approach offers the advantage of hearing preservation in small CPA tumors that do not have extensive IAC involvement. However, the craniotomy and cerebellar retraction used during this procedure are not without their complications. Also, the facial nerve is placed at increased risk of damage when tumors located laterally are removed while not being under direct vision. The retrolabyrinthine approach offers the advantage of seventh and eighth cranial nerve preservation while offering a limited exposure to the CPA. The transcochlear and transotic approaches are useful for selected tumors requiring exposure of the clivus, vertebral and basilar arteries, and petrous carotid arteries. The seventh nerve function is usually preserved during these procedures with the transotic approach avoiding seventh nerve transposition and thus resulting in less postoperative weakness than the transcochlear approach.[69] The middle fossa approach may also be used for lesions located in the petroclival area where hearing is still intact. Temporal lobe retraction and poor access to the CPA and inferior IAC limit the usefulness of this approach to the posterior cranial base.

Complications
FACIAL NERVE

Acoustic neuromas arise from the vestibular nerves and are commonly juxtaposed to the facial nerve in the IAC. The anatomic integrity of the nerve can often be preserved in these cases even though the nerve may be splayed out over a very large tumor. Other CPA tumors such as meningiomas can effect the facial nerve as well. Tumors that may involve the facial nerve more distal than the CPA include glomus tumors, which can involve the nerve in the middle ear and as it exits the stylomastoid foramen. Squamous cell carcinoma of the skull base and adenoid cystic carcinoma of the parotid may also damage the facial nerve. Additionally, trauma such as gunshot and stab wounds as well as temporal bone fractures may also result in facial nerve damage.

The facial nerve (seventh cranial nerve) is responsible for the motor innervation to the mimetic facial musculature, the posterior belly of the digastric, the stylohyoid, and the postauricular muscles. There are also sensory and parasympathetic fibers carried with the motor neurons. The nerve exits the midbrain in the form of two roots: a motor root and a mixed sensory and parasympathetic root known as the nervus intermedius, nerve of Wrisberg, or glossopalatine nerve. The nervus intermedius is a rather small filament lying between the eighth nerve and the voluntary portion of the seventh nerve.[70] At the geniculate ganglion, the greater superficial petrosal nerve is given off. Distal to the ganglion, the branch to the stapedius exits followed by the chorda tympani. After exiting the stylomastoid foramen, the nerve courses through the parotid to the peripheral musculature. The branches to the postauricular muscles, poterior belly of the digastric, and the stylohyoid muscle come off the nerve just as it exits the stylomastoid foramen.

The best technique to avoid surgical damage to the facial nerve is to identify it. Once the nerve is identified, often quite large acoustic neuromas may be dissected from it with preservation of facial function. Some tumors such as primary facial neuromas may invade the facial nerve in addition to the temporal bone and thus require resection. Facial nerve dysfunction in this case is a sequela of surgery and not a surgical complication as such. Facial nerve dysfunction may also be a result of mobilization and retraction such as in the transotic approach. If the nerve is cut, direct reanastomosis is the procedure of choice. The critical factor in primary reanastomosis is the amount of tension on the anastomotic sites.[71] The nerve may be mobilized to gain approximately 0.8 mm of length simply by removing it from the fallopian canal. Retropositioning the parotid gland with a permanent stitch can add another 3 mm of length. Dissecting out and removing a portion of the tympanic bone can add another 5 to 6 mm for a total of 1.7 mm of added length.[72] If primary reanastomosis is not possible, the procedure of choice is a nerve interposition graft. The most common nerve used for grafting is the greater auricular nerve, which offers the advantages of being in the same operative field and being of a similar diameter. An alternative choice if the greater auricular nerve is involved in tumor, has been previously radiated, or is otherwise unavailable is the sural nerve which is removed from the leg. The nerve ends should be cut cleanly and the anastomosis made with epineurally placed 7-0 or 8-0 nylon sutures. Only enough sutures should be used to hold the two stumps in apposition. An adequate length of graft should be used to avoid tension. If the distal nerve is sectioned beyond the pes anserinus, the graft of choice is the sural nerve which can be split. If the nerve is sacrificed distal to a line dropped from the lateral iris, an anastomosis is extremely difficult.

If the nerve has to be taken just as it exits the midbrain facial reanimation procedures are the only options. The goals of facial reanimation procedures include providing eye protection primarily, and cosmetic enhancement secondarily. The most devastating result of facial nerve paralysis is blindness from corneal ulceration secondary to inability to close the eye. Postoperative care providers as well as patients and their family members should be taught how to apply ocular ointment and patch the eye shut at night as well as the importance of instilling artificial tears during the daytime. We now routinely use the implantation of gold weights in the eyelid to aid with blinking. This has helped in preventing corneal dessication; however, it is still difficult to make the blinking motion completely symmetrical with only the use of a gold weight.[73] The preferred method of facial reanimation involves a VII - XII transfer when the resection of the nerve is near the midbrain with preservation of the distal portion. The procedure should be done before 1.5 to 2 years of denervation owing to degeneration of motor endplates on the facial musculature beyond that time. There are other static facial reanimation procedures available but they are beyond the scope of this chapter.

The loss of nonmotor branches of the facial nerve results in much less morbidity. The loss of taste to the anterior two thirds of the tongue when the chorda tympani is sectioned is well tolerated. The loss of parasympathetic innervation to the submandibular gland and glands of the nose does not seem to create much functional disturbance as does the lack of stapedial reflex.

VESTIBULOCOCHLEAR NERVE

The eighth cranial nerve is most frequently involved with tumors that arise in the CPA. The most common tumor in this area is the acoustic neuroma, but other tumors include meningiomas, petrous apex cholesteatomas, cholesterol granulomas, eosinophilic granulomas, and various temporal bone lesions.

The eighth cranial nerve is separated into the vestibular and cochlear components, which are fairly easily identified as the nerve leaves the brain stem. The relationship between the two components is such that the most anteroinferior part is the cochlear nerve and the vestibular nerves are superior and posterior. Acoustic neuromas most commonly arise from the superior vestibular nerve; however, both the vestibular and cochlear components of the eighth nerve must usually be sacrificed in removing acoustic neuromas because of the size that they often attain before presentation. The variable that most often correlates with hearing preservation in acoustic neuroma removal is the size of the tumor.[74-77] At our institution this has also proven to be the case. A retrospective review of acoustic neuroma removal via a retrosigmoid approach revealed a hearing preservation rate of 34% in small (<1.5 cm) tumors, 10% in medium (1.5 to 2.9 cm) tumors, and 0% in large (>2.9 cm) tumors.[78] Thus, the smaller the tumor, the greater the chance of hearing preservation. Other authors have found similar results with hearing conservation more likely if tumors are less than 1.5 cm. In addition to tumor size, Wade and House[79] have suggested that ideal selection criteria for hearing conservation include a speech reception threshold (SRT) better than 30 dB and speech discrimination greater than 70%. Other authors have mentioned the possibility of a relationship between the normality of the ABR and the chance for successful hearing conservation.[77] Thus the more normal the ABR, the greater the chance for hearing preservation. A study by Kemink et al[80] reported an intraoperative ABR loss of wave V to correlate with a profound hearing loss postoperatively. A shift of wave V latency of less than 2 msec, however, was still associated with hearing preservation. These authors suggest monitoring wave V latency intraoperatively as a guideline to hearing preservation. This may be especially useful in cases of an only hearing ear.[80] Another suggestion by Shelton et al[81] is that an abnormal electronystagmogram (ENG) is a better prognostic indicator. They base this on the hypothesis that the caloric response reflects only the superior vestibular nerve function. If the calorics are not hypoactive, they more highly suspect an inferior vestibular nerve tumor as opposed to a superior vestibular nerve tumor. If the tumor lies on the inferior vestibular nerve, the chance of successful hearing conservation surgery is lower in their hands, probably owing to trauma to the adjacent cochlear nerve or interuption of cochlear blood supply.

The importance of attempting hearing preservation has been underscored in a study by Shelton et al[75] showing that hearing in the operative ear decreases more quickly over time than hearing in the nonoperative side. The loss of hearing due to either sectioning of the cochlear nerve or interruption of the blood supply to the cochlea or the cochlear nerve is not regainable. Some patients who require the ability to localize sound may be offered a CROS (contralateral routing of sound) hearing aid. If thay have a hearing loss on the contralateral side, a BI-CROS aid may be indicated.[77,80]

The symptom caused by sectioning the vestibular nerve is dizziness. This is caused by asymmetrical peripheral vestibular input to the brain; however, this is rather quickly compensated for in the otherwise healthy patient. Generally, the peripheral vestibular function will be somewhat hyoactive for quite a while before the patient goes to surgery as evidenced by the fact that most patients claim to be at least slightly unsteady for greater than 6 months prior to their diagnosis.[75,81,82] Patients with a long history of deteriorating vestibular function have time to adjust to decreased unilateral input from their semicircular canals. Indeed, there may not be much function left and removing the tumor may not have a significant impact on their dizziness if the vestibular nerve was not functioning at all prior to surgery. It is important to remind these patients to not walk in the dark without a light until they are very well compensated (Table 21–3).

GLOSSOPHARYNGEAL NERVE

The glossopharyngeal nerve is often involved in skull base tumors, but rarely to the exclusion of other neurovascular structures at the skull base. The glossopharyngeal nerve exits the skull through the jugular foramen. It is the most anterior

Table 21–3. Complications of Acoustic Neuroma Surgery

TYPE	INCIDENCE
Sensorineural hearing loss*	17–100%
Facial nerve paralysis*	1.5–40%
CSF leak	10–35%
Meningitis	1–10%
Intracranial hemorrhage	0.5–2%
Miscellaneous	Variable
Other cranial nerve palsy	
Cerebellar dysfunction	
Headaches	
Pneumocephalus	
Air embolism	
SIADH	
Contralateral hearing loss	
Air embolism	

SIADH, syndrome of inappropriate antidiuretic hormone.
*Dependent on tumor size and operative approach.

of the three nerves exiting this foramen (IX, X, and XI). The nerve usually lies in a groove in the anterior part of the jugular foramen and is separated from the other neurovascular structures in the foramen by a band of fibrous tissue. Occasionally, this fibrous tissue will ossify, creating a "pseudocanal" for the nerve. just outside the jugular foramen, the inferior petrosal sinus, often the most anterior structure in the foramen, usually passes between the ninth and tenth nerves to enter the superior bulb of the internal jugular vein. This relationship, however, is variable.[83] The glossopharyngeal nerve carries motor fibers to the stylopharyngeus muscle and preganglionic parasympathetic fibers arising from the inferior salivatory nucleus and traveling via Jacobson's nerve to anastomose in the otic ganglion to provide parasympathetic innervation to the parotid gland. The sensory fibers of the ninth nerve go to the middle ear, the eustachian tube, the lateral and posterior pharyngeal walls, the tonsillar fossa, and the posterior third of the tongue. There is also a limited region of the external acoustic meatus and ear that is involved. The glossopharyngeal nerve, as it emerges from the jugular foramen, lies anterolateral to the vagus and spinal accessory nerves, medial to the internal carotid artery, and anteromedial to the jugular bulb. Just after leaving the jugular foramen, it passes laterally between the jugular vein and the internal carotid artery and then forward between the internal and external carotid lying deep to the styloid process and its attached muscles. At this point, it is most easily located by looking on the medial border of the stylopharyngeus muscle. It curves around from the medial to the lateral aspect of the stylopharyngeus and then arborizes into a lingual and tonsillar branch as it enters the posterior aspect of the tongue medial to the hyoglossus. The glossopharyngeal nerve also has a branch that goes to the carotid sinus. This branch descends between the internal and external carotid and unites with the carotid branch of the vagus to supply the carotid body and sinus.[83] Care should be taken when working around these nerves, the carotid sinus, and carotid body to avoid brady-cardia and subsequent hypotension. If this occurs, a small amount of 1% lidocaine without epinephrine can be injected into the carotid bulb to prevent reflex bradycardia. Although one would expect a large area of numbness in the pharynx due to isolated sectioning of the ninth nerve, as well as possible dysphagia from dysfunction of the stylopharyngeus, clinically this has not been a large problem when isolated division of the glossopharyngeal nerve is performed. However, when the ninth nerve is sectioned in conjunction with the vagus nerve, these problems can be severe. The loss of the gag reflex is also more associated with sectioning of the tenth nerve than with the ninth nerve despite the theoretical loss of the afferent limb of this reflex. Apparently, both the ninth and tenth nerves supply sensation to the pharynx and their sensory distributions overlap.

VAGUS NERVE

The loss of the ninth and tenth cranial nerves together presents a very high degree of morbidity to patients undergoing cranial base surgery and necessitates tracheostomy and gastrostomy tube placement. Before an operation with this possible outcome is undertaken, patients and their family must be thouroughly counseled. We recommend that only if the patient can expect a reasonably long life after such and operation should this option be considered. Tumor behavior and histology along with location and intracranial invasion must be considered as well.

The tenth nerve passes through the anterior portion of the jugular foramen parallel to the accessory nerve. As the nerve passes through the jugular foramen it has a small superior ganglion from which arise the first branches of the vagus: the auricular and meningeal branches. Just outside the jugular foramen the nerve expands to form the inferior or nodose ganglion. Just below the inferior ganglion, the pharyngeal branch exits to combine with the pharyngeal branch of the ninth nerve. This supplies primary motor innervation to the pharynx. A small number of fibers are given off to the carotid artery, but this is primarily innervated by the glossopharyngeal nerve. The next branch of the vagus is the superior laryngeal nerve that branches into the internal and external laryngeal nerves after picking up sympathetic fibers from the superior cervical ganglion. The internal laryngeal nerve supplies sensation to the supraglottic larynx while the external laryngeal nerve supplies motor innervation to the cricothyroid muscle and a small part of the inferior pharyngeal constrictor. The recurrent laryngeal nerves then exit the vagus just distal to crossing the subclavian artery on the right and the aorta on the left. They then ascend the neck in the tracheoesophageal groove to supply motor innervation to the intrinsic muscles of the larynx with the exception of the cricothyroid muscle. The relationship of the vagus nerve to the internal jugular vein and the internal carotid artery is such that the vagus initially lies medial to both, but as it descends, the vessels shift slightly so that the vein comes to lie lateral to the artery and behind and somewhat between the two.[84]

The morbidity of dividing the vagus nerve in skull base surgery differs from that of only dividing the recurrent laryn-

geal nerve. Although aspiration is a significant risk when either is divided, the loss of the entire vagus function results in the inability to sense food in the supraglottic larynx combined with inability to adduct the vocal fold. Additionally, with division of the vagus proximal to the superior laryngeal branch, the cricothyroid muscle can no longer contribute to vocal fold adduction. Dysphagia is also a result as the constrictor muscles are no longer functioning and the cricopharyngeus fails to relax with swallowing. Along with aspiration and dysphagia, hoarseness is a third complication of dividing the vagus nerve.

If the vagus nerve must be divided owing to the tumor location, immediate postoperative management includes placing a large nasogastric tube for gastric decompression and performing a tracheostomy at the time of surgery. The large nasogastric tube may be replaced by a softer smaller caliber feeding tube once the danger of gastric outlet obstruction has passed. The risk for aspiration will be highest immediately postoperatively and this will be the time when the patient will need monitoring closely in an intensive care unit. The tracheostomy cuff should be left inflated until the contralateral vocal fold begins to compensate. If the contralateral cord fails to compensate with time, a medialization procedure of the paralyzed vocal fold is indicated. Often, a cricopharyngeal myotomy must be performed.

Bilateral vagus nerve loss results in bilateral vocal fold paralysis, which is usually treated with a tracheostomy. The patient's voice may actually be quite good if the site of the division is below the superior laryngeal nerve owing to the adduction provided by the cricothyroid muscles. However, if the lesion is above these branches, the voice may be poor. The patient should also be treated with a palatal obturator immediately postoperatively with long-term treatment including a pharyngeal obturator.[44]

Rehabilitation after, sectioning the vagus nerve includes modifiying the diet including foods that are less likely to be aspirated such as semisolid or thickened liquids. A rehabilative speech therapist can be very helpful in training the patient postoperatively. Often these patients use the "supraglottic" swallow where they take a breath, double swallow, and then cough at the end of deglutition.[44] Vocal fold paralysis can also be treated with a variety of medialization procedures. These procedures include the injection of Teflon paste into the paralyzed vocal fold. This procedure is usually performed with direct laryngoscopy with topical anesthesia while the patient is sedated, or with jet ventilation under general anesthesia. Transcutaneous Teflon injection in the office has also been described.[85] Another method of vocal cord medialization is thyroplasty type I as described by Isshiki et al.[86] This involves excising a small strut of cartilage from the lateral ala of the thyroid cartilage and inserting this lateral to the true cord in such a fashion as to push the true cord medially. Silastic blocks can also be fashioned in such a way as to provide variable amounts of medialization. The amount of medialization can be evaluated while the operation is being performed under local anesthesia using direct vision with a fiberoptic nasopharyngoscope and asking the patient to phonate during the procedure. Once the ideal location for the implant has been determined, it is secured. This procedure offers the advantage of being reversible and avoids possible tissue reaction seen occasionally with Teflon. Recently, Montgomery et al[87] have proposed an implant that is available in different sizes for male and female larynges and they have also introduced measuring devices and a thyroplasty saw blade to help standarize laryngeal framework surgery. An arytenoid adduction procedure may be helpful at the time of surgery if the level of the vocal folds is quite disparate or if there is a posterior glottic chink.[88] The topic of laryngeal rehabilitation remains an evolving one. Kuriloff and coworkers[89] have used a canine model to evaluate vocal cord medialization using an implanted miniature tissue expander. In theory this would allow fine vocal adjustments to be made after implantation.

Spinal Accessory Nerve

The most posterior of the three nerves traversing the jugular foramen is the spinal accessory nerve. This cranial nerve is responsible for motor innervation to the sternocleidomastoid and trapezius muscles. On exiting the skull base, the nerve is medial to the jugular vein between the internal jugular and the internal carotid arteries, and usually passes between the vein and artery to cross the lateral surface of the vein. Occasionally the spinal accessory nerve may be found medial to the jugular vein. This can be explained embryologically as the internal jugular vein forms a ring around the nerve. If the lateral ring persists instead of the medial ring then the spinal accessory will be medial to the internal jugular vein. Anatomic studies have estimated the incidence of this variation to be 20 to 30%; however, clinically, this appears to be less frequent.[90] The nerve then passes inferolaterally to the neck through, or occasionally deep to, the sternocleidomastoid muscle. A branch to this muscle exits before traversing the posterior cervical triangle to enter the trapezius. Division of the spinal accessory nerve leads to denervation of the sternocleidomastoid and trapezius muscles. This results in difficulty raising the shoulder and pulling it back. There is also concomitant strain placed on supporting shoulder muscles related to loss of the trapezius. This can lead to a chronic pain syndrome for which intensive physiotherapy regimens have been devised. When the spinal accessory nerve is known to be severed at surgery, immediate postoperative physiotherapy can prevent subsequent disability and pain.

HYPOGLOSSAL NERVE

The twelfth cranial nerve exits the skull through the hypoglossal canal and is usually accompanied by a venous plexus connecting the marginal sinus with the vertebral vein. This plexus can be quite large in cases where the occipital sinus is large.[91] As the nerve exits the hypoglossal canal it is medial to the internal jugular and internal carotid arteries. It then passes inferolateral and posterior to the vagus nerve. It courses under the sternocleidomastoid branch of the occipital artery and then proceeds medial to the posterior belly of the digastric on its way to providing motor innervation to the intrinsic muscles of the tongue.

Although the hypoglossal nerve exits the cranial base in the posterior cranial fossa, it is most frequently injured owing to involvement with tumors arising in the neck. Glomus tumors may become sufficiently large so that sacrifice of the nerve is unavoidable. Other tumors such as squamous cell carcinoma or adenoid cystic carcinoma of the submandibular gland may directly invade the hypoglossal nerve requiring its resection. Extensive retraction at the skull base to remove other tumors in the area may also result in hypoglossal dysfunction. If the hypoglossal nerve is sectioned inadvertently, primary anastomois should be performed. If a large portion of the nerve is removed in an en block resection, primary anastomosis will not be possible. Division of the nerve results in denervation of the ipsilateral intrinsic muscles of the tongue and their eventual atrophy. The amount of dysarthria and dysphagia varies significantly from patient to patient. Conley[92] noted that about 25% of patients progressed to marked atrophy, 53% have moderate atrophy, and the remaining 22% have little or no muscle degeneration. Rubin el al[93] have proposed the technique of tongue Z-plasty, which transposes an innervated flap of tongue muscle from the functioning side to the denervated side. Although this procedure is not used extensively, there does seem to be improvement in muscle tone and symmetrical movement in these patients within a few months.

If the hypoglossal nerves from both sides are sectioned, the resultant defect is devastating. In these patients, deglutition is impossible and a feeding gastrostomy or jejunostomy should be placed. If the loss of hypoglossal function is combined with the loss of cranial nerves IX and X, consideration should be given to a surgical antiaspiration procedure.[44]

Other Complications

Miscellaneous complications of cranial base surgery include neurosurgical complications that are beyond the scope of this chapter. Some of those complications that are worth mentioning include subperiosteal abscess, major cerebral artery occlusion, intracerebral hematoma, subdural hematoma, epidural hematoma, pulsating exophthalmus, cerebral edema, intracranial hematoma, brain stem ischemia and infarction, and hydrochephalus.

REFERENCES

1. Ketcham AS, Wilkins RH, Van Buren JM, Smith RR. A combined intracranial facial approach to the paranasal sinuses. *Am J Surg.* 1963;106:698–703.
2. Ketcham AS, Hoye RC, Van Buren JM, Johnson RH, Smith RR. Complications of intracranial facial resection for tumors of the paranasal sinuses. *Am J Surg.* 1966;112:591–596.
3. Van Tuyl R, Gussack GS. Prognostic factors in craniofacial surgery. *Laryngoscope.* 1991;101:240–244.
4. Terz JJ, Young HF, Lawrence W. Combined craniofacial resection for locally advanced carcinoma of the head and neck; carcinoma of the paranasal sinuses. *Am J Surg.* 1980;140:618–624.

5. Levine PA, Scher RL, Jane JA, et al: The craniofacial resection—eleven-year experience at the University of Virginia: problems and solutions. *Otolaryngol Head Neck Surg.* 1989;101:665–669.

6. Shah JP, Kraus DH, Arbit E, Galicich JH. Craniofacial resection for tumors involving the anterior skull base. *Otolaryngol Head Neck Surg.* 1992;106:387–393.

7. Ketcham AS, Van Buren JM. Tumors of the paranasal sinuses: a therapeutic challenge. *Am J Surg.* 1985;150:406–413.

8. Richtsmeier WJ, Briggs RJ, Koch WM, et al: Complications and early outcome of anterior craniofacial resection. *Arch Otolaryngol Head Neck Surg.* 1992;118:913–917.

9. Sisson GA, Toriumi DM, Atiyah RA. Parailasal sinus malignancy: a comprehensive update. *Laryngoscope.* 1989;99:143–150.

10. Shah JP, Sundaresan N, Galicich J, Strong EW. Craniofacial resections for tumors involving the base of skull. *Am J Surg.* 1987;154:352–358.

11. Sundaresan N, Shah JP. Craniofacial resection for anterior skull base tumors. *Head Neck.* 1988;10:219–224.

12. Stiemberg CM, Bailey BJ, Weiner RL, Weiner RL, Calhoun KH, Quinn FB. Reconstruction of the anterior skull base following craniofacial resection. *Arch Otolaryngol Head Neck Surg.* 1987;113:710–712.

13. Johns ME, Winn HR, McLean WC, Cantrell RW. Pericranial flap for the closure of defects of craniofacial resections. *Laryngoscope.* 1981;91:952–959.

14. Price JC, Loury McCarson B, Johns ME. The pericranial flap for the reconstruction of anterior skull base defects. *Laryngoscope.* 1988;98:1159–1164.

15. Snyderman CH, Janecka IP, Sekhar LN, Sen CN, Eibling DE. Anterior cranial base reconstruction: role of galeal and pericranial flaps. *Laryngoscope.* 1990;100:607–614.

16. Lalwani AK, Kaplan KJ, Gutin PH. The transsphenoethmoid approach to the sphenoid sinus and clivus. *Neurosurgery.* 1992;31:1008–1014.

17. Maniglia AJ. Indications and techniques of midfacial degloving: a fifteen year experience. *Arch Otolaryngol Head Neck Surg.* 1986;112:750–752.

18. Izquierdo R, Origitano TC, Al-Mefty O, Leonetti JP, Anderson DE, Reichman OH. Use of vascularized fat from the rectus abdominis myocutaneous flap territory to seal the dura of basicrania tumor resections. *Neurosurgery.* 1993;32:192–197.

19. Johnson GD, Jackson CG, Fisher J, Matar SA, Poe DS. Management of large dural defects in skull base surgery: an update. *Laryngoscope.* 1990;100:200–202.

20. Baker SR. Surgical reconstruction after extensive skull base surgery. *Otolaryngol Clin North Am.* 1984;17:591–599.

21. Kinney SE. Trauma. In: Cummings CW, Fredrickson JM, Harker LA, et al, eds. *Otolaryngology—Head and Neck Surgery.* St Louis Mo: Mosby Yearbook; 1986;4:3033–3045.

22. Yokoyama K, Hasegawa M, Shiba KS, et al. Diagnosis of CSF rhinorrhea: detection of tau-transferrin in nasal discharge. *Otolaryngol Head Neck Surg.* 1988;98:328–332.

23. Wolman L. The neuropathological effects resulting from the intrathecal injection of chemical substances. *Paraplegia.* 1966;4:97–115.

24. Calcaterra TC. Extracranial surgical repair of cerebrospinal rhinorrhea. *Ann Otol* 1980;89:108–116.

25. Myers DL, Sataloff RT. Spinal fluid leakage after skull base surgical procedures. *Otolaryngol Clin North Am.* 1984;17:601–612.

26. Kirchner JC, Sasaki CT. Reconstructive surgery of the sinuses. In: Thawley SE, Panje WR, eds. *Comprehensive Management of Head and Neck Tumors* Philadelphia, Pa: WB Saunders Co; 1987;1:433–444.

27. Arbit E, Shah J, Bedford R, Carlton G. Tension pneumocephalus: treatment with controlled decompression via a closed water-seal drainage system: case report. *J Neurosurg.* 1991;74:139–142.

28. Westmore GA, Whittam DE. Cerebral spinal fluid rhinorrhea and its management. *Br J Surg.* 1982;69:489.66.

29. Persing JA, Kassell NF, Jane JA. Neurosurgica! perspectives of special perioperative consideration. In: Cummings CW, et al, ed. *Otolaryngology—Head and Neck Surgery.* St. Louis, Mo: CV Mosby Co; 1986: 3383.

30. Kaplan MJ, Deschler DG, Gutin PG, McDermott M, Mamelak A. Complications of anterior and anterolateral skull base surgery. Presented at the North American Skull Base Association Meeting, February 19–23, 1993. Lake Buena Vista, Fla.

31. Roberson GH, Biller H, Sessions DG, Ogura JH. Presurgical internal maxillary artery embolization in juvenile angiofibroma. *Laryngoscope.* 1972;82:1524–1532.

32. Pletcher JD, Newton TH, Dedo HH, Norman D. Preoperative embolization of juvenile angiofibromas of the nasopharynx. *Ann Otol* 1975;85:740–746.

33. Economou TS, Abemayor E, Ward PH. Juvenile nasopharyngeal angiofibroma:, an update of the UCLA experience, 1960–1985. *Laryngoscope.* 1988;98:170–175.

34. Spector JG. Management of juvenile angiofibromata. *Laryngoscope.* 1988;98:179–175.

35. Ward PH, Liu C, Vinuela F, Bentson JR. Embolization: an adjunctive measure for removal of carotid body tumors. *Laryngoscope.* 1988;98:1287–1291.

36. Young NM, Wiet RF, Russell EJ, Monsell EM. Superselective embolization of glomus jugulare tumors. *Ann Otol Rhinol Laryngol.* 1988;97:613–620.

37. Murphy TP, Brackmann DE. Effects of preoperative embolization on glomus jugulare tumors. *Laryngoscope.* 1989;99:1244–1254.

38. Duvall AJ, Moreano AE. Juvenile nasopharyngeal angiofibroma: diagnosis and treatment. *Otolaryngol Head Neck Surg.* 1987;97:534–540.

39. Valavanis A. Preoperative embolization of the head and neck: indications for patient selection, goals, and precautions. *AJNR.* 1986;7:943–952.

40. Perry C, Levine PA, Williamson BR, Cantrell RW. Preservation of the eye in paranasal sinus cancer surgery. *Arch Otolaryngol Head Neck Surg.* 1988;114:632–634.

41. Knox BE, Gates GA, Berry SM. Optic nerve decompression via the lateral facial approach. *Laryngoscope.* 1990;100: 458–462.

42. Sofferman RA. Sphenoethmoid approach to the optic nerve. *Laryngoscope.* 1981;91:184–196.

43. Stankiewicz JA. Blindness and intranasal endoscopic ethmoidectomy: prevention and management. *Otolaryngol Head Neck Surg.* 1989;101:320–329.

44. Sataloff RT, Myers DL, Kremer FB. Management of cranial nerve injury following surgery of the skull base. *Otolaryngol Clin North Am.* 1984;17:577–589.

45. Schuller DE, Goodman JH, Miller CA. Reconstruction of the skull base. *Laryngoscope.* 1984;94:1359–1364.

46. Krespi YP, Sisson GA. Transmandibular exposure of the skull base. *Am J Surg.* 1984;148:534–538.

47. Cocke EW, et al: The extended maxillotomy and subtotal maxillectomy for excision of skull base tumors. *Arch Otol Head Neck Surg.* 1990;116:92–104.

48. Janecka IP, Nuss DW, Sen CN. Midfacial split for access to the central cranial base. *Acta Neurochir Suppl* 1991;53:199–203.

49. House WF, Hitselberger WE. The transcochlear approach to the skull base. *Arch Otolaryngol.* 1976;102:334–342.

50. Glasscock ME, et al. A one-staged combined approach for the management of large cerebellopontine angle tumors. *Laryngoscope.* 1978;88:1563–1576.

51. House WF. Transtemporal bone microsurgical removal of acoustic neuromas: report of cases. *Arch Otolaryngol Head Neck Surg.* 1964;80:617–667.

52. Fisch U. Infratemporal fossa approach to tumors of the temporal bone and base of skull. *J Laryngol Otal.* 1978;92:949–967.

53. Fisch U, Pillsbury HC. Infratemporal fossa approach to lesions in the temporal bone and base of skull. *Arch Otolaryngol Head Neck Surg.* 1979;105:99–107.

54. House WF. Surgical exposure of the internal auditory canal and its contents through the middle cranial fossa. *Laryngoscope.* 1961;71:1363–1365.

55. Osguthorpe JD, Hungerford GD. Transarterial carotid occlusion: case report and review of the literature. *Arch Otolaryngol Head Neck Surg.* 1984;110:694–696.

56. Matas R. Testing the efficiency of the collateral circulation. *JAMA.* 1914;63:1441–1447.

57. Andrews JC, Valavanis A, Fisch U. Management of the internal carotid artery in surgery of the skull base. *Laryngoscope.* 1989;99:1224–1229.

58. Hays RJ, Levinson SA, Wylie EJ. Intraoperative measurement of carotid back pressure as a guide to operative management for carotid endarterectomy. *Surgery.* 1972;72:953–960.

59. Ehrenfeld W, Stomy RJ, Wylie EJ. Relation of carotid stump pressure to safety of carotid artery ligation. *Surgery.* 1983;95:299–305.

60. de Vries EJ, Sekhar LN, Horton JA, et al: A new method to predict safe resection of the internal carotid artery. *Laryngoscope.* 1990;100:85–88.

61. de Vries EJ, Sekhar LN, Janecka IP, Eibling DE. Elective resection of the internal carotid artery without reconstruction. *Laryngoscope.* 1988;98:960–966.

62. Yonas H, Gur D, Goode BC, et al. Stable xenon CT blood flow mapping for evaluation of patients with extracranial/intercranial bypass surgery. *J Neurosurg.* 1985;62:333.

63. Sekhar LN, Schramm VL, Jones NF, et al: Operative exposure and management of the petrous and upper cervical internal carotid artery. *Neurosurgery.* 1986;19:967–982.

64. Munson ES, Paul WC, Perry JC, et al. Early detection of venous air embolism using a Swan-Ganz catheter. *Anesthesiology.* 1975;42:223–226.

65. Everts EC. Surgical complications. In: Cummings CW, Fredrickson JM, Harker LA, et al, eds. *Otolaryngology—Head and Neck Surgery.* St Louis,Mo: CV Mosby; 1986:1411.

66. Maroon JC, Goodman JM, Homer TG, Campbell RL. Detection of minute venous air emboli with ultrasound. *Surg Gynecol Obstet.* 1968;127:1236–1238.

67. Bedford RF, Marshall WK, Butler A, Welsh JE. Cardiac catheters for diagnosis and treatment of venous air embolism. A prospective study in man. *J Neurosurg.* 1981;55:610–614.

68. Hollinshead WH (ed). *Anatomy for surgeons: The Head and Neck.* 3rd ed. Philadelphia, Pa: Harper & Row, 1982;1: 490–492.

69. Nuss DW, Janecka IP. Surgery of the anterior and middle cranial base. In: Cummings CW, Frederickson JM, Harker LA, et al, eds. *Otolaryngology—Head and Neck Surgery.* St Louis, Mo: CV Mosby Co; 1993:3300–3337.

70. Hollinshead WH (ed). *Anatomy for Surgeons: The Head and Neck.* 3rd ed. Philadelphia, Pa: Harper & Row; 1982;1:81.

71. Gantz BJ. Intratemporal facial nerve surgery. In: Cummings CW, Frederickson JM, Harker LA, et al, eds. *Otolaryngology—Head and Neck Surgery.* St Louis, Mo: CV Mosby Co; 1986:3353.

72. Yarbrough WG, Brownlee RE, Pillsbury HC. Primary repair of extensive facial nerve defects: an anatomic study. *Am J Otol.* 1993;14:238–246.

73. Bojrab DI. Upper eyelid gold weight implantation in facial paralysis. *Insights Otolaryngol.* 1989;4:1–8.

74. Mangham CA. Complications of translabyrinthine vs. suboccipital approach for acoustic tumor surgery. *Otolaryngol Head Neck Surg.* 1988;99:396–400.

75. Shelton C, Hitselberger WE, House WF, Brackmann DE. Hearing preservation after acoustic tumor removal: long-term results. *Laryngoscope.* 1990;100:115–120.

76. Shelton C, Brackmann DE, House WF, Hitselberger WE. Middle fossa acoustic tumor surgery: results in 106 cases. *Laryngoscope.* 1989;99:405–408.

77. Glasscock ME, McKennan KX, Levine SC. Acoustic neuroma surgery: the results of hearing conservation surgery. *Laryngoscope.* 1987;97:785–789.

78. Pillsbury HC, Campbell JP, Bernard EJ. Retrosigmoid approach to the acoustic neuroma, The University of North Carolina experience. Presented at the Southern Section meeting of the American Laryngological, Rhinological, and Otologic Society; January 15, 1993; Boca Raton, Fla.

79. Wade PJ, House W. Hearing preservation in patients with acoustic neuromas via the middle fossa approach. *Otolaryngol Head Neck Surg.* 1984;114:85–87.

80. Kemink JL, LaRouere MJ, Kileny PR, Telian SA, Hoff JT. Hearing preservation following suboccipital removal of acoustic neuromas. *Laryngoscope.* 1990;100:597–602.

81. Shelton C, Brackman DE, House WF, Hitselberger WE. Acoustic tumor surgery. *Arch Otolaryngol Head Neck Surg.* 1989;115:1213–1216.

82. Wiegand DA, Fickel V. Acoustic neuroma—the patient's perspective: subjective assessment of symptoms, diagnosis, therapy, and outcome in 541 patients. *Laryngoscope.* 1989;99:179–187.

83. Hollinshead WH (ed). *Anatomy for Surgeons: The Head and Neck.* 3rd ed. Philadelphia, PA: Harper & Row; 1982;1: 490–492.

84. Hollinshead WH (ed). *Anatomy for Surgeons: The Head and Neck.* 3rd ed. Philadelphia, PA: Harper & Row; 1982;1:495.

85. McCaffrey. Transcutaneous teflon injection for vocal cord paralysis. *Otolaryngol Head Neck Surg.* 1993;109:54–59.

86. Isshiki N, Morita H, Okamura H, Hiramoto M. Thyroplasty as a new phonosurgical technique. *Acta Otolaryngol.* 1974; 78:451–457.

87. Montgomery WW, Blaugrund SM, Varvares MA. Thyroplasty: a new approach. *Ann Otol Rhinol Laryngol.* 1993;102:571–579.

88. Isshiki N, Tanabe M, Sawada M. Arytenoid adduction for unilateral vocal cord paralysis. *Arch Otolaryngol Head Neck Surg.* 1978;104:555–558.

89. Kuriloff DB, Goldsher MC Blaugrund SM, Krespi YP. Controlled laryngoplasty for vocal cord medialization: a technique using tissue expansion. *Laryngoscope.* 1990;100:615–622.

90. Hollinshead WH (ed). *Anatomy for Surgeons: The Head and Neck.* 3rd ed. Philadelphia, Pa: Harper & Row, 1982;1:497.

91. Hollinshead WH (ed). *Anatomy for Surgeons: The Head and Neck.* 3rd ed. Philadelphia, Pa: Harper & Row; 1982;1:85.

92. Conley J. Management of facial nerve paresis in malignant tumors of the parotid gland. In: Rubin LR, ed. *Reanimation of the Paralyzed Face: New Aproaches.* St Louis, Mo: CV Mosby Co; 1977:230.

93. Rubin LR, Mishriki YY, Speace G. Reanimation of the hemiparalytic tongue. *Plast Reconstr Surg.* 1984;73:184–192.

22 Rehabilitation of Facial Nerve Injury

Lawrence P.A. Burgess, M.D., F.A.C.S., Richard L. Goode, M.D., F.A.C.S.

Rehabilitation following facial nerve injury attempts to return both function and cosmesis to the face, with both being important. For function, restoration of eye closure is the primary goal. Second is the correction of drooping at the corner of the mouth to restore oral competence. For cosmesis, restoration of symmetry at rest is the primary goal. Second is the generation of symmetrical motion. Often, one has to be satisfied with asymmetrical motion that is too weak or prone to mass movement. In addition, donor sites providing nerves or muscles can contribute to morbidity surrounding the condition.

The reconstructive surgeon is faced with a difficult challenge in balancing these considerations. This is not made any easier with the wide array of surgical techniques that have been described to rehabilitate the paralyzed face, with all procedures not having equal value. In this chapter, the most commonly used techniques will be reviewed for their advantages and disadvantages. Although we will discuss some issues in the evaluation and management of certain acute palsies (0 to 3 months from injury), most of our emphasis will be on the later months of the subacute period (3 to 12 months) and the chronic period (after 12 months). These time periods were chosen arbitrarily, only for the purpose of discussion.

DIAGNOSTIC EVALUATION

The history surrounding a patient's paralysis establishes the time, type, and the degree of injury. Timing is particularly important for cases where the distal facial nerve remains both anatomically and functionally intact with the facial musculature. In this situation, any neural procedure that attempts to provide reinnervation must be performed prior to atrophy of both the distal nerve and musculature.

The type of injury will greatly influence the reanimation procedure utilized. At the histological level, peripheral nerve injury was classified by Seddon into neuropraxia, axonotmesis, and neurotmesis. This was later incorporated by Sunderland into a classification describing 5° of injury[1]: 1° or neuropraxia—Increased intraneural pressure leads to a conduction block of neural impulses, but the distal nerve can still be stimulated electrically. Increased pressure may be from external compression or intraneural edema leading to external bony compression by the fallopian canal. There is no loss of neural structures and recovery is complete if the pressure is relieved. 2° or axonotmesis—If the intraneural pressure causing 1° injury is not relieved, swelling continues leading to disruption of the flow of nutrients from arterioles leading to loss of axons. The endoneural tubes remain intact. With relief of external compression, recovery will still be complete as in 1° injury, but will be slower as axons must regenerate down the open tubes. 3° or neurotmesis—With continued compression, loss of endoneural tubes results. Recovery will be slower and there is potential for synkinesis or faulty reinnervation as proximal axons intended for one muscle group reinnervate several muscle groups. 4°—Partial transection of the nerve with partial loss of intervening neural structures. 5°—Complete transection with complete loss of intervening neural structures. This classification is useful in understanding the nature of nerve injury, but it should be remembered that a combination of several degrees of injury is often present at the same time within the nerve.

At the gross anatomic level, in cases where the distal facial nerve and musculature remain in continuity, reinnervation from the proximal facial nerve is best. If the proximal facial nerve is lost, reinnervation using another motor nerve might be employed. When there has been distal nerve or muscle loss, innervated muscle or another substitute must be brought into the region. In a dynamic transfer, innervated and vascularized muscle is transposed from local or regional sites, or transferred as a microneurovascular free muscle graft. In static procedures, fascia or alloplasts provide correction by static suspension.

The degree of injury and resultant defect will ultimately decide whether total facial reanimation is required, or whether a partial procedure can be used for regional areas of the face. Cases with partial return can be problematic. In this situation, many of the standard reanimation procedures require surgical approaches through regions where facial nerve branches are still functioning. Because these branches are providing partial function or muscle tone, residual function could be lost if the nerve is injured.

Physical examination of facial function and grading of the degree of paralysis is evaluated on the first evaluation and on subsequent visits. The first sign of function is muscle tone. Is there symmetry at rest? How much muscle bulk is present in comparison to the other side? Mimetic function is evaluated with the following maneuvers and documented photographically: at rest, forehead elevation, eye closure—normal and tight, and mouth—smiling, pucker (whistling), and blowing out the cheeks. Motion is graded using the House classification[2] (Table 22-1). Abnormal synkinetic or mass movements are noted, such as eye closure with smiling.

Electrodiagnostic testing is a method of evaluating the status of the nerve and muscle following nerve injury. Although an individual test result is usually indicative of the status of nerve or muscle, the entire test battery should be correlated with the history and physical examination. The most commonly utilized electrical tests are nerve excitability tests, electromyography (EMG), and evoked electromyography (EEMG, electroneuronography).

Nerve excitability testing in the office with the Hilger nerve stimulator (WR Medical Electronics Co, St Paul, MN) is useful in the evaluation of acute paralysis.[3] Main branches of the nerve are stimulated, and the milliamperage (mA) required for stimulation is compared from the normal to paralyzed side. A difference of 3.5 mA indicates a pathologic process. The test is not useful in the first 3 days following injury, as a nerve with complete transaction more proximally will continue to conduct electrical impulses distally for 3 days. A normal result with testing is less reliable than an abnormal result because 42% of patients with a normal response to testing can have residual functional deficits 6 months later.

The main advantage with nerve excitability testing is that it is an office procedure that can be performed sequentially in the early days following injury to evaluate the progression of disease. A significant disadvantage is that it is not sensitive enough to evaluate lesser degrees of nerve transmission that do not result in visible motion of the muscle group. Owing to this lack of sensitivity, the test also has little application in the evaluation of subacute or chronic paralysis.

Electromyography has been a standard in the analysis of facial paralysis beyond 2 weeks,[3-5] and together with EEMG plays an important role in evaluating patients with subacute and chronic paralysis. It evaluates the distal musculature from two different viewpoints. The muscle is analyzed as a separate entity apart from the nerve by evaluating the electrical response to needle insertion. The nerve and muscle are also analyzed together as a motor unit using two parameters: spontaneous activity and action potentials from voluntary muscle contraction. Findings on EMG are reviewed in Figure 22-1.

Insertion of the needle electrode through the skin and into the muscle usually results in a normal amount of electrical activity. Increased activity can be noted in early stages of denervation. However, in chronic paralysis with fibrotic or atrophic muscle, insertional activity is decreased or absent. Muscle biopsy can be used to correlate the degree of fibrosis.

Following needle insertion and cessation of needle movement, there normally is no activity recorded. Spontaneous

Table 22-1. House Facial Nerve Grading System

GRADE	DESCRIPTION	CHARACTERISTICS
I	Normal	Normal facial function in all areas
II	Mild dysfunction	Gross: slight weakness on close inspection; may have minimal synkinesis
		At rest: normal symmetry and tone
		Motion: Forehead—moderate to good
		Eye—complete closure with minimal effort
		Mouth—slight asymmetry
III	Moderate dysfunction	Gross: obvious but not disfiguring difference between two sides; noticeable but not severe synkinesis, contracture, and/or hemifacial spasm
		At rest: normal symmetry and tone
		Motion: Forehead—slight to moderate
		Eye—complete closure with effort
		Mouth—slightly weak with maximum effort
IV	Moderately severe dysfunction	Gross: obvious weakness and/or disfiguring asymmetry
		At rest: normal symmetry and tone
		Motion: Forehead—none
		Eye—incomplete closure
		Mouth—asymmetric with maximum effort
V	Severe dysfunction	Gross: barely perceptible motion
		At rest: asymmetry
		Motion: Forehead—none
		Eye—incomplete closure
		Mouth—slight movement
VI	Total paralysis	No movement

From House.[2]

activity indicates a pathologic process within the nerve, especially if it can be reproduced at two muscle sites. Positive sharp waves and fibrillation potentials occurring spontaneously indicate muscle denervation, and usually appear within 10 to 14 days following injury. Positive sharp waves occur early in the course of denervation, and are replaced by fibrillation potentials by the second to third week.

Although fibrillation potentials indicate that denervation has occurred, the degree of denervation cannot be predicted. Fibrillation potentials can be present in both conduction block and complete nerve disruption, and its presence does not indicate the percentage of nerve fibers affected. The presence of fibrillation potentials should be interpreted as indicating viable denervated muscle awaiting reinnervation.

The motor unit is assessed by having the patient voluntarily contract a muscle group (as with smiling). Absence of action potentials indicates denervation. Acutely, this could be due to conditions ranging from conduction block to nerve disruption. Beyond the acute time period, no activity indicates

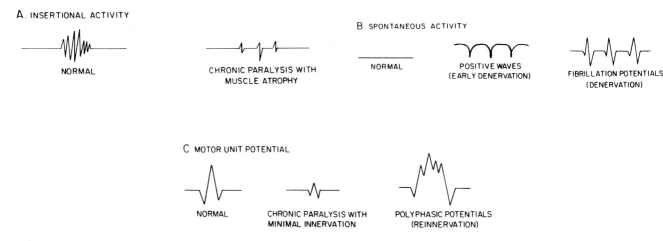

Figure 22–1. Electromyography. Typical results in peripheral facial paralysis as compared with normal are demonstrated. **(A).** Electrical activity on insertion correlates with the amount of viable muscle fibers present, with a decrease of electrical activity indicative of muscle atrophy or fibrosis. **(B).** After cessation of movement following needle insertion, spontaneous activity such as positive sharp waves (<2 weeks of injury) and fibrillation potentials (>2 weeks of injury) indicates viable denervated muscle. **(C).** On voluntary motion by the patient, an action potential indicates innervated muscle, no electrical activity indicates denervation. Polyphasic potentials indicate that reinnervation is proceeding.

denervation at that point in time. A reduction in the amplitude and duration of the motor unit potential is seen when there is a loss of muscle fibers surrounding the motor unit. In cases of chronic paralysis, this would indicate loss of innervated muscle fibers.

Reinnervation is indicated if the action potentials are large polyphasic potentials. A polyphasic potential combines several motor unit potentials that fire at slightly different times, due to latency variability of regenerating motor axons. Although this indicates reinnervation, it is not possible to determine what the clinical degree of functional return will be. The resence of polyphasic potentials is probably the lone test result that should cancel or postpone a potential reanimation procedure, until the degree of clinical return can be determined.

Evoked electromyography has been well reviewed with regards to acute paralysis,[3,6] but is less understood in the evaluation of subacute and chronic paralysis. It evaluates the muscle and nerve together. Using surface electrodes, a stimulating electrode is placed over the main trunk of the nerve after exiting the stylomastoid foramen and a recording electrode placed over the distal musculature. Recording electrodes have been described in the perioral region[6] and over the nasal alae,[3] which may explain differences in results between authors. A supramaximal stimulus is applied at the stylomastoid foramen and the response recorded distally. If intact axons are present over the segment of nerve being tested, an action potential will be generated and recorded distally. If axonal degeneration or nerve transaction has occurred, the ability to transmit an impulse distally will be lost within 5 to 7 days.[3]

Both the normal and abnormal sides are tested, with the amplitude of the evoked summation action potential of the abnormal side expressed as a percentage of the normal side. If the amplitude of the abnormal side is 10% of the normal side, it is expressed that the nerve is 90% denervated (Fig. 22–2). Coker[7] has reviewed nuances of EEMG.

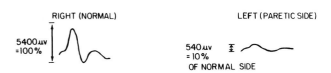

Figure 22–2. Evoked electromyography. Electroneuronography depicting the normal right side with an action potential amplitude of 5400 μV, whereas the paretic left side has an amplitude of 540 μV. Because 540 μV ÷ 5400 μV = .10, the left side has .10 or 10% innervation as compared with the normal side. It is more commonly stated that the left side has undergone 90% denervation as compared with the normal side.

Evoked electromyogram is somewhat similar to the maximal stimulation test (MST), which is a nerve excitability test that applies a supramaximal stimulus to the main trunk and allows visible motion of the face to be observed.[3] A positive MST requires that enough viable axons are present to cause visible motion of the face. An evoked electromyogram is more sensitive and objective because distal electrodes record any electrical activity in the muscle that may or may not be enough to elicit visible facial motion.[8]

For subacute and chronic paralysis, periodic evaluations can help to provide information as to the course of recovery. As Esslen[6] demonstrated in sequential studies, EEMG amplitude shows recovery over time and correlates with functional return. Mild cases of Bell's palsy with 1° and 2° injury recover rapidly by EEMG, whereas more severe cases recover incompletely over a longer period of time. After initial recovery, when amplitude fails to increase on sequential testing, further improvement in electrical testing is unlikely. This would also correlate with a decreasing chance for further clinical recovery.

An EEMG can also help to assess the presence of conduction block occurring more proximal to the site of testing. In the absence of facial movement, supramaximal stimulation may result in visible motion or muscle twitching in cases of maximal conduction block.[9] In cases with smaller amounts of conduction block, visible motion may not be seen, but we suspect that a larger than expected amplitude may be recorded.

Presence of an evoked potential in the second week following injury indicates a good prognosis with partial or complete recovery expected. In chronic total paralysis, the presence of an evoked potential with a large amplitude may indicate an intratemporal nerve decompression or a nerve crossover procedure rather than a muscle transposition or free muscle graft (see "Total Facial Paralysis—Neural Procedures").

Evoked electromyography is often not readily available outside of facial nerve centers. In this situation, a modified EEMG can be obtained, that is, the recording electrode is a needle electrode inserted into the muscle (as for EMG) rather than a surface electrode. Be aware that some physiatrists conducting the study are not familiar with the use of surface electrodes for EEMG. They may inform you that they do perform the EEMG study, when in actuality it is the modified study with needle electrodes that patients are obtaining. A major disadvantage with the needle electrode is that the amplitude of the action potential can change significantly with even slight shifts in needle position.[6] The surface electrode of the standard EEMG provides an average action potential for a larger surface area of the muscle. There is also less reproducibility between sequential tests with the needle electrode because it cannot be reinserted at precisely the same location. This problem can be reduced by taking several readings from different locations within the muscle and averaging the amplitudes. As this modified EEMG technique has not been standardized, the results should be interpreted with caution.

Imaging the facial nerve can be useful in the evaluation of the paralysis patient. With the advent of magnetic resonance imaging (MRI), the diagnosis of tumors affecting the nerve can usually be made. For this reason, an MRI with gadolinium enhancement should be considered in all patients with idiopathic paralysis prior to a reanimation procedure. Magnetic resonance imaging should be combined with high resolution computed tomography (CT) of the temporal bone to examine the course of the facial nerve. In cases of trauma, CT often provides enough bony detail to help localize the site of lesion.

TOTAL FACIAL PARALYSIS— NEURAL PROCEDURES

Procedures that attempt to restore neural input to an anatomically and functionally intact neuromuscular junction give the best results in total paralysis. Restoring impulses from the ipsilateral facial nerve is the first choice. This could result from nerve exploration with removal of adjacent tumor, facial nerve decompression, neurorrhaphy, or cable grafting. Nerve crossover procedures are the second consideration with variations of XII to VII being the most commonly used. Cross-face nerve grafts rank third but has largely been abandoned

owing to the poor results. However, cross-face grafts used with free neurovascularized muscle grafts are gaining some acceptance for midface and oral commissure reanimation.

Facial Nerve Exploration

Based on May's[10] series of 1575 facial palsies seen over a 20-year period, facial paralysis was caused by a primary or secondary tumor involving the facial nerve in 6% of cases. Such tumors often present with progressive facial paralysis. However, 32% of patients with benign tumors and 47% with malignant tumors presented with sudden complete paralysis.

A tumor should also be suspected if there is recurrent ipsilateral facial paralysis. In May's[10] series of 48 patients with recurrent paralysis, the paralysis was due to a tumor in 8 (17%). A tumor is indicated by electrodiagnostic testing if there is no response to MST or EEMG within the first 5 days after onset of paralysis. Facial numbness, twitching with weakness, no recovery after 6 months, other cranial nerve deficits, and segmental paralysis with sparing of other branches are other signs suggesting a tumor.

As previously noted, MRI with gadolinium combined with temporal bone CT will help to diagnose these lesions. However, small facial neuromas may still not be seen by imaging, especially if located extratemporally. Exploration when performed should be conducted both intra and extratemporally if necessary. Janecka and Conley[11] reported a series of 30 patients with primary facial nerve neuromas, with the tumor located extracranially in 17 and involving the main trunk in 12. The 13 remaining lesions were located intratemporally, with 10 cases involving the horizontal or vertical segments.

Facial nerve decompression in the acute stages of Bell's palsy has been well described but is usually not indicated. Fisch[12] recommended decompressing the labyrinthine segment of the facial nerve through a middle fossa approach if denervation by EEMG reached 95% within 2 weeks or 90% within 3 weeks of injury. Exploration and decompression following temporal bone trauma is well accepted when indicated by electrical testing. However, conservative management is often successful when good prognostic results on electrical testing are obtained.[13] Other surgical problems will often delay facial nerve decompression, as these patients are frequently multiple trauma victims. Even following delays that may last weeks to months, one should not be deterred from decompressing a trauma patient when indicated.

Electrical testing as performed in acute facial paralysis is accomplished, with a decision to operate based on the same criteria: total paralysis with greater than 3.5 mA difference between sides and EEMG data as described by Fisch above. Usually, only nerve excitability studies are initially obtainable on these patients at the bedside. An EMG and EEMG can be obtained later to complete the evaluation. As many of these patients have associated hearing loss, an audiogram should be obtained preoperatively.

Most would agree that there is little role for the utilization of facial nerve decompression for patients with subacute and chronic paralysis. However, occasional patients have been described in the literature in whom late decompression was accomplished 4 to 11 months following the onset of paralysis, and facial motion was demonstrated within 24 hours of surgery.[14] Electrical activity was absent preoperatively by MST, with no facial movement noted on stimulation. Evoked electromyography was not utilized at that time and long-term facial motion results were not provided.

For movement to occur so rapidly, a conduction block (1° injury) must have been present in a region of the nerve that was decompressed. If a conduction block was present, one must suspect that some transmission was occurring along the nerve. This would provide some muscle tone, but not enough axonal flow to stimulate the number of motor units necessary to demonstrate any observable facial function on voluntary motion or electrical stimulation of the nerve.

As discussed earlier, EEMG might be helpful to establish the presence of small degrees of conduction block for cases without facial motion. The presence of summation potentials with EEMG indicates viable axons. Depending on the amplitude of the potential in relation to the degree of paralysis present, a larger than expected potential might indicate a conduction block. However, there have been only anecdotal cases with no specific EEMG criteria to clearly determine what action potential amplitude would indicate a conduction block.

Decompression following a chronic traumatic injury can also be successful. Brodsky et al[15] described a temporal bone trauma patient with complete facial paralysis 15 months following injury. Preoperatively, only synkinetic movements of the upper branches were noted. An evoked electromyogram revealed summation potentials and EMG was consistent with muscle denervation. Following nerve decompression, some function was noted immediately in the lower branches. Good return of facial function was noted 5 months following surgery. In our opinion, the presence of summation potentials on EEMG demonstrated the potential benefit of decompression. This would assume a larger than expected amplitude on EEMG, the degree of which was not stated.

Again, with only anecdotal cases, it is not possible to surmise what is a large enough amplitude to indicate that a conduction block is present. Clinically, we suspect conduction block patients would have characteristics similar to those presented: good muscle tone with minimal or no motion.

If it is within the first 3 to 6 months following trauma, a lack of response by EEMG should not exclude a potential nerve decompression. The nerve may still be undergoing regeneration and has not reached a stimulatable state. Brodsky et al[15] decompressed a trauma patient 3 months following injury with absent stimulation by EEMG and denervation by EMG. Good return was noticed within 6 weeks following decompression.

Although evidence for decompression of subacute and chronic total facial paralysis remains anecdotal, the potential for good results makes us consider conduction block as a lingering cause of paralysis. Sequential EEMGs can be helpful in assessing the status of the nerve in these cases, with a larger than expected summation potential possibly indicating a conduction block.

Neurorrhaphy

The timing of neurorrhaphy is the first consideration. The best time for repair is immediately following injury. However, some have considered 21 days following injury to be the optimum repair time, based on theoretical physiological reasons. Barrs[16] reviewed this topic and conducted repair of facial nerves in micropigs from 0 to 90 days after nerve transaction. Results showed no significant differences between operative groups for electrophysiological testing, but a trend towards a lower axon count in the more delayed repairs. This study confirmed the validity of immediate repair and showed that grafting at 21 days did not produce better results. The clinical experience of May[17] supports Barrs' experimental results. He reported that primary neurorrhaphy accomplished within 3 months after injury provided the best results. Beyond this time frame up to 1 year, good results were still obtainable but less predictable.

Surgical repair of the main trunk of the facial nerve can be conducted by either epineural repair or perineural (fascicular) repair. Small distal branches are repaired by epineural sutures. Controversy exists as to which method of repair is better.[18,19] Epineural repair has several advantages (Fig. 22–3A). It is technically easier for the occasional microneurovascular surgeon. Second, there is less surgical trauma to the interior of the nerve than with perineural repair. A disadvantage is an increased likelihood of improperly aligned fascicles. This is partially reduced by ensuring that the nerve is lying in its natural anatomic position prior to suturing.

The number of sutures for epineural repair was studied in distal branches of the facial nerve in rabbits by Szal and Miller.[20] Repairs were undertaken with 10-0 nylon sutures using 3, 7, or 14 stitches. The best functional and histological results were seen in nerves repaired with seven sutures, indicating that between six to eight sutures is probably optimal. Naturally, the size of the nerve will play a role in determining the number of sutures needed.

This study demonstrated that the guiding principle for epineural repair should be good approximation of epineurium to epineurium around the full circumference of the nerve to prevent axon escape with resultant neuroma formation. Good approximation also prevents gaps from forming that would contribute to connective tissue ingrowth into the anastomotic site, also resulting in less axons traversing the wound.

Perineural (fascicular) repair requires removal of 2 to 3 mm of epineurium from the nerve endings (Fig. 22–3B). Individual fascicles are approximated with single 10-0 nylon sutures through the perineurium. Perineural repair is more difficult than epineural repair and requires more technical proficiency by the surgeon. Advantages of perineural repair include direct alignment of fascicles while removing the epineurium from which secondary scar tissue arises. However, Kline et al[21] demonstrated in an experimental study that there was no difference in results whether the previously back dissected epineurium was resected or returned to its original position.

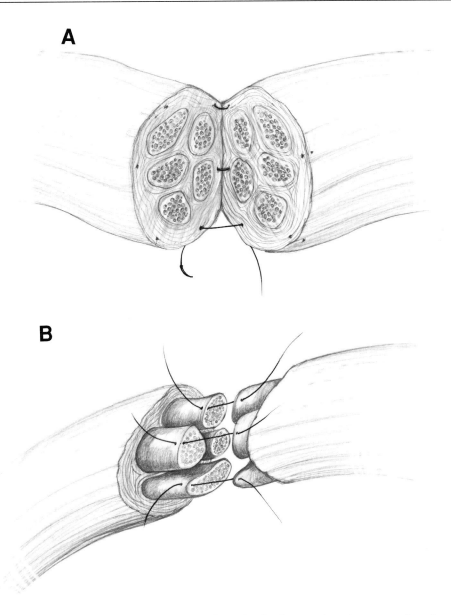

Figure 22–3. Nerve repair. **(A).** Epineural repair is performed under the operating microscope using microneural techniques with 10–0 monofilament nylon. A taper needle is preferred over a cutting needle. A Micro Edge Taper (Xomed, Inc, Jacksonville, FL) is thought to have some advantages.[94,95] The nerve edges are freshened with a microblade on a tongue depressor or microscissors. A standard blue or green silicone 1-mm grid background is used beneath the nerve ends while suturing. Tupper et al[19] described an Acland nerve frame to assist with turning the nerve ends over to suture the underside of the nerve. However, most repairs are usually sutured freehand because a nerve frame requires well-mobilized nerve endings to allow for the space necessary for turning the frame over. Freehand suturing makes the underside of the nerve difficult to expose. Two sutures placed 180° apart are used as traction sutures to expose the underside of the nerve for suture placement. A second alternative is to use a Cobbett type suturing technique that is shown, where the underside of the nerve is sutured first. The needle is passed outside-in then inside-out, leaving the knot external to the nerve. Normally, six sutures are spaced 60° apart placing the underside sutures first. Less sutures could be used for smaller peripheral nerve branches. **(B).** Perineural (fascicular) repair. The adventitia and epineurium are dissected back 2 to 3 mm exposing the fascicles. Excessive removal of the adventitia should be avoided, as this strips the edges of the nerve of its blood supply. The epineurium should only be removed to allow access to the fascicles, as excess removal causes the fascicles to lose their orientation and separate into spaghettilike strands. Protruding endoneurium is trimmed from the edges of the fascicles using microscissors and single 10–0 nylon sutures are used to approximate individual fascicles. The epineurium can then be replaced or resected, with no difference in end results.[21]

Disadvantages of perineural repair include increased surgical trauma to the interior of the nerve with an increase in technical difficulty. As in epineural repair, it is important not to disrupt the fascicle with the needle or suture as this will contribute to neuroma formation.[20] The nerve should also receive only minimal mobilization so that blood supply is not disrupted.

Regardless of the repair method, the degree of tension on the suture line is a critical factor affecting the final result. Increased tension could contribute to wound separation leading to both axon escape with neuroma formation and fibrous ingrowth of scar tissue. Both result in less axons traversing the wound. Millesi[22] demonstrated that more scar tissue resulted when gaps of more than 2 cm were closed primarily, and recommended autografts in this situation. Orf[23] concluded that grafting becomes necessary when the gap distance exceeded 5 to 8% of the total available nerve length, and as low as 4% in certain instances. Kim et al[24,25] repaired sciatic nerve defects in monkeys with grafts of identical or longer lengths as compared with the defect, with better results for the longer grafts with less wound tension.

To increase length intra or extratemporally, the nerve can be rerouted in its horizontal and vertical portion of the temporal bone to gain up to an additional 1 cm of length so that a primary anastomosis can be achieved. Rerouting will deprive the nerve of its blood supply, which could be detrimental to the anastomosis; this is probably better than using a nerve graft with less axon regeneration through two anastomoses. Rerouting can also be combined with grafts following skull base surgery or trauma as reviewed by Fisch and Lanser.[26] For extratemporal defects, the gap is usually too large for rerouting to provide enough nerve to close the gap.

A vast amount of nerve repair research is being conducted in an attempt to improve clinical results.[18,27] Attempts at local hormonal or chemotherapeutic manipulation comprise the bulk of the literature. The second largest area includes technical innovations such as laser repair, fibrin glue, and resorbable nerve couplers. A small segment is looking at the use of nerve conduits as an alternative to nerve grafts.

Nerve Grafts

Nerve grafts are used for defects when a tensionless closure is not possible with primary repair. Regardless of the donor nerve chosen, the proximal-distal orientation of the donor nerve is reversed when possible to prevent regenerating axons from exiting the nerves through neural foramina. For intratemporal grafts, the graft is placed in the fallopian canal abutting the freshened edges of the nerve. Fisch and Lanser[26] recommended fibrin glue to approximate the nerve. Pulec[28] also reviewed basics of intratemporal grafting techniques.

Extratemporal grafting cases commonly follow resection for parotid malignancy. Three grafts are usually placed to each main distal branch. However, Fisch and Lanser[26] reported using only two grafts to the upper and lower branches. They bypass the central branches to help prevent mass movements to the midface, concentrating nerve regeneration to the upper and lower areas of the face. They also clip facial nerve branches to the platysma, digastric muscle, and most buccal branches to concentrate regenerating axons to areas with open pathways.

Two donor nerves are commonly used for facial grafting procedures. For cases with potential malignant neural invasion requiring less than 10 cm, the contralateral greater auricular nerve is used. The ipsilateral nerve can be used for cases without potential tumor invasion from the parotid. If the greater auricular nerve can be traced to three terminal branches, the proximal side can be anastomosed to the pes while the terminal branches are connected to the three main distal nerve branches. In this instance, the proximal-distal orientation of the graft is not reversed. The sural nerve provides up to 35 cm of nerve that can be used in grafting with minimal sensory deficit. This is applicable for large or multiple defects, or for situations such as cross-face grafting.[22,29–33]

Nerve Crossover

In a nerve crossover, another motor nerve provides the neural input to the distal facial nerve and musculature. Advantages include one anastomotic suture line and motion that can resemble mimetic function with practice. Disadvantages include donor site morbidity and mass movement. In general, nerve crossover techniques remain the mainstay of treatment when, for example, the proximal facial nerve has been anatomically or functionally lost and primary repair is not possible. When function or anatomic integrity of the proximal nerve is questionable, the patient's recovery should be evaluated for 6 to 12 prior to attempting a crossover procedure.

The crossover procedure must be accomplished before atrophy of the facial musculature and distal facial nerve has occurred. Clinical experience has shown that crossovers accomplished within 1 year of injury are generally successful in restoring motion. Beyond this time frame, results are less predictable as muscle and nerve atrophy will progress in certain patients. Younger patients tend to have less muscle and nerve atrophy for longer time periods, allowing for crossover several years following paralysis.[34,35]

The type of nerve injury would affect this timing factor. If the nerve is still anatomically intact as in a Bell's palsy or Ramsay-Hunt patient, it is more likely that some axonal flow is present and the distal musculature is receiving some innervation. As previously discussed, electrical testing can help to confirm this. In this situation, crossover could possibly be accomplished several years after the original injury because open tubules are present for axons to grow through.

Muscle bulk is ascertained both clinically and by electrical testing. Clinically, muscle tone is a good prognostic sign indicating some degree of innervation and preservation of muscle bulk. An EMG should show insertional activity, which could be correlated with a muscle biopsy if needed. It may also show spontaneous fibrillation potentials, indicating viable denervated muscle fibers. With voluntary contraction, EMG might show action potentials in some areas indicating partial innervation of viable muscle.

Atrophy of the facial nerve is an equally important consideration. If the distal facial nerve has atrophied, new axons from the donor nerve cannot grow down the endoneural tubes to innervate the muscle. As reviewed by Ylikoski et al,[36] the distal nerve undergoes wallerian degeneration following injury. Schwann cells hypertrophy and form tubelike strands or "bands of Bunger" that guide regenerating axons. If the distal nerve does not become reinnervated, these bands atrophy and are replaced by fibrous tissue. This collagenization of the endoneural tubes makes future reinnervation less likely to succeed because advancing axons have less open tubes to grow through. However, not all severed nerves will collagenize progressively if not reinnervated. In two different human facial nerve specimens at 3 and 30 months postseverance, an equal degree of mild collagenization was present. This indicated that the structural basis for a successful crossover was still present at 30 months from injury in this nerve.

Nerve atrophy can be evaluated electrically and clinically. Action potentials on EMG or EEMG indicate at least a partially functioning nerve with functioning axons and endoneural tubes through which new axons could grow. Yanagihara[37] described five cases of paralysis for which XI-VII crossover with the branch to the sternocleidomastoid muscle was conducted from 2 to 24 years after injury. Direct electrical stimulation (nerve excitability) of distal nerve branches was confirmed at surgery, with some return of tone in all cases and fair results for one patient 17 years following injury. However, best results were for patients who received electrical stimulation less than 3 years from the time of injury. Both the presence of electrical stimulation and the time from injury were considered important factors influencing a positive outcome.

In the absence of electrical activity by EMG or EEMG, Conley[34] believed that atrophy of the nerve could be evaluated grossly at surgery. He reported eight cases where XII-VII crossover was attempted 2 to 33 years following injury. When atrophy was less than 50% of normal, four of five cases had good to excellent results. Two of these also had some response to electrical testing. In three cases with atrophy greater than 50% of normal, results were all poor. Atrophy of the nerve on gross examination probably correlates with the degree of collagenization within the nerve.

Gagnon and Molina-Negro[35] also reported good results when nerve crossover procedures were attempted 2 to 7 years following injury in five cases, without activity in the nerve by EMG or EEMG. As Conley[34] had discussed, they believed that if the distal facial nerve was not atrophic it would still provide a good conduit for axonal regrowth and reinnervation. Although muscle atrophy might also be a limiting factor, like Conley they thought that this occurred over a longer time frame in the face as opposed to the extremities. Younger patients were thought to do better than older patients.

Although nerve crossover beyond 1 year may be conducted without electrical activity in the nerve, success appears more reliable when electrical activity is present in the nerve by EMG or EEMG. The presence of electrical activity in the nerve is a good prognostic sign as new axons can grow through the endoneural tubes of existing axons. The absence of neural atrophy on gross examination at surgery is another good prognostic sign, but of less reliability than electrical activity.

In the absence of electrical activity, we are reluctant to perform a nerve crossover procedure well beyond 1 year. In this situation, one is hoping that significant collagenization has not taken place within the nerve, which would retard axonal

regrowth. Although the nerve may still provide a successful framework for reinnervation several years after injury, results appear to be too unpredictable when electrical activity is absent to use this method routinely, considering potential donor site morbidity.

The hypoglossal nerve (XII) is the most commonly used nerve in crossover procedures (Fig. 22–4A). Classically, XII is traced distally, severed, and rotated to the stump of VII. Based on the experience of Conley and Baker,[38] 95% of patients will have tone and symmetry and 77% will have good facial motion. All will have some degree of mass movement that is described as minimal.

Tongue atrophy will occur, which will lead to mastication problems in 16%, swallowing difficulty in 12%, and speech difficulty in 10%. This was most common with delayed reconstruction. Pensak et al[39] also reported swallowing difficulties in 21% and failure of eye protection in 21%. Rubin et al[40,41] described a Z-plasty to rehabilitate the paralyzed tongue, by interdigitating paralyzed muscle with normal muscle. Cross innervation results, with myoneurotization of the paralyzed muscle from the normal muscle.

May et al[42] described a jump graft from a partially severed XII in 23 patients, with best results obtained when used within 1 year following injury (Fig. 22–4B). One third to one half of the nerve was transferred with a greater auricular nerve graft to the facial nerve branches. Two jump grafts were also used in some cases to selectively innervate the two distal trunks of the facial nerve. Retrograde elevation of the transacted portion of the nerve was not performed, to prevent damage to intertwining axons.

Tongue atrophy occurred in only 13% of cases as opposed to 100% for the classic procedure. Identical facial motion was obtained with the jump graft as compared with historic XII-VII controls. Mass movement, a universal problem with the classic procedure, was not noted in the jump graft procedure. This is probably because less axons are transferred. Facial motion is not as strong and takes longer to develop than with the classical procedure. In 3 of 20 patients, results were superb with the ability to produce mimetic expression while separating eye and mouth movement.

Cross-Face Grafts

Cross-face grafts were first developed in the early 1970s independently by Anderl.[43] Thirty to 50% of peripheral facial nerve branches on the normal side are severed and connected to the corresponding peripheral branches of the paralyzed side with sural nerve grafts. This resulted in no or minimal deformity on the normal side and restoration of symmetry and some movement to the paralyzed side.

The theoretical advantage to this technique is that it attempts to return true symmetrical, mimetic function to the face. However, a significant disadvantage is that the procedure limits the number of axons transposed to the paralyzed side of the face because only a portion of the nerve fibers from the normal side can be used. This results in a smaller force of contraction and less facial movement than desired.

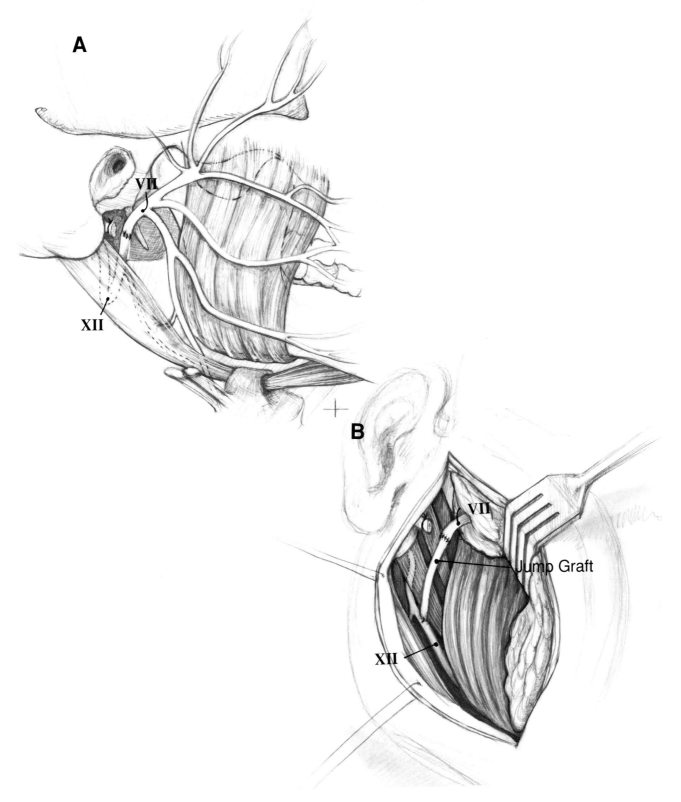

Figure 22–4. XII-VII crossover. **(A).** Through a parotidectomy approach, cranial nerve XII is sectioned, rotated deep to the digastric muscle, and sutured to the pes. The 12th nerve can also be split after sectioning and sutured to the main upper and lower branches of the facial nerve. **(B).** XII-VII crossover with jump graft.[42] Cranial nerve XII is isolated, with a small Penrose drain placed beneath the nerve distal to the take-off of the ansi hypoglossal. This delivers XII toward the surgeon, ensuring that fibers of the ansi hypoglossal are not confused as contributing to the diameter of XII. One third to one half of the nerve is sectioned without back elevation. A greater auricular nerve graft is sutured between the cut segment of XII and VII.

Conley and Baker[38] reported poor results with this procedure in 10 patients. This was compared with the powerful and predictable reanimation obtainable with the classical XII-VII crossover. This less than satisfactory experience with cross-face grafts mirrors the results of others.[44,45]

Although cross-face grafts provided some promise initially, this technique has fallen into disfavor owing to these mixed results. However, cross-face grafts combined with free muscle grafts have gained some acceptance as an alternative to neuromuscular transfers. After a cross-face sural graft is tunneled and anastomosed in the first stage, the free muscle graft is transferred at a second stage 6 to 12 months later. Using standard microneurovascular techniques, the graft's vessels are anastomosed to the temporal or facial vessels and the graft's motor nerve to the end of the sural graft. This is primarily used for reanimation of the corner of the mouth (see "Free Muscle Grafts").

For total facial reanimation, O'Brien et al[46] used a free gracilis muscle flap with cross-face grafts for total paralysis reanimation in 30 patients, with 40% obtaining eye closure. These mediocre results and other local problems around the eye due to the bulky muscle slips caused them to abandon total reanimation with the gracilis. They recommended the gracilis for the lower face with gold weights for eyelid paralysis.

Terzis[47] described a free pectoralis minor flap with cross-face grafts for total paralysis. With its dual nerve supply, innervation of muscle slips to the eye and mouth were independent of one another allowing for individualized movements. This technique was found to yield excellent results for young children with developmental facial paralysis.

Temporalis Transposition

Transposing regional musculature to reanimate the paralyzed face was originally described in the late 1800s and early 1900s. More recently, Rubin[48,49] and Conley and Baker[50] helped to popularize these techniques and May and Drucker[51,52] have provided further refinements. During this evolution, temporalis muscle transposition with an intact neurovascular bundle became one of the mainstays in managing patients with total facial paralysis, when a neural procedure was not possible or likely to succeed. Specific indications include: (1) severe long-standing paralysis greater than 3 to 4 years without a strong likelihood of recovery with a neural procedure, (2) distal facial musculature or nerves atrophied or unavailable for a neural procedure, (3) contraindication to nerve crossover procedure as XII-VII owing to reasons as maintaining voice, swallowing, or because of potential secondary nerve tumors in von Recklinghausen's disease, and (4) partial paralysis of upper lip elevators.

However, despite the use of temporalis transposition in the 1970s and 1980s for total facial reanimation, mixed results with eyelid reanimation have caused May and Drucker[52] and Conley[53] to use the temporalis only for oral reanimation. For orbital reanimation, they now prefer more predictable procedures such as gold weight implantation (see "The Eye").

Most reanimation efforts for total paralysis are currently using this type of dual reanimation, with independent procedures for the eye and oral cavity.

Innervation and strength of the temporalis should be evaluated preoperatively by having the patient bite down on the molars. If a weak muscle is palpated as compared with the opposite side, strengthening exercises such as chewing gum should be initiated. This should be continued for several months prior to transfer of the muscle.

The procedure has been presented in detail by Rubin,[48,49] Baker and Conley,[50] and May and Drucker[51,52] (Fig. 22-5). May prefers Conley's use of pericranium instead of fascia to lengthen the muscle slips, and adds fascia lata if more length is needed. May places two layers of sutures at the oral cavity, with one at the mucocutaneous junction and the other beneath the skin incision at the lip-cheek groove. Rubin has added a third suture line between these two suture lines and also utilized a slip from the masseter muscle for lower lip reanimation at the corner of the mouth.

Patients complain of the muscle bulge overlying the zygomatic arch. A carved or custom Silastic block is usually placed in the defect above the zygoma to improve contour, but this does not diminish the size of the bulge. The arch of the zygoma may be removed to reduce this bulge, but the fulcrum effect is lost and the strength on contraction is reduced.[50]

ORAL COMMISSURE REANIMATION

Reanimation of the oral commissure is the cornerstone to correcting the cosmetic asymmetry of the paralyzed face, as well as improving functional competence of the oral cavity. If neural procedures are not possible, either static or dynamic techniques may be utilized. Static suspension attempts to elevate the corner of the mouth at rest using fascia or alloplastic materials suspended to the zygoma. Dynamic reconstructions with neuromuscular transfers or free muscle grafts with microneurovascular techniques attempt to provide symmetry at rest while providing facial motion as well. Other accessory procedures may be used in both static and dynamic reanimation to enhance results. These often include excision of skin in the lip-cheek groove or preauricular region, suspension of the superficial musculoaponeurotic system (SMAS), and rhytidectomy.

Static Procedures

Static elevation of the corner of the mouth with slings of fascia lata suspended to the zygoma was one of the earlier techniques in oral commissure reanimation and still remains an alternative to more sophisticated procedures.[54-58] The main advantage is that following a basic one-stage procedure, the face returns to symmetry at rest as well as provides functional improvement. The fascia may also be sutured to the temporalis muscle instead of the zygoma to facilitate minimal motion. This procedure can be used for more elderly patients who

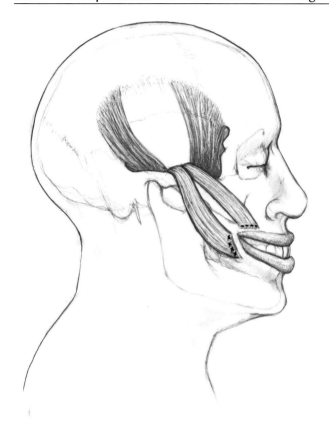

Figure 22–5. Temporalis transposition. The temporalis is approached through a vertical incision over the temporalis region, which can be extended into a preauricular incision if flaccid skin is also to be removed to enhance suspension of the lower face. Two methods may be used to provide length to the temporalis to reach the oral commissure and surround the eye. Rubin[48,49] used the fascia overlying the temporalis. Basing the fascial flap superiorly, the inferior cut is at the level of the outer canthus of the eye and the fascia is dissected in a superior direction off the underlying muscle. When the muscle is elevated off the skull, the fascia is pulled downward to provide the necessary extension. The fascia-muscular junction is reinforced with sutures with a free fascial strip used for backing. In the second method, Baker and Conley[50] used 2 cm of contiguous pericranium for this purpose, and found little difficulty in reaching the insertion sites. May[51] preferred this periosteal methods over the fascial method and added fascia lata if additional length was needed.[52] Removing the arch of the zygoma can also be used to gain an additional 2 cm if necessary as well as to reduce the prominence of the muscle bulge. However, the force of contraction is less as the fulcrum effect from the arch is lost. The muscle is elevated downward to the upper level of the zygomatic arch, where care must be taken as the nerve enters the muscle just below this region. The subcutaneous tunnel overlying the zygomatic arch must be at least two fingerbreadths wide to allow the muscle pedicle to flatten as much as possible. The prominence over the zygoma also accentuates the depression in the region vacated by the temporalis. A carved or custom Silastic rubber implant with several holes for fibrous ingrowth can be used to improve the contour. The pericranium and muscle are now split into two slips as shown. The muscle slips are passed through incisions in the lip-cheek groove and a small curvilinear incision below the lateral commissure. The muscle slips are sutured to the dermis between the mucocutaneous junction and the lip-cheek groove. After undermining the soft tissue off the orbicularis oris, the pericranium or fascia is sutured to the mucocutaneous line with 2-0 braided nylon on a tapered needle.[51] This is identifiable by the smooth tissue on the lip side and the cobblestonelike texture of the minor salivary glands on the mucosa side of the lip. A second line of sutures is placed just medial to the lip-cheek groove, which provides additional security from pulling out while helping to form the groove with smiling. A third line of sutures can be placed between these two lines. The lateral corner of the mouth is overcorrected maximally to allow for the laxity that will occur.

are poor anesthetic risks or who desire not to undergo more complex, staged procedures. A significant disadvantage is the recurrence of laxity over time.

Suspension can also be performed with alloplastic material, which eliminates the need for obtaining fascia grafts. Gore-Tex (W.L. Gore and Assoc, Inc, Flagstaff, Ariz) expanded polytetrafluoroethylene has been described to suspend the corner of the mouth.[59,60] Well known for its success as a replacement graft in vascular surgery, sheets of the material have also been useful in repairing abdominal and inguinal hernia defects.[61] However, May and Drucker[52] noted a 30% delayed extrusion rate when Gore-Tex was used to provide extra length in temporalis transposition and have abandoned its use for facial reanimation.

A unilateral rhytidectomy coupled with SMAS suspension is an adjunct to many procedures attempting to reanimate the oral cavity and lower face. Excess skin is excised and tightened with SMAS suspension providing underlying correction of the deeper structures. This alone is often the procedure of choice in cases of partial paralysis with good facial tone but minimal sagging of the skin and subcutaneous tissues. Excess skin in the lip-cheek groove can also be excised as needed. These procedures may need to be repeated for recurrent laxity over time.

Neuromuscular Transposition

The temporalis can be used for restoration of the corner of the mouth alone or combined with the masseter, as discussed in the "Total Paralysis—Neural Procedures" section. Masseter transfer can also be utilized alone for oral commissure reanimation, and has been a reliable procedure for this purpose. The procedure can be performed either extraorally to transfer the entire muscle belly, or intraorally to transfer the anterior one half (Fig. 22–6). This remains a reliable procedure to help manage lower facial paralysis. Following reconstruction, patients learn to smile by biting down on the molars. With practice in front of a mirror, satisfying results can be obtained.[62]

Conley[63] reported best results with this technique when the entire masseter was transferred at the initial extirpative procedure of the parotid. This was thought to be due to the excellent physiological conditions that existed for neurotization. The exposed muscle surface of the split masseter comes in direct contact with the exposed and denervated facial musculature. This engenders axon budding from the masseter into the denervated neural tubules of the facial musculature. Good results were also obtained when the muscle was transferred for long-standing facial paralysis, but less successfully than with primary reconstruction. For total paralysis, Sachs and Conley[64] described a masseter transfer to the lower face with a cable graft to the eye branches.

There are several disadvantages with the procedure. In patients with thin skin and subcutaneous tissue, the angle of the mandible can become sharply demarcated and visible beneath the skin. Second, the buccal fat pad can bulge excessively owing to the rotated masseter stiffening the cheek

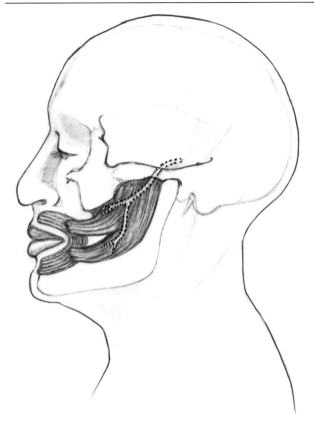

Figure 22-6. Masseter muscle transposition.[50] The masseter originates on the inferior edge of the zygoma and inserts into the angle of the mandible. The blood and neural supply enter from the infratemporal fossa deep to the muscle through the coronoid notch of the mandible. The entire muscle can be rotated to reanimate the corner of the mouth. If partial transposition is desired, it is recommended to separate the muscle at the junction of the anterior two thirds with the posterior one third to preserve the nerve supply.[96] The muscle can be approached externally through a small cervical incision beneath the mandible, or an intraoral approach through an incision in the gingivobuccal sulcus (for partial transposition).[62] The entire muscle with its tendinous insertion is elevated from the inferior border of the mandible up to the glenoid notch using a broad periosteal elevator. These tendinous insertions are carefully preserved, which provide a strong attachment for suturing. The neurovascular bundle coming through the coronoid notch is also preserved. Skin tunnels are dissected to both the upper and lower lip incisions. The upper lip incision is made just medial to the lip-cheek groove and the lower incision is placed in an angular fashion lateral and inferior to the commissure. The muscle is split longitudinally no farther than one-third its length, to preserve the neurovascular supply to both bundles of muscle. Sachs and Conley[97] advocated using the pinch test in this process, where the scissors are used to dissect in the line of the incision with lateral pressure on spreading helping to identify and stimulate motor nerves in the path of the incision. The muscle bundles are passed to the lip incisions and secured with nonabsorbable sutures to the underlying dermis as described for the temporalis (Fig. 22-5). As with temporalis transposition, the lips and commissure are pulled laterally and overcorrected. If the muscle bundles are too short, additional length may be gained by partially releasing the muscle from its origin on the zygoma; this also improves the angle of muscle pull.

and pushing the fat pad up and out.[65] Third, the direction of pull is more lateral than desired, creating a less than natural appearance.

Intraoral transfer is primarily indicated for mild to moderate regional paralysis of the upper lip and commissure because only one half the muscle is transferred. It has advantages of no external incision and does not interfere with regional seventh nerve function, which could allow for spontaneous regeneration. Disadvantages include decreased exposure and an increased risk of bleeding.[62]

Free Muscle Grafts

The term "free muscle grafts" can imply several different scenarios of vascularization and neurotization. Muscle grafts can be transferred either with or without neural and vascular supply. Neural supply can be from ipsilateral functioning nerves, from previously placed cross-face grafts, from a cross-face anastomosis with the nerve pedicled to the muscle graft, or from direct neurotization from exposed normal muscle tissue. Initially, vascular anastomosis was not utilized but it is now routinely utilized to decrease the amount of atrophy to the free graft. Results are dependent on the choice of the donor muscle, as well as the neural and vascular scenario that is utilized.

These procedures have similar indications as for neuromuscular transfer of the temporalis or masseter. Free grafts are often chosen instead of neuromuscular transfer based on preference of the operator. Numerous donor muscles have been described for use as free grafts, both with and without microneurovascular anastomosis. Best results have been obtained when both neural and vascular anastomosis are accomplished (Fig. 22-7). Advantages and disadvantages of the available free muscle flap choices for facial reanimation are reviewed in Table 22-2.[66]

The large number of donor muscles described attests to the fact that this procedure is in its early evolutionary stages. With this in mind, several considerations should be discussed with the patient: the long time period between staged procedures, the expense, and the potential for disappointing results.

Marginal Mandibular Paralysis

The deformity is characterized by elevation of the lower lip on the paralyzed side that is more evident on smiling. It may be approached by correcting the paralyzed side or by decreasing function on the normal side.[67] We do not favor the latter, as potential loss of function may result to the lower lip. With one side paralyzed, the patient is able to compensate. With both sides paralyzed, functional competence may emerge as a new problem.

The depressor on the normal or paralyzed side may be altered. Rubin et al[68] described resecting a portion of a hyperactive depressor on the normal side to lessen the asymmetry. The paralyzed depressor can also be shortened by placation or resection.

The paralyzed lower lip may be reanimated by the anterior belly of the digastric muscle. Edgerton[69] mobilized the muscle from the mandible, with a fascia lata graft lashed to the

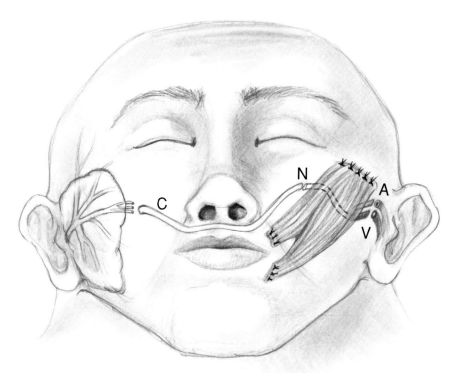

Figure 22–7. Microneurovascular free muscle graft.[43,98] In the first stage, the peripheral branches of the normal side of the face are exposed through a preauricular approach. Other incisions directly over the anastomotic sites or melolabial folds may also be used. Peripheral branches are stimulated electrically (5 to 20 mA) and blocked with local anesthetic to determine the dominant branches to the normal side. These are preserved as the others are severed. In general, 50% of fibers are ideally resected, usually providing six to eight fascicles from the buccal branches. These branches are anastomosed to sural nerve grafts using 10–0 nylon sutures and are crossed to the other side. **(C).** Sural grafts are tunneled with the help of midline incisions in the philtrum and glabella. After tunneling with a pair of Metzenbaum scissors, a red rubber catheter is passed across the face. A metal probe or wire is sutured to the nerve graft and the nerve is pulled into the catheter, after which the catheter is removed while holding the nerve in position.[99] A trochar with a round drain tube attached to it could also be used to tunnel the catheter into position.[32] The end of the graft is brought out beyond the edge of the parotid gland and marked with a colored thread that is brought out through the skin and cut near the surface. During the first 2 to 3 months following the first stage, some weakness of both the eye and mouth on the normal side can result.[32] The second stage is accomplished 6 to 12 months later when the axons have grown to the end of the graft. Axon advancement is followed by the Tinel sign, which is a tingling sensation localized to the position directly over the nerve graft that corresponds to regenerating nerve fibers. The sign is elicited by percussing the denervated nerve trunk from distal to proximal until percussing first produces tingling.[66] At the second stage, the donor muscle such as a free gracilis graft[100-102] is transferred, anastomosing its vessels to the superficial temporal vessels **(A, V)** and its motor nerve **(N)** to the previously placed cross-face graft. An alternative for vascular anastomosis is the facial vessels. Alternatives for neural input include the sectioned facial nerve (acutely), one of its branches, or another ipsilateral motor nerve such as the auriculotermporal (branch of V) or the hypoglossal (XII). The pectoralis minor,[103] latissimus dorsi,[104] rectus abdominis,[105] and serratus anterior[106] have also been described as donor muscles.

muscle and split into two tails. These are passed to the lower lip and lateral commissure, and brought back into the neck and secured with slight overcorrection to the lower lip.

Conley et al[70] modified this technique by leaving the anterior belly of the digastric attached to the mandible, rotating up the digastric tendon that is split and sutured to the lower lip. As with Edgerton's procedure, this will not reconstitute a fully paralyzed oral commissure. It only attempts to provide symmetry at rest and with smiling.

Cheiloplasty is often used as an adjunct in facial paralysis. Glenn and Goode[71] described a technique where wedge resection of the lower lip was combined with vermilion border advancement. This improved oral competence and provided the desired symmetry.

THE EYE

A multitude of procedures have been described regarding paralytic lagophthalmos and ectropion. This usually indicates that a single procedure is not applicable for all indications. As these procedures may be infrequently performed, particularly for the lower lid, we recommend consultation with an ophthalmologist as necessary.

Eye closure may be accomplished by either addressing the upper lid alone or both the upper and lower lids together. Often, only an upper lid procedure is required, as a lower lid with mild laxity does not need to be addressed to effect closure. Procedures that address both the upper and lower lids are indicated in cases of moderate to severe paralysis with

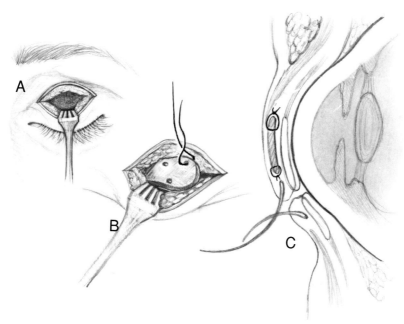

Figure 22–8. Gold weight implantation.[72,75,77,85] **(A).** Twenty-four karat polished gold weights are available in weights ranging from 0.6 to 1.4 g (Meddev Corp, Los Altos, CA). With the patient sitting, these are taped to the upper lid 2 to 3 mm above the lash line over the tarsal plate using double-sided tape on the underside of the weight. The patient is asked to blink, and the weight that provides closure is then selected. The surgical approach is similar to that of upper lid blepharoplasty, with loupes required by the surgeon for suture placement. The gold weight is placed on the upper lid skin 2 to 3 mm above the lash line and the pocket is outlined with a marking pen. Although most prefer the pocket in the midline, some place the implant more medially at the junction between the medial and middle third of the upper lid.[85] Following the infiltration of local anesthetic into the upper lid, an incision is made in the tarsal-supratarsal fold. This is extended down through the skin and orbicularis oculi muscle to the tarsal plate and orbital septum. The pocket is enlarged in this plane. **(B, C).** The gold weight is placed into the pocket and secured with three 8-0 permanent monofilament sutures through the three holes in the implant. For the two superior holes, the suture is secured to the tissue overlying the orbital septum. The suture through the inferior hole is secured to the tissue superficial to the tarsal plate. The wound is closed in layers with interrupted 7-0 Vicryl or 6-0 chromic sutures used for muscle closure and 6-0 nylon or fast-absorbing gut used for skin closure.

Table 22–2. Free Muscle Grafts for Facial Reanimation Using Microneurovascular Techniques

DONOR MUSCLE	BLOOD SUPPLY	NERVE SUPPLY	TWO-TEAMS?	ADVANTAGES	DISADVANTAGES
Extensor digitorum brevis	Dorsalis pedis, venae commitantes, 3–4 cm, reliable	Anterior tibial, nerve 3–4 cm	Yes	—	Inadequate bulk, contraction strength, short pedicle
Gracilis	Profunda femoris branches, 5–8 cm, reliable	Obturator nerve, anterior branch, 10 cm	Yes	Debulk muscle in situ, independent neuromuscular units	Bulky
Latissimus dorsi	Thoracodorsal artery and vein, 8–10 cm, reliable	Thoracodorsal nerve, 13–14 cm	No	Debulk muscle in situ, segmental innervation	Bulky
Pectoralis minor	Axillary (direct branches) or lateral thoracic or thoraco-acromial artery and vein, variable	Medial and lateral pectoral nerve, 4–5 cm	Yes	Dual nerve supply, good form, shape, and bulk	Debulking not possible in situ; short, complex, neurovascular pedicle
Rectus abdominis	Deep inferior epigastric artery and vein, 6–10 cm, reliable	Segmental thoracic intercostal nerve, 3–15 cm	Yes	Tendinous inscriptions, segmental innervation	Bulky
Serratus anterior	Thoracodorsal artery and vein branches, 4–5 cm, reliable	Long thoracic nerve, 9 cm	Yes	Segmental innervation	Bulky

Modified from Aviv and Urken.[66]

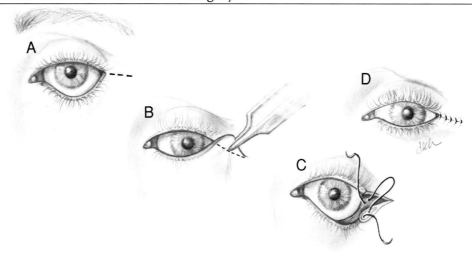

Figure 22–9.   Lateral ectropion repair.[86] **(A).** The procedure is performed under local anesthetic as for blepharoplasty. A corneal protector may be used after topically anesthetizing the cornea. The lateral canthal tendon is exposed with an incision in a horizontal crow's foot. **(B).** Castroviejo forceps are used to grasp the lid to overlap it with the lateral canthal angle, such that the lid is against the globe. A conservative, full thickness excisions of lid is accomplished at the lateral angle to shorten the lid. Total resection may require 3 to 5 mm of lid shortening in cases of facial paralysis. **(C).** The canthus is suspended laterally just superior to the previous position of the canthal tendon on the inner aspect of the lateral orbital rim using a 4-0 coated polyester sutures. Comparison with the other lateral canthus should be made for symmetry. **(D).** The muscle is closed with 5-0 chromic and the skin incision is closed with 6-0 nylon. When complete, the lid will appear tight and will remain this way for several weeks. The amount of scleral show should be slightly overcorrected to allow for some laxity over the ensuing months. If readjustment of the lateral canthus is necessary, the suture may be repositioned at revision surgery.

lower lid laxity leading to ectropion. Owing to preexisting senile changes, ectropion is more common in older patients with facial paralysis. Procedures may consist of encircling techniques that address the upper and lower lids together, or combining procedures that address the upper and lower lids separately.

Upper Eyelid Techniques

Of the available upper lid procedures, gold weight implantation is currently the most popular (Fig. 22–8). Satisfactory results with this technique have been described by several authors,[72–78] mirroring our good results with this procedure.

Advantages include a basic procedure that is readily performed through an upper lid blepharoplasty incision, with May[72] reporting a 91% successful closure rate and 9% unsuccessful rate (lack of closure—4.5%, or overclosure with lid droop—4.5%). One theoretical disadvantage is that the implant may not be effective when the patient is lying down because the gravitational effect is lost. However, May noted that this has not been a problem.[72] Should a problem exist, patients should utilize lubrication and tape their eyes shut during sleep. Other disadvantages include a slow blink, a visible bulge outlining the implant in patients with thin skin, and occasional extrusion.

As compared with gold weight implantation, wire spring placement requires more technical precision by the surgeon. The surgeon constructs the spring from 0.3 mm (0.01 in) orthodontic wire and places it through a blepharoplasty incision. In 101 procedures, May[72] reported success in 87 (87%). Thirteen were removed and 10 replaced. There was one extrusion. May favors this technique for patients with

lid retraction or poor Bell's phenomenon where the cornea does not roll up under the partially closing upper lid.

Advantages include a faster blink with less chance of visibility beneath the skin as with gold weights. This latter advantage over gold weights is preferred by many women because the supratarsal fold is not redundant, which would tend to help camouflage the gold weight. The main disadvantage is the technical expertise required to construct the spring and implant it into the upper lid, with faulty construction and implantation leading to poor function or extrusion. At this time, we do not recommend a spring as a primary treatment modality.

Lower Eyelid Techniques

Lower eyelid techniques specifically address ectropion in the paralysis patient. These are frequently combined with an upper lid technique such as gold weight implantation. For cases with lateral ectropion or scleral show, several options exist.[79]

For most cases, wedge resection combined with rotation of lower lid skin (modified Kuhnt-Szymanowski) is excellent.[79–82] A McLaughlin tarsorrhaphy can also be utilized for further correction, but this will narrow the palpebral fissure.[81]

Some prefer combining wedge resection with placation of the lateral canthal tendon[83] or suturing the lower and upper limbs of the canthal tendon together.[84,85] Variations of the tarsal strip procedure are popular, where the tendon is released, resected, and resutured to the periosteum on the inner surface of the lateral orbital rim (Fig. 22–9).[79,86–89]

A more recent technique reintroduced by May[90] utilizes

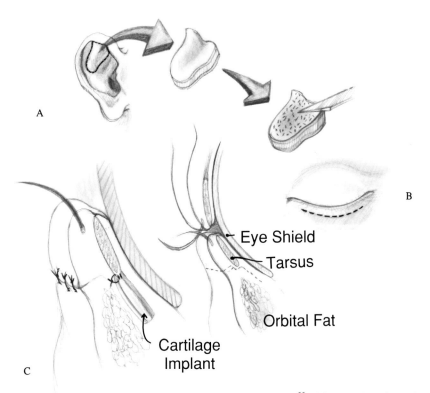

Figure 22–10. Lower lid laxity repair—cartilage implant with lid shortening.[90] This procedure is performed under local anesthetic, with loupes required by the surgeon for suture placement. It is often combined with the Bick procedure, which consists of vertical lid shortening (wedge resection) in the lateral canthus region. The Bick procedure has a similar surgical approach to the canthal tightening procedure (Fig. 22–9), but no adjustment to the lateral canthal tendon is undertaken.[86] **(A).** Cartilage is harvested from the fossa triangularis through a U-shaped flap on the anterior surface of the ipsilateral ear. The cartilage is harvested such that perichondrium is left attached to both surfaces. After removal, the cartilage is trimmed and stippled with a scalpel through the perichondrium and cartilage on the lateral convex surface, but not through the perichondrium on the deep side. The stiffness of the cartilage is reduced by this maneuver. **(B).** A globe protector may be utilized after topically anesthetizing the cornea. A subciliary incision is placed 3 mm below the lash line. The lower border of the tarsus is identified and a plane is developed inferior to the tarsus and superficial to the conjunctiva extending downward towards the conjunctival cul-de-sac at the level of the orbital rim. **(C).** The implant is placed into the pocket, such that the concave side conforms to the curvature of the globe. Interrupted 8-0 nylon sutures are utilized to suture the implant to the inferior border of the tarsus. The skin is closed with 6-0 mild chromic or fast-absorbing gut suture.

conchal cartilage to provide support to the lower lid, combined with a lateral wedge resection of the lid. The cartilage is sutured to inferior edge of the tarsus, just outside the conjunctivae (Fig. 22–10).

If medial ectropion is more of a problem than lateral ectropion, a procedure is necessary to address the medial canthus. Epiphora and conjunctival or corneal irritation are symptoms requiring treatment. For mild medial ectropion where the punctum is visible without grasping the lid, a triangular or elliptic conjunctival excision can help to invert the punctum.[79,82] The punctum may also be enlarged with a one-, two-, or three-snip punctoplasty, where the lacrimal system comes in contact with the conjunctiva.[82,91]

For moderate to severe medial ectropion, the "Lazy-T" technique is recommended.[79,82,88] This combines a wedge resection lateral to the punctum with a horizontal resection of conjunctiva and tarsus to return the punctum inward to the lacrimal lake. A medial canthoplasty is another good alternative. A third alternative is to plicate the medial canthal tendon, combined with medial skin flap rotation.[79,85] If skin

flap rotation is not planned, medial canthal tightening may be combined with the Lazy-T procedure.

Combined Upper and Lower Eyelid Techniques

The following procedures address the upper and lower lids together with the same procedure. Tarsorrhaphy, the method of choice in earlier years, has largely been replaced by more cosmetically acceptable procedures that do not narrow the palpebral fissure resulting in a smaller-appearing eye and decreased lateral vision. Temporary tarsorrhaphy may be accomplished medially or laterally, by denuding opposing epithelium on the lid margins followed by suturing. Unless performed with precision, breakdown is frequent.[82,89] It should be noted that after taking down these adhesions following return of function, localized lid notching and troublesome trichiasis can result.[89] More sophisticated temporary procedures have been described.[89]

Permanent tarsorrhaphy of the lateral palpebral fissure may be accomplished by one of several methods. The McLaughlin tarsorrhaphy maintains the lashes of the upper lid while denuding lashes of the lower lid.[80,81] The Soll tarsorrhaphy interdigitates a flap of lower conjunctiva with a corresponding resected area of conjunctiva in the upper lid.[79,82] It has the advantage of preserving the lashes of both the upper and lower lids, potentially making it reversible without sequela.

Utilization of temporalis muscle slips with attached fascia or pericranium was frequently chosen in the past when the temporalis transfer was used to reanimate the lower face. However, this technique is plagued by disappointing success rates due to stretching of the fascia or periosteum.[85] May[51] cited mixed results for eye closure owing to several reasons: failure to overcorrect, failure to fix the periosteal muscle slips to the muscle, and failure to bring in the slips laterally at a level above the lateral canthus. Mass motion or eye closure associated with other facial movements is also a problem. More recently, May and Drucker[52] and Conley[53] have abandoned this procedure for eye reanimation due to these problems.

Silastic threads have been described to encircle the eye, but this technique is largely of historic interest.[78,92] Another alloplastic implant, Gore-Tex, has also been used to encircle the eye,[59] but more experience is needed with this material.

The Eyebrow

Brow ptosis can be prominent in patients with facial paralysis causing significant asymmetry. Correction of the ptosis is accomplished with a unilateral direct or mid-forehead brow lift. Rubin et al[68,93] also utilized a slip of contralateral normal frontalis muscle to provide some motion and correction to the medial brow.

Restoring the brow to a higher position usually will adversely effect eye closure as the upper lid is positioned more superiorly. With predictable upper lid procedures like gold weight implantation, there is less of a concern with this adverse effect than in the past. However, conservative brow elevation is recommended. If a brow lift and gold weight implantation are planned for the same surgery, preoperatively the brow should be corrected manually and held in position while checking various gold weights taped to the upper lid. Failure to do this may result in using a lighter weight than needed.

REFERENCES

1. May M. Microanatomy and pathophysiology of the facial nerve. In: May M, ed. *The Facial Nerve,* New York, NY: Thieme; 1986:63–74.
2. House J. Facial nerve grading systems. *Laryngoscope.* 1983;93:1056–1069.
3. Blumenthal F, May M. Electrodiagnosis. In: May M, ed. *The Facial Nerve.* New York, NY: Thieme; 1986:241–263.
4. Kimura J. Type of abnormality. In: *Electrodiagnosis in Diseases of Nerve and Muscle: Principles and Practice.* Philadelphia, Pa: FA Davis Co; 1989:249–274.
5. Post BS. Diagnosing the site of nerve disruption by electronic methods. In: Rubin LR, ed. *Reanimation of the Paralyzed Face. New Approaches.* St Louis, Mo: CV Mosby Co; 1977:81–97.
6. Esslen E. *The Acute Facial Palsies.* New York, NY: Springer-Verlag; 1977.
7. Coker NJ. Facial electroneurography: analysis of techniques and correlation with degenerating motoneurons. *Laryngoscope.* 1992;102:747–759.
8. Fisch U. Maximal nerve excitability testing vs electroneuronography. *Arch Otolaryngol Head Neck Surg.* 1980; 106:352–357.
9. Harris JP, Davidson TM, May M, Fria T. Evaluation and treatment of congenital facial paralysis. *Arch Otolaryngol Head Neck Surg.* 1983;109:145–151.
10. May M. Tumors involving the facial nerve. In: May M, ed. *The Facial Nerve.* New York, NY: Thieme; 1986:455–467.
11. Janecka IP, Conley J. Primary neoplasms of the facial nerve. *Plast Reconstr Surg.* 1987;79:177–185.
12. Fisch U. Surgery for Bell's palsy. *Arch Otolaryngol Head Neck Surg.* 1981;107:1-11.
13. May M. *The Facial Nerve,* New York, NY: Thieme; 1986.
14. McCabe BF. Some evidence for the efficacy of decompression for Bell's palsy: immediate motion postoperatively. *Laryngoscope.* 1977;87:246–249.
15. Brodsky L, Eviatar A, Daniller A. Post-traumatic facial nerve paralysis: three cases of delayed temporal bone exploration with recovery. *Laryngoscope.* 1983;93:1560–1565.
16. Barrs DM. Facial nerve trauma: optimal timing for repair. *Laryngoscope.* 1991;101:835–848.
17. May M. Management of cranial nerves I through VII following skull base surgery. *Otolaryngol Head Neck Surg.* 1980;88:560–575.
18. Sunderland Sir S. End-to-end nerve repair. In: *Nerve Injuries and Their Repair. A Critical Appraisal.* New York, NY: Churchill Livingstone; 1991:439–465.
19. Tupper JW, Crick JC, Matteck LR. Fascicular nerve repairs. A comparative study of epineurial and fascicular (perineurial) techniques. *Orthop Clin North Am.* 1988;19:57–69.
20. Szal GJ, Miller T. Surgical repair of facial nerve branches. *Arch Otolaryngol.* 1975;101:160–165.
21. Kline DG, Hudson AR, Bratton BR. Experimantal study of fascicular nerve repair with and without epineurial closure. *J Neurosurg.* 1981;54:513–520.
22. Johns ME, Crumley; RL. *Facial Nerve Injury, Repair, and Rehabilitation.* 2nd ed. Washington, DC: American Academy of Otolaryngology—Head & Neck Surgery Foundation Inc; 1984.
23. Orf G. Critical resection length and gap distance in peripheral nerves. *Acta Neruochir Suppl (Wien)* 1978;26:1-
24. Kim DH, Connolly SE, Gillespie JT, Voorhies RM, Kline DG. Electrophysiological studies of various graft lengths and lesion lengths in repair of nerve gaps in primates. *J Neurosurg.* 1991;75:440–446.
25. Kim DH, Connolly SE, Voorhies RM, Beuerman RW, Kline DG. Initial evaluation of variable graft lengths and lesion lengths in the repair of nerve gaps. *J Reconstr Microsurg.* 1990;6:311–316.
26. Fisch U, Lanser MJ. Facial nerve grafting. *Otolaryngol Clin North Am.* 1991;24:691–708.
27. Wong BJF, Mattox DE. Experimental nerve regeneration. A review. *Otolaryngol Clin North Am.* 1991;24:739–752.
28. Pulec JL. Facial nerve grafting. *Laryngoscope.* 1969;79: 1562–1583.
29. Hill HL, Vasconez Lo, Jurkiewicz MJ. Method of obtaining a sural nerve graft. *Plast Reconstr Surg.* 1978;61:177–179.
30. Hankin FM, Jaeger SH, Beddings A. Autogenous sural nerve grafts: a harvesting technique. *Orthopedics.* 1985;8:1160, 1161.
31. Ortiguela ME, Wood MB, Cahill DR. Anatomy of the sural nerve complex. *J Hand Surg.* 1987;12A:1119–1123.
32. Mackinnon SE, Dellon AL. Technical considerations of the latissimus dorsi muscle flap: a segmentally innervated muscle transfer for facial reanimation. *Microsurgery.* 1988;9: 36–45.

33. Sunderland Sir S. Nerve grafting and related methods of nerve repair. In: *Nerve injuries and their Repair. A Critical Appraisal.* New York, NY: Churchill Livingstone; 1991:467–497.

34. Conley J. The treatment of long-standing facial paralysis—a new concept. *Trans Am Acad Ophthalmol Otol.* 1974;78: 386–392.

35. Gagnon NB, Molina-Negro P. Facial reinnervation after facial paralysis: Is it ever too late? *Arch Otorhinolaryngol* 1989; 246:303–307.

36. Ylikoski J, Hitselberger WE, House WF. Degenerative changes in the distal stump of the severed human facial nerve. *Acta Otolaryngol (Stockh).* 1981;92:239–248.

37. Yanagihara N. Rehabilitation of the face by VIIth nerve substitution. In: Fisch U, ed. *Facial Nerve Surgery.* Amstelveen, The Netherlands: Kugler Medical Publication BV; 1977:237–241.

38. Conley J, Baker DC. Hypoglossal-facial nerve anastomosis for reinnervation of the paralyzed face. *Plast Reconstr Surg.* 1979;63:63–72.

39. Pensak ML, Jackson CG, Glasscock ME, Gulya AJ. Facial reanimation with the VII-XII anastomosis: analysis of the functional and psychologic results. *Orolaryngol Head Neck Surg.* 1986;94:305–310.

40. Rubin LR, Mishriki YY, Speace G. Reanimation of the hemiparalytic tongue. *Plast Reconstr Surg.* 1984;73:184–194.

41. Rubin LR. Reanimation of the hemiparalytic tongue. In: Rubin LR, ed. *The Paralyzed Face.* St Louis, Mo: Mosby Year Book; 1991:228–233.

42. May M, Sobol SM, Mester SJ. Hypoglossal-facial nerve interpositional-jump graft for facial reanimation without tongue atrophy. *Otolaryngol Head Neck Surg.* 1991;104:818–825.

43. Anderl H. Cross-face nerve grafting—up to 12 months of seventh nerve disruption. In: Rubin LR, ed. *Reanimation of the Paralyzed Face.* St Louis, Mo: CV Mosby Co; 1977;241–277.

44. Gary-Bobo A, Fuentes JM. Long-term follow-up report on cross-facial nerve grafting in the treatment of facial paralysis. *Br J Plast Surg.* 1983;36:48–50.

45. Fisch U. Cross-face grafting in facial paralysis. *Arch Otolaryngol Head Neck Surg.* 1976;102:453–457.

46. O'Brien BM, Pederson WC, Khazanchi RK, Morrison WA, MacLeod AM, Kumar V. Results of management of facial palsy with microvascular free-muscle transfer. *Plast Reconstr Surg.* 1990;86:12–24.

47. Terzis JK. Pectoralis minor: a unique muscle for correction of facial palsy. *Plast Reconstr Surg.* 1989;83:767–776.

48. Rubin, L. Temporalis and masseter muscle transposition. In: May M, ed. *The Facial Nerve.* New York, NY: Thieme; 1986;665–680.

49. Rubin LR. Reanimation of tital unilateral facial paralysis by the contiguous facial muscle technique. In: Rubin LR, ed. *The Paralyzed Face.* St Louis, Mo: Mosby Year Book; 1991;156–177.

50. Baker DC, Conley J. Regional muscle transposition for rehabilitation of the paralyzed face. *Clin Plast Surg.* 1979; 6:317–331.

51. May M. Muscle transposition for facial reanimation. Indications and results. *Arch Otolaryngol Head Neck Surg.* 1984; 110:184–189.

52. May M, Drucker C. Temporalis muscle for facial reanimation. A 13-year experience with 224 procedures. *Arch Otolaryngol Head Neck Surg.* 1993;119:378–382.

53. Conley J. Discussion: temporalis muscle for facial reanimation, M. May and C. Drucker. *Arch Otolaryngol Head Neck Surg.* 1993;119:383, 384.

54. Blair VP. Further observation upon the compensatory use of live tendon strips for facial paralysis. *Ann Surg.* 1930;92: 694–703.

55. Gillies H. Experiences with fascia lata grafts in the operative treatment of facial paralysis. *Proc R Soc Med.* 1934;27: 1372–1384.

56. Brown JB, McDowell F. Support of the paralyzed face by fascia. *JAMA.* 1947;135:18–20.

57. Brown JB, McDowell F, Fryer MP. Facial paralysis supported with autogenous fascia lata. *Ann Surg.* 1948;237:858–862.

58. McLaughlin CR. Surgical support in permanent facial paralysis. *Plast Reconstr Surg.* 1953;11:302–314.

59. Petroff MA, Goode RL, Levet Y. Gore-Tex implants: applications in facial paralysis rehabilitation and soft-tissue augmentation. *Laryngoscope.* 1992;102:1185–1189.

60. Konior RJ. Facial paralysis reconstruction with Gore-Tex soft-tissue patch. *Arch Otolaryngol Head Neck Surg.* 1992;118: 188–1194.

61. Bauer JJ, Salky BA, Gelernt IM, Kreel I. Repair of large abdominal wall defects with expanded polytetrafluoroethylene (PTFE). *Ann Surg.* 1987;206:765–769.

62. Sachs ME, Conley J. Intraoral masseter muscle transposition: use with reconstruction of regional facial paralysis. *Arch Otolaryngol Head Neck Surg.* 1982;108:397–400.

63. Conley J. Mimetic neurotization from masseter muscle. *Ann Plast Surg.* 1983;10:274–283.

64. Sachs ME, Conley J. Dual simultaneous systems for facial reanimation. *Arch Otolaryngol Head Neck Surg.* 1983;109: 137–139.

65. Casler JD, Conley J. Simultaneous 'dual system' rehabilitation in the treatment of facial paralysis. *Arch Otolaryngol Head Neck Surg.* 1990;116:1399–1403.

66. Aviv JE, Urken ML. Management of the paralyzed face with microneurovascular free muscle transfer. *Arch Otolaryngol Head Neck Surg.* 1992;118:909–912.

67. Clodius L. Selective neurectomies to achieve symmetry in partial and complete facial paralysis. *Br J Plast Surg.* 1976; 29:43–52.

68. Rubin LR, Lee GW, Simpson RL. Reanimation of the long-standing partial facial paralysis. *Plast Reconstr Surg.* 1986; 77:41–49.

69. Edgerton MT. Surgical correction of facial paralysis: a plea for better reconstructions. *Ann Surg.* 1967;165:985–998.

70. Conley J, Baker DC, Selfe RW. Paralysis of the mandibular branch of the facial nerve. *Plast Reconstr Surg.* 1982;70: 569–577.

71. Glenn MG, Goode RL. Surgical treatment of the "marginal mandibular lip" deformity. *Otolaryngol Head Neck Surg.* 1987;97:462–468.

72. May M. Gold weight and wire spring implants as alternatives to tarsorrhaphy. *Arch Otolaryngol Head Neck Surg.* 1987; 113:656–660.

73. Jobe RP. A technique for lid loading in the management of the lagophthalmos of facial palsy. *Plast Reconstr Surg.* 1974; 53:29–32.

74. Neuman AR, Weinberg A, Sela M, Peled IJ, Wexler MR. The correction of seventh nerve palsy lagophthalmos with gold lid load (16 years experience). *Ann Plast Surg.* 1989;22: 142–145.

75. Sobol SM, Alward PD. Early gold weight lid implant for rehabilitation of faulty eyelid closure with facial paralysis: an alternative to tarsorrhaphy. *Head Neck.* 1990;12:149–153.

76. May M. Surgical rehabilitation of facial palsy: total approach. In: May M, ed. *The Facial Nerve.* New York, NY: Thieme; 1986:695–777.

77. Kartush JM, Linstrom CJ, McCann PM, Graham MD. Early gold weight eyelid implantation for facial paralysis. *Otolaryngol Head Neck Surg.* 1990;103:1016–1023.

78. Levine RE. Eyelid reanimation surgery. In: May M, ed. *The Facial Nerve.* New York, NY: Thieme; 1986:681–694.

79. Bosniak SL. Ectropion. In: Smith BC, Della Rocca RC, Nesi, FA, Lisman RD, eds. *Ophthalmic Plastic and Reconstructive Surgery.* St Louis, Mo: CV Mosby Co; 1987;1:562–579.

80. Smith MFW, Goode RL. Eye protection in the paralyzed face. *Laryngoscope.* 1979;89:435–442.

81. Hatt M. *Ophthalmic Plastic and Reconstructive Surgery*. New York, NY: Thieme; 1986:30–47.
82. Rathbun JE. Ectropion. In: *Eyelid Surgery*. Boston, Mass: Little, Brown & Co; 1990:71–110.
83. Schaefer AJ. Lateral canthal tendon tuck. *Ophthalmology*. 1979;86:1879–1882.
84. Tenzel RR. Treatment of lagophthalmos of the lower lid. *Arch Ophthalmol*. 1969;81:366–368.
85. Freeman MS, Thomas JR, Spector JG, Larrabee WF, Bowman CA. Surgical therapy of the eyelids in patients with facial paralysis. *Laryngoscope*. 1990;100:1086–1096.
86. Wesley RE, Collins JW. McCord procedure for ectropion repair. *Arch Otolaryngol Head Neck Surg*. 1983;109:319–322.
87. Lisman RD, Rees T, Baker D, Smith B. Experience with tarsal suspension as a factor in lower lid blepharoplasty. *Plast Reconstr Surg*. 1987;79:897–905.
88. Smith B. The "Lazy-T" correction of ectropion of the lower punctum. *Arch Ophthalmol*. 1976;94:1149, 1150.
89. McCord CD, Tanenbaum M, Dryden RM, Doxanas MT. Eyelid malpositions: entropion, eyelid margin deformity and trichiasis, ectropion, and facial nerve palsy. In: McCord CD, Tanenbaum M, eds. *Oculoplastic Surgery*. New York, NY: Raven Press; 1987: 279–324.
90. May M, Hoffmann DF, Buerger GF Jr, Soll DB. Management of the paralyzed lower eyelid by implanting auricular cartilage. *Arch Otolaryngol Head Neck Surg*. 1990;116:786–788.
91. Hatt M. *Ophthalmic Plastic and Reconstructive Surgery*. New York, NY: Thieme; 1986:74–96.
92. Arion HG. Dynamic closure of the lids in paralysis of the orbicularis muscle. *Int Surg*. 1972;57:48–50.
93. Rubin LR. Reanimation of the paralyzed eyelid. In: *The Paralyzed Face*. St Louis, Mo: Mosby Year Book; 1991: 234–242.
94. Horn KL, Crumley RL. The physiology of nerve injury and repair. *Otolaryngol Clin North Am*. 1984;17:321–333.
95. Pitt TTE, Humphries NLM. Microarterial anastomoses in the rat: the influence of different suture materials on the patency, strength and the electron microscopic appearance of the vessels. *Br J Plast Surg*. 1982;35:150–155.
96. De Castro Correia P, Zani R. Masseter muscle rotation in the treatment of inferior facial paralysis. Anatomical and clinical observations. *Plast Reconstr Surg*. 1973;52:370–373.
97. Sachs ME, Conley J. The pinch scissors technique for motor nerve dissection. *Laryngoscope*. 1981;91:822–825.
98. Anderl A. Rehabilitation of the face by VIIth nerve substitution. In: Fisch U, ed. *Facial Nerve Surgery*, Amstelveen, The Netherlands: Kugler Medical Publications BV; 1977:245–249.
99. Dellon AL, Mackinnon SE. Gentle passage of nerve grafts. *J Hand Surg [Am]*. 1983;8:108–109.
100. Harii K, Ohmori K, Torii S. Free gracilis muscle transplantation, with microneurovascular anastomoses for the treatment of facial paralysis. A preliminary report. *Plast Reconstr Surg*. 1976;57:133–143.
101. Harii K. New concepts in rehabilitation of the long standing facial paralysis. In: Fisch U, ed. *Facial Nerve Surgery*. Amstelveen, The Netherlands: Kugler Medical Publications BV; 1977:258–268.
102. Harii K. Microneurovascular free muscle transplantation. In: Rubin LR, ed. *The Paralyzed Face*, St Louis, Mo: Mosby Year Book; 1991:178–200.
103. Harrison DH. The pectoralis minor vascularized muscle graft for the treatment of unilateral facial palsy. *Plast Reconstr Surg*. 1985;75:206–213.
104. Dellon AL, Mackinnon SE. Segmentally innervated latissimus dorsi muscle, Microsurgical transfer for facial reanimation. *J Reconstr Microsurg*. 1985;2:7–12.
105. Hata Y, Yano K, Matsuka K, Ito O, Matsuda H, Hosokawa K. Treatment of chronic facial palsy by transplantation of the neurovascularized free rectus abdominis muscle. *Plast Reconstr Surg*. 1990;86:1178–1189.
106. Buncke HJ. Facial paralysis. In: *Microsurgery: Transplantation-Replantation*, Philadelphia, Pa: Lea & Febiger; 1991:487–506.

23 Complications of Anesthesia for Otolaryngology–Head and Neck Surgery

Eileen P. Tyler, M.D.

The methods recomended in the ensuing pages are based upon the following basic considerations: that relief from pain and discomfort is an essential part of the modern practice of medicine; that anesthetic techniques offer this opportunity; that these techniques, improperly employed, may be a danger instead of a blessing; and, that an improved mutual understanding of the common problems between anesthesiologist and surgeon should greatly facilitate the provision of more adequate medical care for the patient.

Donald F. Proctor, Preface of
Anesthesia and Otolaryngology, 1957

According to the 1985 (2nd) edition of *The American Heritage Dictionary*, the medical definition of *complication* is: "a condition occurring during another disease and aggravating it." The aggravating condition can be common or uncommon, expected or unexpected, mild or severe, acceptable or unacceptable. Furthermore, its occurrence (in the procedures highlighted within this specific textbook on otolaryngology) may be "credited to" the anesthetic/the anesthetist, the surgery/the surgeon, and, not infrequently, both.

The close interaction between surgeon and anesthetist characteristic of all ear, nose, and throat (ENT) surgical procedures has been emphasized many times in the anesthesia literature. There is perhaps no other single surgical subspecialty that so proudly and so frequently trespasses upon the territory of the anesthesiologist! There is perhaps no other surgeon-anesthesiologist pair who can demonstrate so completely the necessity for mutual communication and cooperation in the operating room.

Oftentimes the surgeon and anesthesiologist seem to share responsibility for the occurrence of adverse events (eg, laryngospasm in a freshly operated larynx, nausea and vomiting following middle ear surgery, airway fires during (carbon dioxide) laser procedures on the larynx or trachea). Historically most, if not all, of these perioperative situations have been labeled "anesthetic complications." To debate the absolute accuracy of this assignation is neither productive nor desirable. In keeping with history, I shall review here some of the more common complications associated with otolaryngological surgery performed under general anesthesia.

Regardless of who claims their ownership, they are conditions aggravating the patient with otolaryngological disease. They are conditions with which the student of anesthesia and the student of ENT surgery should become familiar.

THE ART OF COMPLICATIONS
Anticipation

Although many anesthetic complications are unforeseen and unavoidable, just as many may be predictable and amenable to prevention. The first rule in dealing with complications is to avoid them; this can be accomplished only by awareness. To coin a phrase, a "dash" of anticipation precedes an ounce of prevention. For instance, consider the patient with an unanticipated difficult airway: an imprudent choice of muscle relaxant could cause a disastrous cascade of events. The anesthesiologist must anticipate the likelihood of a given complication and plan the anesthetic technique accordingly. It is helpful to develop an algorithmic style of thinking so that decisions at crossroads will come to mind quickly.

Recognition

Second, it matters little that one is "loaded for bear" if one is looking the other way when the beast presents itself. As an example, exotic preoperative arrangements for technique and equipment may be designed to manage the patient who is suspected to be malignant hyperthermia (MH) susceptible. Failure to recognize the earliest warning signs of this condition intraoperatively can delay life-saving treatment.

Treatment

Finally, it is intuitively obvious that an anticipated complication that occurs despite all known methods for prevention must be appropriately treated as soon as it's recognized. Imagine the scenario of the postoperative "bleeding tonsil." Hemorrhage should always be anticipated and steps taken to prevent it, but occasionally it's going to happen despite the very best surgical technique. Timely, skillful anesthetic management is critical as the patient returns to the operating room.

SPECIFIC COMPLICATIONS
Respiratory/Airway Complications

Adverse respiratory outcomes are a significant cause of patient morbidity and financial liability in anesthetic practice. Multiple studies have documented respiratory complications as a primary cause of patient injury.[1-4] Additional evidence for the magnitude and persistence of complicating respiratory events is found in the closed claims analysis conducted by the Committee on Professional Liability of the American Society of Anesthesiologists (ASA). Adverse outcomes resulting from respiratory events accounted for 34% (522 of 1541) of the closed claims collected from 1985 to 1990. This class of injury emerged as the single leading cause of patient morbidity.[5] Three fourths of the respiratory events fell into one of these three categories: inadequate ventilation (38%), esophageal intubation (18%), or difficult tracheal intubation (17%). Most disturbingly, 85% of respiratory-related claims resulted in death or permanent brain damage.

The limitations of clinical signs (chest excursion, breath sounds, skin color, reservoir bag motion, etc) as indicators of respiratory insufficiency are well known. Hemodynamic derangements such as bradycardia, hypotension, and asystole are late findings in the setting of esophageal intubation, and, once evident, are probably indicative of some degree of irreversible damage. Therefore, routine clinical signs and hemodynamic parameters are notoriously unreliable in the timely recognition and correction of causes of inadequate ventilation. Because most of the adverse claims incidents occurred between 1975 and 1985,[5] it is likely that our now commonplace use of quantitative ventilatory measurement (ie, pulse oximetry, capnometry) was not a standard feature of anesthetic management. Presumably these adjunctive monitors will enable earlier detection of inadequate ventilation and prevention of devastating sequelae.

Other respiratory complications associated with anesthetic administration include laryngospasm, postobstructive pulmonary edema, and aspiration pneumonitis. Although each one of these accounts for less than 1% of respiratory insults as registered in the closed claims analysis,[5] the incidence of each is by no means that rare an occurrence. One might conclude that the recognition and timely management of these events are responsible for the fact that sequelae of death, brain damage, or other significant morbidity are frequently avoided. However, it is their frequency of occurrence and the potential for disastrous outcome that dictates a discussion of these complications in this chapter.

Laryngospasm
DESCRIPTION

Laryngospasm is a common occurrence complicating the airway management during many general anesthetics. The incidence of laryngeal spasm has been reported to be as high as 0.9% in the general population and 1.7% in the pediatric surgical population.[6] Although this form of airway obstruction is usually readily corrected, inappropriate (or appropriate

but unsuccessful) treatment will occasionally lead to disastrous sequelae. Failure to relieve total airway obstruction inevitably results in hypoxia, which, when severe and prolonged, can precipitate cardiac arrest. If additional resuscitation efforts prove ineffective, the usual aftermath of circulatory collapse can ensue, the most significant of those being cerebral and/or myocardial infarction and even death.

Closure of the larynx results from malfunction of either the intrinsic or extrinsic muscles of the larynx, or both. Fink's[7] discussion of the etiology and treatment of laryngeal spasm provides the clearest and most functional explanation for the varied clinical signs associated with laryngospasm. Depending on which laryngeal muscles are involved, differing degrees of glottic closure occur. The heralding signs of laryngospasm are specific to the degree/mechanism of glottic closure. It is important to recognize this distinction because the treatment for the varieties of laryngospasm are different.

According to Fink, airway obstruction involving the larynx occurs by two mechanisms:

1. Shutter mechanism—adduction and approximation of true vocal cords.
2. Ball-valve mechanism—adduction and approximation of true vocal cords and false cord adduction that foreshortens the larynx, inverts the glottic aditus, and presses the rounded pre-epiglottic soft tissues against the upper surface of the vocal cords.

Clinically, the shutter mechanism is manifested as either inspiratory or expiratory stridor. Inspiratory stridor (passive closure at the glottis) is actually not laryngospasm at all, but a natural condition of air flow that is worsened by the presence of anesthesia. Air flow through the narrow glottis may create a force drawing the cords together (Bernoulli's theorem). In the unanesthetized patient, this adduction is countered by abduction of the vocal cords, and the flow of air is not restricted. With the progressive loss of skeletal muscle tone and relaxation of soft tissues accompanying general anesthesia, laryngeal muscles are weakened, the supportive abduction of cords does not occur, and the characteristic pitch of inspiratory stridor is heard. Expiratory stridor (reflex closure of the glottis), on the other hand, signifies active adduction (spasm) of vocal cords as a reflex to noxious stimuli. A "singing" sound is heard during expiration. In both cases, because there is audible air movement, the obstruction is incomplete. Other respiratory efforts are heightened as compensation. Inspiratory and expiratory stridor are mediated by the intrinsic muscles of the larynx.

The classic picture of laryngospasm is complete obstruction produced by the ball-valve mechanism in response to noxious stimuli. Respiratory efforts are dramatic and spastic with obvious contraction of abdominal muscles during the obstructed expiratory phase. There is no air movement with this complete closure of the larynx, and no sound is heard. Although there is no support in the literature, otolaryngology—head and neck surgery is more likely to be associated with laryngospasm because of the high number of pediatric cases, blood in the airway, and avoidance of muscle relaxants.

Inspiratory stridor is most often seen on induction of general anesthesia but frequently on emergence as well. Almost every patient having an inhalation induction will reach the point of inspiratory stridor unless the anesthetist provides some assistance in maintaining airway patency. Pertinent airway adjuncts and suction must be readily available.

Expiratory stridor is precipitated by noxious stimuli in the presence of light anesthesia. "Noxious" is a broad adjective and encompasses a surprisingly wide range of stimuli. Classic teaching included the following as common initiating factors: excessive stimulation or manipulation of the airway, accumulation of secretions, blood, or mucus in the pharynx, irritation of respiratory passage by acrid anesthetic vapors, and premature insertion of oral airways. Keep in mind that any uncomfortable sensory input may precipitate vocal cord spasm as well. Attempts to start intravenous (IV) lines and cycling of the noninvasive blood pressure monitor are two other common peri-induction stimuli that can cause problems. One study evaluated the laryngospasm prophylaxis of 4% lidocaine, 4 mg/kg, sprayed on the larynx and pre-epiglottic area at the time of tracheal intubation in tonsillectomy patients.[8] It was concluded that this regimen significantly reduced postoperative stridor and laryngospasm in the patient group studied. Advance preparation of the oropharynx with a topical local anesthetic spray may blunt the afferent limb of the laryngeal reflex. There are conflicting reports on the efficacy of intravenous lidocaine as prophylaxis against laryngospasm as well. Expiratory stridor occurs on induction or emergence with about equal frequency.

Reflex laryngeal closure occurs in response to stimulation of visceral nerve endings in the pelvis, abdomen, thorax, or larynx itself.[6] Although there may be occasions where procedures involving this type of stimulation are carried out under general anesthesia with a mask, the majority of these cases occur with an endotracheal tube in place. Complete obstruction secondary to laryngospasm cannot occur in the presence of an endotracheal tube. In my experience, this type of laryngospasm generally occurs during emergence and immediately postextubation when the patient is not fully awake. Blood or secretions stimulate the larynx and compound a preexisting partial obstruction, producing complete laryngeal closure.

TREATMENT

Inspiratory stridor is relieved by any maneuver that will relieve upper airway soft tissue obstruction and/or abduct the vocal cords. Neck extension and jaw thrust positioning often improve ventilation dramatically. Insertion of an oral airway moves the tongue forward from the posterior pharynx. Gentle, continuous positive pressure with bag and mask will provide necessary airway distention. Finally, lightening the anesthetic will help restore tone to vocal cord abductors (but lightening the anesthetic may not be desirable). Depending on the patient's condition, high inspired fractions of oxygen

can be supplied to maintain adequate tissue oxygen saturation. If adequate ventilation cannot be regained by cutting back the anesthetic and attempting to alleviate upper airway obstruction, intubation of the trachea will secure the airway. This is not the time to use muscle relaxants because adequate ventilation by bag and mask has not been successfully demonstrated. Spontaneously breathing patients, difficult to mask ventilate, stridulous as they may be, are in a much safer place than paralyzed patients should it be found that intubation is difficult/impossible. Because deep anesthesia is a primary condition in producing inspiratory stridor, unless the patient has actually been awakened again, the anesthetic depth is probably appropriate for intubation without relaxation.

The treatment of expiratory stridor is similar to that for inspiratory stridor with one very notable exception: to treat successfully one must increase the depth of anesthesia while eliminating any noxious stimuli. Constant positive pressure is also generally helpful in this situation. Again, endotracheal intubation will provide a secure airway. Short-acting muscle relaxants (1 mg/kg succinylcholine) will abolish the reflex vocal cord spasm but this should be administered based on the level of confidence that intubation will be accomplished.

The ball-valve type of laryngeal obstruction is more critical and more difficult to manage. These are the instances that most frequently demand administration of succinylcholine, and more rarely, tracheostomy or cricothyroidotomy if intubation is not possible. Positive pressure ventilation is likely to be of no value, given the anatomic and physiological variables at play. Cessation of any noxious stimulus as well as head extension and extreme jaw thrust may alleviate the obstruction partially. Again IV lidocaine (1 to 2 mg/kg) has proven useful in some reports. It is said that profound hypoxia and hypercapnia may actually terminate laryngospasm, but the wisdom of testing that hypothesis as a first-line treatment is questionable.

The cornerstone of managing laryngospasm is anticipation and early prevention. Advance preparation and vigilance during the specific times it is most likely to occur will help avoid this complication. The common denominator is inadequate anesthesia usually. Ensuring that blood and secretions are cleared and avoiding any unnecessary stimuli while the patient is lightly anesthetized without an endotracheal tube in place is the key. A calm, organized, efficient demeanor goes a long way should severe laryngospasm present itself. Table 23–1 summarizes the information found in Fink's review of laryngospasm.

Postobstructive Pulmonary Edema (POPE)

DESCRIPTION

The occurrence of negative pressure pulmonary edema in association with airway obstruction has been described by multiple observers. It has been documented during acute episodes of laryngospasm, epiglottitis, and croup,[9–12] and during chronic airway obstruction of varying etiologies.[13,14] Although many reports describe this complication in children,

Table 23-1. Summary of the Etiology and Treatment of Laryngeal Spasm

Type of Glottic Closure	Clinical Signs	Mechanism	Muscles Involved	Treatment
"shutter" approximation of vocal cords during inspiration (*accentuated upper airway obstruction*)	incomplete obstruction - inspiratory stridor of pathognomonic pitch Active respiratory efforts	[a] Bernoulli effect at glottis accentuated by "negative" pressure of inspiration-cords drawn together unopposed by abduction of cords due to anesthetic induced loss of skeletal muscle tone [b] active adduction of cords	intrinsic	gentle continuous positive pressure by bag and mask; lightening the plane of anesthesia to restore abductor tone; remove noxious stimuli 100% O_2 endotracheal tube
"shutter" approximation of vocal cords during expiration	incomplete obstruction - expiratory stridor similar to singing active respiratory efforts	adduction of vocal cords	intrinsic	removal of noxious stimuli deepening the plane of anesthesia endotracheal tube
"ball-valve" pre-epiglottic body (tissue softens from hyoid to notch of thyroid) becomes rounded and presses against upper surface of false cords	complete obstruction no sound made- no air movement vigorous respiratory efforts		extrinsic thyrohyoid sternohyoid sternothyroid	jaw thrust maneuver remove noxious stimuli positive pressure may aggravate

From Fink.[7]

adults with airway obstruction are likewise at risk.[15-17] Characteristically, the onset of pulmonary edema is noted following alleviation of the airway obstruction. Clinical signs and symptoms of edema are usually evident simultaneously with reestablishing the airway or shortly thereafter. In some cases, however, there may be a lag of several hours before respiratory difficulty ensues.

The physiological mechanisms favoring transudation of fluid into the alveoli when an obstructed airway is rendered unobstructed have been described. The primary pathogenetic factor is believed to be negative intrathoracic pressure.

In the setting of significant upper airway obstruction, changes occurring in the Starling forces operating within the lung balance each other, so that a compensated state is reached. While the obstruction persists, there is no pulmonary edema. As soon as the airway is cleared hydrostatic and interstitial pressure gradients, which function during expiration to counteract the negative transpulmonary intrathoracic pressures resulting from inspiration against obstruction, are now unopposed, favoring transudation of fluid into the alveoli. This is best illustrated in the schematic diaphragm offered by Galvis et al[18] (Fig. 23-1).

ANTICIPATION

A high index of suspicion for the advent of POPE may well serve to attenuate or even avoid its clinical presentation. Quite simply, all patients with a history of upper airway obstruction will be at risk for the development of pulmonary edema once the airway obstruction has been relieved. Common causes of chronic obstruction include patients with a history of any cancer in the head or neck impinging on the airway at various levels, smoldering subclinical infectious processes obstructing breathing passages, obstructive sleep apnea, hypertrophied tonsils/adenoids, airway stenoses secondary to previous surgery/tracheostomy for airway pathology, and recurrent vocal cord polyps or papillomata obstructing airflow. Most cases will fall into this realm of chronic or subacute pathology. Acute airway obstruction is primarily represented by aspirated foreign bodies, abscesses, epiglottitis/croup, and pronounced airway obstruction (including laryngospasm) during induction of, or emergence from, anesthesia.

RECOGNITION

Postobstructive pulmonary edema has the classic clinical hallmarks of pulmonary edema arising from any other etiology. Its onset is almost immediate following the relief of upper airway obstruction, although it may be slightly more insidious, progressing over 20 to 60 minutes later. The patient will be tachypneic and dyspneic, with a cough productive of pink, frothy sputum. Pulse oximetry and arterial blood gas measurements will document significant hypoxia and hypoxemia. The chest radiograph typically reveals a diffuse bilateral alveolar infiltration. In the setting of recent alleviation of airway obstruction, the respiratory distress described is quite easily diagnosed.

Complications of Anesthesia 375

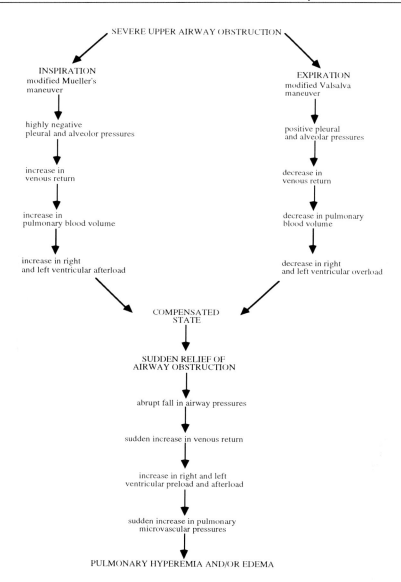

Figure 23-1. Schematic representation of physiological changes leading to pulmonary edema following treatment for acute upper airway obstruction (from Galvis et al[18]).

TREATMENT

Although maintenance of airway obstruction will surely preclude the possibility of POPE by allowing the continued balance of inspiratory and expiratory pressure gradients, that option is clearly a nonsensical approach. Continued airway obstruction takes its toll eventually in profound hypoxia, hypercapnia, acidosis, and ultimately, cardiovascular collapse and death. The obstruction, of course, is to be relieved. A period of watchful waiting and prompt response should pulmonary edema ensue will compress the time frame of distress.

The mainstays of treatment are supplemental oxygen, positive airway pressure, and diuretics. Although some case reports describe the use of steroids in this setting, there is no good evidence that steroids are indicated in treating the pulmonary congestion. There may be other attendant features in patients at risk for the development of POPE that dictate the use of steroids (such as edematous airway passages of any etiology, at any level).

Depending on the nature of airway obstruction and the resultant individual clinical scenarios, the patient may or may not have an artificial airway in place at the time that pulmonary edema presents itself. For example, in the case of pulmonary edema following an episode of treated laryngospasm periextubation at the conclusion of surgery, the patient would be using no airway adjuncts. On the other hand, the patient who is intubated to alleviate airway obstruction secondary to acute epiglottitis would quite obviously have an endotracheal tube in place. Method of continuous positive airway pressure (CPAP) and supplemental oxygen delivery may thus be either mask or endotracheal CPAP, 5 to 15 cm H_2O. At some point it may become necessary to decide if the patient on mask CPAP requires endotracheal intubation to improve oxygen delivery. The dose of furosemide is variable, but generally small amounts (40 mg or less) are effective.

Although pulmonary edema developing soon after relief of airway obstruction is most likely related, it is prudent to keep in mind that there is a differential diagnosis, and that other entities may present in very similar fashion. The two most common conditions to consider are aspiration and fluid overload. Other causes of acute pulmonary edema that occur on emergence from general anesthesia include cardiac failure precipitated by extreme hypertension, cardiac failure secondary to coronary artery disease, and cardiac failure resulting from mitral valve dysfunction. It may take a few hours to make the diagnosis, and even then both aspiration pneumonitis and primary pulmonary edema may respond favorably in much the same way as POPE.

Fortunately cases of POPE exhibit rapid resolution once therapy is underway. Steady marked improvement and clearing of the lungs typically ensue over the course of a few hours. The use of positive airway pressure can be discontinued once the patient demonstrates respiratory stability during a 20 to 30-minute trial with no distending pressure.

The Difficult/Failed Intubation

Few head and neck surgical procedures can be successfully conducted under local anesthesia (with or without adjunctive IV sedation): general anesthesia is the rule. Given the location of surgical sites, and the positioning required to facilitate surgical exposure, the patient's head (airway) is often at some distance from the anesthetist, and it is not readily accessible. Therefore, the majority of otolaryngological procedures, in addition to requiring general anesthesia, also require endotracheal intubation.

Before the patient ever approaches the operating room, a plan is formulated concerning the safest and most desirable technique for placement of the endotracheal tube. The plan derives from a thorough assessment of each individual's physical examination (anatomy and pathology), medical/surgical history, and subjective symptomatology—specifically as these factors pertain to the airway. The majority of difficult airways will be readily detected by conscientious preoperative assessment. Modification of equipment, techniques, and anesthetic agents can all be planned for and prepared in advance.

Anticipated problem airways tend not to result in complications. Because the problem is anticipated, management is tailored to avoid the problem, and immediate treatment is readily available should difficulty be encountered. On the contrary, more disastrous adverse outcomes are associated with the unanticipated problem airway. It is every anesthetist's nightmare to be challenged suddenly and unexpectedly by an airway they cannot control.

This section will therefore focus only on the management of an airway that suddenly declares itself unmanageable.

ANTICIPATION

The most reliable predictor of a straightforward airway is written documentation within the patient's medical record of a previous uncomplicated general anesthetic that included airway manipulation. This has become affectionately labeled a "proven airway." Even if certain anatomic features of the

patient (described subsequently in this section) arouse concern about the ease of intubation, actual verification that this patient had no difficulty the last time, and that all things are still equal, virtually ensures repeated success. One must ascertain, however, that the previous intubation success involved an airway manager with skills equivalent to the endoscopist who is about to perform the upcoming intubation. That is to say, an intubation considered easy by a seasoned, experienced anesthetist may not be as easy in the hands of a neophyte.

In addition, there are clinical examinations that can be performed preoperatively to assist in the prediction of intubation difficulty. The first of these evaluates the size of the tongue in relation to the size of the oral cavity. The airway is classified according to how much the tongue obscures pharyngeal structures.[1] With the patient's mouth opened as widely as possible, and the tongue maximally protruded, the examiner notes the visibility of anatomy as follows: (1) class I, soft palate, fauces, uvula, anterior and posterior tonsillar pillars visualized; (2) class II, soft palate, fauces, uvula visualized; (3) class III, soft palate, base of uvula visualized; and (4) class IV, soft palate not visible at all (Fig. 23–2).

There is a correlation between ease of laryngoscopy and the Mallampati classification of the airway.[19,20] Class I airways are associated with a grade I laryngoscopic view 99 to 100% of the time.[21] Class IV airways produce a grade II-IV view 100% of the time (Fig. 23–3). Unfortunately, airways evaluated as class II and class III were associated with a rather equal frequency of all grades of laryngoscopic views.[19,22] Other factors (eg, degree of neck mobility, size of the mandibular space, and interobserver variability) are not considered in the Mallampati classification, and this may account for false positives and false negatives.

Second, evaluation of the patient's ability to assume the "sniffing" position affords some idea of degree of difficulty in intubation. It has long been appreciated that the sniffing

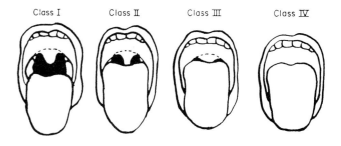

Figure 23–2. Classification of the upper airway in terms of tongue size and pharyngeal structures visible upon mouth opening (from Mallampati et al[19]).

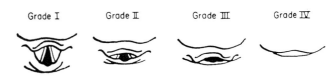

Figure 23–3. Correlation between ease of laryngoscopy and the Mallampati classification of the airway.

position (neck flexed on chest plus head extended on neck) aligns the oral, pharyngeal, and laryngeal axes, providing a direct view of the larynx on endoscopy. Patients with limited atlanto-occipital joint extension will be less able to optimize anatomy, and intubation will be more difficult.

The third measurement commonly employed in evaluating the airway for ease of intubation is the thyromental or hyomental distance and/or the horizontal length of the mandible. A thyromental distance greater than 6 cm and a horizontal mandibular length greater than 9 cm correlate with a low tongue/pharyngeal size classification (Mallampati), strongly suggesting that visualization of the larynx by direct laryngoscopy will be relatively easy.[23-25]

Although not foolproof, the combination of these three simple clinical assessments provides a reliable prediction of the degree of airway difficulty in the majority of patients. According to Cobley and Vaughan,[26] "unfortunately, a small number of patients appear to be normal at clinical examination but subsequently present an extremely difficult or even impossible airway to intubate." It is this small subset of patients who will experience complications, at least during their first exposure. Presumably, conscientious documentation of unexpected airway problems in the medical record will convert them from an unanticipated challenge to an anticipated one before subsequent encounters.

RECOGNITION AND TREATMENT

The scenario of unexpected airway difficulty occurs usually in one of three ways:

1. Anesthesia induced in the usual (IV) fashion → mask ventilation attempted and successful → muscle relaxants administered → intubation attempted but unsuccessful.
2. Anesthesia induced in the usual (IV) fashion → mask ventilation attempted but inadequate or impossible → intubation attempted but unsuccessful.
3. Anesthesia induced in the usual (IV) fashion → mask ventilation not attempted or not guaranteed → muscle relaxants administered → intubation attempted but unsuccessful.

In all three situations, the patient is impossible to intubate by conventional methods. The potential for serious sequelae hinges on the drugs administered and the ability to mask ventilate the patient.

In the first instance, as long as the ability to ventilate is maintained (and not worsened or obliterated by repeated attempts at intubation), there is more cause for annoyance than alarm. If the surgical procedure necessitates intubation, it will most likely have to be postponed until a time when a plan and the necessary equipment are on hand for less conventional intubation techniques. The patient faces no danger. Manual ventilation must be maintained until anesthetic agents and muscle relaxants have either worn off or been reversed by pharmacological antagonists. The duration depends on the characteristics and doses of agents given (ie, short-acting muscle relaxant vs intermediate-acting relaxant, dose of nar-

cotic, presence or absence of inhalational agents). The patient must remain sedated while still under the influence of muscle relaxants. Reversal of paralyzing agents cannot be forced before enough receptors are available at the neuromuscular junction—and this is a function of time, specific for each individual agent.

The second scenario describes an anesthetized patient who cannot be adequately ventilated by mask and who cannot be intubated in the usual fashion (standard laryngoscopy, intubation under direct vision). An organized approach to diagnose the cause for inadequate mask ventilation may prove helpful. Upper airway obstruction may be relieved by oronasal airways or readjustment of the patient's head into a better sniffing position. If laryngospasm is the primary cause for inability to ventilate, continuous positive airway pressure and/or the use of succinylcholine will be corrective. Reactive airway disease may involve bronchospasm significant enough to prevent adequate mask ventilation, and oftentimes deepening the anesthetic (with or without adjunctive use of aerosol or intravenous bronchodilators) is effective. Other causes of difficult mask ventilation are not readily remediable. Anatomic derangements in airway patency secondary to intrinsic mass lesions in the pharynx, larynx, trachea, and bronchi or extrinsic mass lesions in close proximity to the airway (thyroid tumors, massive lymphadenopathy, mediastinal masses, neck abscesses, etc) will require surgical correction.

If mask ventilation cannot be improved (regardless of the cause), the patient is at risk for the development of hypoxia, hypercapnia, and the sequelae thereof. That risk will be determined by the patient's baseline medical condition, the degree to which partial oxygenation/ventilation is possible, and the length of time inadequate ventilation persists. Until patients awaken and maintain spontaneous ventilation with the ability to support their own airway, they remain at risk. Fortunately standard IV induction agents are usually of short duration (thiopental, methohexital, propofol). Longer-acting narcotics or sedatives can often be reversed by antagonists (naloxone, flumazanil). Inhalation agents are fairly quickly eliminated by the lungs (but of course this necessitates some ventilation, and the worse the ventilation, the longer it will be before the patient awakes from these volatile agents).

The only saving grace in this situation is that the patient has not received a neuromuscular blocking drug. Some degree of spontaneous respiration usually persists, and no "bridges have been burned." Again, for elective surgical procedures, awakening the patient and returning to the operating room at some future date seems prudent. Advanced warning of the need for alternative airway management techniques should facilitate a more successful outcome.

The third type of unanticipated failure to intubate is the worst. The patient is unconscious, the patient is paralyzed, the anesthetist can't ventilate the patient by mask, and endotracheal intubation proves impossible. Even in cases where succinylcholine was the muscle relaxant given, one cannot merely wait for its metabolism and the resumption of spontaneous respiration. Immediate action must be taken to provide oxygenation, or severe hypoxia with irreversible sequelae is certain. The ASA's Task Force on the Difficult Airway (see Fig. 23–4) recommends transtracheal jet ventilation at this juncture. Once ventilation is guaranteed, a decision can be made concerning further airway invasion (cricothyroidotomy or alternative intubation techniques) versus awakening the patient and rescheduling the surgical procedure.

For all three scenarios, the elective or emergent nature of the surgical procedure will greatly determine the extent to which the difficult airway algorithm (Fig. 23–4) is completed. Cases that cannot be postponed will obviously result in more drastic interventions and surgical airways (particularly in otolaryngological surgery where mask ventilation is not a practical consideration even if it is possible).

Postoperative Nausea and Vomiting (PONV)
DESCRIPTION

Of all the complications associated with anesthesia, significant nausea and vomiting in the recovery phase play a pivotal role in engendering dread or fear of anesthesia in many patients. A history of perioperative emetic episodes is remarkably easy to elicit—the information is usually volunteered,

coupled with a plea for prevention the next time around. The patient's concern is legitimate. Even in mild forms postoperative nausea, retching, and vomiting are distressing discomforts. Severe or intractable emesis can result in a host of other consequences: serum electrolyte imbalances, dehydration, wound disruption, increased bleeding at the surgical site. Indeed, nausea and vomiting could conceivably become life-threatening in situations where residual anesthetics maintain depressed levels of consciousness, placing the patient at risk for aspiration.

Despite the major strides in other areas of anesthetic management during the last several decades, there seems to have been little or no progress made in reducing the occurrences of PONV.[27] The incidence of emetic sequelae after an anesthetic without use of antiemetics still hovers around 30%.[28]

ANTICIPATION

The literature on this topic does offer some assistance in isolating patients who may be at particular risk for postoperative sickness. Once these patients are identified, then

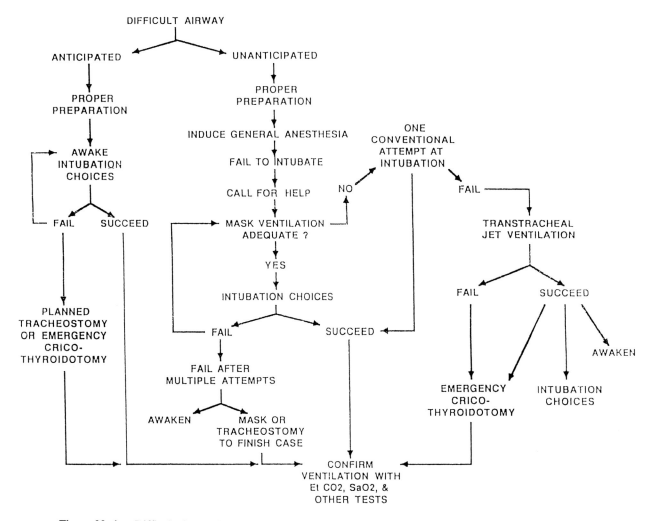

Figure 23–4.   Difficult airway algorithm. Developed by the Difficult Airway Task Force of the Committee on Patient Safety and Risk Management, American Society of Anesthesiologists, November 1990.

antiemetic prophylaxis can be attempted. The development of PONV is multifactorial. The main categories of factors influencing the problem include patient factors, anesthetic management, and surgical procedures (Table 23–2).

Patient Factors

Similar to the wide variation observed in gag reflexes, there is a spectrum of individual response to emetic stimuli. Some segments of the general population will experience nausea and vomiting at even the slightest provocation. This group of patients presents the greatest management challenge, and they will probably have some difficulty no matter how we try to tailor perioperative care to that specific need. Patients who have suffered previous postoperative vomiting were noted in one study to have a threefold increase in risk of vomiting in the first 24 hours.[29] This most likely reflects those patients' low threshold for vomiting. Furthermore, patients who give a history of motion sickness also seem to have a higher incidence of postoperative emetic symptoms.[28,29]

Most investigators report a significantly higher incidence of nausea and vomiting in women than in men.[30-32] Bellville[33] postulated that this increased incidence may be related to elevated plasma gonadotrophin and progesterone levels.[33] This idea may be supported by the observation that emetic symptoms are seen in equal numbers among male and female children.[34] Children exhibit twice the incidence of PONV when compared with adults.[34] Although there is some conflict in data, most investigators noted the tendency for decreasing postoperative emesis with increasing age.[31]

Obesity has been reported to increase the risk of PONV. The reasons are not entirely clear, but this correlation was borne out in an article by McKenzie et al.[35] Their study of patients undergoing first trimester abortions shows that the heaviest patients had a higher incidence of emesis.

It would seem intuitive that any patients with preexisting or concurrent conditions that involve emesis are more likely to have a higher incidence of postoperative vomiting than those who did not have such symptoms. Generally such patients will be undergoing emergent surgery that cannot be postponed until their emesis abates. The most common examples of this are patients with acute appendicitis or small bowel obstruction or acute gastrointestinal bleeding. In these cases the surgical procedure should effect a long-term cure, but these patients will be at particular risk during emergence and in the immediate recovery period. More germane to otolaryngology and head and neck surgery is the posttonsillectomy patient who is bleeding. There is no choice but to return to the operating room. Unfortunately the repeat anesthetic occurs in the setting of a stomach full of swallowed blood, a setting that entails a significant risk of regurgitation during the peri-induction period and upon emergence from anesthesia and an increased risk of continued emesis into the postoperative period. Other more subacute conditions that may involve preoperative nausea or emesis include cases of increasing intracranial pressure or metabolic disturbances or toxicity due to drugs or alcohol.

Table 23–2. Common Factors Increasing the Risk of Postoperative Nausea and Vomiting

Patient factors
  Individual predisposition (variability in vomiting reflex threshold)
  Previous history of postoperative nausea and vomiting
  History of motion sickness
  Gender
  Age
  Weight
  Concurrent illness
  Gastric volume
Anesthetic management
  Premedication
  Anesthetic agents
  Anesthetic technique
  Use of nasogastric tube
Surgical procedures
  Laparoscopy
  Ophthalmologic procedures (especially strabismus repair)
  Middle ear procedures
  Urologic procedures (especially testicular)
  Gastrointestinal procedures

Finally, any patient with increased gastric volume will be at increased risk for perioperative regurgitation and emesis. Pregnant women, diabetics with delayed gastric emptying, patients noncompliant with "nothing by mouth" restrictions, and severely anxious individuals are some examples of this predisposing factor.

Anesthetic Management
PREMEDICATION

Premedication in general seems to have fallen by the wayside in daily anesthetic practice, primarily because the majority of our patients are not in house the night before their surgery. Spending a restful night in their own homes with their friends and families nearby is probably as anxiolytic as any pill or injection. The desirability of sedating patients preoperatively (without specific indication) is questionable. Should the need for premedication arise, however (and it frequently does arise in the pediatric population), some consideration can be given to the class of premedicant in an effort to minimize any potentiation of PONV. For example, Riding[36] demonstrated clearly the well-known problems with morphine in this regard. Only 22.4% of women undergoing uterine dilatation and curettage experienced nausea, retching, or vomiting when they were unpremedicated. However, the incidence of postoperative symptoms rose to 67% when morphine was added. On the other hand, low-dose meperidine intramuscularly (<1 mg/kg [IM]) was found by Bellville[33] to be antiemetic. The emetic and antiemetic properties of opiates have led to the proposal of an antiemetic center in the brain wherein enkephalins are the neurotransmitters.[37] The different effects of opiates may be explained by the presence of different opiate receptors at this center[38] (Fig. 23–5).

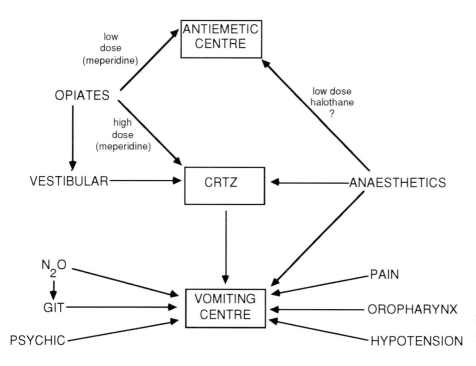

Figure 23–5. Sites of action of stimuli related to anaesthesia (from Palazzo and Strunin[27]).

In my opinion, a narcotic is the premedication of choice only when the patient is in pain and analgesia is required to achieve the desired tranquil state. Otherwise there is a complete menu of assorted sedatives, hypnotics, and tranquilizers from which to select a satisfactory preoperative drug. Most anesthesia practices have a standard favorite drug and route of administration. Examples are Midazolam/Tylenol or Pediprofen elixir for children (orally) and midazolam for adults (IM, IV, occasionally orally as for children). The message is: if premedication is indicated, select one that serves the purpose, trying to avoid compounds that will stimulate the chemoreceptor trigger zone. If such compounds cannot be avoided, consider adjunctive agents or measures that will offset the undesirable effects (see "Treatment of PONV").

ANESTHETIC AGENTS

Beyond premedication, maintenance anesthetic choices can also contribute to postoperative sickness. It seems that almost every agent, IV or inhalational, has been implicated at some time in some way.

The reports on N_2O are confusing and inconclusive. One can find data that discourage its use in patients prone to emesis,[39] but one can just as easily find studies that claim there is no association between its use and the development of PONV.[40] We do know that N_2O possesses characteristics that intuitively would seem to increase the chance of emesis. It has a central effect, stimulating the CRTZ in the brain while peripherally acting to distend the bowel. Gastric distention associated with the use of N_2O could very likely result in more problems postoperatively with nausea and/or vomiting.

The other inhalational agents have also been scrutinized in an effort to determine the least likely offender in postanesthetic vomiting. Most of these studies are conducted on outpatients in whom avoidance of protracted postoperative

emesis is critical for a successfully efficient, smoothly functioning ambulatory surgery unit. Again the data are somewhat conflicting, but the most consistent conclusion seems to be that isoflurane is associated with more PONV than either halothane or enflurane. There are no good studies yet on the two newest agents, desflurane and sevoflurane.

Some of the IV agents have a reputation for causing nausea (etomidate, ketamine, propranidid), and these are best avoided in patients at risk. When the N_2O relaxant-narcotic technique was compared with the nitrous-isoflurane method, the patients receiving narcotics had a higher incidence of nausea and vomiting. The newer drugs (fentanyl, alfentanil, sufentanil) seemed to be worse than meperidine.[41] When droperidol (as an antiemetic) was added to the narcotic techniques, there was a comparable incidence of nausea and vomiting between the two groups.[41] Of the newer IV agents, midazolam and propofol appear least associated with postoperative emesis. Propofol was noted to have a significantly lower incidence of vomiting when compared with N_2O-methohexital, N_2O-enflurane, and isoflurane.[42–44]

For the sake of completeness, I will only mention that regional anesthesia (spinal, epidural) is a more attractive alternative to general anesthesia when the surgical procedure is suitable. Although there is a decreased incidence of regional-associated nausea/vomiting, it is still by no means a rare occurrence. The arterial hypotension frequently seen with spinal anesthesia can result in decreased cerebral blood flow and stimulation of the vomiting center. In addition, increased gastrointestinal peristalsis results from the preganglionic sympathetic blockade, and this further contributes to nausea/vomiting.

ANESTHESIA TECHNIQUE

As influential as the choice of agent(s) is in avoiding emetic complications, care and concern in performing basic anesthetic procedures or maneuvers are also very important. The anesthetist must be skillful in airway management, for example. Avoidance of overly aggressive mask ventilation (which can distend the stomach) and proper timing when it comes to suctioning the oropharynx or removing the oral airway will go a long way in preventing gagging and retching. Careful transport of patients to the postanesthesia care unit (PACU), eliminating rapid, sharp turns, is another way to safeguard them from emetic stimuli. Finally, the use of a nasogastric tube to decompress the stomach and remove swallowed blood and gastric contents has definitely been shown to reduce the incidence of postoperative vomiting. It is wise to remove the nasogastric tube before the patient awakens and the nasopharyngeal stimulation activates the gag reflex.

SURGICAL PROCEDURES

Once again there is a lack of universal opinion concerning which surgical procedure(s) results in the highest incidence of nausea and vomiting. Conflicting conclusions are presented in the literature because there seems to be inadequate standardization of patients and too wide a variation in anesthetic techniques. The most repetitive finding, though, seems to be that the incidence of nausea and vomiting is highest after middle ear procedures and gastrointestinal surgery.

TREATMENT

Nothing needs to be said about the recognition of this complication—most medical personnel feel quite confident in their ability to diagnose vomiting. Measures of prophylaxis and treatment do warrant some discussion.

PROPHYLAXIS

Because we have the appropriate pharmacology at our disposal, and because some antiemetic agents are notably devoid of adverse clinical side effects, some would suggest that all patients who present with a constellation of risk factors for emesis should receive prophylaxis. Keats[45] stated that "80–90% of patients given prophylactic antiemetics will have been treated unnecessarily because vomiting would not have occurred in 70% of the patients and another 10–20% will vomit even though they were treated." Because women have a 1.5 to three times higher incidence of nausea/vomiting than men, should antiemetic prophylaxis be used for all women?

It would seem that the relative weight(s) of the risk factor(s) present should determine whether or not the patient receives antiemetics preoperatively. For instance, if a woman with a past history of postoperative vomiting presented for thyroid surgery, I might be more likely to use prophylaxis than I would for a young boy having a tonsillectomy. I believe that certain surgical procedures entail a high enough risk for associated vomiting (viz, strabismus repair, middle ear surgery, laparoscopy) that all patients undergoing these should

receive prophylaxis. I believe that patients with a history of motion sickness or previous postoperative vomiting should be prophylaxed even if they are having a bunionectomy under spinal anesthesia.

The drugs commonly used for antiemetic prophylaxis include anticholinergic agents (eg, scopolamine, hyoscine), antihistamines (eg, hydroxyzine, promethazine), butyrophenones (eg, droperidol), and dopamine receptor antagonists (eg. metoclopramide). In recent years some have utilized sympathomimetics (eg, ephedrine), and currently a selective serotonin 5-hydroxytryptamine type-3 (5-HT$_3$) receptor antagonist named ondansetron is under investigation as a prophylactic antiemetic for surgical patients (ondansetron has been approved for the prevention of nausea and vomiting occurring with emetogenic cancer chemotherapy). Of all these drugs, the three proving efficacious with acceptable side effects are droperidol, metaclopramide, and ondansetron.

Droperidol is administered IV at the outset of surgery in a dose of 15 to 35 μg/kg. It has proven quite effective in these doses, but occasionally a total of 50 μg/kg is required to counteract nausea in the postoperative period. Sedation then is a common, usually undesirable side effect, and dysphoria is also frequently reported. Droperidol is antidopaminergic and acts centrally at the CRTZ. By comparison, metoclopramide is also antidopaminergic, but is a peripherally active gastrokinetic agent that decreases residual gastric volume.[28] Prophylactic metoclopramide may be given by mouth (10 mg preoperatively) or by IV route (0.15 mg/kg) at the end of surgery, just before entering the PACU. According to the early reports on ondansetron, a selective serotonin 5-HT$_3$ antagonist, this drug may be administered by oral route (4, 8, or 16 mg) preoperatively or IV (4 or 8 mg) at the beginning of surgery.[46,47] It seems likely that combining two of these agents that have different sites of action will increase the chances of successful antiemetic therapy.

Although many anesthesiologists also add histamine receptor blockers when facing a patient at risk for perioperative vomiting, cimetidine and ranitidine are not antiemetic. The rationale for their use is that they will decrease gastric acidity ($\uparrow$ pH) so that if the potential for aspiration is realized, the aspirate will be (hopefully) less of an insult.

MANAGEMENT OF ACTIVE VOMITING

As mentioned earlier, there is that small segment of patients who will vomit perioperatively despite every precautionary measure exercised. We can only hope that their discomfort was at least attenuated by prophylactic antiemetics, exquisite airway management, and conscientious gastric decompression. We can continue to provide supportive care, encourage slow, deep breathing, and minimize movement of the patient. If the patient is experiencing pain, an analgesic (even an opiate) should be administered because pain is not infrequently the cause of the nausea in the early postoperative period. Some patients will not experience relief of nausea until their pain is controlled. Ketorolac (a nonsteroidal antiinflammatory agent) has gained widespread popularity as an analgesic throughout our hospital, and it is a satisfactory alternative if one wishes to avoid the potential emetogenic side effects of opiates.

In summary the problem of PONV is multifactorial, and in any given patient there is likely to be more than a single cause. Therefore, it is likely that more than one therapeutic maneuver will be required. In addition to the use of antiemetics (both prophylactic and during acute vomiting episodes), skillful anesthetic techniques and attention to detail are mandatory. Close follow-up to ensure pain control, adequate hydration, and avoidance of hypotension will prevent further aggravation/accentuation of nausea and vomiting.

Awareness during Anesthesia

DESCRIPTION

It is now a well-recognized fact that some patients can experience varying levels of awareness of intraoperative events. That is, some patients will be able to recall specific details of occurrences that took place during their surgery at a time when they were considered to be unconscious. A significantly larger percentage of patients may experience dreams and/or hallucinations under the influence of anesthetic agents, but awareness appears to be associated with sequelae of greater distress and discomfort.

Furthermore, concern over waking up in the middle of the operation is a common finding during preoperative interviews with patients. In a recent evaluation of the causes of preoperative anxiety in 247 patients,[48] approximately 50% feared they would not be asleep during surgery. More than one half of these were still worried postoperatively about not being asleep during future operations, even though they had just undergone surgery without any such misadventure.

To discuss the incidence of awareness, one must first define the term. Unfortunately, there is variability throughout the anesthetic literature, and the words "awareness," "memory," and "recall" are used inconsistently and often interchangeably. The *Oxford English Dictionary* (1989) defines *awareness* as "the quality or state of being aware; ie, watchful, vigilant, informed, cognizant, or conscious." *Recall* is "remembering what was seen or heard during the period of awareness; a deliberate recollecting of events, sights or sounds," Some patients will spontaneously recall intraoperative events whereas others will do so only after prompting (even hypnosis).[49]

Most estimates of incidence of awareness during anesthesia depend on the patients' ability to recall events when interviewed postoperatively. One study reported a 2% incidence of recall when 500 patients anesthetized with only N_2O (70%)/O_2 (30%) were evaluated.[50] A similar incidence of 2 to 4% was noted when the concentration of N_2O was reduced slightly (60 to 70%).[51] Still others, using a variety of anesthetic techniques on patients having a variety of surgical procedures, have estimated the incidence to be 0.2%[52] to 1.2%.[53,54] A much higher incidence of awareness and recall has been reported in those situations that require light

anesthesia. For example, in obstetric cases where minimal exposure of the fetus to anesthetic agents is desirable, awareness can range from 7 to 28%.[55] During major trauma cases in which severe hemodynamic instability permits little or no anesthesia, recall may be as high as 34%.[56]

Equipment failures/factors may result in inadequate concentrations of anesthesia being delivered to the patient. The level of anesthesia may be purposely kept light (eg, trauma, obstetrics). Some patients may have increased requirements for anesthetics, similar to the variability of responses seen for most drugs. These are the three primary reasons for the cause of awareness during anesthesia. Whichever one applies, awareness occurs because the anesthesia is inadequate, and because the inadequacy cannot by detected by the anesthesiologist.

Recognizing that the patient is aware during anesthesia is the key to preventing intraoperative awareness and recall. After 145 years of anesthetic care, we are struck by the realization that it is not always possible to determine with absolute certainty whether a given patient is unconscious during surgery. Many methods for testing wakefulness have been explored, but each one has fallen short in expectations. There is no (or very low) correlation between responses to command under anesthesia (arm isolated from muscle relaxation[57]) and clinical signs of light anesthesia, for example, increase in blood pressure, heart rate, sweating, or lacrimation. Physical signs are neither predictive nor reliable as an indication of wakefulness. Quite often these signals occur without subsequent complaints of awareness from patients. Furthermore, these signals may be masked or attenuated by the concomitant use of muscle relaxants, β-blockers, narcotics, and vasodilators or vasoconstrictors. Although many studies have attempted to use the electroencephalograph (EEG) as a monitor for anesthetic depth, this too has not proved to be of practical value in identifying consciousness with or without postoperative recall.[58] Some EEG patterns always indicate unconsciousness, but there are no patterns that prove that consciousness is present.[59] Similarly, other physiological measurements have proven to be of little use in predicting anesthetic depth. Sensory evoked responses, auditory evoked potentials, surface electromyography, lower esophageal contractility, and skin conductance responses have all been investigated to determine their utility in predicting consciousness. To date, no one of these emerges as a reliable monitor in the prevention of awareness.

What remains then is to practice prevention of the known causes of awareness. Compulsive check-out of anesthesia equipment, continuous monitoring of inspiratory and expiratory gases, and constant vigilance during an anesthetic will generally eliminate unintended delivery of inadequate concentrations of anesthesia. When feasible, premedicating patients with amnestic drugs such as scopolamine or benzodiazepines will provide an additional safeguard. Supplementation of N_2O/opioid anesthetics with volatile agents intraoperatively will also provide further amnesia. Finally, the use of headphones or earplugs has been advocated by some as one more precautionary measure.

In the unfortunate event that a patient does experience recall of intraoperative events, an appreciation of the potential for extreme distress will facilitate management. Patients who are aware during anesthesia display variable symptoms, but Blacker[60] noted several cases of a traumatic neurotic syndrome in patients who awakened from anesthesia but were rendered paralyzed by muscle relaxants. In these patients there was a high frequency of repetitive nightmares, generalized anxiety, preoccupation with death, and reluctance to discuss their feelings for fear of being considered insane. Remarkable relief was obtained by frank discussion and admission that it is possible to awaken during the course of an anesthetic. Reassurance that they were not insane, and an explanation of how awareness may have occurred were often sufficient to eliminate the neurotic symptoms.

Despite the best efforts at prevention, until there exists a dependable means of documenting unconsciousness, intraoperative awareness is likely to occur in the frequency of 2 to 4% of cases. It is critical that surgeons and anesthesiologists avoid blanket guarantees to patients when discussing this concern preoperatively. Of course honest admission that awareness in the operating room is in fact possible must be at least evenly balanced with a supportive, nurturing demeanor. The intent is not to undermine a patient's confidence in a safe successful surgical outcome.

Malignant Hyperthermia

DESCRIPTION

Perhaps the anesthetic complication to strike the most fear in the most hearts of anesthesiologists (and surgeons) is MH. Although its occurrence is rare (approximately 1:60,000 general anesthetics when succinylcholine is used and 1:220,000 general anesthetics when succinylcholine is avoided[61]), the full-blown syndrome is a catastrophic event never to be forgotten once experienced. Fortunately, remarkable progress has been made in the recognition and treatment of MH crises, specifically in the form of dantrolene therapy. Mortality rates have declined from 80% in the 1960s to less than 10% in the 1980s.[62]

Malignant hyperthermia is described as a skeletal muscle defect, genetic in origin, that results in a hypermetabolic state when triggered by specific anesthetic agents. The principal triggering drugs are succinylcholine and all the volatile anesthetics. The details of the biochemical lesion are not completely understood, but there is an abnormal release of calcium from the sarcoplasmic reticulum resulting in a marked elevation of intracellular calcium.[63] This elevation of calcium activates the cell's contractile apparatus and metabolic processes, with consumption of O_2 and hydrolysis of adenosine triphosphate (ATP), producing heat, carbon dioxide (CO_2), and lactic acid (Fig. 23–6). As ATP levels fall, the lack of energy substrate for basal metabolic processes results in loss of functional integrity of the cell and release of intracellular contents (CPK, K^+, Ca^{++}, myoglobin). Eventually the calcium delivered to the myoplasm overwhelms the

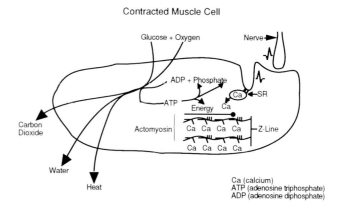

Contracted Muscle Cell

Ca (calcium)
ATP (adenosine triphosphate)
ADP (adenosine diphosphate)

Figure 23–6. In an MH reaction, the muscle cells remain "locked" in the contracted state, producing large amounts of CO_2, H_2O, and heat (from Britt[74]).

energy-dependent calcium-sequestering processes and muscle contracture is prolonged. According to Muller,[64] "If the local temperature elevation coincident with this rapid synthesis and breakdown of high energy phosphate bonds is severe enough, contracture can be perpetuated in a calcium-independent manner, and irreversible contracture ensues."

ANTICIPATION

It is commonly accepted that malignant hyperthermia susceptibility (MHS) is an inherited disorder, usually with familial involvement, but no single pattern of genetic transfer universally applies to all reported cases. The majority are clearly autosomal dominant and the next largest group probably autosomal dominant, both together accounting for approximately 50% of cases.[65] The remainder suggest recessive or multifactorial inheritance, or no genetic pattern at all. Furthermore, even in apparently dominant cases, MH crises are not seen in all susceptible patients in all presumably triggering circumstances. It would seem that there are additional influential factors that must coincide at the same time and place with the inherited disposition to result in an MH event.

Because of the confusing inheritance patterns, it is difficult to select those family members who should undergo preoperative MHS testing. There are some evaluations that may shed light on the susceptibility of any given patient. The most reliable of these is muscle biopsy with in vitro halothane and halothane-caffeine testing, but it is expensive, time-consuming, and inconvenient. Because it is not 100% reliable (and patients with negative muscle biopsy tests have gone on to develop MH syndrome) many anesthesiologists treat all patients with a positive family history as MH susceptible, regardless of the results of muscle biopsy testing. Plasma creatine kinase (CK) levels are still used in an attempt to predict MHS, but both false negatives and false positives make decision-making as arbitrary as if the CK results were not obtained.

The desire for a reliable diagnosis of MH susceptibility preoperatively is based on (1) the desire to provide more accurate preoperative counseling to patients and their families concerning risks, outcomes, planned management, and expectations; (2) the desire to avoid the use of dantrolene sodium (however benign) if its use is not necessary; (3) the desire to avoid invasive monitoring (central venous lines, arterial lines, Foley catheters, etc) if these are not truly indicated; and (4) the desire to select more routine anesthetic agents and equipment. Until the day when preoperative diagnosis is more reliable, it seems advisable to treat MH "suspicious" patients as if they are susceptible. Therefore, after careful history-taking, one should anticipate the possibility of MH in any patient who has either a personal past history suggestive of MH or who has a close family member with a history suggestive of MH.

In addition, certain neuromuscular disorders are noted to have an association with MH. These include Duchenne muscular dystrophy, myotonia congenita, central core disease, Evan Syndrome, King Syndrome, and ocular strabismus. It has been advocated that a patient carrying one of these diagnoses be presumed to be MH susceptible.

RECOGNITION

One of the earliest warning signs is masseter muscle rigidity (MMR), which is a contraction of masseter muscles following a dose of succinylcholine. It may be seen in adults but is more commonly seen in children who have undergone an inhalational induction with halothane followed by IV succinylcholine to facilitate intubation. There is a gradation of jaw tightness, and those patients who exhibit masseter spasm but whose mouths can still be opened for laryngoscopy and intubation (even if difficult) are probably normal. In one investigation, approximately 1% of children experienced masseter contraction of this moderate degree.[65] Those children whose masseter spasm prevented their mouth from being opened were most worrisome. Over one half of these children had muscle biopsies consistent with MH.[66] Those children with jaws tight enough to preclude intubation are appropriately designated as exhibiting MMR.

Should MMR occur, all investigators advise the prudence of immediately discontinuing the offending triggering agents and aborting an elective surgical procedure.[66–69] There are no available data to support the suggestion that converting to a nontriggering anesthetic technique is a safe alternative (although it may be the only alternative during emergency surgery that must continue). Patients exhibiting MMR should then be referred for muscle biopsy and in vitro contracture tests in addition to serial CK enzyme levels (Tables 23–3, 23–4).

An MH crisis may occur without the prelude of masseter muscle spasm, particularly when the halothane-succinylcholine combination is not utilized (see Fig. 23–8). The increased metabolic rate will result in signs similar to light anesthesia, that is, a hyperdynamic circulation with tachycardia and hypertension. The earliest reliable sign is an inappropriate increase in CO_2 production. This will be detected by rising end-tidal CO_2 concentration (capnometry is fairly standard during the administration of all general

Table 23–3. Masseter Muscle Rigidity—Elective Surgery

1. Stop triggering drugs.
2. Abort procedure.
3. Ventilate with clean machine or Mapleson system with high flow.
4. Monitor: ECG, BP, T° (core), skin color, muscle tone, ABG/VBG, CK, BUN, Cr, Lytes, CA^{++}, lactate, urine color (myoglobin).
5. Hold dantrolene if stable.
6. Monitor in ICU × 24 h. Force diuresis with fluids, CK at 6, 12, 24 h. Other labs PRN.
7. CK at 6, 12, 24 h. Look for CK > 20 000 IU/L; other labs PRN.
8. Family counseling—muscle biopsy.

BP = blood pressure, ABG/VBG = arterial blood gas/venous blood gas, CK = creatinine kinase, BUN = blood urea nitrogen, Cr = creatinine, PRN = as needed.
From Kaplan.[62]

Table 23–4. Masseter Muscle Rigidity—Emergency Surgery

1. Stop triggering drugs.
2. Hyperventilate by mask.
3. MH machine and extra personnel.
4. Monitor: EKG, BP, T° (core) muscle tone, ABG/VBG, CK.
5. Use safe agents.
6. Dantrolene 2.5 mg/kg IV.
7. Monitor in ICU × 24 h as per no. 4.
8. Family counseling—muscle biopsy.

MH = malignant hyperthermia, BP = blood pressure, ABG/VBG = arterial blood gas/venous blood gas, CK = creatinine kinase.
From Kaplan.[62]

anesthetics) in the patient whose ventilation is controlled. The spontaneously breathing patient will increase minute ventilation to eliminate the CO_2 (temporary compensation may result in stable end-tidal CO_2 until the crisis is more advanced). The canister containing CO_2-absorbent on the anesthesia machine may be noted to be warm or rapidly exhausted. Fever is a later sign, and its presence is rather inconsistent. The temperature elevation *per se* probably reflects the magnitude of the MH reaction, and is roughly correlated with mortality[64] (Fig. 23–7). Other disturbing elements frequently seen in the full-blown MH crisis include cardiac dysrhythmias, respiratory **and** metabolic acidosis, cyanosis or mottling, and myoglobinuria. There may be late complications of a severe MH episode, such as rhabdomyolysis, disseminated intravascular coagulation (DIC), cerebral edema, renal failure, and pulmonary edema (Table 23–5).[62]

TREATMENT

Prevention. For patients with a positive or suspicious history of MHS, anticipation and prevention of an MH crisis is the preferred treatment. All patients with a known history of a previous MH episode or positive *in vitro* muscle contracture test should receive IV dantrolene (2.5 mg/kg) 30 minutes prior to induction, if the surgical procedure is determined to be particularly physiologically stressful or longer than 2

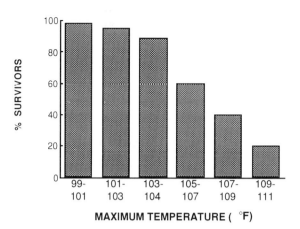

Figure 23–7. Correlation of the survival of MH patients with maximal temperature elevation (from Mueller[64]).

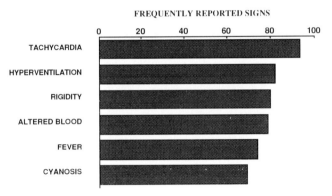

FREQUENTLY REPORTED SIGNS

Figure 23–8. Clinical signs that may indicate the onset of MH (from Mueller[62]).

Table 23–5. Signs of Malignant Hyperthermia

Tachycardia*	Metabolic acidosis*
Tachypnea*	Respiratory acidosis*
Fever*	Central venous desaturation*
Rigidity*	Central venous hypercarbia*
Arrhythmias	↑ End-tidal CO_2*
Cyanosis	Hyperkalemia
Skin mottling	Myoglobinemia
Massetter muscle rigidity	↑ CK
Sweating	Unstable BP

CK = creatinine kinase, BP = blood pressure.

From Kaplan.[62]

*Primary signs of malignant hyperthermia.

hours in duration.[62] Even if the procedure is brief and of minimal physiological insult, patients who are MH susceptible **and** who have other underlying conditions (coronary artery disease, cerebrovascular disease, renal failure), which would cause them to poorly withstand even mild hypermetabolism, should also receive dantrolene prophylaxis.[62] A vapor-free anesthesia machine should be used during the surgery and an MH cart containing all the necessary drugs, fluids, and equipment essential in treating an MH crisis should be at

hand. Mandatory monitoring includes all routine anesthetic monitors and specifically, capnography and temperature probe (at many institutions and hospitals, these also are customary and routine monitors). Indwelling arterial lines or central venous lines are indicated based on the patient's general health and the nature and duration of the proposed procedure.

The general anesthetic technique employed should be MH trigger-free. With the exception of succinylcholine and all the volatile anesthetic agents except N_2O (halothane, enflurane, isoflurane, methoxyflurane), most of the commonly used drugs are safe to use. Some controversy surrounds amide local anesthetics (prilocaine, lidocaine, mepivocaine, bupivacaine, etidocaine) but continuing experience with these agents indicates that amides may be safe as well. Should a full-blown MH crisis occur, treatment is based on the recommendation published by the Malignant Hyperthermia Association of the United States (MHAUS), as indicated in Figure 23–9.

It is critical to maintain a urine output of at least 2 mL/kg/h. The mannitol in the dantrolene preparation combined with recommended IV fluid therapy should establish a brisk diuresis. Furosemide may be added to the resuscitation if urine volume is too low. Sinus tachycardia is tolerated because cardiac output must be adequate to allow for increased heat and gas production/exchange accompanying this hypermetabolic state. A specific caution against the use of verapamil in patients who have received dantrolene is warranted. Verapamil and dantrolene have been reported to precipitate hyperkalemia and cardiovascular collapse in some experiments.[70,71] As indicated by the MHAUS recommendations, patients who have experienced an acute MH episode should be observed in an intensive care setting as continued treatment of delayed complications may be required.

CONCLUSION

Despite tremendous advances in technology, pharmacology, and anesthetic techniques, anesthetic complications continue to occur today and *will* continue to occur in the future. More sophisticated monitoring has enabled anesthesiologists to detect impending mishaps more easily and at earlier stages, but the ever-increasing age and complex pathology of our patients present continuously changing dilemmas in the nature and extent of adverse events. The potential for unintended insult remains a trademark of all invasive subspecialties in the practice of medicine.

We can take great pride in the accomplishments made over the years in the management of untoward events. Consider the following exerpt from the *Medical Times and Gazette* in 1856:

> On one occasion, while I was removing a scirrhous tumor, the patient, who was rather advanced in life, got an overdose of chloroform, . . . and I do believe that her recovery was owing entirely to injecting a glass of brandy and water into the rectum. The accident happened owing to the gentleman who had charge of the chloroform getting so interested in the dissection that he forgot to raise the towel off her face till respiration had become imperceptible.[72,73]

LOOK FOR • tachycardia • muscle stiffness • hypercarbia • tachypnea • cardiac dysrhythmias • respiratory metabolic acidosis • fever • unstable/rising blood pressure • cyanosis/mottling • myoglobinuria

Emergency Therapy for
Malignant Hyperthermia
Revised 1993
ACUTE TREATMENT

1. Immediately discontinue all volatile inhalation anesthetics and succinylcholine. Hyperventilate with 100% oxygen at high gas flows; at least 10l/min. The circle system and CO_2 absorbent need not be changed.
2. Administer dantrolene sodium 2-3 mg/kg initial bolus rapidly with increments up to 10 mg/kg total. Continue to administer dantrolene until signs of MH (e.g. tachycardia, rigidity, increased end-tidal CO_2, and temperature elevation) are controlled. Occasionally, a total dose greater than 10 mg/kg may be needed. Each vial of dantrolene contains 20 mg of dantrolene and 3 grams mannitol. Each vial should be mixed with 60 mL of sterile water for injection USP without a bacteriostatic agent.
3. Administer bicarbonate to correct metabolic acidosis as guided by blood gas analysis. In the absence of blood gas analysis, 1-2 mEq/kg should be administered.
4. Simultaneous with the above, actively cool the hyperthermic patient. Use IV iced saline (not Ringer's lactate) 15 mL/kg q 15 min. X 3.
   a. Lavage stomach, bladder, rectum and open cavities with iced saline as appropriate.
   b. Surface cool with ice and hypothermia blanket.
   c. Monitor closely since overvigorous treatment may lead to hypothermia.
5. Dysrhythmias will usually respond to treatment of acidosis and hyperkalemia. If they persist or are life threatening, standard anti-arrhythmic agents may be used, with the exception of calcium channel blockers (may cause hyperkalemia and CV collapse).
6. Determine and monitor end-tidal CO_2, arterial, central or femoral venous blood gases, serum potassium, calcium, clotting studies and urine output.
7. Hyperkalemia is common and should be treated with hyperventilation, bicarbonate, intravenous glucose and insulin (10 units regular insulin in 50 mL 50% glucose titrated to potassium level). Life threatening hyperkalemia may also be treated with calcium administration (e.g. 2-5 mg/kg of $CaCl_2$).
8. Ensure urine output of greater than 2 mL/kg/hr. Consider central venous or PA monitoring because of fluid shifts and hemodynamic instability that may occur.
9. Boys less than 9 years of age who experience sudden cardiac arrest after succinylcholine in the absence of hypoxemia should be treated for acute hyperkalemia first. In this situation calcium chloride should be administered along with other means to reduce serum potassium. They should be presumed to have subclinical muscular dystrophy.

POST ACUTE PHASE

A. Observe the patient in and ICU setting for at least 24 hours since recrudescence of MH may occur, particularly following a fulminant case resistant to treatment.
B. Administer dantrolene 1 mg/kg IV q 6 hours for 24-48 hours post episode. After that, oral dantrolene 1 mg/kg q 6 hours may be used for 24 hours as necessary.
C. Follow ABG, CK, potassium, calcium, urine and serum myoglobin, clotting studies and core body temperature until such time as they return to normal values (e.g. q 6 hours). Central temperature (e.g. rectal, esophageal) should be continuously monitored until stable.
D. counsel the patient and family regarding MH and further precautions. Refer the patient to MHAUS. Fill out and Adverse Metabolic Reaction to Anesthesia (AMRA) report available through the North American Malignant Hyperthermia Registry (717) 531-6936.

CAUTION: This protocol may not apply to every patient and must of necessity be altered according to specific patient needs.

Names of on-call physicians available to consult in MH emergencies may be obtained 24 hours a day through:

MEDIC ALERT
FOUNDATION INTERNATIONAL
(209) 634-4917
Ask for: INDEX ZERO

For Non-Emergency or Patient Referral Calls:
MHAUS
(203) 847-0407
P.O. Box 191
Westport, CT 06881-0191

Figure 23–9. 1993 MHAUS revision of emergency therapy for MH (from MHAUS[75]).

Modern therapy has improved considerably! Resuscitation for respiratory arrest today would entail quite different maneuvers. The unchanging aspect of that scenario though, as crucial today as it was over a century ago, is the necessity for vigilance on the part of the anesthetist. Not conversation nor loud music nor even the intrigue of fascinating surgery can be permitted to distract attention from the patient's welfare. And so our task remains to anticipate, to recognize, and then to treat the complications always attendant to procedures and drugs that so drastically alter basic physiology.

Acknowledgement. Figure 23–6 was reproduced from the *Canadian Journal of Anaesthesia* (1985;32:669). Figure 23–9 was reproduced from MHAUS.

REFERENCES

1. Harrison GC. Death attributable to anaesthesia: a ten-year survey, 1967–1976. *Anesthesiology.* 1990;72:828–833.
2. Utting JE, Gray TC, Shelly FC. Human misadventure in anaesthesia. *Can J Anaesth.* 1979;26:472–478.
3. Holland R. Anaesthesia related mortality in Australia. *Int Anesthesiol Clin.* 1984;22:61–71.
4. Keinan RL, Bovan CP. Cardiac arrest due to anesthesia. A study of incidence and causes. *JAMA.* 1985;253:2373–2377.
5. Caplan RA, Posner KL, et al. Adverse respiratory events in anesthesia: a closed claims analysis. *Anesthesiology.* 1990;72:828–833.
6. Olsson GL, Hallen B. Laryngospasm during anesthesia: a computer-aided incidence study in 136,929 patients. *Acta Anaesth Scand.* 1984;28:567.

7. Fink BR. The etiology and treatment of laryngeal spasm. *Anesthesiology.* 1956;17:569–577.

8. Staffel JG, Weissler MC, Tyler EP, Drake AF. The prevention of postoperative stridor and laryngospasm with topical lidocaine. *Arch Otolaryngol Head Neck Surg.* 1991;117:1123–1128.

9. Lee KWT, Downes JJ. Pulmonary edema secondary to laryngospasm in children. *Anesthesiology.* 1983;59:347–349.

10. Travis KW, Todres ED, Shannon DC. Pulmonary edema associated with croup and epiglottitis. *Pediatrics.* 1977;59:695.

11. Soliman MG, Richer P. Epiglottis and pulmonary edema in children. *Can J Anaesth.* 1978;25:270.

12. Cozanitis DA, Leijala M, Pesonen E, et al. Acute pulmonary edema due to laryngeal spasm. *Anaesthesia.* 1982;37:1198, 1199.

13. Luke MJ, Mebrizi A, Giger GM Jr, et al. Chronic nasopharyngeal obstruction as a cause of cardiomegaly, corpulmonale, and pulmonary edema. *Pediatrics.* 1966;37:762.

14. Oswalt E, Gates A, Holmstrom MG. Pulmonary edema as a complication of acute airway obstruction. *JAMA.* 1977;238:1833–1835.

15. Melnick BM. Postlaryngospasm pulmonary edema in adults (letter). *Anesthesiology.* 1984;60:516, 517.

16. Jackson FN, Rowland V, Corssen C. Laryngospasm-induced pulmonary edema. *Chest.* 1980;78:819–821.

17. Lorch DG, Sahn SA. Post-extubation pulmonary edema following anesthesia induced by upper airway obstruction. *Chest.* 1986;90:802–805.

18. Galvis AG, Stool SE, Bluestone CD. Pulmonary edema following relief of acute upper airway obstruction. *Ann Otol.* 1980;89:124–128.

19. Mallampati SR, Gatt SP, Gugino LD, et al. A clinical sign to predict difficult tracheal intubation: a prospective study. *Can J Anaesth.* 1985;32:429–434.

20. Samson GLT, Young JRB. Difficult tracheal intubation: a retrospective study. *Anesthesia.* 1987;42:487–490.

21. Cormack RS, Lehane J. Difficult tracheal intubation in obstetrics. *Anaesthesia.* 1984;39:1105–1111.

22. Cohen SM, Zaurito CE, Segil LJ. Oral exam to predict difficult intubations: a large prospective study (abstract). *Anesthesiology.* 1989;71:A937.

23. Finucane BT, Santora AH. *Evaluation of the Airway Prior to Intubation: Principles of Airway Management.* Philadelphia, Pa: FA Norris Co; 1988:69–83.

24. Mathew M, Hanna LS, Aldrete JA. Preoperative indices to anticipate a difficult tracheal intubation. *Anesth Analg.* 1989;68:5187.

25. Patil VU, Stehling LC, Zauder HL, Techniques of endotracheal intubation. In: *Fiberoptic Endoscopy in Anaesthesia.* Chicago, Ill: Year Book Medical Publishers, Inc; 1983:79.

26. Cobley M, Vaughan RS. Recognition and management of difficult airway problems. *Br J Anaesthesia.* 1992;68:90–97.

27. Palazzo MGA, Strunin L. Anaesthesia and emesis. I: etiology. *Can J Anaesth.* 1984;31:178–187.

28. White PF, Shafer A. Nausea and vomiting: causes and prophylaxis. *Semin Anesth.* 1987;4:300–308.

29. Purkis IE. Factors that influence postoperative vomiting. *Can J Anaesth.* 1964;11:335–353.

30. Burtles R, Peckett BW. Postoperative vomiting. *Br J Anaesth.* 1957;29:114–123.

31. Bellville JW, Bross IDJ, Howlands WS. Postoperative nausea and vomiting. Five factors related to postoperative nausea and vomiting. *Anesthesiology.* 1960;21:186–193.

32. Knapp MR, Beecher HK. Postanaesthetic nausea vomiting and retching. *JAMA.* 1960;160:376–385.

33. Bellville JW. Postanaesthetic nausea and vomiting. *Anesthesiology.* 1961;22:773–780.

34. Vance JP, Neill RS, Norris W. The incidence and etiology of postoperative nausea and vomiting in a plastic surgical unit. *Br J Plast Surg.* 1973;26:336–339.

35. McKenzie R, et al. Antiemetic effectiveness of intramuscular hydroxyzine compared with intramuscular droperidol. *Anesth Analg.* 1981;60:783–788.

36. Riding JE. Postoperative vomiting. *Proc R Soc Med.* 1960;53:671–677.

37. Costello DJ, Borison HL. Naloxone antagonizes narcotic self blockade of emetics in the cat. *J Pharmacol Exp Ther.* 1977;203:223–230.

38. Harris AL. Cytotoxic therapy induced vomiting is mediated via enkephalin pathways. *Lancet.* 1982;1:714–716.

39. Lonie DS, Harper NJN. Nitrous oxide anaesthesia and vomiting. *Anaesthesia.* 1986;41:703–707.

40. Muir JJ, Warner MA, et al. Role of nitrous oxide and other factors in postoperative, nausea and vomiting; a randomized and blinded prospective study. *Anesthesiology.* 1987;66:513–518.

41. Pollard J. Clinical evaluation of intravenous vs. inhalational anesthesia in the ambulatory surgical unit: a multicenter-study. *Curr Ther Res.* 1984;36:617–626.

42. Doze VA, Westphal LM, White PF. Comparison of Propofol with methohexital for outpatient anaesthesia. *Anesth Analg.* 1986;65:1189–1195.

43. Korttila K, Östman PL, et al. Randomized comparison of outcome after Propofol-nitrous oxide or Enflurane-nitrous oxide anaesthesia in operations of long duration. *Can J Anaesth.* 1989;36:651–657.

44. Doze VA, White PF. Comparison of Propofol with thiopental-isoflurane for induction and maintenance of outpatient anesthesia. *Anesthesiology.* 1986;65:A544.

45. Keats AS. Preoperative use of antiemetics (editorial). *Anesthesiology.* 1960;21:213.

46. Scuderi P, Wetchler B, et al. Treatment of postoperative nausea and vomiting after outpatient surgery with the 5-HT$_3$ antagonist Ondansetron. *Anesthesiology.* 1993;78:15–20.

47. McKenzie R, Kovac A, et al. Comparison of Ondansetron vs. placebo to prevent postoperative nausea and vomiting in women undergoing ambulatory gynecologic surgery. *Anesthesiology.* 1993;78:21–28.

48. McCleane GJ, Cooper R. The nature of preoperative anxiety. *Anaesthesia.* 1990;45:153–155.

49. Levinson BW. States of awareness during general anaesthesia. *Br J Anaesth.* 1965;37:544–546.

50. Utting JE. Awareness. In: Rosen M, Lunn JN, eds. *Clinical Aspects, Consciousness, Awareness, and Pain in General Anaesthesia.* London: Butterworths; 1987:171–179.

51. Brice DD, Hetherington RR, Utting JE. A simple study of awareness and dreaming during anaesthesia. *Br J Anaesth.* 1970;42:535–542.

52. Lui WHD, Thorp TAS, Graham SG, Aitkenhead AR. Incidence of awareness with recall during general anaesthesia. *Anaesthesia.* 1991;46:435–437.

53. Wilson SL, Vaughan RW, Stephen CR. Awareness, dreams and hallucinations associated with general anesthesia. *Anesth Analg.* 1975;54:609–616.

54. Hutchinson R. Awareness during surgery: a study of its incidence. *Br J Anaesth.* 1969;33:463–469.

55. Bogod DG, Orton JK, Yau HM, Oh TE. Detecting awareness during general anaesthetic cesarean section. An evaluation of two methods. *Anaesthesia.* 1990;45:279–284.

56. Bogetz MS, Katz JA. Recall of surgery of major trauma. *Anesthesiology.* 1984;61:6–9.

57. Breckenridge J, Aitkenhead AR. Isolated forearm technique for detection of wakefulness during general anaesthesia. *Br J Anaesth.* 1981;53:665–666,.

58. Ghoneim MM, Block RI. Learning and consciousness during general anesthesia. *Anesthesiology.* 1992;76:279–305.

59. Plourde G. Depth of anaesthesia (editorial). *Can J Anaesth.* 1991;38:270–274.

60. Blacker RS. On awakening paralyzed during surgery: a syndrome of traumatic neurosis. *JAMA*. 1975;234:67, 68.

61. Ording H. Incidence of malignant hyperthermia in Denmark. *Anesth Analg*. 1985;64:700.

62. Kaplan RF. Hypothermia/hyperthermia. In: Gravenstein N, ed. *Manual of Complications During Anesthesia*. Philadelphia, Pa: JB Lippincott Co; 1991:121–150.

63. Lopez JR, Acamo L, et al. Intracellular ionized calcium concentration in muscles from humans with malignant hyperthermia. *Muscle Nerve*. 1985;8:355.

64. Mueller RA. How to identify malignant hyperthermia. In: Vaughan, Kirby, Brown, eds. *Problems in Anesthesia, Perioperative Problems/Catastrophes*. Philadelphia, Pa: JB Lippincott Co; 1987:233–244.

65. Carroll JB. Increased incidence of masseter spasm in children with strabismus anesthetized with halothane and succinylcholine. *Anesthesiology*. 1987;67:559.

66. Fleivellen EH, Nelson TE. Masseter spasm induced by succinylcholine in children: contracture testing for malignant hyperthermia: report of six cases. *Can J Anaesth*. 1982;29:42.

67. Ellis FR, Halsall PJ. Suxamethonium spasm: a differential diagnostic conundrum. *Br J Anaesth*. 1984;56:381–383.

68. Fleivellen EH, Nelson TE. Halothane-succinylcholine induced masseter spasm: indicative of malignant hyperthermia susceptibility? *Anesth Analg*. 1984;63:693–697.

69. Rosenberg H, Reed S. *In vitro* contracture tests for susceptibility to malignant hyperthermia. *Anesth Analg*. 1983;62:415–420.

70. Saltzman LS, Kates RA, Corke BC, et al. Hyperkalemia and cardiovascular collapse after verapamil and dantrolene administration in surine. *Anesth Analg*. 1984;63:473.

71. Gallant WM, Foldes FF, Rempel WE, et al. Verapamil is not a therapeutic adjunct to dantrolene in porcine malignant hyperthermia. *Anesth Analg*. 1985;64:601.

72. Lyman HM. *Artificial Anaesthesia and Anaesthetics*. New York, NY: William Wood and Co; 1881:57.

73. Lyman HM. Artificial anaesthesia and anaesthetics. *Med Times Gazette*. 1856:652.

74. Britt BA. Malignant hyperthermia. *Can Anaesth Soc J*. 1985;32:669.

75. MHAUS. *1993 Revision of Emergency Therapy for Malignant Hyperthermia*. MHAUS: 1993.

24 Complications of Head and Neck Imaging

Mauricio Castillo, M.D., Patricia A. Hudgins, M.D.

The complications of imaging procedures performed to evaluate pathology of the head and neck reflect those encountered in radiology in general as multiple imaging modalities are employed for these patients. This chapter begins by addressing complications from the simplest procedures such as contrast swallows and sialography. Contrast swallows are especially important in the postsurgical patient. Sialograms are only rarely performed, as computed tomography and magnetic resonance imaging have become the mainstays in the evaluation of salivary gland pathology. Complications associated with computed tomography are mostly related to the administration of iodinated contrast material, which, for practical purposes, is needed in most patients with head and neck pathology. Magnetic resonance is becoming important in head and neck pathology and is now considered the imaging method of choice in the evaluation of carcinomas arising above the soft palate. Invasive procedures in head and neck include cisternograms and diagnostic and therapeutic angiograms. Transcatheter embolizations are now done routinely before surgery for nasopharyngeal angiofibromas, arteriovenous malformations, and some base of the skull meningiomas.

ORAL CONTRAST SWALLOWS

Complications of oral contrast agents are rare and are related to either contrast media aspiration or to the extravasation of contrast into an extraluminal location; (Figs. 24–1 to 24–3). Patients who aspirate or have a perforation will usually have an underlying history of aspiration pneumonias.

Barium sulfate is the contrast agent used for esophageal and upper gastrointestinal examinations. Mediastinitis and mediastinal empyema are extremely serious complications of the extravasation of barium sulfate. Therefore, if extravasation is suspected, a water-soluble iodinated contrast agent should be used. Extravasation of water-soluble iodinated contrast material into the mediastinum results only in a mild inflammatory reaction.[1] However, water-soluble agents are hypertonic and, if aspirated, may lead to acute pulmonary edema.[1] If forewarned about the potential for aspiration or

for a tracheobronchial fistula, the radiologist will choose a barium-based contrast agent for the esophageal swallow.

SIALOGRAPHY

Although sialography is no longer a commonly performed procedure, it continues to be the only imaging method capable of diagnosing abnormalities of the salivary ductal system (ie, chronic sialadenitis, sialosis, and immune-mediated disorders).[2] Radiation exposure from either a conventional radiographic sialogram or a computed tomographic (CT) sialogram is insignificant (fluoroscopy: 2 to 3 R/min to the surface of the skin).[1]

The exact number of patients who will suffer an allergic reaction to the contrast media utilized for sialography is not known, but from our personal experience it tends to be extremely low. Patients with known sensitivity to iodinated compounds are therefore better evaluated with noncontrast enhanced CT or magnetic resonance imaging (MRI). A documented allergy to radiographic contrast materials is considered by most authorities to be a contraindication to sialography.[2–4] If a patient reports a tendency to faint, the physician performing the sialogram should be prepared to treat a vagal-mediated reaction. Administration of intravenous fluids and atropine intramuscularly (0.6 to 1.2 mg) will generally suffice.[4]

Sialography should not be performed in the presence of an active infection or inflammation of the salivary glands. Propagation of the infection is likely, besides the majority of these patients are in pain and will not tolerate the examination. Under these conditions the examination will generally be of suboptimal quality. The fragility of the ductal epithelium makes extravasation of contrast material likely, therefore increasing the risk of disseminating the infectious/inflammatory process.

Extravasation of contrast material has been implicated in the formation of granulomas.[5] This problem seems to be related to the use of earlier oily contrast media (particularly Ethiodol, Lipiodol, and Pantopaque)[2] and in our experience it is not seen when newer water-soluble contrast materials

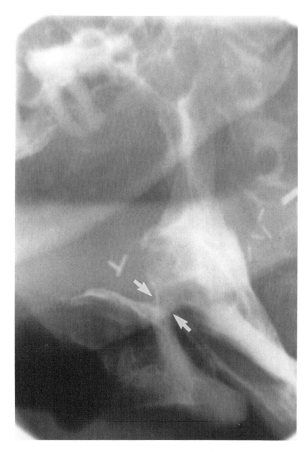

Figure 24–1. Oblique view from the barium swallow in a case of postoperative fistula. Middle-aged male following cervical esophageal bypass with small bowel for laryngeal cancer. Arrows point to postoperative fistula.

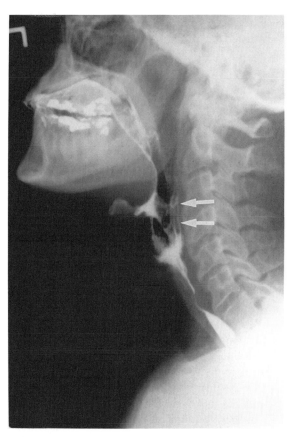

Figure 24–2. Lateral view from the esophagogram in a patient with hypopharyngeal perforation following rigid endoscopy. Notice contrast tracking dorsal to hypopharynx in prevertebral soft tissues (arrow).

(Renografin, Hypaque, or ideally Sinografin) are used. Of the lipid-based contrast media, Lipiodol and Pantopaque have a much higher incidence of eliciting foreign body salivary parenchymal reactions.[2] However, this type of reaction is only seen if a perforation has occurred. If a CT study is to follow the sialogram, lipid-based contrast media are desirable as water-soluble contrast media tend to give less opacification and do not remain in the ductal system for very long. Some patients complain of localized discomfort and/or pain for a few hours after the procedure. These symptoms are probably related to the distention of the salivary ductal system or to a minor and sterile inflammatory reaction to the contrast material (Fig. 24–4). Occasionally, iodinated contrast material (especially lipid-based ones) may be retained within the gland and interfere with future thyroid function tests.[4] During the cannulation of the ducts, the person performing the examination must be careful and gentle as application of undue force will certainly result in perforations with subsequent extravasation of the contrast material into the subcutaneous tissues. De novo infections following sialography are rare occurrences. Most infections are probably due to the inadvertent injection of contrast material into a gland that is subclinically infected.[3] As stated before, patients may experience mild discomfort in the immediate hours that follow a sialogram.

If increasing discomfort, swelling, and dull aching are present 24 to 36 hours after the examination, the patient should contact the referring physician who will probably prescribe a short course of antibiotics.

COMPUTED TOMOGRAPHY

When a patient undergoes a conventional radiographic study, the surface of the body located directly in front of the x-ray tube receives the maximum radiation exposure. Conversely, the surface of the body opposite the source of x-ray receives the least amount of radiation. During CT scanning, the x-ray tube rotates and therefore every area of the patient's skin is exposed and will receive a maximum amount of radiation.[6] In CT studies, both the skin and midbody radiation doses are higher than those received during conventional radiographic procedures.[7] This is secondary to the higher energy of the radiation used for CT, which is achieved by heavy filtration. However, the integral dose for CT studies is lower than that received during other x-ray procedures owing to the small area of tissue radiated during the acquisition of each slice. For comparison purposes, a CT study delivers approximately 8 rads (0.08 Gy) per examination whereas a chest radiograph delivers 0.05 rads (0.0005 Gy) a barium enema 15 to 20 rads

Table 24–1. Summary of Complications Related to Diagnostic Imaging Procedures of the Head and Neck

PROCEDURE	LOCAL COMPLICATIONS	SYSTEMIC COMPLICATIONS
Contrast swallow	Mediastinitis, mediastinal abscess, pulmonary edema (with water-soluble agents)	Allergic reaction (extremely rare)*
Sialogram	Acinarization, extravasation, granuloma formation, infection, abscess	Vagal reaction, allergic reaction†
CT	Extravasation of contract media at site of injection, aspiration pneumonia‡	Allergic reaction,† renal toxicity†
Cisternography	CSF leak	Headache, allergic reaction,† alteration of mental status
MRI	Aspiration pneumonia,‡ damage to or by ferromagnetic devices	Claustrophobia, allergic reaction§
Angiography (including therapeutic procedures)	Pain, intimal tear, subintimal hematoma, arterial thombosis, pseudoaneurysm or fistula formation, dissection, arterial rupture, groin hematoma, temporary or permanent neurological deficit, skin necrosis, infection	Allergic reaction,† vagal reaction, renal toxicity†

* Related to either iodine or barium-based contrast agents.
† Related to iodinated contrast media.
‡ Related to inability to handle secretions in supine position.
§ Related to Gadolinium-DTPA.

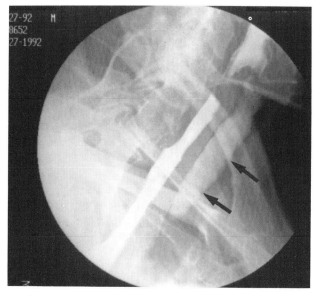

Figure 24–3. Oblique view from a barium swallow showing marked tracheal aspiration. Opacification of trachea (arrows) during an esophageal swallow performed for dysphagia.

(0.15 to 0.2 Gy) and most angiographic procedures deliver more than 75 rads (0.75 Gy).[7]

A CT study performed for the evaluation of head and neck disease usually lasts approximately 10 to 15 minutes. Spiral or volumetric CT shortens acquisition time to 30 to 40 seconds. During this time, patients will be on their back and it is conceivable that the inability to swallow secretions may lead to coughing spells or aspiration. In our experience, this is not a significant problem, especially if spiral CT is available.

The major concerns during a CT study are those related to the administration of iodinated contrast compounds. All patients undergoing a conventional CT study of the neck receive a relatively large dose of contrast material (150 to 200 mL, 60% iodine) to opacify the vessels and differentiate them from adjacent structures, mainly lymph nodes. For spiral CT studies, one may achieve good vessel opacification with only one third of the above dose.

Conventional contrast media are hyperosmolar (five to eight times the osmolality of plasma).[8] Even the new so-called "low-osmolar" iodinated contrast materials have an osmolality two to three times higher than that of plasma.[8] Injection of large volumes of contrast media is generally required for conventional CT imaging and may result in a shift of extravascular water into the intravascular space. Adverse effects related to this shift of water include vasodilation, hemodilution, hypervolemia, and crenation of erythrocytes.[8] Moreover, immediately following the injection of conventional contrast media, there may be a 10% to 15% increase in the total blood volume leading to increased cardiac venous return.[9] This effect may lead to changes in cardiac output, tissue anoxia, and systemic hypotension.[8] Low-osmolar contrast agents reduce systemic vasodilation and are recommended for patients with compromised cardiac output.[9] Rapid intravenous injection of contrast media (generally required in the ear, nose, and throat [ENT] patient) may produce damage to the endothelial cells of the lung capillaries leading to the release of substances that may precipitate a severe reaction.[10] All of the above-described effects can be reduced by using low-osmolar contrast materials or spiral CT and reducing the dose.

Contrast materials inhibit the thrombin-fibrinogen reaction as well as platelet aggregation.[11] This effect is probably clinically insignificant but does play an important role during angiography. In vitro, nonionic low-osmolar contrast media have a lesser anticoagulant effect than conventional radiographic contrasts and thus may lead to the formation of clots in angiographic catheters and wires.[12]

All conventional iodinated contrast agents are ionic. Ion toxicity may lead to brain and heart conduction abnormalities.[8] These problems can be avoided by utilizing several of the low-osmolar contrast agents that are also nonionic.

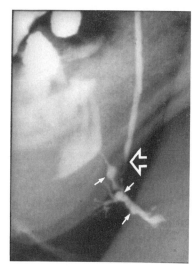

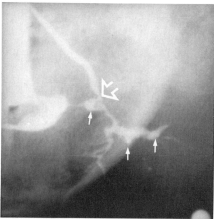

Figure 24–4. Two views showing acinarization (small arrows) due to the application of high pressure during a sialogram. A proximal stenosis (open arrow) in Wharton's duct is present.

Because a patient being studied for a neck neoplasm will occasionally have an associated acute cerebral infarction, the neurotoxic effects of contrast media will be briefly addressed here. Normally, radiographic contrast media do not diffuse into the brain parenchyma. During a stroke, the blood-brain barrier (BBB) loses its integrity and brain cells will then become exposed to circulating contrast material. Contrast media are mildly neurotoxic and therefore it may injure an already damaged brain. Ideally, contrast should not be administered in the presence of acute cerebral infarctions. In these cases, the administration of contrast material is usually a risk-versus-benefit situation and should be approached on an individual case basis.

One of the most important issues is that of renal toxicity. More than 99% of the total dose of radiographic contrast media is excreted by the kidneys.[13] The actual degree of renal toxicity is unknown, however, both glomerular and tubular toxicities may occur.[8] The incidence of contrast-induced renal failure has increased in the last few years. This observation is probably a reflection of the greater number of patients undergoing radiographic studies and of the more liberal use of contrast media in the elderly or seriously sick

patient. Overall, renal toxicity is lower with the newer low-osmolar nonionic contrast materials. In the majority of patients who suffer contrast-induced acute renal failure, the prognosis is favorable and complete resolution may be expected within 1 to 2 weeks.[8] However, on rare occasions, death from uremia has been reported.[8] The presence of renal disease, diabetes, and cardiac disease worsen the prognosis. In these cases, low-osmolar nonionic contrast material is definitely advantageous.[14] Patients with ENT carcinomas may have a decreased fluid intake so it is important to remember that, if dehydration is present, it must be corrected first because it represents a risk factor for nephrotoxicity. Some authors list advanced patient age as another risk factor.[8] In our experience, older patients may safely receive contrast media if they are adequately hydrated and if their renal function tests are normal. Hydration is extremely important in patients with multiple myeloma.[15]

Anaphylactoid reactions are not uncommon and are probably related to a combination of antigenic reactions (antibody mediated), release of cellular mediators (mainly histamine), psychogenic factors, and to the activation of vasoactive compounds such as complement and kinins.[16] Adverse allergic reactions may be classified into minor, intermediate, and severe. In one large series, 2.5% of patients receiving conventional iodinated contrast media manifested minor reactions (nausea, vomiting, and/or limited urticaria).[17] The incidence of minor reactions dropped from 2.5% to 0.58% when the newer nonionic contrasts were used. Intermediate reactions (severe vomiting, faintness, extensive urticaria, dyspnea, bronchospasm, chest or abdominal pain, and/or severe headache) occurred in 1.2% and 0.11% of the patients receiving conventional and nonionic contrasts, respectively. Severe reactions (loss of consciousness, cardiac arrest, shock, or symptomatic heart arrhythmias) were seen in 0.4% of patients receiving conventional contrast media; no patients receiving the newer contrasts experienced a severe reaction. It has been well documented that the newer contrast materials will induce not only less significant reactions, but produce a smaller number of them.[18,19] One of the most important predisposing factors leading to an anaphylactic reaction is a history of previous allergic reaction to contrast media. If administration of radiographic contrast media is considered essential in such a patient, it is prudent to use a premedication regimen. We prefer to use prednisone, 20 mg orally every 6 hours for three doses, before the procedure. Once the patient is placed on the CT table and is about to receive the iodinated contrast material, 30 to 50 mg of Benadryl are given intravenously. We do not routinely use cimetidine. One must always be ready to provide resuscitative measures in these patients. The overall incidence of repeat contrast-induced reactions varies between 5% to 40%.[8]

Accidental extravasation of contrast agents at the site of injection has been reported to occur in approximately 0.04% of patients undergoing CT examinations.[20] Most extravasations involve small volumes of contrast material and are not clinically significant. Extravasation of large quantities of contrast media may lead to skin ulceration and necrosis.[20] This is particularly true when conventional contrast media are involved. Extravasation of nonionic contrast materials is generally well tolerated. In our experience, warm compresses, elevation of the extremity involved, and analgesics generally suffice. Late adverse reactions to nonionic contrast media occur in approximately 8% of patients.[21] These are usually mild and self-limiting and consist of headaches and vomiting.

CISTERNOGRAPHY

Cisternography is performed primarily to determine the site of cerebrospinal fluid (CSF) leak. The cisternogram technique consists of performing a lumbar puncture (LP) under fluoroscopy and placing 2 to 5 mL of nonionic contrast medium (180 to 200 mg iodine/mL) within the subarachnoid space. The patient is then placed head-down for 1 to 2 minutes and the contrast is allowed to flow cranially. Pre- and postcisternogram thin-section CT scans in the axial and coronal planes are obtained through the areas of interest. Pooling of the high-density contrast on the CT within the middle ear, paranasal sinuses, or nasal vault suggests the location of the leak. The examination can be performed as an outpatient procedure with few complications.

When they occur, complications are related to either the LP or to the administration of contrast media, and although the complication rates for cisternography alone have not been reported, rates for myelography are available and we believe both are probably similar. For complications related to contrast dosage, the rates for cisternography may be lower than those for myelography because a very low dose of intrathecal contrast is used. Headache is the most common complication of myelography with nonionic contrast media and occurs in 25% to 44% of patients.[22-25] The incidence of headaches may be reduced by careful technique, use of a small (22 to 25 g) LP needle diameter, and adequate patient hydration following the procedure. Even with the most careful technique, headache may occur. Lumbar puncture or myelographic-related headaches tend to resolve within several days following the procedure, but occasionally patients will require placement of an autologous epidural blood patch. Nausea is less common, occurring in 3% to 10% of patients undergoing myelography.[22-25] Neurotoxic side effects such as seizures, clinically apparent psychological changes, or meningeal irritation are uncommon.

Overpressure cisternography has been used for the purpose of improving the detection of CSF leaks.[26] In this technique, artificial CSF is infused into the subarachnoid space to elevate the intracranial pressure. Theoretically, this technique reduces the time of examination and improves localization of the site of CSF leak. We have seen one patient who developed severe mental status changes following overpressure cisternography. Because the majority of CSF leaks may be identified by using a combination of iodinated contrast/radiotracer cisternography, at this time, we do not recommend the use of overpressure cisternography on a routine basis.

MAGNETIC RESONANCE IMAGING

Magnetic resonance imaging has had an enormous impact on imaging in the extracranial head and neck. Lesions best evaluated with MRI include acoustic neuroma, malignancies of the paranasal sinuses, nasopharynx, oropharynx, parotid glands, skull base and orbits, cranial neuropathies, and labyrinthitis.

Although MRI uses no ionizing radiation, it exposes patients to three separate types of electromagnetic fields: a static magnetic field, a gradient or varying field, and radio frequency pulses.[27] Some of this power could potentially be absorbed by the patient, with subsequent changes in physiological parameters. Changes in tissue and body temperature and vital signs have been measured at field strengths and in head coils commonly used in daily practice. Changes in skin temperature are variable and although they may be as high as 3.5 °C, they do not appear to be clinically significant.[28,29] No clinically significant changes in blood pressure, heart rate, or respiratory rate have been noted.[28,30]

Claustrophobia occurs in 15% to 20% of patients undergoing MRI examinations. This is a higher rate than for CT, probably because the bore of the magnet is longer, encompasses the whole body, and is of a smaller diameter. Surface coils, which improve signal-to-noise ratios and result in better images, may contribute to the feeling of claustrophobia especially if they wrap around the head and neck. The quality of MRI studies on patients with head and neck lesions may be compromised, as these patients often have difficulty with excessive secretions, or may be short of breath due to airway compromise or chronic lung disease. Motion during an MRI study compromises all images obtained during that sequence. We have found that careful patient education prior to beginning the examination is helpful. The technologist positions the neck in neutral position or slight hyperextension, advises the patient against exaggerated respiratory or swallowing attempts, frequently stops to allow the patient to relax, and offers help with pooled secretions.

Because the MRI unit has a strong magnetic field, a ferromagnetic structure (iron, nickel, or cobalt) brought into the field has the potential to deflect and align with the magnetic field. Materials extrinsic to the patient, such as hair clips, belt buckles, ventilators, or other life support equipment, may be pulled into the bore of the magnet. This may result in damage to the instrument or injury to the patient. Therefore, patients must be carefully screened for the presence of ferromagnetic foreign bodies.

Seriously ill patients requiring life-support equipment can undergo an MRI, but great care must be taken to assure that all devices are MRI compatible. Nonferromagnetic ventilator, endotracheal tubes, multilumen catheters, halos, traction systems, and other support equipment are now available.[31-33]

The presence of a cardiac pacemaker is a definite contraindication for MRI examination, as the pacemaker may become dislodged or may malfunction. Some intracranial aneurysm clips are ferromagnetic and could potentially move or become displaced within the MRI unit.[34-36] Most neurosurgeons now use nonferromagnetic aneurysm clips, but if the type of clip is not known, the MRI should not be performed. Intraocular metallic foreign body is another contraindication to having an MRI. There has been one reported case of vitreous hemorrhage with blindness caused by deflection of an intraocular metallic fragment.[37] Patients should be carefully screened about occupational or exposure history. Sheet metal workers, in particular, are at risk for harboring small ocular foreign bodies. Plain films or axial thin-section CT scan of the orbits should be performed to screen for any ocular foreign bodies. If a metal fragment is found, the MRI should not be performed.

Cochlear implants will torque and become magnetized if exposed to the magnetic field of the MRI unit, potentially causing harm to the patient by affecting the proper function of the implant.[38,39] No other currently available otologic implant has been reported to deflect or torque within magnetic field strengths commonly used in medical imaging. Implants that are considered safe include ventilation tubes, stapes and incus prostheses, and ossicular wires.[38-41] Older otologic implants have not been thoroughly tested.[39]

Patients with surgical wires, skin staples, clips, orthopedic metallic devices, and intracranial shunt devices may safely undergo MRI examinations.[42] However, a typical artifact appearing as a focal area of signal void surrounded by a crescent of high signal intensity results from these devices and may obscure the underlying tissues (Fig. 24–5).

Metallic bullet fragments located near important neurovascular structures represent potential risk by deflecting in the soft tissues. Commercial sporting ammunition is usually nonferromagnetic, as are most domestically manufactured bullets and shotgun pellets.[43] BBs made by both Daisy and Crosman have been reported to deflect.[31] Shrapnel made outside the United States or older bullets dating to World War II may deflect within the MRI field.[44] Most patients with retained ballistic metallic fragments can be studied safely. However, if a fragment of unknown make or vintage is located near an important neurovascular structure, the MRI should be deferred.

The rapid alterations of the currents within the gradient coils of the magnet result in vibration and produce a loud banging sound. The amplitude of this sound varies between 65 and 95 dB and depends on the magnet itself or the type of sequence being performed.[45] Temporary hearing loss, which resolved after 15 minutes, of less than 15 dB at one frequency has been reported in as many as 43% of patients undergoing an MRI.[46] Earplugs have been shown to markedly decrease the incidence of this mild temporary hearing loss and should be offered to every patient undergoing an MRI examination.[46]

Gadopentetate Dimeglumine (Gd-DTPA, Magnevist; Berlex) is the intravenous paramagnetic contrast agent that has been available for clinical use with MRI since the mid-1980s. It is used to improve lesion conspicuity and to assess integrity of the BBB. Clinical trials have shown Gd-DTPA to be safe with only rare severe side effects. Over 1 million doses of the contrast agent have been administered worldwide, with less than 10 reported anaphylactoid reactions.[47] Reported adverse reactions possibly related to Gd-DTPA include headache (3.6%), coldness at the injection site (3.6%), and nausea (1.5%). Hypotension and/or a vasovagal reaction have been reported in less than 0.5% of patients.[48] Clinically insignificant hemolysis, which occurs immediately after Gd-DTPA administration, probably accounts for the transient elevation of serum iron and bilirubin in some patients.[48] Hemoglobin, hematocrit, and red blood cell values do not change after Gd-DTPA administration. Gadolinium is excreted via glomerular filtration by the kidneys. Nephrotoxicity, which may be a serious side effect of conventional iodinated contrast, is not a reported side effect of Gd-DTPA at the standard dose of 0.1 mmol/kg body weight.[49] Recently introduced MRI contrast agents, such as Gadodiamide (Omniscan, Sanofi-Winthrop) and gadoteridol (Prohance, Squibb Diagnostics) provide a safety margin even greater than gadolinium-DTPA.

ANGIOGRAPHY
Diagnostic

Complications of diagnostic angiography may be related to the administration of radiographic contrast media and/or to catheter manipulation. When compared with the more common intravenous route, adverse reactions to radiographic contrast agents tend to be less common when these drugs are administered intra-arterially. The exact explanation for this

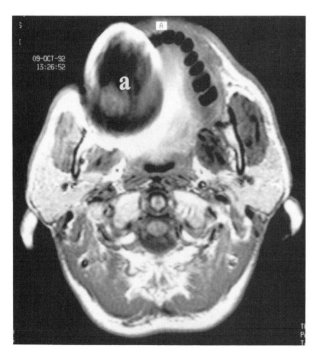

Figure 24–5.   Axial T1-weighted image in a patient with a floor of mouth tumor. The tumor is obscured by the large artifact (a) arising from metallic dental fillings.

phenomenon is unknown. Complications arising from the use of contrast media have been discussed in the section dealing with CT and will not be addressed here. It is important to remember that some angiographic procedures require the administration of large doses of contrast media, thus increasing the incidence of several of the risks previously described. Also, when the external carotid arteries are injected with constant media, the majority of patients will experience marked pain. The severity of this pain can be lessened by utilizing low-osmolar nonionic media and digital subtraction techniques that require the injection of only small amounts of contrast material.

Local complications of angiography are not uncommon. Inadvertent intra-arterial injections of local anesthetics (particularly lidocaine) may produce seizures.[50] Allergic reactions to local anesthetics may also occur.[50] Damage to the intima is not uncommon in elderly patients, especially those with generalized arteriosclerotic disease.[51] In our experience, if dissection of the iliac artery occurs, the wire or catheter should be immediately removed and careful observation of the peripheral pulses is all that is needed. In the majority of patients, these dissections are generally asymptomatic and do not require treatment. Intimal tears and subintimal hematomas occur in approximately 0.6% of angiograms. Arterial thrombosis is a serious complication occurring at the site of insertion of the catheter. Excessively long angiographic procedures, low cardiac output, subcutaneous hematoma, and arterial spasm are important predisposing factors.[52] Because loss of limbs has been reported, immediate surgical exploration of the puncture site and thrombectomy may be indicated if arterial thrombosis is suspected. Groin hematomas are reported in up to 10.7% of patients.[53] Most hematomas do not require surgical evacuation. In our opinion, a rapidly expanding groin hematoma, a hematoma suspected to contain more than 250 mL of blood, or a hematoma leading to compromise of the distal arterial perfusion should be treated surgically. Other less common vascular injuries include the formation of arteriovenous fistulae or false aneurysms at puncture sites[50] (Fig. 24–6). These two rare entities may remain asymptomatic for several weeks after the initial procedure.

Nerve damage is more commonly seen when the puncture site is in the brachial or the axillary arteries. Infection at puncture sites is very uncommon.

Catheter manipulation in the neck may on rare occasions lead to injuries of the carotid arteries or to cerebral complications (Fig. 24–7), which include new deficits or exacerbation of preexisting ones. The rate of death or permanent neurological deficits varies from 0.16 to 2.4% when conventional angiography is performed.[50–53] With the use of digital subtraction angiography, this risk can be reduced.[54]

Angiography of the external carotid artery is less painful when performed with low-osmolality contrast materials. However, these contrast agents are more prone to incite the formation of intracatheter clots than their conventional counterparts.[55] Therefore, the risk of thromboembolism may be potentially higher when using the newer low-osmolality contrast media.

Therapeutic

The main risks of embolization of head and neck pathology include: (1) passage of embolic materials from the external into the internal carotid artery with subsequent development of cerebral ischemia and/or infarctions, (2) occlusion of branches from the external carotid artery may lead to cranial nerve dysfunctions, and (3) embolization of cutaneous branches that may produce delayed skin healing, necrosis, and/or infection.[56]

Of particular importance is the development of neurological or ophthalmologic deficits that have been reported in 0.5 to 1% of all head and neck embolizations.[57] When deficits occur, some authors recommend the use of plasma volume expanders, antihypertensive medication, and/or arterial bypasses.

Swelling usually begins within 24 hours after an embolization procedure. If the lesion is located close to the airway, respiratory compromise should be anticipated and dealt with in an expeditious manner. Inability to open the mouth due to postembolization edema may require the insertion of nasogastric or orogastric tubes. The eyes must receive proper care if closing of the eyelids is prevented by swelling. In severe cases, steroid administration may alleviate the swelling.

Skin necrosis usually requires only local hygiene and spontaneous healing generally occurs. However, grafting may be needed in some patients.

Preoperative embolization of paragangliomas deserves special mention due to the well-known risk of inducing an acute hypertensive crisis secondary to the release of catecholamines.[58] The exact number of patients in whom this complication occurs is not known (we have never personally witnessed this complication.) Standby anesthesia and the use of nonionic contrast agents and alpha-blockers (phentolamine or phenoxybenzamine) are advisable if this complication is foreseen. Postembolization swelling of carotid body tumors may produce bradycardia.[59] If tachycardia occurs, beta-blockers may be needed.

Test Balloon Occlusions

Test balloon occlusions are generally performed before resection or permanent occlusion of the internal carotid arteries. Because the circle of Willis is completely intact in only 21% of the adult population, a significant number of patients will not tolerate permanent ligation of one internal carotid artery.[59] The study is performed using a nondetachable latex balloon fixed to the tip of a catheter. The artery may be damaged by the tip of the catheter or by the relatively stiff balloon. We have seen one case in which the internal carotid artery was ruptured by overinflation of the balloon (Fig. 24–8).

Approximately 5% to 20% of patients who show no neurological deficit during test occlusion will develop a cerebral infarction after permanent internal carotid occlusion.[59] Recent data suggest that the systemic injection of a radiotracer (99mTc- HMPAO) improves the sensitivity of the balloon test occlusion.[59–61] Imaging with single photon emission computed tomography (SPECT) will detect abnormalities of cerebral perfusion in some patients who have passed the balloon test occlusion. Permanent occlusion of the one internal carotid artery is not well tolerated by these patients.

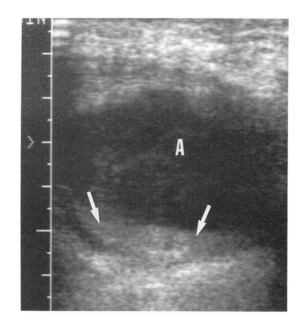

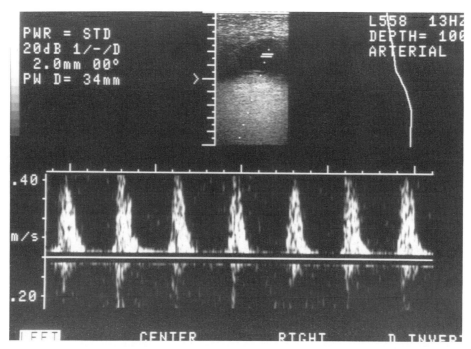

Figure 24–6. **(A).** Groin ultrasound in patient who presented with a left pulsatile mass following an angiogram. A 3 × 5 cm pseudoaneurysm arising from the left common femoral artery is present and contains thrombus (arrows) in its posterior aspect. **(B).** Doppler tracing with probe positioned in the mid portion of the aneurysm lumen shows a pattern typical of arterial flow.

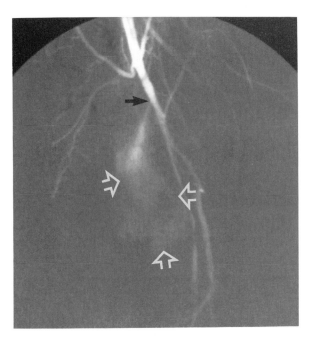

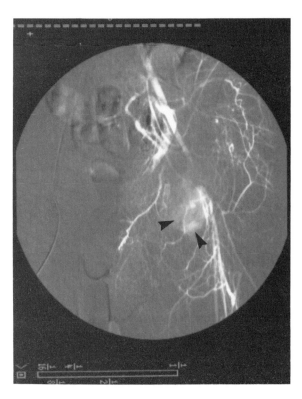

C

D

Figure 24–6   (continued). (C). Frontal digital subtraction view during the early part of the left common femoral angiogram. There is a jet of contrast medium (black arrow) into the pseudoaneurysm (open arrows) that shows early filling. **(D).** Later phase of the angiogram in the same patient shows filling of the lumen of the pseudoaneurysm (arrowheads).

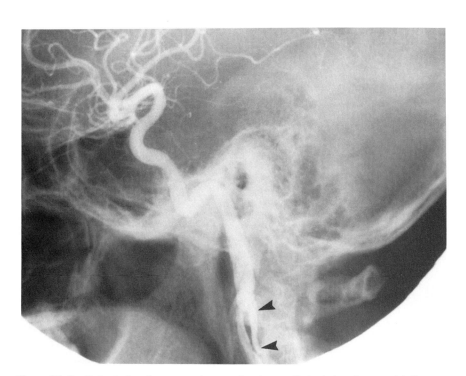

Figure 24–7.   Lateral view from an angiogram showing a catheter-induced segmental dissection (arrowheads) of the internal carotid artery. The patient did not manifest any symptoms but was placed on anticoagulants for 6 weeks.

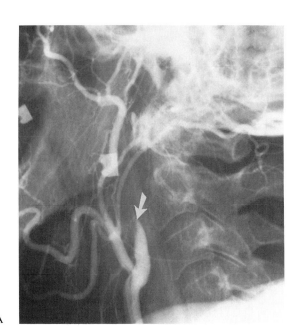

A

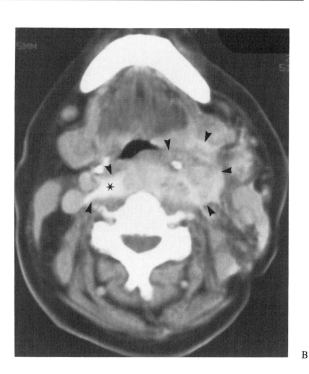

B

Figure 24–8. **(A).** Lateral view from the common carotid angiogram following test balloon occlusion of the internal carotid artery performed for a lesion located in the petrous apex. Immediately afer inflation of the balloon, the patient complained of severe neck pain, dysphagia, and shortness of breath. In this view, the internal carotid artery is occluded (arrow) just beyond the bulb. **(B).** CT in the same patient obtained immediately after angiography. The left carotid artery and jugular vein are indistinct and surrounded by the hyperdensity of the extravasated contrast (arrowheads). Contrast can be seen crossing the midline along the retropharyngeal space. Fresh contrast (star) in the medial right carotid-jugular space is also present.

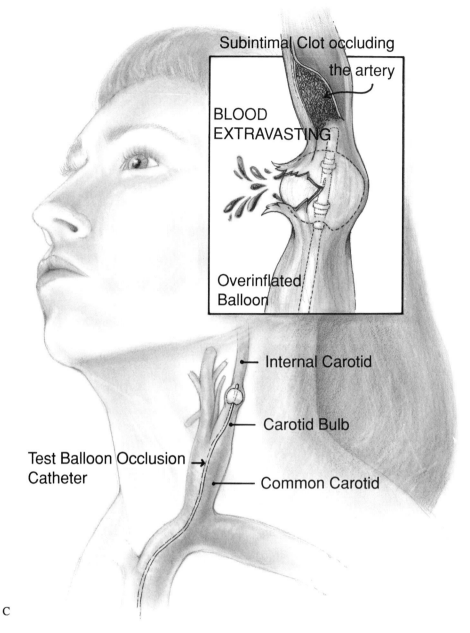

Figure 24–8 (continued). (C). Drawing depicts rupture of the internal carotid artery secondary to overinflation of a test balloon occlusion catheter.

REFERENCES

1. Gelfand DW, Ott DJ. Gastrointestinal contrast agents. In: Taveras JW, Ferrucci JT, eds. *Radiology. Diagnosis-Imaging-Interventional.* Philadelphia, Pa: JB Lippincott Co; 1988:6–7.

2. Som PM. Salivary glands. In: Som PM, Bergeron RT, eds. *Head and Neck Imaging.* 2nd ed. St Louis, Mo: Mosby Year Book; 1991:284–286.

3. Hanafee WN. Sialography. In: Valvassori GE, Potter GD, Hanafee WN, Carter BL, Buckingham RA, eds. *Radiology of the Ear, Nose, and Throat.* Philadelphia, Pa: WB Saunders Co; 1984:312–332.

4. Meine FJ, Woloshin JH. Radiologic diagnosis of salivary gland tumors. *Radiol Clin North Am.* 1970;8:475–485.

5. Rankow RM, Polayes IM. Surgical treatment of salivary gland tumors. In: Rankow RM, Polayes IM, eds. *Diseases of the Salivary Glands.* Philadelphia, Pa: WB Saunders Co; 1976: 239–283.

6. Ter-Pogossian MM. Computerized cranial tomography: equipment and physics. *Semin Roentgenol.* 1977;12:13–25.

7. Ter-Pogossian MM. Physical principles and instrumentation. In: Lee JKT, Sagel SS, Stanley RF, eds. *Computed Body Tomography.* New York, NY: Raven Press; 1983:7.

8. Stolberg HO, McClennan BL. Ionic versus nonionic contrast use. *Curr Probl Diagn Radiol.* 1991;20:1–88.

9. Grainger RG. Osmolality and osmolality-related side effects. In: Felix R, Fisher HW, Kormano M, et al, eds. *Contrast Media from the Past to the Future.* Stuttgart: Georg Thieme Verlag; 1987:25–32.

10. Walton JN. *Brain's Diseases of the Nervous System.* 8th ed. Oxford: Oxford University Press; 1977:317.

11. Stormorken Hl Skalpe IO, Testart MC. Effects of various contrast media on coagulation, fibrinolysis, and platelet function. An in vitro and in vivo study. *Invest Radiol.* 1986;21:348–354.

12. Stormorken H. Effects of contrast media on the hemostatic and thrombotic mechanisms. *Invest Radiol.* 1988;23S:308–325.

13. Dawson P. Aspects of contrast agent nephrotoxicity. In: Felix R, Fisher HW, Kormano M, et al, eds. *Contrast Media from the Past to the Future*. Stuttgart: Georg Thieme Verlag; 1987: 137–148.
14. McClennan BL. Ionic and nonionic iodinated contrast media: evolution and strategies for use. *AJR*. 1990;155:225–233.
15. McCarthy CS, Becker JA. Multiple myeloma and contrast media. *Radiology*. 1992;183:519–521.
16. Lasser EC. Adverse systemic reactions to contrast media. In: *Handbook of Experimental Pharmacology*. Heidelberg: Springer Verlag; 1984:73.
17. Wolf GL, Arenson RL, Cross AP. A prospective trial of ionic vs nonionic contrast agents in routine clinical practice: comparison of adverse effects. *AJR*. 1989;152:939–944.
18. Palmer FJ. The RACR survey of intravenous contrast media reactions final report. *Australas Radiol*. 1988;32:426–428.
19. Katayama H, Yamaguchi K, Kozuka T, et al. Adverse reactions to ionic and nonionic contrast media. A report from the Japanese committee on the safety of contrast media. *Radiology*. 1990;175:621–628.
20. Cohan RH, Dunnick NR, Leder RA, Baker ME. Extravasation of nonionic radiologic contrast media: efficacy of conservative treatment. *Radiology*. 1990;176:65–67.
21. Yoshikawa H. Late adverse reactions to nonionic contrast media. *Radiology*. 1992;183:737–740.
22. Moschini L, Manara O, Bonaldi G, et al. Lopamidol and metrizamide in cervical myelography: side effects, EEG, and CSF changes. *AJNR*. 1983;4:848–850.
23. Latchaw RE, Hirsch WL Jr, Horton JA, Bissonette D, Shaw DD. Iohexol vs. metrizamide: study of efficacy and morbidity in cervical myelography. *AJNR*. 1985;6:931–933.
24. Bannon KR, Braun IF, Pinto RS, et al. Comparison of radiographic quality and adverse reactions in myelography with iopamidol and metrizamide. *AJNR*. 1983;4:312–313.
25. Trevisan C, Malaguti C, Manfredini M, Tampieri D. Iopamidol vs metrizamide myelography: clinical comparison of side effects. *AJNR*. 1983;4:306–308.
26. Curnes JT, Vincent LM, Lowalsky RJ, McCartney WH, Staab EV. CSF rhinorrhea: detection and localization using overpressure cisternography with TC-99M-DTPA. *Radiology*. 1985;154:795–799.
27. Davis PL, Crooks L, Arakawa M, et al. Potential hazards in NMR imaging: heating effects of changing magnetic fields and RF fields on small metallic implants. *AJR*. 1981;137:857–860.
28. Shellock FG, Crues JR. Temperature, heart rate, and blood pressure changes associated with clinical MR imaging at 1.5T. *Radiology*. 1987;163:259–262.
29. Shellock FG, Crues JV. Temperature changes caused by MR imaging of the brain with a head coil. *AJNR*. 1988;9:287–291.
30. Kido DK, Morris TW, Erickson JL, Plewes DB, Simon JH. Physiologic changes during high field strenth MR imaging. *AJR*. 1987;148:1215–1218.
31. Shellock FG, Curtis JS. MR imaging and biomedical implants, materials, and devices: an updated review. *Radiology*. 1991;180:541–550.
32. Dunn V, Coffman CE, McGowan JE, Ehrhardt JC. Mechanical ventilation during magnetic resonance imaging. *Magn Reson Imaging*. 1985;3:169–172.
33. Mirvis SE, Borg U, Belzberg H. MR imaging of ventilator-dependent patients: preliminary experience. *AJR*. 1987;149:845–846.
34. Dujovny M, Kossovsky N, Kossowsky R, et al. Aneurysm clip motion during magnetic resonance imaging: in vivo experimental study with metallurgical factor analysis. *Neurosurgery*. 1985;17:543–548.
35. Holtas S, Olsson M, Romner B, et al: Comparison of MR imaging and CT in patients with intracranial aneurysm clips. *AJNR*. 1988;9:891–897.
36. Becker RL, Norfray JF, Teitelbaum GP, et al. MR imaging in patients with intracranial aneurysm clips. *AJNR*. 1988;9: 885–889.
37. Kelly WM, Paglen PG, Pearson JA, San Diego AG, Soloman MA. Ferromagnetism of intraocular foreign body causes unilateral blindness after MR study. *AJNR*. 1986;7:243–245.
38. Mattucci KF, Setzen M, Hyman R, Chaturvedi G. The effect of nuclear magnetic resonance imaging on metallic middle ear prostheses. *Otolaryngol Head Neck Surg*. 1986;94:441–443.
39. Shellock FG, Schatz CJ. Metallic otologic implants: in vitro assessment of ferromagnetism at 1.5T. *AJNR*. 1991;12:279–281.
40. Leon JA, Gariele OF. Middle ear prosthesis: significance in magnetic resonance imaging. *Magn Reson Imaging*. 1987;5: 405–406.
41. Applebaum EI, Valvassori GE. Effects of magnetic resonance imaging fields on stapedectomy prostheses. *Arch Otolaryngol Head Neck Surg*. 1985;111:820–821.
42. Laakman RW, Kaufman B, Han JS, et al. MR imaging in patients with metallic implants. *Radiology*. 1985;157:711–714.
43. Gieszl R, Williams KD, Drayer BP, Keller PJ. Magnetic resonance imaging and ferromagnetic bullets. *Assoc Firearm Tool Mark Examiners*. 1989;21:595–605.
44. Teitelbaum GP, Yee CA, Van Horn DD, Kim HS, Colletti PM. Metallic ballistic fragments: MR imaging safety and artifacts. *Radiology*. 1990;175:855–859.
45. Kanal E, Shellock FG, Talagala L. Safety considerations in MR imaging. *Radiology*. 1990;176:593–606.
46. Brummett RE, Talbot JM, Charuhas P. Potential hearing loss resulting from MR imaging. *Radiology*. 1988;169:539–540.
47. Tishler S, Hoffman JC Jr. Anaphylactoid reactions to IV Gadopentetate Dimeglumine. *AJNR*. 1990;11:1167.
48. Goldstein HA, Kashanian FK, Blumetti RF, et al: Safety assessment of Gadopentetate Dimeglumine in U.S. clinical trials. *Radiology*. 1990;174:17–23.
49. Haustein J, Niendorf HP, Krestin G, et al: Renal tolerance of Gadolinium-DTPA/Dimeglumine in patients with chronic renal failure. *Invest Radiol*. 1992;27:153–156.
50. Howieson J. Complications of cerebral angiography. In: Newton TH, Potts DG, eds. *Radiology of the Skull and Brain Angiography*. Great Neck NY: Medibooks; 1974:1034–1046.
51. Vitek JJ, Powell DF, Anderson RD. Damage of brachiocephalic vessels due to catheterization. *Neuroradiology*. 1975;9:63–67.
52. Osborn AG. *Introduction to Cerebral Angiography*. Philadelphia, Pa: Harper and Row; 1980:21–22.
53. Olivecrona H. Complications of cerebral angiography. *Neuroradiology*. 1977;14:175–181.
54. Waugh JR, Sacharias N. Arteriographic complications in the DSA era. *Radiology*. 1992;182:243–246.
55. Casalini E. Role of low-osmolality contrast media in thromboembolic complications: scanning electron microscopy study. *Radiology*. 1992;183:741–744.
56. Valvanis A. Preoperative embolization of head and neck: patient selection, goals, and precautions. *Am J Neuroradiol*. 1986;7:943–952.
57. Lasjaunias P, Berenstein A. *Surgical Neuroangiography. Endovascular Treatment of Craniofacial Lesions*. Berlin: Springer-Verlag; 1987:56.
58. Eskridge JM. Interventional neuroradiology. *Radiology*. 1989;172:992–1006.
59. Peterman Brothers S, Taylor A, Hoffman JC. Improved detection of cerebral hypoperfusion with internal carotid balloon occlusion and 99mTc-HMPAO cerebral perfusion SPECT imaging. *Am J Neuroradiol*. 1991;12:1035–1041.
60. Moody EB, Dawson RC, Sandler MP. 99mTc-HMPAO SPECT imaging in interventional neuroradiology: validation of balloon test occlusion. *Am J Neuroradiol*. 1991;12:1043,1044.
61. Monsein LH, Jeffrey PJ, van Heerden BB, et al. Assessing adequacy of collateral circulation during balloon test occlusion of the internal carotid artery with 99mTc-HMPAO SPEC. *Am J Neuroradiol*. 1991;1045–1051.

25 Complications in the Critical Care Unit

William R. Blythe, M.D., Fuad Ramadan, M.D., David Smith, M.D., Samir M. Fakhry, M.D., F.A.C.S.

Many patients undergoing major head and neck surgical procedures are admitted to a critical care unit for postoperative care and observation. The majority of these patients have an uneventful stay in the critical care unit. Complications may occur in patients who have serious preexisting medical conditions, elderly patients, or those who have operative misadventures. In this chapter, we review a variety of complications that may be encountered in the critical care setting and discuss diagnosis and management options. Complications specific to particular operative procedures are covered in other chapters.

CARDIAC DYSFUNCTION
Congestive Heart Failure

Congestive heart failure (CHF) may manifest in a number of ways, ranging from congested organs to hypoperfused tissue. In early compensated CHF, resting cardiac output (CO) is normal. Any stress such as fever, surgery, exercise, pain, or sepsis results in an inadequate CO, and the severity of the symptoms becomes more pronounced. Many factors can lead to myocardial dysfunction and CHF, but the most common causes in the surgical intensive care unit (ICU) are ischemic dysfunction and myocardial infarction (MI) secondary to coronary artery disease, hypotensive/hypoxemic episodes, and, less commonly, valvular disease. In the patient undergoing head and neck surgery, myocardial dysfunction and MI are most often related to atherosclerotic coronary artery disease.

Successful management depends on early identification of the syndrome. An acute increase in the pulmonary capillary wedge pressure (PCWP) is associated with early CHF. A decrease in stroke volume (SV) results, and the heart rate increases in an attempt to compensate for the drop in SV. In some patients the tachycardia fails to compensate for the decreased SV and the patient goes from compensated CHF to uncompensated CHF with a rise in the systemic vascular resistance (SVR). End organ perfusion is diminished with the increase in SVR, and the mixed venous oxygen saturation begins to fall.

The bedside echocardiograph is useful in making the diagnosis of right versus left ventricular failure. Right ventricular failure can resemble cardiac tamponade and is usually seen with an increased central venous pressure (CVP) that is usually greater than or equal to the PCWP. In left ventricular failure the PCWP is usually elevated and is greater than the CVP.[1]

THERAPY

The primary goal of therapy in left ventricular failure is to improve CO and prevent pulmonary edema. The main guide to therapy is the PCWP. There is no single PCWP that is ideal for all patients. The ideal PCWP maximizes CO without pulmonary edema. The first goal is to optimize the preload. If preload is low, then volume infusion is required to improve CO because pharmacological intervention will be of little benefit when the diastolic filling is suboptimal. If the filling pressure, that is, PCWP, is optimal and the patient remains hypotensive, then pharmacological therapy is indicated. The drug of choice in this setting is dopamine, which has dopaminergic effects, beta inotropic effects, and alpha adrenergic effects (Table 25–1). In the patient with a normal blood pressure, optimal PCWP, but low CO, the drug of choice is dobutamine.[3] Dobutamine is less useful in the hypotensive patient. If the patient is hypertensive with low CO and an optimal PCWP, either nitroprusside or dobutamine may be useful as the initial drug therapy. Nitroprusside may precipitate significant hypotension in some patients. The use of dobutamine causes a decrease in SVR with an improvement of the CO caused by its inotropic effect. If myocardial ischemia is suspected, intravenous nitroglycerin is indicated. Sublingual or dermal nitrates can be used initially while adequate venous access is obtained.

Cardiac Dysrhythmias

Cardiac dysrhythmias occur commonly in patients admitted to surgical critical care units. Isolated or short-lived dysrhythmias may not require therapy, especially if they are supraventricular (eg, atrial premature beats, short-lived

Table 25–1. Recommended Doses for Drug Therapies in CHF

DRUG	DOSE	ACTION
Dobutamine	2.5–20 μg/kg/min	Inotrope/vasodilator
Dopamine	1–5 μg/kg/min (dopaminergic)	
	5–10 μg/kg/min (beta)	Inotrope
	10–20 μg/kg/min (alpha)	Vasoconstrictor
Nitroprusside	0.5–10 μg/kg/min	Vasodilator
Nitroglycerin	1–50 μg/min	Venodilator
	>50 μg/min	Vasodilator

Table 25–2. Recommended Doses of Antiarrhythmic Agents

Lidocaine	1 mg/kg loading; 2 mg/min maintenance drip. Titrate to adequate levels
Verapamil	1 mg/min IV up to 10 mg/min until rate slows.
Diltiazem	Load with 0.25 mg/kg; may repeat with 0.35 mg/kg if needed, then IV drip 5–15 mg/h. Titrate to effect
Adenosine	6 mg IV push, then 12 mg 2 min later, then 12 mg again if no results
Digitalis	12–15 μg/kg LBM: 1/2 the dose initially, then 1/4 dose every 6 h × 2. Maintenance: 0.125–0.375 mg/d IV or PO
Atropine	0.5 mg IV, up to 2 mg total

LBM, lean body mass; IV, intravenous.

supraventricular tachycardia). They may be signs of electrolyte abnormalities (eg, hypokalemia or hypomagnesemia), hypoxia, or myocardial ischemia and therefore should prompt an evaluation of these possible etiologies.

The decision to treat abnormal electrical activity of the heart present without hemodynamic compromise should be carefully weighed because all pharmacological treatments have a negative inotropic effect and in some instances may precipitate a worse dysrhythmia. Pertinent questions include: Does the patient require therapy? When should therapy be instituted? What therapy is indicated?

THERAPY

Treatment decisions are based on patient stability and the origin of the dysrhythmia. All stable patients should have an electrocardiogram (ECG) prior to treatment to document the dysrhythmia and its type. All dysrhythmias associated with hemodynamic instability, except asystole, should be treated immediately by cardioversion. The goal of cardioversion is to reorganize cardiac electrical activity. In an emergency situation, as with an unstable patient, one should perform cardioversion with 100 J and rapidly increase to 400 J until cardioversion is successful.[4]

In the stable patient who is bradycardic, atropine 0.5 to 1 mg intravenously is the drug of choice (Table 25–2). A total of 2 mg (the vagolytic dose) may be given. If the patient continues to require atropine to maintain an adequate heart rate, then an external or transvenous pacemaker may be used to maintain an acceptable rate. Profound resistant bradycardia may be treated with epinephrine. If epinephrine is required, the patient is likely to become hemodynamically unstable and this type of bradycardia is frequently preterminal.

For rapid ventricular rates in stable patients, treatment is guided by the ECG and rhythm strip. The most important information obtained from the ECG is the duration of the QRS complex. Normal electrical conduction in the heart is very fast because the atrial impulse is transmitted to the ventricles via the Purkinje fibers and the QRS complex is not longer than 0.08 seconds. If the electrical impulse is generated by an ectopic ventricular focus then the impulse cannot access the Purkinje fibers and the QRS is prolonged to greater than 0.08 seconds. Wide complex tachycardia (ventricular

tachycardia) is treated by cardioversion followed by a lidocaine, 1 mg/kg, intravenous bolus. Continuous infusion of lidocaine starting at 2 mg/min should be instituted and serum lidocaine levels monitored.

For patients with a narrow QRS complex (0.08 seconds or less), the ECG should be examined for P waves to distinguish between atrial fibrillation, atrial flutter, and sinus tachycardia. If no P waves can be identified and the rate is irregular, then the patient is in atrial fibrillation. If the ventricular rate is high, the patient can be initially treated with a calcium channel blocker such as verapamil or diltiazem. Calcium channel blockers produce an arteriovenous (AV) nodal blockade. Verapamil may be associated with significant hypotension due to peripheral vasodilatation.[4] Hypotension is less commonly seen with diltiazem, and therefore it may become the drug of choice for treating paroxysmal supraventricular tachycardias (PSVT). When hypotension is seen secondary to the administration of calcium channel blockers, it can be treated with the administration of calcium intravenously. Digitalis is usually used for longer-term treatment of atrial fibrillation. The ventricular rate should first be controlled with a calcium channel blocker. At the same time, the patient may be loaded with digitalis and then begun on a daily dose as needed, checking levels to help prevent digitalis toxicity.

Adenosine causes conduction delay through the AV node and can also be used for treatment or diagnosis of supraventricular tachycardia. It is extremely effective in decreasing heart rate and in fact occasionally produces asystole or other dysrhythmia. These rhythm changes are very short lived and require no additional therapy. The half-life of adenosine is less than 10 seconds and its onset of action is almost immediate. Because adenosine will slow most PSVT, it is useful in diagnosis by making the slowed rhythm easier to identify. However, the physiological abnormalities that led to the onset of the PSVT are likely to remain after treatment with adenosine, and therefore the rhythm disorder is likely to recur after the drug is metabolized, usually in 2 minutes or less. An initial dose of 0.6 mg of adenosine intravenously is recommended. A repeat dose can be used if the desired response is elicited. Subsequent dosing with 1.2 mg can also be done over a period of 20 minutes.

Myocardial Infarction

Postoperative MI in patients undergoing noncardiac surgery is a significant cause of morbidity and mortality, particularly in patients with a history of tobacco and/or ethanol abuse. The mortality for postoperative MI approaches 50% overall.[5] Perioperative cardiac risk can be estimated based on criteria proposed by Goldman in 1983.[6] These factors include presence of underlying heart failure (greatest risk for postoperative cardiac death), recent MI, history of significant dysrhythmia, aortic valve disease, age, and overall medical condition. An additional risk factor is the type of procedure performed.

In patients who have had a recent MI, elective surgery should be postponed for at least 6 months following the MI owing to the significantly increased risk of reinfarction. Following MI, the risk for reinfarction is over 30% for procedures performed in less than 3 months, falls to 15% between 3 and 6 months, and levels off at 5% after 6 months. In high-risk patients intraoperative and occasionally preoperative pulmonary artery catheterization may be useful in patient management.

DIAGNOSIS

The diagnosis of MI postoperatively may be difficult because chest pain is often masked or not present. Myocardial infarction must be suspected in any postoperative patient who develops a new dysrhythmia, altered mental status, hypotension, or a labile blood pressure. The diagnosis is made on the basis of ECG changes and cardiac isoenzymes. The greatest risk of postoperative MI occurs on postoperative day 3 and most MIs occur by day 6. Patients with an ECG suggestive of MI should be admitted to a critical care unit.

THERAPY

In patients with chest pain, prompt pain relief is important and is achieved using intravenous morphine and nitroglycerin. Intravenous morphine can be started at 1 to 5 mg and given every few minutes or a drip started, as long as the patient is not oversedated. Intravenous nitroglycerin is usually started at 10 to 50 mg/min and titrated by 10-mg increments every 5 to 10 minutes until pain relief is achieved, or until mean blood pressure is decreased 10% in normotensive patients, or 30% for patients with blood pressure > 140/90.[7] Nitroglycerin is usually continued for 24 to 36 hours, or longer if needed. Both of these treatments may cause significant hypotension and the patients may require close hemodynamic monitoring. Prophylactic lidocaine treatment for acute MI is controversial and probably not required unless the patient has significant ectopy.[8] All patients should be on supplemental oxygen. Thrombolytic therapy has clearly been shown to improve survival in patients with an acute MI; however, an absolute contraindication to thrombolytic therapy is recent major surgery.[8]

Cardiogenic Shock

Cardiogenic shock is a severe complication of acute MI associated with 80% mortality. The development of cardiogenic shock implies the loss of a large amount of myocardium, usually 30 to 40%. The diagnosis is made on the basis of hypotension, often following an MI, and elevated left atrial filling pressures or PCWP (greater than 15 mm Hg for nonintubated patients). Dopamine is the drug of choice, and dobutamine may also be beneficial in these patients. In some patients an intra-aortic balloon pump may be life saving because it decreases myocardial oxygen requirements by decreasing afterload and increasing coronary filling.[5] The balloon pump may stabilize the patients who are candidates for coronary revascularization long enough so that they may be taken for emergent coronary artery bypass grafting.

ACUTE RENAL FAILURE

The kidney plays a key role in the elimination of metabolic waste products and the excretion of many drugs as well as the maintenance of normal homeostasis by regulating water, electrolyte, and acid-base balance. Through its synthetic capacity, it is involved in numerous regulatory pathways, involving blood pressure, red blood cell mass, and calcium metabolism.

Acute renal dysfunction is an infrequent but devastating complication of surgery. With the continuing advances in perioperative monitoring and management of critically ill patients, the incidence of acute renal failure has decreased over the past 50 years; however, despite the availability of dialysis, the mortality of severe renal failure (requiring dialysis) has not changed. Indeed, postsurgical acute renal failure continues to be associated with mortality rates ranging from 33 to 100%.[9] The morbidity and mortality of many surgical procedures are closely related to the status of the patient's renal function.

The fundamental goal in the management of acute renal failure is its prevention, or at least limiting its severity. This requires timely recognition of the high-risk situation and rapid intervention. A thorough understanding of the various types of renal dysfunction, their etiologies, clinical characteristics, and pathophysiology is crucial in the ICU.

Acute Renal Failure Syndromes

For therapeutic, as well as prognostic reasons, it is convenient to classify acute renal dysfunction by broad etiologic categories of prerenal, renal, and postrenal types.[10] Prerenal azotemia usually results from a drop in glomerular filtration rate (GFR) secondary to a decrease in renal perfusion or an increase in renal vascular resistance. In the surgical patient, this is the most common cause of renal dysfunction and is most often due to hypovolemia.[11] Less likely causes include impaired cardiac function or renal vascular obstruction. With the drop in renal blood flow and the concomitant reduction in GFR, there is increased proximal tubular reabsorption of sodium and water leading to hypertonic urine. This is reflected by a low urinary sodium (less than 10 mEq/L) and a renal failure index and fractional excretion of sodium of less than 1.

Postrenal azotemia usually results from obstruction of the urinary tract. It presents as total anuria reslting from bladder neck obstruction or bilateral ureteral obstructions. The prognosis for recovery from obstructive uropathy depends on the extent and duration of obstruction. The need for timely diagnosis and intervention is evident.

Parenchymal disease can be divided into two major categories: hemodynamically mediated (ischemic) and nephrotoxic. The former can result from intraparenchymal vasomotor dysfunction, which is believed to be prostaglandin mediated, and leads to intrarenal redistribution of blood flow. Sepsis and the hepatorenal syndrome are examples of clinical situations where this type of renal dysfunction occurs.[12] A number of substances ranging from aminoglycosides and radiographic contrast agents[13] to endogenous pigments (such as myoglobin)[14] have been recognized as nephrotoxic and can lead to parenchymal renal dysfunction. The various types of renal dysfunction, their relative frequencies, etiologies, and diagnostic findings are summarized in Table 25–3.

DIAGNOSIS

Renal insufficiency can be a subtle process. Because of various compensatory mechanisms, significant deterioration in renal function can develop before the onset of symptoms. A high level of awareness should be maintained with regard to patients at increased risk for renal dysfunction. These include patients with prolonged shock or severe injury, as well as the elderly and patients with preexisting renal insufficiency.

Acute renal dysfunction in the surgical patient usually presents with a decrease in urine output, or a rise in serum creatinine, or both. Because the reciprocal relationship between serum creatinine and GFR (as measured by creatinine clearance) is not linear, a 50 to 75% loss in nephron mass and creatinine clearance must occur before a rise in serum creatinine level is detected. Therefore, a rise in serum creatinine level of 1 mg/dL over baseline indicates about a 50% drop in GFR.

Oliguria is defined as urine output of 100 to 400 mL/d or less than 0.5 mL/kg per hour in adults (1 mL/kg/h in children weighing less than 10 kg). Anuria occurs when urine output falls below 100 mL/d. The cause of the oliguria should be determined and promptly addressed. Most patients with renal dysfunction will not progress to renal failure if properly managed. Because the prognosis for recovery depends on the duration of dysfunction, every effort should be made to identify reversible causes and intervene in a timely fashion. Therefore signs of hypovolemia, CHF, and urinary obstruction should be sought. Renal hypoperfusion as well as urinary obstruction may be readily correctable. Prompt diagnosis and treatment may limit the damage from nephrotoxic agents. It is therefore useful to determine whether a prerenal or postrenal,

component exists. The fractional excretion of sodium (FE_{Na}) remains the most reliable means of distinguishing between prerenal and other causes of acute renal dysfunction.

A reduction in renal perfusion pressure leads to an increase in renin secretion by the juxtaglomerular apparatus, resulting in elevated levels of angiotensin II, a potent stimulus of aldosterone production. As a consequence, reabsorption of sodium is maximized and urine sodium concentration drops to minimal values. Therefore a urine sodium concentration less than 20 mEq/L is strongly suggestive of a prerenal etiology, whereas a concentration greater than 40 mEq/L suggests parenchymal or postrenal causes.[10] More accurate is FE_{Na}, which reflects the fraction of the filtered sodium that is actually excreted in the urine. As would be expected from the preceding discussion, this fraction would be very small in prerenal situations. Indeed, FE_{Na} has been shown to be the most effective noninvasive test for the differential diagnosis of acute renal failure.[15] Except for acute glomerulonephritis, an FE_{Na} less than 1 is seen only with prerenal azotemia. Acute glomerulonephritis is virtually unheard of in the immediate postoperative setting and is nevertheless easily distinguishable from prerenal azotemia by clinical manifestations. An FE_{Na} greater than 1 is only seen with renal parenchymal or postrenal causes of renal dysfunction. The FE_{Na} is calculated as follows:

$$FE_{Na} = \frac{U_{Na}/P_{Na}}{U_{Cr}/P_{Cr}} \times 100$$

where U_{Na} and P_{Na} are the urine and plasma concentrations of sodium, respectively, and U_{Cr} and P_{Cr} are those concentrations for creatinine. It is important to remember that urinary sodium concentrations and excretions become meaningless and lose their diagnostic value with the use of diuretics.

Diagnosis of postrenal causes of renal dysfunction is fairly straightforward once suspected. Obstructive uropathy will manifest as hydronephrosis that is easily seen on ultrasonography. This can even be performed at the bedside in patients too critically ill to transport. Bladder outlet obstruction can be easily ruled out and sometimes relieved by placement of a Foley catheter.

The diagnosis of the renal or parenchymal type of acute renal failure is one of exclusion and can only be made after prerenal and postrenal causes have been ruled out. Frequently the clinical setting is helpful in making this diagnosis and identifying the cause. In certain cases, such as in the presence of nephrotoxic drugs, myoglobinuria, or sepsis, such information can be useful in stopping the offending agent and limiting the injury. Urine microscopy may be useful in revealing tubular, red, or white blood cell casts, which would suggest an ischemic or inflammatory etiology.

The severity of the renal dysfunction can be quantitated by creatinine clearance, which closely approximates GFR. It is calculated as $V \times U_{Cr}/P_{Cr}$, where V is the urine volume for the collection period and U_{Cr} and P_{Cr} are the urine and plasma concentrations of creatinine, respectively.

Table 25–3. Types of Acute Renal Dysfunction

TYPE	INCIDENCE	ETIOLOGY	FE$_{Na}$
Prerenal	50%–90%	Hypovolemia Cardiac failure Renovascular obstruction	≪1
Renal	10%–30%	Ischemia: sepsis, hepatorenal syndrome Toxicity: aminoglycosides, contrast media, myoglobin inflammation	≫1 (except in AGN: ≪1)
Postrenal	1%–15%	Bladder outlet obstruction Ureteral obstruction (bilateral)	≫1

AGN, acute glomerulonephritis.

Creatinine clearance is normalized to a body surface area of 1.73 m². It is a more sensitive and more accurate measure of GFR than serum creatinine determinations, although more cumbersome to obtain.

THERAPY

The goals in management are prevention and timely diagnosis to try to limit renal damage and minimize complications. As mentioned earlier, acute renal dysfunction, when recognized in a timely fashion and aggressively managed, rarely progresses to failure. In most surgical patients, acute oliguria or a rise in serum creatinine level can be assumed to result from renal hypoperfusion and should be empirically treated with fluid administration. Numerous studies suggest that adequate hydration with salt and water loading has a protective effect in preventing acute tubular necrosis (ATN) or blunting its course. Even in cases where the underlying cause is not prerenal, maintenance of adequate renal perfusion is still essential.[16] The first therapeutic measure should be an attempt at reexpansion of intravascular volume unless there is clear evidence of volume overload. Liberal use of invasive monitoring should assist in making this determination. The fact that postoperative or severely injured patients may have significant depletion of their intravascular volume despite massive peripheral edema and weight gain cannot be overemphasized. In the surgical setting, it is more harmful to withhold fluid administration than the reverse. In some patients, the use of low-dose dopamine (<5 mg/kg/min) may have a significant effect on restoration of urine output, and should be considered when fluid administration alone does not produce the desired response.[17] In rare situations, cardiac dysfunction will require the additional use of inotropes, but this should follow the establishment of adequate preload with volume replacement and the use of invasive monitoring to guide therapy.

The use of mannitol as a protective agent has theoretical appeal but has not been shown to affect prognosis. It presumably reduces cellular edema in the glomerulus and tubule, and helps prevent the "no reflow" phenomenon.[18] Mannitol should be used judiciously to avoid abrupt increases in plasma volume that could precipitate pulmonary edema.

Diuretics are frequently used in an attempt to "convert" the oliguric to a nonoliguric form, and hence simplify fluid management and reduce associated complications. However, their effectiveness is also unproved and they do not seem to affect the natural course of acute renal failure, nor do they improve survival.[19] It is more likely that a response to diuretics simply identifies a subpopulation of patients with a lesser degree of renal damage and better prognosis, rather than representing true conversion of oliguric to nonoliguric renal failure.[20]

Additional measures should be directed at the specific cause. All nephrotoxic agents should be identified and discontinued. If rhabdomyolysis is present, clearance of the pigment load should be accomplished by establishing a brisk diuresis until the urine is clear. In situations where the evolving renal dysfunction is due to sepsis, septic foci should be aggressively searched for and eliminated. The management of postrenal dysfunction depends on the location of the obstruction, and can range from insertion of a urethral or suprapubic catheter for bladder outlet obstruction to placement of nephrostomy tubes for ureteral obstructions.

Once oliguria sets in and is not reversible, careful attention to fluid management and electrolyte abnormalities is essential to maintain normal homeostasis. In addition, drug dosages and dosing intervals should be adjusted and guided by monitoring serum drug levels. Adequate nutritional support should be provided. Dialysis should be used for the management of fluid overload, metabolic derangements, or encephalopathy. Its early use has been associated with improved survival, especially in young trauma patients. Absolute creatinine levels are not indications for dialysis. Patients with fluid overload but no other metabolic indication for dialysis can be managed with ultrafiltration, which may be useful in patients with hemodynamic instability who cannot tolerate dialysis.[21]

PROGNOSIS

Although the incidence of acute renal failure has decreased over the past 50 years, the mortality from severe renal failure (requiring dialysis) has not changed.[9] This seems to be directly related to the increasing presence of associated multiorgan failure (MOF). Isolated renal failure has a significantly better prognosis than that associated with sepsis or multiorgan dysfunction.[22] Patients with nonoliguric acute renal failure have a significantly lower mortality than those with oliguric acute renal failure. Additionally, they have a lower incidence of complications such as gastrointestinal (GI) hemorrhage, sepsis, and metabolic derangements. The prognosis of acute renal failure in medical and obstetric patients is significantly better than in surgical patients. This is mainly due to the presence of comorbid conditions in surgical patients, such as sepsis, GI bleeding, pulmonary insufficiency, wound complications, and malnutrition. Despite improvements in monitoring and dialysis, the mortality from acute postsurgical renal failure has remained high, ranging from 30 to 80%, depending on the underlying cause and associated complications. Infectious complications, most commonly pneumonia, are the leading cause of death in these patients. Among survivors, the chance of recovery of renal function is best in younger patients with nonoliguric renal failure. Overall, up to one third of survivors may have complete recovery, and another one half may have partial return of renal function.[23]

SEPSIS AND MULTIPLE ORGAN FAILURE

Sepsis and MOF are the leading causes of death of patients admitted to an ICU in the United States. Approximately 400,000 patients develop sepsis annually with a mortality rate between 20 and 50%.[24] Approximately one half of all patients who develop sepsis will develop shock. Between 60 and 80% of patients who develop septic shock succumb.[25] Although the term sepsis implies the presence of infection in a patient, some confusion has developed with respect to the terminology that describes the conditions encountered clinically.[26-28] "Bacteremia" is the presence of bacteria in the blood confirmed by culture. "Septicemia" implies bacteremia with clinical manifestations of infection. "Sepsis" refers to infection with a characteristic systemic response. The term "sepsis syndrome" describes a constellation of findings in a patient suggestive of infection, which in most cases is gram-negative infection (Table 25–3). It is important to recognize that many patients with signs and symptoms of sepsis syndrome will not have an identifiable source of infection and their cultures will remain negative.[26,29] This uncontrolled inflammation has been termed the systemic inflammatory response syndrome (SIRS). Although patients with sepsis syndrome generally suffer from impaired organ perfusion, they are often not overtly hypotensive. As long as the patient is able to compensate for the effects of sepsis the blood pressure may be normal. Once the septic process progresses, or the patient's ability to compensate is exceeded, frank hypotension occurs and results in septic shock. It is important to point out, however, that evidence of organ dysfunction often appears without frank hypotension. Signs of impaired organ perfusion include abnormalities of mentation, decreased urine output, hypoxemia, and elevated liver function tests. The successful management of patients who develop

sepsis and MOF requires early recognition of the process and the identification of any reversible factors before the onset of advanced organ dysfunction.

Pathophysiology

Significant advances in our understanding of the pathophysiology of sepsis and MOF have occurred in the past 10 years but the precise mechanisms are still incompletely understood. The sepsis syndrome is most commonly associated with gram-negative bacteria, especially *Escherichia*, *Klebsiella*, and *Pseudomonas*. Other gram-negative organisms, gram-positive bacteria, fungi, viruses, and many other organisms are known to produce signs and symptoms indistinguishable from gram-negative infection. The syndrome will also develop after shock, multiple trauma, pancreatitis, burns, and crush injury.[29] In many of these patients no definitive source of infection will be identified even at autopsy. Endotoxin released by gram-negative bacteria is known to initiate a cascade of events that results in the full picture of the sepsis syndrome. These affects are triggered by the release of tumor necrosis factor (TNF) from macrophages exposed to endotoxin.[29,30] Other stimuli can also initiate the release of TNF from macrophages and thus simulate the entire syndrome.[31,32] In addition to TNF, other inflammatory mediators or cytokines have been implicated in the pathophysiology of sepsis and MOF. These include interleukin-1 (IL-1) and interleukin-6 (IL-6), platelet activating factor (PAF), interferon gamma, and numerous other inflammatory mediators. These inflammatory mediators are responsible for many of the effects seen in the sepsis syndrome and likely contribute to the development of MOF. The cytokines mediate their effects through a variety of substances such as growth factors, acute phase proteins, eicosanoids, nitric oxide, and other cytokines. Three general hypotheses have been invoked to explain the progression from sepsis to MOF. These have been recently reviewed[31] and include the macrophage hypothesis involving the elaboration of cytokines and other mediators; the microcirculatory hypothesis involving underperfusion of tissues with subsequent reperfusion and generation of oxygen radicals and activated neutrophils with injury to tissues and the microvascular system; and the gut hypothesis wherein underperfusion of the GI tract associated with the lack of oral intake results in the translocation of bacteria from the lumen of the GI tract into the lymphatics and blood stream with resultant systemic sepsis.

Systemic Effects of the Sepsis Syndrome

Organ dysfunction is commonly associated with the onset of the sepsis syndrome. In the early stages of sepsis, organ dysfunction may be relatively mild. However, if the septic process is not brought under control and the inflammatory response does not subside, organ dysfunction progresses and becomes the major cause of mortality (Table 25–4).

With the onset of the sepsis syndrome, significant leakage of intravascular fluid into the interstitium occurs. This results

Table 25-4. The Sepsis Syndrome

Fever or hypothermia
Tachycardia
Tachypnea and dyspnea
Elevated white cell count
Hypotension and decreased SVR
Increased (as long at the patient is well compensated)
Decreased organ perfusion
Lactic acidosis
Evidence of MOF: ATN, ARDS, hepatic failure, stress gastritis, CNS dysfunction

CNS, central nervous system.

in hypovolemia, which if not corrected will lead to septic shock. The leakage of fluid results from damage to the capillary-endothelial barrier. This effect is not mitigated by fluid restriction. On the contrary, in most cases fluid restriction in this setting will only worsen the underperfusion of tissues and result in progressive organ dysfunction.

Renal dysfunction is evident early in the course of the sepsis syndrome, especially when associated with shock. Acute tubular necrosis will result if the process is not reversed and continues to carry a high mortality rate despite dialysis. It is manifest by oliguria or anuria and will usually respond to volume resuscitation early in the course of sepsis. Progressive organ dysfunction will ultimately lead to a rise in serum creatinine level with renal shutdown in many patients. Once the creatinine level begins to rise the kidneys have already sustained significant damage.

The effects of the sepsis syndrome on the lung are manifested clinically as adult respiratory distress syndrome (ARDS). This is discussed in more detail in a subsequent section. The response of the lung, like the response of other organs to the systemic process, is likely mediated by inflammatory substances such as the cytokines. Neutrophils also play an important role in the lung injury that results in ARDS. The alveolar capillary membrane is damaged with resultant leakage of fluid and proteins into the interstitium. As the lung parenchyma fills with fluid and protein, hypoxemia results and compliance of the lungs worsens. This is manifested clinically as dyspnea, tachypnea, and hypoxemia. Sepsis or the sepsis syndrome is the cause of ARDS in up to 80% of patients. The development of ARDS should prompt an aggressive workup for a source of sepsis to avoid irreversible lung damage.

In addition to renal and pulmonary dysfunction, many patients will develop evidence of hepatic dysfunction and may progress to liver failure. Certain subgroups of patients, in particular those who have a source of sepsis within the abdomen, may develop liver dysfunction at an earlier stage than other patients with the sepsis syndrome. A gradual rise in the serum bilirubin level may be the earliest manifestation of liver dysfunction. The Kupffer cells within the liver release IL-6 in response to stimulation by endotoxin or TNF. Interleukin-6 shifts the synthetic function of the hepatocyte to the production of acute phase reactants and mediators of inflammation.

This will ultimately result in protein deficiency and a low serum albumin. As the septic process continues patients develop progressive immune dysfunction associated with anergy, decreased T-cell function, and a variety of other immunologic deficiency states. Gastrointestinal bleeding may develop late in the course of sepsis and MOF, and likely represents underperfusion of the gastric mucosa with resultant erosion and bleeding.

An altered mental status is commonly encountered in the patient with advanced sepsis syndrome. Derangements in mental status in critically ill patients should therefore be regarded as possible early signs of sepsis and should be differentiated from other causes of neurological abnormalities.

Patients with sepsis have been shown in a variety of settings to have depressed cardiac function. The major effect appears to be on diastolic function and may ultimately result in cardiac failure. In the early stages of the sepsis syndrome, however, the majority of patients develop a hyperdynamic state with an increased CO and a decreased SVR. This is quite typical of the early compensated phase of sepsis and results in the "warm shock" state that is identified in patients. If cardiac function deteriorates, or if the patient is unable to maintain an increase in CO, peripheral vasoconstriction with "cold shock" develops and is associated with worsening organ function. A high CO in response to the septic process is associated with a better prognosis. Whether increasing the CO of patients with "inadequate" cardiac function will result in improvement in survival remains controversial.[33]

Treatment

The most effective treatment for sepsis is prevention. Efforts to minimize the risk of developing sepsis in the critical care setting include removing central lines as quickly as possible, minimizing the time of intubation and mechanical ventilation, early ambulation, optimizing nutritional support, using the enteral route whenever possible for nutritional support, aggressive debridement of wounds and drainage of infected sites, early repair of fractures in the injured patient, and adhering to strict hygienic protocols such as hand washing and gloving.

The patient who develops sepsis or sepsis syndrome in the critical care unit is at an increased risk for organ failure as outlined above. It is therefore imperative that the early care of such patients include aggressive volume resuscitation to replace intravascular losses into the interstitium. This is most often accomplished using a crystalloid solution. Colloids are also used for volume expansion. The choice of crystalloid is more cost-effective. Neither crystalloids nor colloids have been demonstrated to be more effective in the resuscitation from shock. Proportionally more crystalloid solution would be required than colloid solution to achieve the same end points of adequate tissue perfusion. Although crystalloid solutions will leak to a significant degree from the intravascular space, the resultant tissue edema does not in itself bode for a worse prognosis and crystalloid resuscitation does not result in pulmonary insufficiency or ARDS as had been suggested in the past. It is the process of sepsis, especially if inadequately treated, that will ultimately result in lung dysfunction. The end point for resuscitation should be the return of adequate tissue perfusion. This can be assessed by the return of adequate urine output, normal mentation, vital signs that are within the normal range, capillary refill, and the resolution of acidosis. It has been suggested that these "traditional end points" may be inadequate in some patients and that more aggressive resuscitation is warranted. It is still unclear whether such "supranormal" resuscitation materially affects survival.[33] Patients who achieve high CO with return of organ perfusion tend to have the best prognosis.

Once resuscitation has been initiated, a search for the source of sepsis is indicated. If a source of sepsis can be identified, it should be treated aggressively. This may include drainage of purulent collections, debridement of necrotic tissue, therapy for pneumonia or other infectious processes, or the removal of infected catheters or other devices. Many patients will not have a source of sepsis located. These patients should be screened periodically for the source of sepsis with cultures and other diagnostic tests as appropriate. Empirical broad spectrum antibiotic therapy is justified in the setting of sepsis or sepsis syndrome. Antibiotic therapy should in general be adjusted based on the results of cultures once these are available. Patients who do not appear to be responding to antibiotic therapy should not be maintained indefinitely on these drugs. Discontinuing antibiotic therapy and repeating cultures may in some cases result in the identification of a source of infection.

In addition to resuscitation, antimicrobial therapy, and the management of septic foci, the critically ill patient with sepsis syndrome will require aggressive nutritional management. In most cases this should be initiated if a patient is expected to be unable to take oral nutrition within approximately 5 days. The GI tract should be used whenever possible and feeding tubes should be passed beyond the pylorus to minimize the chance of aspiration, or beyond the ligament of Treitz if possible. Total parenteral nutrition represents an acceptable alternative if enteral feedings are not possible, but carries significantly higher risks and involves greater costs. The composition of the nutritional formulas used in this setting have undergone important changes in recent years. A smaller caloric load is currently advocated (approximately 126 kJ/kg/d). In addition, a higher protein content (1.5 to 2 mg/kg/d) and a smaller proportion of calories as fat (20 to 30%) is recommended.[34]

As our understanding of the pathophysiology of the sepsis syndrome has improved, several novel therapies have been advocated for the treatment of these patients. These have included the use of monoclonal antibodies directed against endotoxin.[32] Double-blind randomized clinical studies have been conducted with encouraging results, but the clinical use of monoclonal antibody against endotoxin will require further study before it can be recommended. Therapies directed against IL-1 have included monoclonal antibody to IL-1, as well as IL-1 receptor antagonists. Clinical trials currently underway will define the role of these agents in clinical prac-

tice. In addition, a monoclonal antibody against TNF has been generated and is currently in clinical trials. The cost of these agents is substantial, but if their efficacy can be demonstrated they could represent an important advance in the management of the patient with sepsis, especially for the subgroup with septic shock.

ADULT RESPIRATORY DISTRESS SYNDROME

In 1967 Ashbaugh et al[35] described 12 patients with respiratory failure of varied etiologies characterized by dyspnea, tachynea, hypoxemia, stiff lungs, and diffuse lung infiltrates on chest radiograph. This syndrome was later called the ARDS. It currently affects an estimated 150,000 people in the United States each year, with mortality rates exceeding 50% in most series. It can be defined by a combination of clinical findings (Table 25–5). These clinical findings represent a syndrome resulting from direct or indirect damage to the lungs with demonstrated respiratory distress, hypoxemia, stiff lungs, and chest radiograph findings of bilateral pulmonary infiltrates. Cardiogenic pulmonary edema should be ruled out in this situation.

Many pseudonyms exist for ARDS. These include DaNang lung, shock lung, white lung, posttraumatic lung, adult hyaline membrane disease, etc. The list of conditions associated with ARDS is lengthy and includes shock, sepsis, burns, fat emboli, pulmonary contusion, a variety of infectious processes, oxygen toxicity, aspiration, numerous medications, pancreatitis, postcardiopulmonary bypass, disseminated intravasular coagulation (DIC), and carcinomatosis. Although the conditions associated with ARDS are numerous, the clinical manifestations are quite similar. A variety of risk factors for ARDS have been identified. Systemic sepsis is by far the most commonly associated condition. Patients who have ARDS should be investigated carefully for the presence of sepsis.

Pathophysiology

The pathophysiology of ARDS involves direct or indirect damage to the lung. This can be precipitated by any of the conditions mentioned above. Whatever the mechanism of pulmonary damage, the initial injury appears to be to the alveolar capillary membrane. Once the alveolar capillary membrane is damaged, increased permeability results in the

Table 25–5. ARDS: Definition

Predisposing condition causing direct or indirect damage to the lungs
Dsypnea
Tachypnea
Hypoxemia (POa2/ FiO$_2$ < 250; A-a gradient smaller than 350)
Diffuse bilateral pulmonary infiltrates
Stiff lungs (total static compliance < 50 mm/cm H$_2$O)
Noncardiogenic pulmonary edema (PCWP <20)

collection of fluids, proteins, and cellular elements in the lung interstitium. This includes activated leukocytes that can further the damage through their toxic oxygen metabolites. As the fluid content of the interstitium increases and overwhelms the ability of the pulmonary lymphatics to clear it, fluid appears in the alveolar spaces and the picture of pulmonary edema ensues. Because of the increased fluid content in the interstitium and in the intralveolar spaces, the lungs' functional residual capacity (FRC) is decreased and compliance is reduced. A significant intrapulmonary shunt exists in patients with ARDS because of perfusion of poorly ventilated areas of the lung. In addition to the above changes, injuries to the type 2 cells lining the pulmonary air spaces occur. These are replaced by type 1 cells that are incapable of synthesizing surfactants. This surfactant deficiency worsens the insult and results in a greater tendency to pulmonary edema, as well as a greater tendency to alveolar collapse and reduced FRC.

Damage to the lung is mediated by several mechanisms. Cytokines play an important role, including the interleukins, TNF, and interferon. Complement, bradykinin, and coagulation proteins also play a role. Platelet activating factor, leukotrienes, prostaglandin, and serotonin are also known to contribute to the progressive lung injury. Increased pulmonary artery pressures, activation of leukocytes, endothelial cell damage with leakage of fluid and protein into the interstitium, bronchial spasm, and intrapulmonary shunting result from the elaboration of these inflammatory mediators. Leukocytes play an important role in the lung injury, and the presence of receptors for leukocytes on the endothelial surface of the small vessels in the lung may account for the propensity of the lung to sustain damage while other tissues are relatively spared.

In the early stages of ARDS an exudative phase occurs (the first 5 days). Interstitial and alveolar edema, poor compliance, and high intrapulmonary shunts are apparent. This results in hypoxemia, which is resistant to increases in the fractional inspired concentration of oxygen (FiO_2). If the process does not abate, the injury progresses to a stage of proliferation and ultimately fibrosis. This results in organization of the hyaline membranes and the alveolar septae. A restrictive fibrotic pattern of healing occurs in the lung and is associated with hypercapnia. As the patient progresses from hypoxemia to hypercapnia the prognosis tends to worsen and the likelihood of weaning from mechanical ventilation decreases. Surfactant deficiency is known to play a role in the development and progression of ARDS. Clinical trials are currently in place to determine the exact role of exogenous surfactant in the treatment of this disorder.

Treatment

Early management of the patient who develops ARDS consists of the institution of supplemental oxygen and the support of hemodynamic function. If a source of sepsis can be identified and treated, it is possible to ameliorate the syndrome. Patients who have further progression generally require mechanical ventilation for respiratory distress. Fluid management in such patients should focus on optimizing oxygen delivery and supporting organ function. This can generally be accomplished without exacerbating the pulmonary dysfunction if care is taken to titrate the fluid therapy to acceptable end points. In patients who have significant cardiopulmonary disease who are at greater risk for complications, placement of a pulmonary artery catheter can be extremely helpful in clinical management. The use of a pulmonary artery catheter will allow for more accurate titration of fluid to ensure organ perfusion without excessive fluid loading. In many critically ill patients the ability to assess volume status by standard noninvasive clinical parameters is quite limited.[36] The use of a portable chest x-ray can be misleading and result in inappropriate decisions with regards to fluid management. Although some have advocated fluid restriction in the management of ARDS, most surgical patients require significant volume resuscitation and can achieve organ perfusion without exacerbating the lung injury.

The early management of hypoxemia is often by increasing FiO_2 by the use of a face mask. Most patients who have ARDS will require intubation and mechanical ventilation. The use of FiO_2 below 0.6 is recommended to avoid oxygen toxicity. To achieve this goal it is often necessary to add positive end-expiratory pressure (PEEP) to the mechanical ventilation regimen. This will allow the restoration towards normal of FRC by "recruiting alveoli." This improves ventilation/perfusion mismatching and decreases intrapulmonary shunting. Compliance may improve. Using levels of PEEP > 15 cm H_2O is often associated with significant decreases in venous return with a resultant drop in the CO. Such patients should generally be managed with invasive monitoring using a pulmonary artery catheter to ensure that there is adequate preload. Such patients often require further volume loading to maintain their CO. The use of high levels of PEEP has been associated with an improvement in outcome in selected groups of patients.[37]

Patients with ARDS generally receive volume ventilation using techniques such as intermittent mandatory ventilation (IMV). Patients with severe ARDS may require high levels of PEEP with IMV. In some instances the use of inverse ratio pressure control ventilation (IR-PCV) has been beneficial and allows patients to be managed at lower peak pressures. Other methods of mechanical ventilation such as high frequency ventilation have been proposed and may be of benefit in some patients. A variety of novel therapeutic measures are being currently evaluated. These include the use of exogenous surfactant, inhaled nitric oxide,[38] the use of the intravenacaval oxygenator (IVOX), liquid breathing, and adult extracorporeal oxygenation (ECMO).[39] Inhaled exogenous surfactant (EXOSURF, Burroughs-Wellcome Co) is currently being tested in a large double-blind clinical trial and may prove to be of benefit in ameliorating the lung injury. The use of nitric oxide has been associated with improvement in hypoxemia and reduction of intrapulmonary shunting. Nitric oxide is inhaled along with the mechanically delivered breaths. It is a very short-acting vasodilator and is carried into open, functioning alveoli. Nitric oxide therefore causes selective vasodilatation of blood vessels to open alveoli, improving VQ matching and decreasing intrapulmonary shunting. Further clinical trials are underway to determine its exact role in patients with ARDS. The use of adult ECMO has recently generated interest because it may represent an important salvage therapy for many cases of severe ARDS.[39] Difficulties associated with the use of adult ECMO include the high cost and significant resource allocation necessary for its successful implementation, as well as the relatively high rates of bleeding encountered in some series.

Conclusion

The onset of ARDS in the critically ill patient represents a significant complication because mortality rates have remained around 50% for many years. An aggressive search for a source of sepsis or other initiating condition should be conducted and once identified aggressive therapy implemented. Adult respiratory distress syndrome is one element in the spectrum of MOF. Successful therapy of ARDS using aggressive supportive measures does not guarantee the patient's survival if the underlying condition is not controlled. A variety of novel approaches to the management of ARDS are now being evaluated. The traditional approach to the management of ARDS currently involves the use of mechanical ventilation and other supportive measures while the underlying cause of the lung injury is treated or subsides.

CLOSTRIDIUM DIFFICILE COLITIS

Clostridium difficile colitis is a condition that occurs occasionally in patients receiving broad spectrum antibiotics. Because of its early association with the use of clindamycin, it was formerly called clindamycin-associated colitis.[40] The term antibiotic-induced colitis or diarrhea is currently preferred, as the condition has been shown to occur in association with many antibiotics in addition to clindamycin.[41] Ampicillin and cephalosporins are considered to be the most common causes today, with an incidence between 5 and 25%.[41,42] Because patients in ICU are very likely to receive antibiotics, the the condition is seen disproportionately in this setting.[40] The condition is also seen in association with chemotherapeutic medications. Table 26-6 lists commonly implicated agents. Dosage and duration of therapy are only weakly predictive of its occurrence.

Etiology

C difficile colitis is caused by a pair of toxins produced by C difficile species.[40,43,44] Toxin A is an enterotoxin and toxin B is a cytotoxin, the two of which combine to cause damage to and malfunction of the colonic mucosa.[45] C difficile is an anaerobic gram-positive bacillus present in the normal colonic flora of a small percentage of patients.[42,46] This subgroup is somewhat predisposed to the development of diarrhea and colitis.[43,46] However, the pathogenic bacteria may

Table 25-6. Agents Implicated as Causes of C difficile Pseudomembranous Colitis or Diarrhea

General classification and specific agent

Penicillins
  Methicillin, nafcillin, oxacillin, cloxacillin, diclosacillin
  Penicillin G, penicillin V
  Ampicillin
  Amoxicillin
  Carbenicillin, ticarcillin
First-generation cephalosporins
  Cephalothin
  Cefazolin
  Cephradine
  Cephalexin
Second-generation cephalosporins
  Cefamandole
  Cefoxitin
Third-generation cephalosporins
  Moxalactam
  Cefotaxime
  Cefizoxime
  Cefoerazone
  Imipenem
Lincosamides
  Lincomycin
  Clindamycin
Macrolides/tetracyclines
  Erythromycin
  Spiramycin
  Tetracycline
Miscellaneous antimicrobials
  Chloramphenicol
  Metronidazole
  Sulfisoxazole
  Sulfamethaxazole-trimethoprim
  Sulfasalazine
  Rifampin
  Aminoglycosides (given orally)
  Amphotericin
  Miconazole
Cancer Chemotherapeutics
  Adriamycin
  Cyclophosphamide
  5-Fluorouracil
  Methotrexate

From George.[44]

be spread between patients, which is an important concern in the close accommodations of the ICU. The organism is resistant to most antibiotics, allowing for its overgrowth as the normal colonic flora is altered.[46] The elaborated toxins directly damage the mucosa, leading to fever, diarrhea, and abdominal distention.

Presentation

The clinical syndrome commonly presents with the triad of fever, abdominal distention, and bloody diarrhea.[41,43] Most commonly, the diarrhea develops 5 to 10 days after the initiation of antimicrobial therapy.[43,46] In 20 to 40% of cases, however, the diarrhea starts after the offending antibiotic has been discontinued, which may confuse the association.[40,46]

The diarrhea is occasionally profuse and this may lead to dehydration if GI losses are not replaced. The alert patient will often complain of severe colicky abdominal pain, but this important symptom is absent in the obtunded or sedated patient. Therefore, increased stool volume may be the clinician's earliest warning of the development of C difficile colitis. In extreme cases, toxic megacolon and colonic perforation may develop and lead to sepsis and possibly death.[43,46]

The spectrum of clinical presentations has led to a variety of names given to this disorder. Antibiotic-associated enterocolitis is the preferred general term for the disorder, as it indicates the central role of antibiotic administration in its development.[46] This nomenclature also accounts for those cases of diarrhea that occur in association with antibiotics that are caused by bacteria other than clostridia species. Pseudomembranous colitis represents a subgroup of antibiotic-associated colitis that is more severe and by definition is diagnosed by colonoscopy and biopsy.[46]

Diagnosis

A high index of suspicion is essential for the early diagnosis of C difficile colitis. Any patient who develops diarrhea during or following antibiotic therapy should be suspected of having the syndrome. White blood cell count will be elevated, especially in the more severe cases.[46] Stool should be examined microscopically to eliminate the possibility of parasitic colonization and disease. Microscopic examination of the stools of patients with C difficile colitis will reveal only leukocytes and red blood cells.[14] The present standard of diagnosis is assay for C difficile toxin in the stool by latex agglutination tests.[44] These tests are rapid and sensitive, although many false positives have been reported, especially in immunocompromised patients.[44] Culture of C difficile is difficult and time-consuming, so this is usually reserved for confirmation of unusual cases. However, stool should be routinely cultured for enteropathogens other than clostridium.

Sigmoidoscopy or colonoscopy is occasionally employed for diagnosis and assessment of the colonic mucosal condition. This is useful in severe and protracted episodes, but is usually not necessary in milder cases. Mucosal changes may range from simple erythema to frank pseudomembrane formation.[40,41] Histologically, the pseudomembranes are composed of neutrophils, fibrin, and epithelial debris.[40] Barium enema is also occasionally used for diagnosis.

Treatment

Treatment of C difficile colitis is supportive and medical. Most importantly, the offending antibiotic is discontinued. The condition generally resolves spontaneously within 7 days of discontinuation of the antibiotic.[40,41,43] However, patients with a late diagnosis or those who develop the condition after a complete course of antibiotics may have a more severe and prolonged clinical course.[40] If the patient is in need of continued antibiotic therapy, a replacement should be chosen that

has a lesser association with pseudomembranous colitis. Metronidazole is an excellent choice because it is infrequently associated with colitis and has excellent activity against Clostridium species.[46] Oral vancomycin is a very effective definitive therapy for C difficile.

Careful attention must be paid to the patient's volume status until the diarrhea resolves. Colonic losses may predispose the patient to hypoalbuminemia, hypovolemia, electrolyte disorders, and pH imbalances.[41,46] These conditions must be monitored closely and corrected as indicated. Anridiarrheal agents are discouraged, as continued bowel activity will evacuate the offending organisms and toxins.[43,46] Careful attention to supportive therapy while the organism is eradicated is the most important principle of management.

Recent attention has focused on the prevention of C difficile colitis, especially in the ICU. A primary concern has been the avoidance of interpatient spread of the offending organisms. Careful attention must be given to strict hand washing and isolation techniques in the care of a patient with proven or suspected C difficile colitis.[40,43] Selective decontamination of the GI tract has been considered in order to reduce the incidence of nosocomial pneumonia and antibiotic-associated colitis. The results of selective digestive tract decontamination have been controversial. Currently, the best method of prevention is careful avoidance of cross-contamination from infected patients, close monitoring of patients on broad spectrum antibiotics, and avoidance of unnecessary antimicrobial therapy.

UPPER GASTROINTESTINAL HEMORRHAGE

Gastrointestinal hemorrhage is a relatively common cause of morbidity and mortality in the intensive care setting. Overall, acute GI hemorrhage carries a mortality rate of approximately 10%.[42] In the setting of the ICU, however, the associated mortality may be as much as threefold higher.[45] The combination of postoperative stress, preexisting risk factors, and concomitant medical illness increases the incidence and severity of GI hemorrhage in the critically ill patient.

Many sources of hemorrhage are found in the upper GI tract. These include esophageal varices, peptic ulcers, tumors, and mucosal tears. The primary concern in the postoperative patient, however, is stress-related hemorrhagic gastritis. This potentially preventable disorder occurs in a large percentage of critically ill patients and carries a high morbidity and mortality. Prevention and expedient treatment of GI bleeding should be a prime consideration in the management of patients in the ICU.

Etiology

Certain risk factors predispose patients to the development of GI bleeding, and many of these are combined in the postoperative head and neck surgery patient. Tobacco and alcohol abuse are well-known predisposing habits for head and neck cancer. They also predispose the patient to upper GI hemorrhage from peptic ulcer disease, hemorrhagic gastritis, Mallory-Weiss tears, and esophageal varices. Stress is a major risk factor, whether it be secondary to trauma, burns, or a major surgical procedure.[47] Medications that are associated with risk of GI hemorrhage include steroids, aspirin, and other nonsteroidal anti-inflammatory agents. Transient hypotension commonly precipitates acute hemorrhagic gastritis. Severe liver and renal disease and sepsis also predispose patients to the development of GI bleeding.[50]

Presentation

Upper GI hemorrhage is surprisingly asymptomatic in many patients. Abdominal pain is a rare feature. Some patients will complain of nausea and anorexia prior to the development of hematemesis, but this symptom is not reliable. Otherwise, the physician must be cued into signs that may indicate subclinical GI blood loss. A falling hematocrit value may be an indication, especially if the clinician is certain that this is not secondary to hemodilution or losses into the surgical wound. An increased blood urea nitrogen (BUN) to creatinine ratio above 20 may also indicate bleeding into the digestive tract.

Melenic stool is the most common feature of upper GI hemorrhage. Melena is over three times more common than hematochezia as a sign of upper GI bleeding.[45] Generally, hematochezia as a result of hemorrhage proximal to the ligament of Treitz occurs only in the face of massive bleeding. Thus, red stools are an ominous sign in the patient with acute GI hemorrhage. Hematemesis, usually of red or maroon-colored blood, occurs in over one half of cases.[42,48] Red or coffee-ground nasogastric aspirates are also common presenting signs.

Diagnosis

The initial diagnostic procedure is esophagogastroduodenoscopy by a qualified endoscopist. The source of bleeding can be determined by initial endoscopy in over 85% of cases, and repeat endoscopy will determine the source in up to 70% of the residual cases.[42] Endoscopy provides the additional benefit of immediate therapy by variceal sclerosis or constriction and coagulation of arterial sources. Endoscopic diagnostic failures are generally due to variceal hemorrhage, which may provide little evidence of recent hemorrhage.[42]

Standard barium contrast radiological evaluation of the upper GI tract has a high failure rate, and is reserved for difficult cases and endoscopic failures in stable patients. Angiography is useful in the diagnosis of arterial hemorrhages, but the bleeding must be brisk for the technique to be effective. Bleeding varices are suboptimally diagnosed by conventional angiography, but the diagnosis can occasionally be inferred from the absence of an arterial source. Radionuclide-labeled red blood cell scanning is used less often.[49]

Treatment

The initial management of GI hemorrhage is the support of acute intravascular volume loss and possible airway compromise. Patients with upper GI bleeding are likely to have hematemesis with a resultant risk of aspiration.[48] As with other emergencies, airway control and support is paramount. The patient should be intubated if obtunded or having voluminous hematemesis. A nasogastric tube should be placed promptly to evacuate and decompress the stomach. This will further protect the airway and allow for estimation of blood loss.

Adequate intravenous access must be established immediately. Initial volume resuscitation should commence with a crystalloid, such as lactated Ringer's solution or normal saline. Fluids should be administered in volumes sufficient to support blood pressure and perfusion while blood is being prepared for transfusion. If the patient is actively exsanguinating, type-specific blood can be transfused immediately. If the patient has a concomitant coagulopathy or thrombocytopenia, appropriate blood products should be judiciously replaced.

Specific therapy for GI hemorrhage depends on the source. Endoscopic sclerotherapy is the current mainstay of initial variceal treatment. It is very effective in the management of acute variceal bleeding, but repeated sclerosis is required to prevent recurrence.[49] Intravenous or selective arterial vasopressin is used to reduce splanchnic arterial flow and thus portal venous pressure. This has been shown to transiently control acute bleeding, but it has many potentially serious systemic side effects. A Sengstaken-Blakemore tube may be used to temporarily tamponade esophageal and gastric varices that are refractory to the above measures. Surgical therapy is a last resort and is aimed at resection of varices and relief of portal hypertension.

Many patients have postoperative emesis, and many have nasogastric or nasoduodenal tubes. These factors predispose them to mucosal tears at the gastroesophageal junction. Mallory-Weiss tears are relatively uncommon sources of upper GI hemorrhage and require only supportive measures until their spontaneous resolution.

Peptic ulcer disease is a common cause of upper GI bleeding in the ICU. As with variceal hemorrhage, initial therapy may be performed at the time of endoscopy. Active bleeding sites or exposed vessels may be treated with electrocautery or epinephrine injection, usually with good results.[42] If the patient undergoes diagnostic arteriography, embolization of arterial bleeders may be accomplished. This therapy is generally effective, but the patient is at risk for local organ necrosis.[50] Antacids and H_2 blockers have been proven efficacious in the prevention of initial hemorrhage from peptic ulcer disease, but they are not useful in stopping acute bleeding or preventing recurrence.[51] Surgery is reserved for treatment of life-threatening or recurrent hemorrhage. Definitive therapy for peptic ulcer disease is usually carried out at the time of laparotomy.[48]

Hemorrhagic gastritis is the major cause of upper GI bleeding in critically ill patients. Clinically significant stress-related gastric hemorrhage has been reported to occur in 20 to 50% of all ICU patients, and acute gastric mucosal erosions have been shown endoscopically in 85 to 100%.[52] Risk factors for the development of acute gastritis include alcoholism, stress of severe illness or trauma, age over 65 years, hypotension, and sepsis.[48,53] Patients with more than one predisposing risk factor have a higher incidence of hemorrhage and a higher mortality rate.[48]

To prevent the development of hemorrhagic gastritis in the seriously ill patient, most should be placed on prophylactic therapy with antacids, H_2 blocking agents, or sucralfate.[47,48] All of these agents have proven to be effective in decreasing the incidence of stress ulceration.[53] Sucralfate has been shown to be as effective as antacid, and it has the added benefit of a low cost and ease of administration.[47] In some studies, these medications have been shown to be even more effective when used in combination. The incidence of acute upper GI hemorrhage can be reduced to 10% or less with prophylaxis using these agents.[53]

Once stress-related hemorrhage has occurred, the mainstay of treatment is conservative support, acid suppression, and reversal of inciting factors. Maintaining a gastric pH of 3.5 or greater decreases the concentration of hydrogen ions and inhibits the proteolytic activity of pepsin.[53] Major stress-related gastric hemorrhage carries an overall mortality rate approaching 30%. Surgery is avoided in all but the most extreme cases, as it is associated with a mortality rate of 40 to 60%.[48]

Outcome and Prognosis

Major stress-related gastric hemorrhage carries an overall mortality rate approaching 30%.[49] Studies have shown a fourfold higher incidence (32%) of hemorrhage-related mortality when GI hemorrhage develops in the hospital setting as compared with bleeding occurring in an outpatient.[45] Patients over 60 years of age and those with multiple medical problems have a higher mortality rate as well. The presence of liver, renal, or pulmonary disease causes a dramatic increase in morbidity and mortality. These points emphasize the need for prophylaxis and early recognition of GI hemorrhage.

MENTAL STATUS CHANGE

Mental status change occurs commonly in the critically ill patient and is related to many factors. It may manifest as delirium, anxiety, agitation, confusion, or psychosis. The causes are numerous and the patient's outcome is dependent on an expedient diagnosis. Acute mental status change should be considered a medical emergency, with the clinician's efforts directed at determining and correcting the underlying cause.

Delirium is a term used to described an acute, transient change in mental function.[54] It is an organic mental syndrome[55] and a manifestation of an insult to brain function. The hallmark of delirium is fluctuating cognition, with the patient showing varying degrees of confusion at different times. It occurs commonly, with an incidence of 10 to 50% in acutely ill patients.[54] Its serious nature is reflected in the fact that the mortality rate for hospitalized patients who develop delirium may approach 30%.[56]

Manifestation

As mentioned, delirium is an organic mental syndrome with the hallmark of acute, fluctuating changes in cognition and attention. These changes may be expressed as confusion, agitation, apathy, rage, or depression. The disoriented, inappropriate, and agitated patient is easy to recognize, but others may present less obviously. A change in sleep pattern or mood may be the earliest symptom,[55] and this is seen frequently in the postoperative ICU patient. Changes in memory and attention span may be very subtle unless they are specifically tested.

The manifestations of delirium are diverse and graded. At the extreme, a patient may become acutely psychotic. Incoherent, fragmented speech and motor disturbances may occur. Altered perception may lead to illusions or hallucinations.[55] These patients are at risk of harming themselves by pulling out lines and drains, and by attempting to get out of bed. Many will misinterpret the actions of the nurses or physicians and become aggressive toward them. It is important to recognize these actions as the product of delirium and not personal attacks on the health care team.

Risk Factors

There are definite factors that predispose critically ill patients to the development of delirium. Children and elderly patients are at increased risk. Patients with the sepsis syndrome, severe burns, brain injuries, or human immunodeficiency virus (HIV) infection also have an increased incidence of acute confusion. Drug abusers, including alcoholics, are well known to develop delirium in the critical care setting, and these patients must be observed for withdrawal reactions and drug interactions. Patients on multiple medications and those with preexisting severe medical conditions are also predisposed. The relative importance of these factors is not well known, and many patients will have a combination of risk factors.

Diagnosis

Evaluation of the acutely confused patient should be prompt and thorough. Assessment of the postoperative patient is complicated by administration of sedatives and analgesics, both of which may cause an intentional or inadvertent change in mental status. However, the clinician must be cautious in attributing confusion and delirium solely to the administration of medications. Recognition of the early signs and symptoms of confusion may provide the best opportunity to correct underlying factors that have caused an acute deterioration in brain function.

The mini-mental status exam will define the nature and extent of the confusion. This will usually show disorientation, dysnomia, dysgraphia, and constructional apraxia.[57] Serial mental status exams are important owing to the fluctuating nature of delirium. The physical exam should be directed toward neurological evaluation, vital signs, and general state of health. The patient may show signs of sympathetic discharge, including tachycardia, diaphoresis, hypertension, and pallor. These signs are particularly frequent in postoperative patients, who may have pain and anticholinergic medications as complicating factors.[54]

Laboratory studies should include serum electrolytes and glucose, liver enzymes and function tests, thyroid function tests, arterial blood gas tests, and urinalysis. Cultures and other laboratory tests are obtained as indicated by the primary evaluations. Sepsis may be manifested by mental status change and this may be the earliest sign of infection in the critically ill patient. Discussion with the family will help confirm changes in baseline mental status.

Medications are a common source of confusion. The "polypharmacy" applied to the critically ill patient creates the potential for serious drug interactions. The list of medications that have been associated with mental status change is extensive, and includes many medications commonly used in the ICU. Many antibiotics, analgesics, diuretics, anticholinergics, sedative-hypnotics, antidepressants, and other medications are frequently associated with the development of confusion.[54]

Further studies, including computed tomographic (CT) and magnetic resonance imaging (MRI) scans, electroencephalogram (EEG), lumbar puncture, and other invasive studies should be ordered as indicated by the preliminary studies. The EEG may show slowing, especially in the lethargic patient. Agitated or anxious patients have a more variable pattern on EEG. Delirium must be differentiated from other psychiatric disorders such as schizophrenia, depression, or dementia. It should be remembered that patients with underlying psychiatric disturbances are at greater risk for the development of acute confusional states.

Treatment

The principal goal of management is to establish a prompt and accurate diagnosis and to correct any reversible causes. All abnormalities discovered on laboratory evaluation should be treated appropriately. Unnecessary medications should be discontinued, especially if they are commonly associated with confusion. Thiamine and folate should be administered to the suspected alcohol abuser. Antibiotics should be administered as indicated by white blood cell count, cultures, and clinical suspicion of sepsis. Providing aural and visual stimulation may help the patient become reoriented.

Acutely confused patients must be managed aggressively to prevent them from harming themselves. Pharmacological agents should be used selectively and sparingly, but in adequate dosage to aid in the control and comfort of the patient. Benzodiazepines are the medication of choice for suspected alcohol or benzodiazepine withdrawal, and should be used prophylactically in patients with a history of abuse. Narcotics are essential for the management of postoperative pain, but they should not be used for sedation of the angry or confused patient. Haloperidol is the antipsychotic medication of choice for the delirious or psychotic patient.[58] It is very effective and has little anticholinergic or hypotensive actions. Its effects are accentuated by low doses of benzodiazepines, which may also be necessary for control of acute confusional states.

COMPLICATIONS OF MONITORING DEVICES

Systemic Arterial Catheters

Arterial lines are usually the most common invasive monitoring devices used in the ICU.[59] They provide a continuous read-out of the patient's blood pressure, as well as a graphic representation of the pressure waveform. In addition, they allow easy access for repeated blood sampling. In most institutions, insertion and use of arterial lines are restricted to the intensive care setting, the operating room, or the recovery room because of maintenance needs and the danger of disconnection and exsanguination.

The indications for placement of a systemic arterial catheter include the need for frequent blood sampling, especially arterial blood gases, as well as the need for continuous monitoring of arterial blood pressure. Use of arterial lines is particularly useful in patients with hemodynamic instability, in patients requiring inotropic or pressor support, or those on vasodilator therapy.

A 2 to 2.5-in, 20 or 22-gauge catheter is usually employed for arterial cannulation in the adult. Arterial lines are commonly placed in the radial artery. Alternate sites include the femoral artery (in patients without atherosclerotic disease) and the dorsalis pedis artery. The axillary artery has been proposed as an alternate site, but has not gained popularity because of the awkward location of the vessel and the proximity of neural structures. If the radial artery is selected, a modified Allen test should be performed.[60,61] The modified Allen test consists of draining blood from the hand by elevating and repeatedly clenching the fist. Both the radial and ulnar arteries are then occluded with digital pressure. The extremity is returned to the neutral position and pressure is released from the ulnar artery. A rapid blush of the hand occurs if the ulnar artery is the dominant blood supply to the palmar arch. This occurs in the majority of patients. If a blush does not occur within a few seconds, then the radial artery is presumed to be the dominant blood supply to the hand and should not be cannulated, given the risk of ischemic changes in the hand.

The brachial artery is rarely used for arterial cannulation because of the lack of collateral blood supply around it and the high incidence of complications associated with its use. Placement of a femoral arterial line is associated with a relatively low complication rate. Patients with lower extremity atherosclerosis, however, are more likely to develop problems such as thrombosis of the vessel with distal ischemia, creation of intimal flaps, or plaque embolization as a result of attempts at femoral artery catheterization. It is thus advisable to avoid repeated attempts at femoral artery cannulation in a patient with atherosclerosis. Use of the femoral artery for arterial cannulation in patients who are confined to bed and have no significant lower extremity atherosclerosis is associated with complication rates that compare favorably with those of radial artery cannulation.[62]

A number of complications are associated with arterial catheters (Table 25-7). A significant percentage of radial arteries that are cannulated develop subsequent thrombosis. Some of these vessels recannulate. The introduction of continuous heparin infusion through the catheter has decreased the incidence of catheter and proximal artery thrombosis to less than 5%.[63] Other complications associated with the use of radial artery catheters include hematoma, pseudoaneurysm, arteriovenous fistula, and cerebral air embolism. Cerebral air embolus may occur when a radial arterial line is flushed for an extended interval at high pressure forcing air retrograde up the extremity into the carotid circulation. This can be avoided by manual flushes of the arterial line using relatively small volumes (2 to 5 mL) of heparinized saline instead of opening the arterial line to a pressure bag system at 300 mm Hg, as occurs when one withdraws the rubber plunger present on most commercial systems.

Catheter-related infection occurs relatively infrequently with systemic arterial lines. The two most commonly used sites, the radial artery and the femoral artery, both have infection rates of between 3 and 5%.[62] The incidence of catheter-related infection is insignificant if the catheter is removed by 48 hours from the time of placement. As the duration of cannulation increases, the infection rate gradually rises. The majority of infections are related to skin flora, predominantly *Staphylococcus aureus*. Routinely changing an arterial catheter that exhibits no signs of mechanical complications or local infection is probably unwarranted. Once the clinical utility of an arterial line is no longer apparent it should be removed. The availability of an arterial line may lead to excessive arterial blood gas determinations simply because of its presence.[59]

Systemic arterial catheters allow access for blood sampling and provide a digital and graphic display of the patient's blood pressure. The systolic and diastolic pressures measured at different sites will vary (the systolic being higher and the diastolic being lower) the further the monitoring site is from the ascending aorta.[64,65] Systolic pressure measured in the radial artery will thus be higher and diastolic pressure lower than in the ascending aorta or the axillary artery, for example. The mean pressure, however, should be the same at any site. In addition to the site of arterial monitoring, errors can

Table 25-7. Complications of Systemic Arterial Catheters

Thombosis
Distal embolization
Hematoma
Pseudoaneurysm
Arteriovenous fistula
Cerebral air embolism
Catheter-related infection

be introduced because of mismatching between the vessel and the monitoring system and because of "catheter whip" artifact.[64,66] Excessively stiff monitoring tubing can result in amplification (hyperresonance) of the pressure waveform. The recorded systolic pressure will be higher than the true value and the diastolic lower. If excessively compliant tubing is used, dampening occurs and the recorded systolic pressure will be lower and the diastolic pressure higher than the actual value. Dampening can also occur if the tubing is excessively long, has a clot or air bubble in it, or is kinked. In most cases the mean pressure should be accurately recorded. The "snap test" can be used to assess the recording system. The recording system is opened to the pressure bag by pulling the tab on the transducer housing and a plateau reading generated on screen. The tab is then released quickly. If the system is hyperresonant, the waveform will overshoot the baseline before returning to the arterial tracing. If the system is too compliant, the waveform slowly returns to baseline with a dampened waveform. The pressure recording system should incorporate short, stiff, noncompliant tubing. If the resulting system is hyperresonant, a commercially available dampening device may be employed. This is preferable to a system that causes dampening for which no adjustment can generally be made. These considerations and others apply to all pressure monitoring systems discussed. This will be discussed further in regards to pulmonary artery catheters.

Central Venous Catheters

Central venous catheters are commonly employed in the care of critically ill patients. Indications for their placement include monitoring central venous pressure, intravenous access for the administration of fluids and medications, administration of total parenteral nutrition, and the administration of medications that may irritate or damage smaller vessels. A large number of catheter sizes are available, 16 and 18 gauge being satisfactory for most cases. The use of polyvinyl catheters has given way to Silastic and polyurethane, which provide superior performance properties.

The internal jugular vein and the subclavian vein are most frequently used for percutaneous placement of central venous catheters for monitoring. Central venous lines can also be placed percutaneously through the femoral vein by threading a long catheter into position above the diaphragm or by cutdown from antecubital or external jugular veins passing the catheter into the thoracic cavity.

A number of complications are associated with placement and use of central venous catheters (Table 25–8). Mechanical complications include pneumothorax, hemothorax, dysrhythmias, malposition of the catheter tip, catheter shearing and embolism, laceration of the great vessels in the chest cavity, pericardial tamponade, brachial plexus injury, laceration of the trachea or esophagus, air embolism, and injury to the thoracic duct. Nonmechanical complications include catheter-related infection and central vein thrombosis. Percutaneous central vein catheterization complication rates varying from less than 1 to 12% have been reported from teaching hospitals.[67,68] Experience of house officers in percutaneous line placement appears to be a major determinant of complications. House officers who had placed over 50 catheters percutaneously experienced no complications in placing percutaneous subclavian catheters in one study.[69]

The most common complication of percutaneous subclavian vein catheterization is pneumothorax, which occurs in between 0.5 and 6% of cases.[68] Another common complication of subclavian vein catheterization is hematoma formation secondary to subclavian artery puncture. Because it is not possible to place direct pressure over the subclavian artery in the chest, these hematomas may enlarge significantly and appear on the chest radiograph as an apical cap. In patients with coagulopathy or thrombocytopenia, puncture of the subclavian artery or other vessels in the thorax can result in life-threatening exsanguination. Perforation of the vena cava, the aorta, or the heart with subsequent pericardial tamponade is potentially rapidly lethal. This complication was associated with a mortality rate of 67% in one series.[70]

Percutaneous catheterization of the internal jugular vein is associated with a lower incidence of pneumothorax than subclavian catheterization. Puncture of the carotid artery is the most common complication of internal jugular catheterization.[71] Given the small size of the needle usually employed, this can generally be controlled by firm pressure. If puncture of the carotid artery is not recognized and a larger catheter is introduced, the complication rate increases. If a large bore catheter such as an 8-French introducer is placed into the carotid artery, it may be necessary to have this removed in the operating room with repair of the carotid artery under direct vision. The use of ultrasound guidance has been shown to increase the success rate and shorten the time to successful internal jugular and subclavian cannulation.[72,73]

Malposition of the tip of the central venous catheter into the pleural cavity can result in the administration of fluids, blood products, and medications into the pleural space. Shearing of the catheter and possible embolization of a fragment can occur, especially using the older catheter-through-needle technique. The incidence of this complication should be minimal using the Seldinger technique: a small bore needle (16 gauge or smaller) is used to enter the vein, a flexible wire is passed through the needle, the needle is removed, and a catheter passed over the wire into position in the vein. Catheter malposition can occur with any technique of central venous catheterization. A chest radiograph should be obtained after each insertion to document that the catheter tip

Table 25–8. Complications of Central Venous Catheterization

MECHANICAL	NONMECHANICAL
Pneumothorax	Catheter-related infection
Hemothorax	Central vein thrombosis
Dysrhythmia	
Malposition of catheter tip	
Catheter shearing and embolism	
Laceration of thoracic great vessels	
Pericardial tamponade	
Brachial plexus injury	
Laceration of trachea or esophagus	
Air embolism	
Thoracic duct injury	

is in the desired position, usually the superior vena cava just above the right atrium. Postinsertion chest radiographs obtained routinely will help in the detection of the majority of complications of central venous catheterizations.

Air embolism can occur with all forms of central vein catheterization. This can be minimized by maintaining the patient in the Trendelenburg position throughout the insertion procedure. Air embolism can also occur if the patient takes a deep breath while the catheter tip is within the venous system and the other end is open to the atmosphere. Catheters should always be maintained capped or digitally occluded during manipulations. The advent of Luer-Lock type connectors has decreased the incidence of accidental disconnection and subsequent air embolism in patients with central vein catheters. Air embolism can occur rapidly. A pressure gradient of 4 mm Hg can cause 90 mL of air to enter the venous circulation per second, which may be sufficient to cause death in 1 second.[74]

Nonmechanical complications of central venous catheterization include catheter-related infection and thrombosis. The most common pathogens cultured in catheter sepsis are skin-borne organisms, predominantly *S aureus* and other gram-positive bacteria.[75] Gram-negative bacteria and fungal species are increasingly isolated in catheter sepsis in the ICU and are associated with high mortality especially if the catheter is not removed promptly. Hematogenous seeding and contamination from infusates are other sources of catheter sepsis. A number of criteria have been proposed singly or in combination to establish the diagnosis including: positive blood cultures, positive quantitative or semiquantitative cultures of the catheter tip,[76] positive gram stain of the catheter,[77] and resolution of the clinical manifestations of infection with catheter removal and antibiotic treatment. The diagnosis of catheter-related sepsis can be difficult to establish and in a critically ill patient high clinical suspicion may be adequate reason to remove the catheter.

The duration of catheterization is directly related to infection rate. Catheters in place less than 4 days have a relatively low infection rate, but this rises rapidly once catheterization exceeds 72 hours.[75,78] Controversy continues regarding the need and timing for catheter removal or exchange. The

Centers for Disease Control (CDC) states that "the proper frequency for changing central lines, including those used for pressure monitoring, is not known."[79] All lines placed emergently using less than optimal sterile technique should be removed within 24 hours. Seven days appears to be a reasonable cut-off for removing or exchanging central lines based on the available data. The exchange of an indwelling catheter over a guidewire in a nonseptic patient has been demonstarted to reduce subsequent infection rates.[75,80] Controversy continues regarding techniques of insertion site dressing care.[75,79,81]

The incidence of central venous thrombosis associated with indwelling venous catheters has been reported to be in the range of 20 to 50%.[82] Only about 5% are clinically apparent. Although generally underdiagnosed, intrathoracic vein thrombosis can be the source of a pulmonary embolus at rates similar to pelvic and lower extremity thrombus.

Pulmonary Artery Catheters

The technique of bedside cardiac catheterization was developed in 1970 with the introduction of a balloon-tipped catheter by Swan and Ganz.[83] Their innovation built on the work of Lategola and Rahn.[84] The technique involves the introduction of the catheter into the central circulation by cutdown or percutaneous puncture. The balloon at the catheter tip is then inflated and the catheter is advanced such that the blood flow "floats" it through the right atrium, into the right ventricle and through the pulmonary outflow tract. The location of the catheter tip is determined by observing the pressure waveform transduced from its tip obviating the need for fluroscopy. Once in the pulmonary artery, the catheter is advanced into a small arterial branch until it is "wedged." The catheter tip will then record the PCWP (or occlusion), which reflects left ventricular filling pressure. Although CVP also reflects filling pressures in the heart, it is imprecise in predicting left ventricular end diastolic pressures, particularly in patients with myocardial or pulmonary disease.[85]

Since its introduction, the Swan-Ganz catheter has undergone a variety of changes. Pulmonary artery catheters are available with multiple lumens for simultaneous recording of pressures from different sites and for fluid or drug infusion. The catheter incorporates a heat sensor for thermodilution measurement of CO and may contain electrodes for intracardiac pacing. Catheters may also contain an oximeter for continuous mixed venous oxygen saturation measurements. The Swan-Ganz catheter is available in several sizes including pediatric ones. The 7-French size is most commonly used in adults.

The indications for hemodynamic monitoring with a pulmonary artery catheter include:

1. Assessement of left ventricular filling pressure (preload).
2. Determination of CO by thermodilution.
3. Evaluation of treatment and titration of inotropes and vasoactive drugs.

4. Management of fluids in patients with severe cardiac or pulmonary dysfunction who are hemodynamically unstable.
5. Obtaining hemodynamic data for preoperative or prognostic evaluation.

Patients with hemodynamic instability or signs of CHF are candidates for early intervention with a pulmonary artery catheter. Monitoring ventricular filling pressure is useful both during the treatment of pulmonary edema and during fluid resuscitation of hypovolemic patients to avoid either inadequate or excessive fluid administration. A major indication for monitoring using a pulmonary artery catheter is the determination of a patient's fluid status. Although the clinician can often identify signs and symptoms that suggest the presence of fluid overload or hypovolemia, discrepancies between clinical and hemodynamic assessments have been well documented.[9,22,86] In patients with preexisting cardiac or pulmonary disease it may be particularly difficult to assess volume status. Patients with abnormal ventricular compliance have filling pressures that are higher than normal and pulmonary artery catheters can be very helpful in establishing optimal filling pressures needed to generate adequate CO.

The value of monitoring with a pulmonary artery catheter has led to concerns over potential overuse of the procedure.[87,88] Placement of pulmonary artery catheters is associated with all the potential complications of central venous line placement. A variety of additional complications are associated with Swan-Ganz catheter placement (Table 25-9). Serious dysrhythmias such as sustained ventricular ectopy or tachycardia occur in up to 50% of patients.[89] The ectopy occurs predominantly during insertion and removal of the catheter. A physician capable of managing dysrhythmias should therefore be at the bedside during either maneuver. Ventricular dysrhythmias are much less common once the catheter is in place and while it is stationary. Prophylactic administration of lidocaine has been shown to be of no benefit in preventing ventricular dysrhythmias during insertion and removal.

Perhaps the most serious complication resulting from pulmonary artery catheters is perforation of the pulmonary artery.[85,89,90] This complication is fortunately rare but carries a very high mortality. Risk factors include age greater than 60 years, anticoagulation, pulmonary hypertension, distal migration of the catheter tip, overdistension of the balloon, and eccentric inflation of the balloon. Hemoptysis is a common early sign. Patients with significant hemoptysis (>30 mL) should be suspected of having pulmonary artery perforation. If the patient is stable and hemoptysis subsides, the balloon is deflated and the catheter withdrawn a few centimeters. A chest radiograph may show a density near the tip of the catheter. Positive end-expiratory pressure appears to be beneficial in patients being observed and bronchoscopy may be helpful in establishing the source of the hemoptysis. If hemoptysis continues or the patient develops a pleural effusion, a wedge arteriogram may demonstrate intraparenchymal

Table 25–9. Complications Specific to Pulmonary Artery Catheterization

Dysrhythmias
Pulmonary artery perforation
Endocardial lesions and vegetations
Valvular damage
Catheter knotting and entanglement
Catheter embolization

bleeding requiring thoracotomy. Patients with massive hemoptysis or hemodynamic instability should be taken for thoracic exploration emergently. The use of a double-lumen endotracheal tube is recommended.

Intracardiac injury secondary to pulmonary artery catheter placement includes valvular injury, endocarditis and vegetations, and thrombus.[89,91–93] The passage of the catheter can cause damage to the valves or the chordae.[91] The areas in contact with the catheter are subjected to trauma from the constant motion of the device. Thrombi and vegetations form on the injured areas. These may become infected and embolize into the lung with high morbidity. The pulmonic valve is most often affected,[93] but the tricuspid valve, the right atrium, and the right ventricle are also at risk. The majority of these lesions remain asymptomatic.

Intracardiac knotting of the pulmonary artery catheter has been reported as having a variety of techniques for untying the knot.[89] Central venous lines and pulmonary artery catheters have become entangled.[94] Withdrawing a catheter that is knotted can result in uncontrolled hemorrhage. Knotting occurs with repeated attempts at passage of the catheter into an enlarged right ventricle. Review of the chest radiograph will confirm the presence of catheter knotting and entanglement as well as catheter embolization. Embolization should be a rare complication with the use of materials that are more resistant to shearing and breakage such as polyurethane.

CLINICAL UTILITY OF PULMONARY ARTERY CATHETERS

The pulmonary artery catheter provides two clinically useful values: PCWP and CO. The relationship between left ventricular end diastolic volume and CO is described by the Frank-Starling relationship. Unfortunately, this relationship is variable and the ability to predict CO based on PCWP is limited.[95] These limits relate to the ventricular function curve and the ventricular pressure volume curve: when the end diastolic pressure is in the normal or upper-normal range, it is a relatively insensitive index of end diastolic volume. Large changes in ventricular stroke work, or in ventricular end diastolic volume, may be associated with relatively small changes in ventricular end diastolic pressure. Patients with increased ventricular stiffness due to hypertrophy or MI develop scarring and stiffening of the ventricular wall. In these patients, the ventricular end diastolic pressure may be

markedly elevated in the presence of a reasonably normal end diastolic volume.[96] Despite these acknowledged limitations, interpretation of left ventricular and diastolic pressure remains a routinely used clinical tool.

Data from our ICU suggest that in a diverse general surgical population requiring pulmonary artery catheterization, there is no consistent relationship between either CVP or PCWP or CO (Fakhry SM, et al, unpublished data). The accurate determination of CO thus requires a specific measurement.

A number of interventions and practices employed in the ICU can introduce error into pulmonary artery catheter readings.[89] The increased intrathoracic pressure resulting from mechanical ventilation and PEEP may be variably transmitted to the pulmonary artery tracing and cause erroneous results. Changes in position cause variation in pressure readings. The previously described considerations for pressure monitoring systems also apply in this setting. Caution should be exercised in the interpretation of isolated wedge pressure readings and other clinical data should be considered in the clinical decision-making process.

PITFALLS IN HEMODYNAMIC MONITORING

A number of errors may occur with the measurement and interpretation of hemodynamic data, some of which were discussed in relation to arterial catheters. Problems include inadequate system frequency response, improper calibration, improper balancing of the transducer to the amplifier system (a problem that is now much less common), improper zero reference, dampening, catheter movement with cardiac function, catheter tip occlusion, external influences such as respiratory variation, increased intrathoracic pressure from positive pressure ventilation, and improper catheter tip location in the chest.

Inadequate frequency response refers to the attenuation or loss of certain high frequency events in the pressure wave form. The frequency response of presently available catheters is adequate and this is not a clinically significant problem for most of the measurements for which the catheter is used. Dampening problems, particularly overdampening, can be caused by even a small amount of blood or air in the connecting tubing. Improper zero and calibration errors can be avoided by attention to the details of the setup procedure. A common problem in patients with hyperdynamic circulations and underdampened catheter systems is the presence of catheter "whip." Excessive motion of the catheter tip within the pulmonary artery results in a cyclic movement of fluid within the catheter causing significant alterations in measurement. Partial occlusion of the catheter cannula tip by thrombus or a vessel wall may also cause abnormalities in pressure measurements. Interpretive errors are also important. The accuracy and reproducibility of the thermodilution technique for determination of CO have been studied and measurement errors in the range of 10 to 20% documented.[97] Significant error can be introduced by variation in the injection volume or temperature and the duration of injection.

CONCLUSION

Complications in the critical care setting have potentially serious implications. They are often difficult to treat and result in an increase in resource utilization and cost. Prevention is clearly desirable but not always possible. Careful observation and early, aggressive management of problems encountered in the critical care unit will result in the lowest rate of complications. Early ambulation, aggressive nutritional support, judicious use of antibiotics, prompt removal of invasive monitoring devices, and regular review of clinical practice should contribute to optimal results in these patients. Close collaboration with a critical care service can provide important support for optimal care of the more complex patient problems that may be encountered.[98]

It is currently standard practice at many institutions to routinely admit patients undergoing major head and neck procedures to an ICU.[99] The relatively low morbidity and mortality rates in such patients at our institution suggested that they could be managed in other settings such as a step-down unit or telemetry ward (ref 100 and Fakhry SM, et al. unpublished data). This results in significant savings in cost without compromising the quality of care delivered to these patients. Individual institutions should regularly review their experience and determine their morbidity and mortality rates. Such continuous quality improvement activities can help establish the appropriate level of postoperative care for optimal patient care with the lowest complication rates and maximal cost savings.

REFERENCES

1. Cohn JN, Gulha NH, Broder MI, et al. Right ventricular infarction: clinical and hemodynamic features. *Am J Cardiol.* 1974;33:209–214.
2. Marino PL. *The ICU Book.* Lea & Febiger; 1991.
3. Leier CV, Unverferth DV. Diagnosis and treatment: drugs five years later—dobutamine. *Ann Intern Med.* 1983;99:490–496.
4. Wilmore DW, Brennan MF, Harken AH, et al. *American College of Surgeons: Care of the Surgical Patient. Vol 1, Critical Care.* New York, NY: Scientific American, Inc,; 1988–1993.
5. Lyerly HK. *The Handbook of Surgical Intensive Care: Practices of the Surgery Residents at the Duke University Medical Center.* Chicago, Ill: Year Book Medical Publisher, Inc. 1989.
6. Goldman L. Cardiac risks and complications of noncardiac surgery. *Ann Surg.* 1983;198:780.
7. Herling IM. Intravenous nitroglycerin: clinical pharmacology and therapeutic considerations. *Am Heart J.* 1984;108:141–149.
8. Civetta JM, Taylor RW, Kirby RR. *Critical Care.* 2nd ed. Philadelphia, Pa: JB Lippincott Co; 1992.
9. Finn W. In: Brenner B, Lazarus J, eds. *Acute Renal Failure.* Philadelphia, Pa: WB Saunders Co; 1983.
10. Miller T, Anderson, R, Linas S. Urinary diagnostic indices in acute renal failure: a prospective study. *Ann Intern Med.* 1978;89:47.
11. Finn A, WJ, Gottschalk C. Pathogenesis of oliguria in acute renal failure. *Circ Res.* 1975;36:675.
12. Lucas C. Renal considerations in the injured patient. *Surg Clin North Am.* 1982;62:133.
13. Byrd L, Sherman R. Radiocontrast-induced acute renal failure: clinical and pathophsiologic review. *Medicine (Baltimore).*

14. Braun S, Weiss F, Keller A. Evaluation of renal toxicity of hemeproteins and their derivatives: a role in the genesis of acute tubular necrosis. *J Exp Med.* 1970;131:443.
15. Espinel C, Gregory AW. Differential diagnosis of acute renal failure. *Clin Nephrol.* 1980;13:73–77.
16. Anderson S, Meyer T, Brenner B. The role of hemodynamic factors in the initiation and progression of renal disease. *J Urol.* 1985;133:363.
17. Parker S, Carlon G, Isaacs M. Dopamine administration in oliguria and oliguric renal failure. *Crit Care Med.* 1981;9:630.
18. Warren S, Blantz R. Mannitol. *Arch Intern Med.* 1981;141:1981.
19. Levinsky N, Bernard D, Johnston P. In: Brenner B, Lazarus J, eds. *Acute Renal Failure.* Philadelphia, Pa: WB Saunders Co; 1983.
20. Anderson R, Linas SL, Berns AS. Nonoliguric acute renal failure. *N Engl J Med.* 1977;296:1134.
21. Mault J, Dechert R, Lees P. Continuous arteriovenous filtration: an effective treatment for surgical acute renal failure. *Surgery.* 1987;101:478.
22. Routh G, Briggs J, Mone J. Survival from acute renal failure with and without multiple organ dysfunction. *Postgrad Med J.* 1980;56:244.
23. Spurney R, Fulkerson W, Schwab S. Acute renal failure in critically ill patients: prognosis for recovery of kidney function after prolonged dialysis support. *Crit Care Med.* 1991;19:8–15.
24. Increase in national hospital discharge survey rates for septicemia—United States, 1979-1987. *MMWR.* 1990;39:31.
25. Taylor RW. Civetta JM, Kirby RR. Sepsis, sepsis syndrome and septic shock. In: *Critical Care.* 2nd ed. Philadelphia, Pa: JB Lippincott Co; 1992.
26. Bone RC. Lets agree on terminology: definition of sepsis. *Crit Care Med.* 1993;19:973.
27. Sprung CL. Definition of sepsis—have we reached a consensus? *Crit Care Med.* 1991;19:849.
28. Bone RC, Balk RA, Cerra FB, et al. Definitions for sepsis and organ failure and guidelines for the use of innovative therapies in sepsis. *Chest.* 1992;101:1644–1655.
29. Beutler R, Mahoney J, LeTrang L, et al. Purification of cachectin, a lipoprotein lipase-suppressing hormone secreted by endotoxin-induced RAW 264.7 cells. *J Exp Med.* 1985;161:984–995.
30. Tracey KS, Beutler N, Lowry SF, et al. Shock and tissue injury induced by recombinant human cachectin. *Science.* 1986;234:470–474.
31. Deitch EA. Multiple organ failure: pathophysiology and potential future therapy. *Ann Surg.* 1992;216:117–134.
32. Fong Y, Lowry SF. Cytokines and cellular response to injury and infection. In: Wilmore DW, ed. *Care of the Surgical Patient.* New York, NY: Scientific American, Inc; 1992.
33. Barone JE, Lowenfels AB. Maximization of oxygen delivery: a plea for moderation. *J Trauma.* 1992;33:651–653.
34. Gubler KD, Jurkovich GJ. Nutritional support of the critically ill and injured patient. In: Maull KI, ed. *Advances in Trauma and Critical Care.* Vol 8. St Louis, Mo: CV Mosby; 1993.
35. Ashbaugh DG, Bigelow DB, Petty TL, et al. Acute respiratory distress in adults. *Lancet.* 1967;2:319–323.
36. Byrne K, Sugerman H. Experimental and clinical assessment of lung injury by measurement of extravascular lung water and transcapillary protein flux in ARDS: a review of current techniques. *J Surg Res.* 1988;44:185–203.
37. Miller RS, Nelson LD, DiRusso SM, et al. High-level positive end-expiratory pressure management in trauma-associated adult respiratory distress syndrome. *J Trauma.* 1992;33:284–291.
38. Rossaint R, Falke KJ, Lopez F, et al. Inhaled nitric oxide for the adult respiratory distress syndrome. *N Engl J Med.* 1993;328:399–405.

39. Bartlett RH. Extra corporeal life support for cardio-pulmonary failure. *Curr Probl Surg*. 1990;27:623–705.
40. Tedesco FJ, Barton R, Alpers DH. Clindamycin-associated colitis. *Ann Intern Med*. 1974;81:429.
41. Nickols RL. Bacterial infectious disease considerations in the surgical patient. In: Civetta JM, Taylor RW, Kirby RR, eds. *Critical Care*. 2nd ed. Philadelphia, Pa: JB Lippincott Co; 1992:798–799.
42. Dagradi AE, Arguello JF, Weingarten ZG. Failure of endoscopy to establish a source for upper gastrointestinal bleeding. *Am J Gastroenterol*. 1979;72:395.
43. Butler T. Gastrointestinal infections. In: Hall JB, Schmidt GA, Wood LD, eds. *Principles of Critical Care*. New York, NY: McGraw Hill, Inc; 1992:1351–1353.
44. Hussain Qadri SM, Akter J, Ostrawski S, Qadri SGM, Cunha BA. High incidence of false positives by latex agglutination test for the diagnosis of *Clostridium* difficile-associated colitis in compromised patients. *Diagn Microbiol Infect Dis*. 1989;12:291–294.
45. Silverstein FE, Gilbert DA, Tedesco FJ, et al. The national ASGE survey on upper gastrointestinal bleeding: II. Clinical prognostic factors. *Gastrointest Endosc*. 1981;27:80.
46. George L. Antimicrobial-associated diarrhea in adult humans. In: Rolfe RD, and Finegold SM, eds. *Clostridium difficile: Its Role in Intestinal Disease*. San Diego, Calif: Academic Press Inc; 1988:31–41.
47. Borrero E, Bank S. Margolis, I, Schulman ND, Chardavoyne R. Comparison of antacid and sucralfate in the prevention of gastrointestinal bleeding in patients who are critically ill. *Am J Med*. 1985;79(suppl 2C):62, 63.
48. Hubert JP, Kiernan PD, Welch JS, ReMine WH, Beahrs OH. The surgical management of bleeding stress ulcers. *Ann Surg*. 1980;191:672–677.
49. Hanan IM. Gastrointestinal hemorrhage. In: Hall JB, Schmidt GA, Wood LD. eds. *Principles of Critical Care*. New York, NY: McGraw Hill, Inc; 1992:2001–2011.
50. Shapiro N, Brandt L, Sprayregan S, et al. Duodenal infarction after therapeutic Gelfoam embolization of bleeding duodenal ulcer. *Gastroenterology*. 1981;80:176.
51. Zuckerman G, Welch R, Douglas A, Troxell R, et al. Controlled trial of medical therapy for active upper gastrointestinal bleeding and prevention of rebleeding. *Am J Med*. 1984;76:361–366.
52. Bank S, Misra P, Mausner D, et al. The incidence, distribution, and evolution of stress ulcers in surgical intensive care patients (abstr). *Am Gastroenterol*. 1980;74:76.
53. Tryba M, Zevounou F, Torok M, et al. Prevention of acute stress bleeding with sucralfate, antacids, or cimetadine: a controlled study with pirenzepine as a basic medication. *Am J Med*. 1985;79(suppl 2C):55.
54. Lipowski ZJ. Delirium (acute contusionai states). *JAMA*. 1987;258:1789.
55. American Psychiatric Association. *Diagnostic and Statistical Manual of Mental Disorders*. 3rd ed. Washington, DC: American Psychiatric Association; 1987.
56. Rabins PV, Folstein MF. Delirium and dementia: diagnostic criteria and fatality rates. *Br J Psychiatry*. 1982;140:149–153.
57. Folstein MF, Folstein SE, McHugh PR. "Mini-mental state": A practical method for grading the cognitive state of patients for the clinician. *J Psychiatr Res*. 1975;12:189.
58. Steinhart MJ. The use of haloperidol in geriatric patients with organic mental disorder. *Curr Ther Res*. 1983;33.132–143.
59. Muakkassa FF, Rutledge R, Fakhry SM, et al. ABGs and arterial lines: the relationship to unnecessarily drawn arterial blood gases. *J Trauma*. 1990;30:1087–1093.
60. Allen EJ. Thromboangiitis obliterans: methods of diagnosis of chronic occlusive arterial lesions distal to the wrist with illustrative cases. *Am J Med Sci*. 1929;178:237.
61. Erjup B, Fischer B, Wright RS. Clinical evaluation of blood flow to the hand: the false positive Allen test. *Circulation*. 1966;33:778.
62. Thomas F, Burke JP, Parker J, et al. The risk of infection related to radial versus femoral sites for arterial cannulization. *Crit Care Med*. 1983;11:807.
63. Weiss BM, Gattiker RI. Complications during and following radial artery cannulation: a prospective study. *Intensive Care Med*. 1986;12:424.
64. Sladen A. Complications of hemodynamic monitoring in the intensive care unit. *Curr Probl in Surg*. 1988;25.
65. Bedford RF. *Invasive Blood Pressure Monitoring*. New York, NY: Churchill-Livingstone; 1985.
66. Abrams JH, Cerra F, Holcroft JW. Cardiopulmonary monitoring. In: Wilmore DW, ed. *Care of the Surgical Patient*. New York, NY: Scientific American, Inc; 1988–1991.
67. Feliciano DV, Mattox KL, Graham JM, et al. Major complications of percutaneous subclavian vein catheters. *Am J Surg*. 1979;138:869.
68. Herbst CA. Indications, management and complications of percutaneous subclavian catheters. *Arch Surg*. 1978;113:1421–1425.
69. Bernard RW, Stahl WM. Subclavian vein catheterization: a prospective study: I non-infectious complications. *Ann Surg*. 1971;173:184.
70. Aldridge HE, Jay AWL. Central venous catheters and heart perforation. *Can Med Assoc J*. 1986;135:1082.
71. Hermosura B, Vanags L, Dicket NW. Measurement of pressure during intravenous therapy. *JAMA*. 1986;195:321.
72. Koski EMJ, Suhonen M, Mattila MAK. Ultrasound facilitated central venous cannulation. *Crit Care Med*. 1992;20:424–426.
73. Sukigara M, Yamazaki T, Hatanaka M, Nagashima N, Omoto R. Ultrasound real time guidance, for subclavian puncture. *Surg Gynecol Obstet*. 1988;167:239–242.
74. Conahan TJ. Air embolization during percutaneous Swan-Ganz catheter placement. *Anesthesiology*. 1979;50:360.
75. Bozzetti F. Central venous catheter sepsis. *Surg Gynecol Obstet*. 1985;161:293–301.
76. Maki DG, Weise C, Sarafin HW. A semiquantitative culture method for identifying intravenous catheter related infection. *N Engl J Med*. 1977;296:1305–1309.
77. Cooper GL, Hopkins CC. Rapid diagnosis of intravascular catheter associated infection by direct gram staining of catheter segments. *N Engl J Med*. 1985;312:1142–1147.
78. Ullmaln RF, Gurveich I, Schoch PE, et al. Colonization and bactremia related to duration of triple lumen intravascular catheter placement. *M J Infect Control*. 1990;18:201–207.
79. Simons BP. Guideline for prevention of intravascular infections. *M J Infect Control*. 1983;11:183–193.
80. Norwood S, Jenkins AB. An evaluation of triple lumen catheter infection using a guidewire exchange technique. *J Trauma*. 1990;30:706–712.
81. Maki DG, Ringer M, Alvarado. Prospective randomized trial of povidone-iodine, alcohol, and chlorhexidine for prevention of infection associated with central venous and arterial catheters. *Lancet*. 1991;338:339–343.
82. Bozzetti F, Scarpa D. Terno G, et al. Subclavian venous thrombosis due to indwelling catheters: a prospective study on 52 patients. *JPEN*. 1983;7:560.
83. Swan HJC, Ganz W, Forrester J, et al. Catheterization of the heart in man with the use of flow-directed balloon-tipped catheter. *N Engl J Med*. 1970;283:447.
84. Lategola M, Rahn H. A self-guiding catheter for cardiac and pulmonary arterial catheterization and occlusion. *Proc Soc Biol Med*. 1953;84:667.
85. Swan HJC, Ganz W. Use of balloon floatation catheters in critically ill patients. *Surg Clin North Am*. 1975;55:501.

86. Forrester JS, Diamond G, Chatterjee K, et al. Medical therapy of acute myocardial infarction by the application of hemodynamic subsets. *N Engl J Med*. 1976;295:1356–1404.

87. Shoemaker WC. Use and abuse of the ballon tip (Swan Ganz) catheter: are patients getting their money's worth? [Editorial]. *Crit Care Med*. 1990;18:1294–1296.

88. Robin ED. The cult of the Swan Ganz catheter. Overuse and abuse of pulmonary flow catheters. *Ann Intern Med*. 1985:103:445.

89. Lipp H. O'Donoghue K, Resnekov L. Intracardiac knotting of a flow directed balloon catheter. *N Engl J Med*. 1971;284:220.

90. Barash PG, Nardi D, Hammond G, et al. Catheter induced pulmonary artery perforation: mechanisms, management and modifications. *J Thorac Cardiovasc Surg*. 1981;82:5–12.

91. Lange HW, Galliani CA, Edwards JF. Local complications associated with indwelling Swan Ganz catheters: autopsy study of 36 cases. *Am J Cardiol*. 1983;52:1108.

92. Ducatman BS, McMichan JC, Edwards WD. Catheter induced lesions of the right side of the heart. *JAMA*. 1985;253:791.

93. Rowley KM, Clubb KS, Smith JGW, et al. Right sided infective endocarditis as a consequence of flow-directed pulmonary catheterization. *N Engl J Med*, 1984;311:1152.

94. Graff J, Gong R, Byron R, et al. Knotting and entanglement of multiple central venous catheters. *J Parenter Ent Nutr*. 1986;10:319.

95. Braunwald E, Ross J Jr. The ventricular end-diastolic pressure: appraisal of its value in the recognition of ventricular failure in man. *Am J Med*. 1963;34:147.

96. Folse R, Braunwald E. A method for the determination of the fraction of left ventricular volume ejected per beat and of the ventricular end-diastolic and residual volumes. *Circulation*. 1962;25:674.

97. Levett JM, Replogle RL. Thermodilution cardiac output: a critical analysis and review of the literature. *J Surg Res*. 1979;27:392–404.

98. Fakhry SM, Buehrer JL, Sheldon GF, et al. A comparison of intensive care unit care of surgical patients in teaching and nonteaching hospitals. *Ann Surg*. 1991;213:19–23.

99. Blythe WR, Harper A, Fakhry SM, et al. Trends in postoperative management of head and neck surgery patients. Presented at the annual meeting of the American Academy of Otolaryngology–Head and Neck Surgery; September 19, 1994; San Diego, Calif.

100. Muakkassa FF, Fakhry SM, Rutledge R, et al. Cost-effective use of microcomputers for quality assurance and resource utilization in the surgical intensive care unit. *Crit Care Med*. 1990;18:1243–1247.

Index

(Numbers in italics indicate references to tables and figures.)

Adenoma, pleomorphic, recurrent, salivary gland surgery complications, 179–180
Adriamycino, 236
Aesthetic facial surgery, 248–278. See also Facial surgery, aesthetic
Air embolism, 344–345
  neck surgery complication, *132*, 133–135, *134*, 134t
Anatomy, 342–343
Anesthesia
  complications of, 371–388
  facial nerve injury, rehabilitation of, complications, 371
  hyperthermia, malignant, 383–385
  intubation, difficult/failed, 376–378
  laryngospasm, 372–373
  nasal/sinus surgery, 75–76, *76*
  nausea and vomiting, postoperative, 378–379
  postobstructive pulmonary edema (POPE), 373–376
  premedication, 379–380, *380*
  prophylaxis, 381
  respiratory/airway complications, 372
  surgical procedures, 381
  vomiting, management of, 381–382
Antibiotics, prophylactic, 159–171, *168*
  basilar skull fractures, 164
  bites, 164–165, 165t
  cost, 159
  cranial base, 162
  facial fractures, 164
  head surgery, 160t, 165–168, 166t, *168*
  laryngotracheal injuries, 164
  neck surgery, 125, 160t, 165–168, 166t, *168*
  neurotology, 162
  otology, 161–162
  prosthetics, 168
  rhinology, 161
  route, 160–161
  timing, 160–161
  tonsillectomy, 163
  trauma, 163–164
  wounds, classification of, 159–160, 160t
Anticoagulation, 21, 22–23, 23t, 24
  acute/chronic, 20–24
  coumadin, 22–24
    complications of, 23t, 23–24
  defibrotide, 24
  dermatan sulfate, 24
  dihydroergotamine, 24
  heparin, 21–22
    complications of, 22
  pentasaccharide, synthetic, 24
  pharmacokinetics dose and clinical use, 21–22

pulmonary embolism, 40
Antidiuretic hormone, inappropriate secretion of. See SIADH
Anti-flammatory drugs, nonsteroidal, 24–25
Arteriovenous malformation, neck surgery complications, 152
Aspirin, and nonsteroidal anti-flammatory drugs, 24–25
Auditory canal, external, related to, salivary gland surgery complications, 178
Autoimmune thrombocytopenia, 10t, 10–11

Bites, antibiotics, prophylactic, 164–165, 165t
Bleeding
  endoscopic sinus surgery, 90–91
  postoperative, 4
  time, hemostasis, 8–9
Bleomycin, 234–235
Blindness, neck surgery complications, 146–147
Blood smear, hemostasis, 9
Brachial plexus injury, neck surgery complications, 145, *145*
Bronchoscopy complications, 60–62, 61t, *62*

Caldwell-Luc operation, 81–82
Cancer, recurrent/persistent, neck surgery complications, 147–148
Carboplatin, 234
Cardiovascular system, sickle hemoglobinopathies, 20
Carotid artery, 343–344
  complications, neck surgery complications, 130–133
Carotid sinus sensitivity, neck surgery complications, 133, *133*
Cascade, coagulation, 5t, 5–6, *6–7*
Central nervous system, sickle hemoglobinopathies, 19
Central venous catheter complications, neck surgery complications, 135–136
Cerebrospinal fluid, leak, 338–340
  endoscopic sinus surgery, 92
Cervical esophagus
  complications, 94–96
    exposure, due to, 95
    repair, due to, 95–96
    resection, due to, 95, *96*
  general principles, 94
  indications, 94
  surgery for neoplasms of
    complications of, 94–106
    sequelae vs. complications, 94, 94t
  tumors of, surgery for, 102–104
Cervical nerve, neuromas, neck surgery complications, 145–146

Cervical sympathetic truck, 345, 345t
Chemotherapy, head and neck cancer, 230–231t, 230–247, 233–234, 235, 236, 237–238
  adjuvant therapy, 240–241
  biologicals, 243
  bleomycin, 234–235
  carboplatin, 234
  chemoprevention, 243
  cisplatin, 233–234
  combination chemotherapy, 238–241
    for advanced head and neck cancer, 241
  combined chemoradiotherapy, 241–243
  cyclophosphamide, 236–237
  doxorubicin, 236
  edatrexate, 238
  5-FU, 235–236
    and leucovorin, 236
  hydroxyurea, 236
  ifosphamide, 237–238
  induction therapy
    with bleomycin and cisplatin, 238–240
    with bleomycin and drugs other than cisplatin, 238
    with cisplatin, 240
    with 5-FU, 240
    overview of toxicities, 238
  infectious complications, 244
  intra-arterial chemotherapy, 243
  late sequelae of chemotherapy, 244
  methotrexate, 231–233
  mitomycin, 237
  mucositis, 243
  oral complications, 243–244
  taxol, 237
  toxicity
    management, 243–244
    specific agents, 231–233
  vinblastine, 236
Chest x-rays, postoperative, 4
Chewing, complications related to, salivary gland surgery complications, 179
Chondronecrosis, laryngeal, laryngeal surgery, 203, 203t
Christmas disease, 14
Chyle leak
  intraoperative, neck surgery complications, 128–129
  neck surgery complications, 127–130
  postoperative, neck surgery complications, 130, *131–132*
Chylothorax, neck surgery complications, 130, *132*
Cisplatin, 233–234
Clavicle disorders, neck surgery complications, 152
Clotting time, activated, 9
  hemostasis, 9

CO_2 laser surgery, complications of, 65–66, *66*
Coagulation, 5–6, 5–30
    anticoagulation, 21, 22–23, 23t, 24, 40
        acute/chronic, 20–24
        coumadin, 22–24
            complications of, 23t, 23–24
        defibrotide, 24
        dermatan sulfate, 24
        dihydroergotamine, 24
        heparin, 21–22
            complications of, 22
        pentasaccharide, synthetic, 24
        pharmacokinetics dose and clinical use, 21–22
    aspirin, 24–25
    cascade, 5t, 5–6, *6–7*
        defects, in liver failure, 16
    disorders, 13–19
        hemophilia A, 13t, 13–14
        treatment, 13–19
    inhibitors of, 18–19
        lupus anticoagulants, 18
        specific factor inhibitors, 19
    intravascular
        clinical manifestations, 17, 17t
        disseminated, 17–18
        laboratory diagnosis, 17
        pathogenesis, 17, 17t
        treatment, 18
    nonsteroidal anti-flammatory drugs, 24–25
Computed tomography evaluation, salivary gland surgery complications, 172–173
Continuous wave Doppler, portable, deep venous thrombosis, 32
Corneal injury, neck surgery complications, 146, *147*
Cost, antibiotics, prophylactic, 159
Coumadin, deep venous thrombosis, 33–34, 34t
Cranial base
    anterior, 336–342
    antibiotics, prophylactic, 162
    surgery, complications of, 336–351, 342–345, 349
        air embolization, 344–345
        anatomy, 337, 342–343, 345
        anterior cranial base, 336–342
        carotid artery, 343–344
        cervical sympathetic truck, 345, 345t
        complications, 338–342, 339t, 343–345, 345–349
        CSF leak, 338–340
        facial nerve, 345–346
        glossopharyngeal nerve, 347–348
        hemorrhage, 341–342
        hypoglossal nerve, 349
        meningitis, 340–341
        ocular complications, 342
        operative approaches, 343, 345
        pneumocephalus, 340, *341*
        posterior cranial base, 345–349
        prognostic factors, 337
        spinal accessory nerve, 349
        surgical approach, 337–338
        vagus nerve, 348–349
        vestibulocochlear nerve, 346–347, 347t
Cranial nerve complications, neck surgery complications, 136–143
Critical care unit, complications, 401–421, 410, 418, 419
    arterial catheters, systemic, 414–415, 415t
    cardiac dysfunction, 401–403
    cardiogenic shock, 403
    central venous catheters, 415–417, 416t

clostridium difficile colitis, 410–411
    congestive heart failure, 401
    dyshythmias, cardiac, 401–402
    gastrointestinal hemorrhage, upper, 411–413
    hemodynamic monitoring, pitfalls in, 418
    mental status change, 413–414
    monitoring devices, complications of, 414–418
    myocardial infarction, 403
    pulmonary artery catheters, 417–418, 418t
    renal failure, acute, 403–406, 405t
    respiratory distress syndrome, adult, 408t, 408–410
    sepsis
        multiple organ failure, 405t, 406–408
        systemic effects of, 406–407, 407t
Cyclophosphamide, 236–237

Death, endoscopic sinus surgery, 93
Deep venous thrombosis, 31t, 31–37, 52
    combination therapy, 37
    diagnosis, 32
    duplex imaging, 32–33
    elastic stockings, 36
    etiology, 31–32, *32*
    fibrinolytic agents, 34–35
    heparin therapy, 33, 37
    impedance plethysmography, 32
    mechanical prophylaxis, 36
    pharmacologic prophylaxis, 36–37
    phleborheography, 33
    pneumatic compression hose, 36
    portable continuous wave Doppler, 32
    presentation, 31
    prophylaxis, 36
    surgical thrombectomy, 35
    transvenous vena caval filtration, 35–36
    treatment, 33–37
    triplex scanning, 33
    venography, 33
    warfarin sodium, 33–34, 34t
    warfarin therapy, 37
Doxorubicin, 236
Drug fever, neck surgery complications, 151
Drug-induced thrombocytopenia, 12
Duplex imaging, deep venous thrombosis, 32–33

Edatrexate, 238
Elastic stockings, deep venous thrombosis, 36
Emphysema, subcutaneous, neck surgery complications, 152
Endoscopic sinus surgery complications, 90t, 90–93, 93
    bleeding, 90–91
    cerebrospinal fluid, leak, 92
    death, 93
    epiphora, 92
    orbit, 92
        hemorrhage, 91t, 91–92
    restenosis, 92–93
Endovascular treatment, pulmonary embolism, 41–42
Epiphora, endoscopic sinus surgery, 92
Esophagoscopy complications, 59–60
    flexible, 59
    rigid, 59–60, *60–61*
Esophagus
    cervical, tumors of, surgery for, 102–104
    motility, alterations in, laryngeal surgery, 114
Esthetic deformity, salivary gland surgery complications, 178–179

Ethanol-related thrombocytopenia, 12–13
Ethmoidectomy, 82–84
    external, *84*, 84–85
Eye, injury to, in laser surgery, 72

Facial fractures
    antibiotics, prophylactic, 164
    complications of surgery for, 290–322, 317
        ankylosis, of temporomandibular joint, 297, *297*
        aspiration, 290
        canalicular injury with epiphora, 292–295, *294*
        cerebrospinal fluid leak, 311–313, 313–314, *316*, 316–317, *318–319, 320*
        cervical spine injury, 290
        chondritis
            of ear, 295
            of septum, 295
        coronoid impingement, 305–306, *306*
        enophthalmos, hypophthalmos, and diplopia, 306–308
        facial nerve injury, 291, *293*
        facial skeleton injuries, 295–317
        frontal bone fractures, 313–316
        hematoma, 295
        infraorbital nerve compression, 305
        lacerations/abrasions, 290–291, *292*
        malar fractures, 301–306
        malunion, 296–297, 298–301, *300*, 301–305, *302–303, 304–305*, 315–316
        mandible fractures, 295–298
        maxillary fractures, 298–301
        mucocele, 314–315, *318–319*
        nasal fractures, 308, *309*
        nasal orbital/ethmoid fractures, 308–313
        nonunion, 295, *296*
        orbital fractures, 306–307, *307*
        parotid duct injury, 291–292, *294*
        respiratory obstruction, 290
        soft tissue injuries, 290–295
        sphenoid bone fractures, 316–317
        telecanthus
            dacryocystitis, 310–311, *314–315*
            epiphora, 308–310, *311–313*
        tooth injuries, 297–298, *298–299*
        traumatic optic neuropathy, 317, *321*
Facial nerve, 345–346
    injury, rehabilitation, 352–370
        cross-face grafts, 359–361
        diagnostic evaluation, 352–355, 353t, *354*
        eye, 364–367
        eyebrow, 367
        eyelid techniques
            lower, 365–366, *367–368*
            upper, 365, *366*
            upper/lower, combined, 366–367
        facial nerve exploration, 355–356
        facial paralysis/neural procedures, 355–361
        free muscle grafts, 363, *364*, 365t
        marginal mandibular paralysis, 363–364
        nerve crossover, 358–359, *360*
        nerve grafts, 358
        neuromuscular transposition, 362–363, *363*
        neurorrhaphy, 356–358, *357*
        oral commissure reanimation, 361–364
        static procedures, 361–362
        temporalis transposition, 361
    neck surgery complications, 138, *139*
Facial surgery, aesthetic, complications, 248–278, 249–250

aesthetic complications, 254–257
allergic reactions, 267
alloplastic materials, 274–275
alopecia, 264
anesthesia, 249
anthelical deformity, 268
asymmetry, 261
autologous materials, 274, *275*
bleeding, 249
blepharoplasty, 257–263, *260*
bony framework, 254, *255–256*
cartilaginous vault, 254–255, *257–258*
chemexfoliation, 269–271
compromise of adjacent structures, 274
conchal deformity, 268
conjunctival lymphedema, 260
contour irregularities, 264
corneal injury, 260–261
cysts/tunnels, 260
dermabrasion, 271–272
diplopia, 261
dog ear, 264
earlobe deformity, 264
early complications, 266–267
ectropion, 261
edema and ecchymosis, 263
edema/ecchymosis, 250
epiphora, 260
eyelashes, loss of, 260
facial nerve injury, 265–266
glaucoma, 262
hematoma, 264–265, 266
hematomas, small, 263
hemorrhage, 249–250
hypertrophic scars, 260
hypertrophic scars and keloids, 267
hypesthesia and paresthesia, 263
implant
    exposure, 273
    failure, 273
    filler agents, 274–275
infection, 249, 250, *251*, 260, 263,
    266–267, 268, 271, 272, 273
    local disfigurements, 263–264
irregularities/scars, 269
ischemia or necrosis, 273
keratoconjunctivitis sicca, 262
lagophthalmus, 261
late complications, 267–268
major complications, 261–263, 264–266
milia/skin texture changes, 271
minor complications, 259–261, 263
nasal obstruction, 251–254, *253*
nasal tip, 255–257, *258–259*
nerve injury, 269
other minor sequelae, 264
otoplasty, 266–268
pain, 263, 266, 273–274
pigmentary changes, 271–272
pigmentation changes, 270
postoperative wrinkling, 260
psychological intolerance, 273
ptosis, 262
recurrence of deformity, 267–268
retrobulbar hematoma, 262
rhinoplasty, 249–257
rhytidectomy, 263–266
scarring, 270, 272
scars, *258*, 263–264
sensory deficits, 267
seroma/hematoma, 268–269
skin
    abnormalities, 271
    discoloration, 269
    excess, 269

necrosis, 267
    side effects on, 272
    slough, 262, 265, *266*, 269
suction lipectomy, 268–269
suture granuloma or extrusion, 267
systemic complications, 270
telangiectasias, 260
telephone deformity, 268
thermal injury, 272
tissue expander, 272–274
traumatic complications, 250–254, *252*
visual loss, 262–263
wound separation, 260
Factor inhibitors, inhibitors of coagulation,
    19
Factor VIII, hemophilia, inhibitors of, 14
Fever, postoperative, 44–45, 46–47, 47–48,
    48, 49, 49t, 50–51, *51*, 51–52, 52,
    53–54, 54
    atelectasis, 46–47
    blood transfusion, 46
    consequences of, 44–45
    deep venous thrombosis, 52
    drug fevers, 54
    evaluation of, 45
    5 to 10 days postoperatively, 53–54
    malignant hyperthermia, 45–46
    necrotizing wound infection, 47
    pathophysiology of, 44–45
    phlebitis, 52
        catheter related, 52
    pneumonia, 50–52
    pulmonary embolism, 52–53
    during surgery, or immediately post-
        operative, 45–46
    temperature, regulation of, 44, *45*
    toxic shock syndrome, 48
    2 to 4 days postoperative, 49–53
    urinary tract infection, 49–50
    wound infection, 53–54
    0 to 2 days postoperative, 46–48
Fibrinolytic agents, deep venous thrombosis,
    34–35
Fine-needle aspiration biopsy evaluation,
    salivary gland surgery complications,
    173–174
Fires, in laser surgery, 65t, 66–67, *66–68*
Fistula
    laryngeal surgery, 107–108, *109*
    neck surgery complications, 127, *128*
Flap necrosis, salivary gland surgery com-
    plications, 178
Frey's syndrome, salivary gland surgery
    complications, 179
Frontal sinuses, trephination, 85–86
5-FU, 235–236
    and leucovorin, 236

Glossopharyngeal nerve, 347–348
Gustatory sweating, salivary gland surgery
    complications, 179

Head and neck surgery, antibiotics, prophylac-
    tic, 160t, 165–168, 166t, *168*
Hematoma
    neck surgery complications, 127
    salivary gland surgery complications, 177
Hemophilia
    A
        testing for, 13
        treatment of, 14
    B, 14
    factor VIII in, inhibitors of, 14

Hemorrhage, 341–342
    in laser surgery, 69–71
    orbit, endoscopic sinus surgery, 91t, 91–92
Hemostasis, 5–30
    activated clotting time, 9
    bleeding time, 8–9
    blood smear, 9
    clinical evaluation of, 6–9
    history, 7–8, 8t
    laboratory tests of, 8–9
    mixes, 9
    partial thromboplastin time, 8
    prothrombin time, *6*, 8
    thrombin time, 8
Heparin therapy, deep venous thrombosis,
    33, 37
Hepatobiliary sickle hemoglobinopathies,
    19
Hydroxyurea, 236
Hypertension, following radical neck dissec-
    tion, neck surgery complications,
    150–151
Hyperthermia, malignant, fever, postoperative,
    45–46
Hypoglossal nerve, 349
    neck surgery complications, 142–143, *143*
Hypoparathyroidism, laryngeal surgery, 115
Hypopharynx
    stenosis, laryngeal surgery, 111–114
    tumors of, surgery for, 102–104
Hypothyroidism, laryngeal surgery, 114–115
Hypoxemia, in laser surgery, 71

Ifosphamide, 237–238
Imaging, head and neck, complications of,
    389–400
    angiography, 394–398
    cisternography, 393
    diagnostic, 394–395, *396–397*
    magnetic resonance imaging, 393–394, *394*
    oral contrast swallows, 389, *390–391*
    sialography, 389–390, *392*
    test balloon occlusions, 395–398, *398–399*
    therapeutic, 395
Impedance plethysmography, deep venous
    thrombosis, 32
Incisions
    neck surgery complications, 124, *125*
    skin, plan for, 3
Induction therapy
    with bleomycin and cisplatin, 238–240
    with bleomycin and drugs other than
        cisplatin, 238
    with cisplatin, 240
    with 5-FU, 240
    overview of toxicities, 238
Infection
    laryngeal surgery, 107–108, *109*
    salivary gland surgery complications, 178
Intravascular coagulation
    disseminated, 17–18
    laboratory diagnosis, 17
    pathogenesis, 17, 17t
    treatment, 18

Jaw-neck mandible-splitting procedure,
    101–102
    complications, 101–102
        exposure, due to, 101
        repair, due to, 102
        resection, due to, 101
    general principles, 101
    indications, 101

Jugular vein
  complications, internal, neck surgery complications, 135–136
  thrombosis, neck surgery complications, 135, *136*

Labs, postoperative, 4
Laryngeal nerve, recurrent, neck surgery complications, 138–140
Laryngectomy
  partial, voice after, 119
  total, 107–108, 107–115
    esophageal motility, alterations in, 114
    fistula, 107–108, *109*
    hypoparathyroidism, 115
    hypopharyngeal stenosis, 111–114
    hypothyroidism, 114–115
    infection, 107–108, *109*
    management, 108, *109*
    medical complications of, 115
    nasal physiology, alterations in, 114
    necrosis, 107–108, *109*
    tracheal stomal stenosis, 108–111
      management of, 109–111, *113*
Laryngopharyngectomy, total, with partial/total esophagectomy, 103–104
Laryngoscopy complications, 56–63
  anesthesia, 57
  direct, 57–58, *58–59*
  endoscopy suite, 56, *56*
  equipment, 56–57
  technique, 57
Laryngospasm, 372–373
Laryngotracheal injuries, 164
  antibiotics, prophylactic, 164
Larynx, conservation surgery
  airway obstruction, 118–119
  complications, 115–119
  glottis
    incompetence, 116–118
      management of, 117–118, *118*
    stenosis, 119
  granuloma, redundant mucosa, 118–119
  patient selection, 116
Laryx, surgery complications, 107–121
Laser, surgery, complications of, 64–65t, 64–73
  CO$_2$ laser surgery, 65–66, *66*
  eyes, injury to, 72
  fires, 65t, 66–67, *66–68*
  hemorrhage, 69–71
  hypoxemia, 71
  laser plume, inhalation of, 72
  Nd:YAG laser surgery, 65
  neural tissue, injury to, 71–72
  operative complications, 65–72
  otology complications, 72
  perforation, tracheobronchial tree, 69, *71*
  plume, inhalation of, in laser surgery, 72
  postoperative complications, 72–73, 73t
  skin, burns to, 64t, 68–69, *69–70*
Leucovorin, 236
Lhermitte's sign, 213
Liver disease, 16–17
  coagulation cascade defects in, 16
  laboratory evaluation, 16
  platelet abnormalities in, 16
  treatment, 16–17
Lung scanning, pulmonary embolism, 38–39
Lupus anticoagulants, coagulation, inhibitor, 18
Lymphedema, neck surgery complications, 147
Lynch procedure, Neel-Lake modification of, 86–87

Magnetic resonance imaging evaluation, salivary gland surgery complications, 172–173
Malignant hyperthermia, fever, postoperative, 45–46
Mandible-sparing procedures, 96–99
  laterial pharyngotomy, 96–97
  pull-through procedures, 99
  transhyoid pharyngotomy, 97–99
Mandible-splitting procedures, 99–102
  anterior mandibulotomy, 100–101
  jaw-neck procedure, 101–102
  lateral mandibulotomy, 99–100
Mandibulotomy
  anterior, 100–101
    complications, 100–101
      closure, due to, 101
      exposure, due to, 100–101
      resection, due to, 101
    general principles, 100, *100*
    indications, 100, *100*
  lateral, 99–100
    complications, 99–100
      exposure, due to, 99
      repair, due to, 99–100
      resection, due to, 99
    general principles, 99, *100*
    indications, 99, *100*
Mastoid surgery, complications, 323–325, 326–329, *328, 330*
Maxillectomy, 87
Meningitis, 340–341
Methotrexate, 231–233
Middle ear surgery, complications of, 323–325
Middle/anterolateral cranial base, 342–345
Mitomycin, 237
Monitoring, patient, 3–4, 4t
  overview, 3
Mucosa, burns to
  in laser surgery, 64t, 68–69, *69–70*
Mucositis, 243
Musculoskeletal sickle hemoglobinopathies, 19

Nasal physiology, alterations in, laryngeal surgery, 114
Nd:YAG laser surgery, complications of, 65
Neck dissection, radical, bilateral, neck surgery complications, 148–149
Neck surgery complications, 122–158
  air embolism, *132*, 133–135, *134*, 134t
  anatomy, 128, *129*
  antibiotics, prophylactic, 125
  arteriovenous malformation, 152
  bilateral radical neck dissection, 148–149
  blindness, 146–147
  brachial plexus injury, 145, *145*
  cancer, recurrent/persistent, 147–148
  carotid artery complications, 130–133
  carotid sinus sensitivity, 133, *133*
  central venous catheter complications, 135–136
  cervical nerve, neuromas, 145–146
  chyle leak, 127–130
    intraoperative, 128–129
    postoperative, 130, *131–132*
  chylothorax, 130, *132*
  clavicle disorders, 152
  corneal injury, 146, *147*
  cranial nerve complications, 136–143
  drug fevers, 151
  emphysema, subcutaneous, 152
  facial nerve, 138, *139*
  fistula, 127, *128*
  hematoma, 127

hypertension, following radical neck dissection, 150–151
  hypoglossal nerve, 142–143, *143*
  incisions, 124, *125*
  internal jugular vein complications, 135–136
  jugular vein thrombosis, 135, *136*
  laryngeal nerve, recurrent, 138–140
  lymphedema, 147
  medical complications, 150–151
  nutrition, 123
  ophthalmic complications, 146–147
  osteoradionecrosis, 152
  phrenic nerve injury, 144–145, *145*
  physiology, 128
  pneumothorax, 136, *137*
  radiation, 123
  seroma, 126–127
  SIADH, 151
  spinal accessory nerve, 140–142, *141*
  surgical preparation, 125
  surgical technique, 123
  sympathetic nerve injury, 143–144, *144*
  tobacco use, 123–124
  tracheotomy, 149–150, 150t
  trigeminal nerve, 136–138, *137*
  unusual, 152
  vagus nerve, 138, *140*
  wound
    closure, 125–126
    drainage, 126
    healing, 124
    infection, 124–125
    problems, 124–126
Necrosis, laryngeal surgery, 107–108, *109*
Neel-Lake modification, Lynch procedure, 86–87
Nerve injury, salivary gland surgery complications, 174–177
Neural tissue, injury to, in laser surgery, 71–72
Neurotology, antibiotics, prophylactic, 162
Nonsteroidal anti-flammatory drugs, 24–25
Nose, chondronecrosis, radiotherapy for head and neck neoplasms, 203
Nutrition, neck surgery complications, 123

Ocular complications, 342
Ophthalmic complications, neck surgery complications, 146–147
Oral cavity, surgery for neoplasms of, sequelae vs. complications, 94, 94t
Orbit
  complications, endoscopic sinus surgery, 92
  hemorrhage, endoscopic sinus surgery, 91t, 91–92
Osteoradionecrosis
  mandible/maxilla, radiotherapy for head and neck neoplasms, 199–201
  neck surgery complications, 152
Osteotomy, osteoplastic frontal, and fat obliteration, 86
Otology
  antibiotics, prophylactic, 161–162
  complications, in laser surgery, 72

Parapharyngeal space tumors, transpharyngeal approach, 102
Parathyroid/thyroid surgery complications, 184–193. See also Thyroid
Parotid surgery
  facial nerve injury, salivary gland surgery complications, 174–176, *175*
  greater auricular nerve sacrifice, and neuroma, salivary gland surgery complications, 176

Partial thromboplastin time, 8
Patient
    assessment, for nasal/sinus surgery, 74–75
    monitoring, 3–4, 4t
    overview, 3
Perfusion scans, pulmonary embolism, 38–39
Perioperative period, general considerations
        of, 1–4
Pharyngectomy, partial, with/without total
        laryngectomy, 102–103
Pharyngotomy, lateral
    complications, 96–97
        exposure, due to, 96–97
        repair, due to, 97, 98
        resection, due to, 97
    general principles, 96
    indications, 96
Pharynx, surgery for neoplasms of
    complications of, 94–106
    sequelae vs. complications, 94, 94t
Phleborheography, deep venous thrombosis, 33
Phrenic nerve injury, neck surgery complica-
        tions, 144–145, 145
Pituitary surgery, 80–81
    secondary, 81
Platelet disorders, 9–13
    clinical course, 10–11, 11–12
    drug-induced thrombocytopenia, 12–13
    ethanol-related thrombocytopenia, 12–13
    function, 9–10, 10
    pregnancy, thrombocytopenia in, 13
    in renal disease, 12
    thrombocytopenia, drug-induced, 12
    thrombocytopenic purpura, idiopathic, 10t,
        10–11
    thrombotic thrombocytopenic purpura,
        11–12
    treatment, 10–11
Plethysmography, impedance, deep venous
        thrombosis, 32
Pneumatic compression hose, deep venous
        thrombosis, 36
Pneumocephalus, 340, 341
Pneumonia, fever, postoperative, 50–52
Pneumothorax, neck surgery complications,
        136, 137
Posterior cranial base, 345–349
Postoperative alimentation, plans for, 3
Postoperative fever, 44–55. See also Fever,
        postoperative
Postoperative irradiation, 204–205
Postoperative management, sickle hemo-
        globinopathies, 20
Pregnancy, thrombocytopenia in, 13
Preoperative period, 1t, 1–2
    airway status, 1
    contingency plans, 2, 2
    extent of disease, understanding, 2
    hydration, 1
    nutritional status, 1
    patient care, overall plan for, 2, 2
    preoperative studies, necessity of, 1–2
    sickle hemoglobinopathies, 20
    staging, and understanding of extent of
        disease, 2
    thromboembolic complications, prophylaxis
        of, 2
Pressure equalizing tubes, complications from,
        323–325, 324
Prophylactic antibiotics, 159–171. See also
        Antibiotics
Prosthetics, antibiotics, prophylactic, 168
Prothrombin time, hemostasis, 6, 8
Pterygomaxillary fossa surgery, 82
Pull-through mandible-sparing procedures, 99

complications, 99
    exposure, due to, 99
    repair, due to, 99
    resection, due to, 99
    general principles, 99
    indications, 99
Pulmonary angiography, pulmonary embolism,
        39–40
Pulmonary embolism, 37–40, 40, 52–53
    anticoagulation, 40
    clinical features, 38, 38t
    endovascular treatment, 41–42
    fever, postoperative, 52–53
    lung scanning, 38–39
    perfusion scans, 38–39
    pulmonary angiography, 39–40
    thrombolysis, 40–41
    treatment, 40–42
    vena caval filter, 42
    ventilation scans, 38
Pulmonary system, sickle hemoglobinopathies,
        19–20

Radiation, neck surgery complications, 123
Radiological studies, postoperative, 4
Radiotherapy, for head and neck neoplasms,
        194–229, 200–201, 202, 218–221
    acute effects, 194–197
    anterior lobe, 221–222
    arteries, large, 223–224
    bone exposure, and osteoradionecrosis of
        mandible and maxilla, 199–201
    brain, 217–221
    brain stem, 213–217
    cartilage necrosis, 202–203
    cataracts, radiation, 211
    chondronecrosis
        laryngeal, 203, 203t
        of nose/ear, 203
    conjunctiva, 195, 207–208
    cranial nerves, 221
    ear, 211–213
        chondronecrosis, 203
    erysipelas, 223
    eyelids, 207
    follow-up policy, 222
    lacrimal apparatus, 205–206, 207–208,
        210–211
    larynx, 194–195
    late effects, 197–225
    lens, 211
    Lhermitte's sign, 213
    lung, 223
    lymphedema, 223
    masticatory muscles, 198, 198–199
    mucosal cancer, 224
    mucous membranes, 194–195
    myelitis, transverse, 214
    nasal cavity, 195, 196
    nasolacrimal drainage system, 207
    neoplasia, after therapeutic irradiation,
        224–225
    optic atrophy, 209
    optic nerve, 209–211
        injury, management of, 211
    optic neuropathy, 209–211, 218–219
    oral cavity, 194–195
    parafollicular cells, 222
    paranasal sinuses, 223
    parathyroid gland, 222
    peripheral nerves, 221
    pharyngeal stenosis, 204
    pharynx and larynx, 194–195
    pituitary gland, 221–222

posterior lobe, 222
postoperative irradiation, 204–205
preoperative irradiation, 204
retina, 208–209
retinopathy, radiation, 206, 208–209, 209,
        212–215, 216
salivary tissue, 195–196, 197
salvage surgery, 204
sarcoma, 224–225
sclera, 208
sensorineural hearing loss, 213
serous otitis media, 211–213
sialadenitis, 196–197, 197
skin, 203–204
skin/subcutaneous tissues, 196–197,
        203–204
soft tissue necrosis, 202
soft tissue/bone necrosis, 199–202
spinal cord, 213–217
    injury, time-dose-volume, 216–217, 220t
subcutaneous fibrosis, 204
taste, sense of, 195, 197
teeth, 197–198
temporal bone necrosis, 201, 201–202
temporomandibular joint, 198, 198–199
thyroid, 222
    cancer, 225
transitory CNS syndrome, 217–218
vestibular disorders, 213
visual apparatus, 205–211, 206
wound healing, 204–205
xerostomia, 196, 197
Reconstructive flaps, complications of,
        279–289, 283–284, 284t, 285–286,
        287–288
    axial pattern flaps, 282–283
    cooling, 281–282
    cutaneous and fasciocutaneous flaps,
        286–287
    delay phenomena, 281
    deltopectoral flap, 282–283
    flap viability, 281–282
    grafts, 287
    internal oblique iliac crest, 287
    intrinsic factors affecting, 281
    jejunum, 287
    lateral forearm flap, 286–287
    latissimus dorsi, 285, 287
    malnutrition, 280
    mechanical factors, 281
    microvascular free tissue transfer, 285t,
        285–286
    muscle/musculocutaneous flaps, 287
    musculocutaneous flaps, 283–285
    operative planning, 279–281
    osteocutaneous flaps, 287
    osteomusculocutaneous flaps, 287
    patient selection, 285
    pharmacological manipulation, 281, 281t
    radial forearm flap, 286
    radiation effects, on wound healing,
        280–281
    random pattern flaps, 282
    rectus abdominis, 287
    scapula, 287
    sternocleidomastoid flap, 284
    trapezius myocutaneous flap, 284–285
Renal system
    disease, platelet disorders, 12
    sickle hemoglobinopathies, 19
Restenosis, endoscopic sinus surgery, 92–93
Reticuloendothelial sickle hemoglobinopathies,
        19
Rhinology, antibiotics, prophylactic, 161
Rhinotomy, lateral, 84, 85

Saliva leak, sialocele, salivary gland surgery complications, 178
Salivary gland surgery complications, 172t, 172-183, 173, 178-181
  adenoma, pleomorphic, recurrent, 179-180
  auditory canal, external, related to, 178
  chewing, complications related to, 179
  computed tomography evaluation, 172-173
  esthetic deformity, 178-179
  fine-needle aspiration biopsy evaluation, 173-174
  flap necrosis, 178
  gustatory sweating, 179
  hematoma, 177
  infection, 178
  late complications, 178-181
  magnetic resonance imaging evaluation, 172-173
  nerve injury, 174-177
  overview, 181-182
  parotid surgery
    facial nerve injury, 174-176, 175
      greater auricular nerve sacrifice, and neuroma, 176
  seroma, 177-178
  sialocele, saliva leak, 178
  submandibular surgery, lingual nerve, 176-177
  surgical complications, 174-178
  tumor, malignant, recurrent, 181, 181t
Secretion, antidiuretic hormone. See SIADH
Septal surgery, 76, 77-80, 78, 80
Seroma
  neck surgery complications, 126-127
  salivary gland surgery complications, 177-178
SIADH, neck surgery complications, 151
Sialadenitis, 196-197, 197
Sialocele, saliva leak, salivary gland surgery complications, 178
Sickle hemoglobinopathy, 19-20, 20
  cardiovascular, 20
  central nervous system, 19
  hepatobiliary, 19
  musculoskeletal, 19
  postoperative management, 20
  preoperative management, 20
  pulmonary, 19-20
  renal, 19
  reticuloendothelial, 19
Sinonasal surgery, complications, 74-89
  anesthetic considerations, for nasal/sinus surgery, 75-76, 76
  Caldwell-Luc operation, 81-82
  ethmoidectomy, 82-84
    external, 84, 84-85
  Lynch procedure, Neel-Lake modification of, 86-87
  maxillectomy, 87
  osteotomy, osteoplastic frontal, and fat obliteration, 86
  patient assessment, for nasal/sinus surgery, 74-75
  pituitary surgery, 80-81
    secondary, 81
  pterygomaxillary fossa surgery, 82
  rhinotomy, lateral, 84, 85
  septal surgery, 76, 77-80, 78, 80
  trephination, of frontal sinuses, 85-86
Sinus
  frontal, trephination, 85-86
  surgery, endoscopic. See Endoscopic sinus surgery
Skin, incisions, plan for, 3
Skull fractures, basilar, antibiotics, prophylactic, 164
Spinal accessory nerve, 349

neck surgery complications, 140-142, 141
Stapedectomy surgery, complications of, 330-334, 331-334
Stenosis, stomal, tracheal, laryngeal surgery, 108-111
Stockings, elastic, deep venous thrombosis, 36
Stomal stenosis, tracheal, laryngeal surgery, 108-111
Submandibular surgery
  facial nerve, salivary gland surgery complications, 176-177
  hypoglossal nerve, salivary gland surgery complications, 176-177
  lingual nerve, salivary gland surgery complications, 176-177
Sympathetic nerve injury, neck surgery complications, 143-144, 144

Taxol, 237
Temperature, regulation of, fever, postoperative, 44, 45
Thrombectomy, deep venous thrombosis, 35
Thrombin time, hemostasis, 8
Thrombocytopenia
  autoimmune, 10t, 10-11
  drug-induced, 12-13
  ethanol-related, 12-13
  in pregnancy, 13
  purpura
    idiopathic, 10t, 10-11
    thrombotic, 11-12
  purpura/autoimmune thrombocytopenia, idiopathic, 10t, 10-11
Thrombolysis, pulmonary embolism, 40-41
Thromboplastin time, partial, 8
  hemostasis, 8
Thrombotic thrombocytopenic purpura, 11-12
Thyroid/parathyroid surgery complications, 184-193
  bleeding
    intraoperative, 184
    postoperative, 184-185
  bone hunger syndrome, 190-191
  delayed, chronic, 192
  hypocalcemia
    management of, 189
    postoperative, 187-191
    symptomatic, 189, 189, 190t
  hypocalcemias, asymptomatic, 189-190, 190t
  hypoparathyroidism, 187
    incidence of, 187
    latent, 189-190, 190t
    management of, 189
  laryngeal nerve, superior, injury, 186-187
  parathyroids
    avoiding injury to, 187
    inferior, location of, 187
    superior, location of, 187, 188
  recurrent laryngeal nerve
    injury to, 185-186
      avoiding, 185
    severed, management of, 186
  seroma, postoperative, 184-185
  thyrotoxic storm, 191-192
    prevention of, 191
    treatment of, 191-192
  unusual complications, 192
  vocal cord paralysis, postoperative, 185-186
Timing, antibiotics, prophylactic, and route, 160-161
Tobacco use, neck surgery complications, 123-124
Tonsillectomy, antibiotics, prophylactic, 163
Toxic shock syndrome, fever, postoperative, 48

Tracheal stomal stenosis
  laryngeal surgery, 108-111
    management of, 109-111, 113
    preventions of, 109
  preventions of, 109
  total laryngectomy, 109
Tracheotomy, neck surgery complications, 149-150, 150t
Transfusion
  complications of, 25-28
    immediate, 25
    late, 25-27, 26t
  hepatitis B, 26
  hepatitis C, 26-27
  HIV, 27
  HTLV-I, 27
  HTLV-II, 27
  immunomodulation secondary to, 27-28
  massive, 28
Transhyoid pharyngotomy, 97-99
  complications, 97-99
    exposure, due to, 97
    repair, due to, 99
    resection, due to, 99
  general principles, 97
  indications, 97
Transoral resection, 94-96
Transpharyngeal approach, to parapharyngeal space tumors, 102
Transvenous vena caval filtration, deep venous thrombosis, 35-36
Trauma, antibiotics, prophylactic, 163-164
Trephination, of frontal sinuses, 85-86
Trigeminal nerve, neck surgery complications, 136-138, 137
Triplex scanning, deep venous thrombosis, 33
Tumor, malignant, recurrent, salivary gland surgery complications, 181, 181t
Tympanic membrane surgery, 325-326, 326

Urinary tract infection, fever, postoperative, 49-50

Vagus nerve, 348-349
  neck surgery complications, 138, 140
Vena caval filter, pulmonary embolism, 42
Venography, deep venous thrombosis, 33
Ventilation scans, pulmonary embolism, 38
Vestibulocochlear nerve, 346-347, 347t
Vinblastine, 236
Voice, after partial laryngectomy, 119
Von Willebrand's disease, 6, 13t, 14-16
  clinical manifestations, 14-15, 15t
  laboratory tests, 14-15, 15t
  treatment, 15-16

Warfarin
  sodium, deep venous thrombosis, 33-34, 34t
  therapy, deep venous thrombosis, 37
Wound
  antibiotics, prophylactic, classification of, 159-160, 160t
  closure, neck surgery complications, 125-126
  drainage, neck surgery complications, 126
  healing, 204-205
    neck surgery complications, 124
  infection
    fever, postoperative, 53-54
    neck surgery complications, 124-125
  neck surgery complications, 124-126

Xerostomia, 196, 197